Best Practice in Labour and Delivery

Best Practice in Labour and Delivery

Edited by

Richard Warren
Richard Warren is Consultant Obstetrician and Gynaecologist, Norfolk and Norwich University Hospital NHS Trust, UK.

Sir Sabaratnam Arulkumaran
Sir Sabaratnam Arulkumaran is Professor and Head, Department of Obstetrics and Gynaecology, St Georges, University of London, UK.

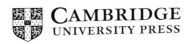
CAMBRIDGE
UNIVERSITY PRESS

CAMBRIDGE UNIVERSITY PRESS
Cambridge, New York, Melbourne, Madrid, Cape Town, Singapore,
São Paulo, Delhi

Cambridge University Press
The Edinburgh Building, Cambridge CB2 8RU, UK

Published in the United States of America
by Cambridge University Press, New York

www.cambridge.org
Information on this title: www.cambridge.org/9780521720687

First published 2009

Printed in the United Kingdom at the University Press, Cambridge

*A catalogue record for this publication is available from the British
Library*

Library of Congress Cataloging-in-Publication Data

Best practice in labour and delivery / edited by Richard Warren,
S. Arulkumaran.
    p. ; cm.
    Includes bibliographical references and index.
    ISBN 978-0-521-72068-7 (pbk.)
  1. Childbirth. I. Warren, Richard. II. Arulkumaran, Sabaratnam.
    [DNLM: 1. Labor, Obstetric. 2. Birth Injuries–prevention & control.
  3. Delivery, Obstetric–methods. WQ 300 B561 2009]
    RG651.B47 2009
    618.4–dc22

                                                                2009024542

ISBN 978-0-521-72068-7 paperback

Contents

List of contributors   vii
Preface   xi
Acknowledgements   xii

1. Pelvic and fetal cranial anatomy and mechanism of labour   1
   Louay S. Louis and Richard Warren

2. The first stage of labour   14
   Sambit Mukhopadhyay and David Fraser

3. Analgesia and anaesthesia in labour   26
   Jason Scott and Geraldine O'Sullivan

4. Intrapartum fetal surveillance   38
   Rohan D'Souza and Sabaratnam Arulkumaran

5. Uterine contractions   54
   Vivek Nama and Sabaratnam Arulkumaran

6. The management of intrapartum 'fetal distress'   66
   Bryony Strachan

7. Nutrition and hydration in labour   76
   David Fraser and Sambit Mukhopadhyay

8. Prolonged second stage of labour including difficult decision-making on operative vaginal delivery and caesarean section   84
   Hajeera Butt and Deirdre J. Murphy

9. Operative vaginal deliveries: indications, techniques and complications   93
   Stergios K. Doumouchtsis and Sabaratnam Arulkumaran

10. Caesarean deliveries: indications, techniques and complications   104
    Lisa Story and Sara Paterson-Brown

11. Breech and twin delivery   116
    Steve Walkinshaw

12. Cord prolapse and shoulder dystocia   131
    Joanna Crofts, Timothy Draycott and Mark Denbow

13. Antepartum haemorrhage   141
    Neelam Potdar, Osric Navti and Justin C. Konje

14. Management of the third stage of labour   153
    Pina Amin and Audrey Long

15. Postpartum haemorrhage (PPH)   160
    Nutan Mishra and Edwin Chandraharan

16. Acute illness and maternal collapse in the postpartum period   171
    Guy Jackson and Steve Yentis

17. Episiotomy and obstetric perineal trauma   182
    Ranee Thakar and Abdul H. Sultan

18. Induction of labour   195
    Devi Subramanian and Leonie Penna

19. Preterm prelabour rupture of membranes (pPROM)   207
    Austin Ugwumadu

20. Preterm labour and delivery   216
    Sarah L. Bell and Jane E. Norman

21. Labour in women with medical disorders   227
    Mandish Dhanjal and Catherine Nelson-Piercy

22. Management of women with previous caesarean section   241
    Rajesh Varma and Gordon C. S. Smith

23. Rupture of the uterus   252
    Nutan Mishra and Edwin Chandraharan

24. Management of severe pre-eclampsia/ eclampsia   262
    James J. Walker

25. Neonatal resuscitation and the management of immediate neonatal problems   273
    Paul Mannix

Contents

26. **The immediate puerperium**   285
    Mahishee Mehta and Leonie Penna

27. **Triage and prioritization in a busy labour ward**   300
    Tracey Johnston and Nina Johns

28. **Risk management related to intrapartum care**   311
    Melissa K. Whitworth and Helen Scholefield

29. **Teamworking, skills and drills**   323
    Dimitrios M. Siassakos and Timothy J. Draycott

30. **Cerebral palsy arising from events in labour**   332
    Julian Woolfson

31. **Objective Structured Assessment of Technical Skills (OSATS) in obstetrics**   341
    S. M. Whitten and M. J. Blott

    Appendix   349

Index   350
Colour plates are to be found between pp. 194 and 195.

Contributors

Pina Amin
Consultant Obstetrician and Gynaecologist
University Hospital of Wales
Cardiff, UK

Sir Sabaratnam Arulkumaran
Professor, Department of Obstetrics and
Gynaecology
St George's Hospital/St George's University
of London
London, UK

Sarah L. Bell
Consultant Paediatric Anaesthetist
Glasgow Royal Infirmary
Glasgow, UK

M. J. Blott
Elizabeth Garrett Anderson and Obstetric
Hospital
University College Hospital NHS Trust
London, UK

Hajeera Butt
Clinical Lecturer in Obstetrics & Gynaecology
Trinity College, University of Dublin
Trinity College Department of Obstetrics
and Gynaecology
Coombe Women and Infants University Hospital
Dublin, Ireland

Edwin Chandraharan
Consultant Obstetrician and Gynaecologist/Lead
Clinician Labour Ward
St. George's Healthcare NHS Trust
London, UK

Joanna Crofts
Specialist Registrar in Obstetrics and Gynaecology
St Michael's Hospital
Bristol, UK

Mark Denbow
Specialist Registrar in Obstetrics and Gynaecology
St Michael's Hospital
Bristol, UK

Mandish K. Dhanjal
Consultant Obstetrician and Gynaecologist
Queen Charlotte's and Chelsea Hospital, London
Honorary Senior Lecturer
Imperial College, London

Stergios K. Doumouchtsis
Senior Specialist Registrar
Department of Obstetrics and Gynaecology
St George's Hospital/St George's University of London
London, UK

Timothy J. Draycott
Consultant Obstetrician and Gynaecologist
Southmead Hospital
Bristol, UK

Rohan D'Souza
Clinical Research Fellow in Obstetrics
and Gynaecology
Division of Clinical Developmental Sciences
St George's University of London
London, UK

David Fraser
Consultant Obstetrician and Gynaecologist
Department of Obstetrics and Gynaecology
Norfolk and Norwich University Hospital
Norwich, UK

Guy Jackson
Obstetric Anaesthetic Fellow
Chelsea & Westminster Hospital
London, UK

Nina Johns
Birmingham Women's Hospital

Edgbaston
Birmingham, UK

Tracey Johnston
Consultant in Fetal Maternal Medicine
Birmingham Woman's Hospital
Birmingham, UK

Justin C. Konje
Consultant Obstetrician and Gynaecologist
Reproductive Sciences Section
Department of Obstetrics and Gynaecology
University of Leicester
University Hospitals of Leicester
Leicester, UK

Audrey Long
Consultant Obstetrician and Subspecialist
in Fetomaternal Medicine
Department of Obstetrics and Gynaecology
University Hospital of Wales
Cardiff, UK

Louay S. Louis
Department of Reproductive Biology
Imperial College London
Faculty of Medicine
London, UK

Paul A. Mannix
Consultant Neonatal Paediatrician
Northwick Park Hospital
Harrow, UK

Mahishee Mehta
Specialist Registrar in Obstetrics and
Gynaecology
King's College Hospital
Denmark Hill
London, UK

Nutan Mishra
Senior Registrar,
St. George's Healthcare NHS Trust
Blackshaw Road,
London, UK

Sambit Mukhopadhyay
Consultant Obstetrician and Gynaecologist
Department of Obstetrics and Gynaecology
Norfolk and Norwich University Hospital
Norwich, UK

Deirdre J. Murphy
Professor of Obstetrics and Gynaecology
Trinity College, University of Dublin
Trinity College Department of Obstetrics
and Gynaecology
Coombe Women and Infants University Hospital
Dublin, Ireland

Vivek Nama
Clinical Research Fellow
Department of Obstetrics and Gynaecology
Division of Clinical Developmental Sciences
St George's University of London
London, UK

Osric Navti
Subspecialty Trainee
Reproductive Sciences Section
Department of Obstetrics and Gynaecology
University of Leicester
University Hospitals of Leicester
Leicester, UK

Catherine Nelson-Piercy
Consultant Obstetric Physician
Guy's and St Thomas' Foundation Trust and
Queen Charlotte's and Chelsea Hospital
London, UK

Jane E. Norman
Professor of Maternal and Fetal Health
University of Edinburgh
Edinburgh, UK

Geraldine O'Sullivan
Dept of Anaesthetics
St Thomas' Hospital
London, UK

Sara Paterson-Brown
Consultant Obstetrician and Gynaecologist
and Labour Ward Lead
Queen Charlotte's and Chelsea Hospital
London, UK

Leonie Penna
Consultant Obstetrician
King's College Hospital
Denmark Hill
London, UK

Neelam Potdar
Clinical Lecturer & Specialist Registrar

Reproductive Sciences Section
Department of Obstetrics and Gynaecology
University of Leicester
University Hospitals of Leicester
Leicester, UK

Helen Scholefield
Health Service Management (Claims Handling
and Risk Management)
Department of Obstetrics
Liverpool Women's NHS Foundation Trust
Liverpool, UK

Jason Scott
Department of Anaesthetics
St Thomas' Hospital
London, UK

Dimitrios M. Siassakos
Specialist Registrar in Obstetrics and Gynaecology
Southmead Hospital, and
Clinical Fellow in Medical Education
North Academy, University of Bristol
Bristol, UK

Gordon C. S. Smith
Professor and Head of Department
Department of Obstetrics and Gynaecology
Cambridge University
The Rosie Hospital
Cambridge, UK

Lisa Story
Clinical Research Fellow
Imperial College
London, UK

Bryony Strachan
Consultant Obstetrician
St Michael's Hospital
Bristol, UK

Devi Subramanian
Specialist Registrar in Obstetrics and Gynaecology
King's College Hospital
London, UK

Abdul H. Sultan
Consultant Obstetrician and Gynaecologist
Department of Obstetrics and Gynaecology
Mayday University Hospital
Croydon
Surrey, UK

Ranee Thakar
Consultant Obstetrician & Gynaecologist
and Urogynaecology Subspecialist
Mayday University Hospital
Croydon, Surrey, UK

Austin Ugwumadu
Consultant Obstetrician and Gynaecologist
St. George's Hospital, London, UK

Rajesh Varma
Consultant Obstetrician and Gynaecologist
Guy's and St. Thomas' NHS Foundation Trust
Directorate of Women's Services
St Thomas' Hospital, London, UK

James J. Walker
Professor, Department of Obstetrics and Gynaecology
St James University Hospital
Leeds, UK

Steve Walkinshaw
Consultant in Maternal and Fetal Medicine
Liverpool Women's Hospital
Liverpool, UK

Richard Warren
Consultant Obstetrician and Gynaecologist
Norfolk and Norwich University Hospital
Norwich, UK

Melissa Whitten
Consultant in Feto-maternal Medicine
University Hospital NHS Trust
London, UK.

Melissa K. Whitworth
University of Liverpool
Department of Reproductive and Developmental
Medicine
Liverpool Women's NHS Foundation Trust
Liverpool, UK

Julian Woolfson
Consultant Obstetrician and Gynaecologist
Independent Sector
London, UK

Steve Yentis
Consultant Anaesthetist
Chelsea & Westminster Hospital
London, UK

ix

Preface

Those privileged to look after women during their labours and deliveries have a duty to practise to the highest standards. A clear understanding of what constitutes best practice will help to ensure the safety and health of mothers and babies through parturition.

Whilst the encouragement of normality is implicit, abnormality in labour must be recognized promptly and, when necessary, must be appropriately managed to ensure best outcome.

An understanding of normality and when and how to intervene are the keys to good clinical care. This textbook is an encompassing reference covering all the essential information relating to childbirth; it offers clear practical guidance across the width of labour and delivery.

We are very grateful to those well-known leading experts who, despite their busy lives, have made such excellent contributions to this definitive text. Each chapter offers a modern authoritative review of best practice with the evidence base for good clinical care necessary to optimize outcome through appropriate clinical management and justifiable intervention.

Whilst this is an ideal textbook for those training or taking examinations in labour ward practice, it offers all those professionals caring for the labouring woman a modern, evidence-based approach, which will help them understand and deliver the best possible clinical care. The importance of team working, prioritizing and the organization of maternity care receive appropriate emphasis with clear guidance and practical advice.

Guided by appropriate, clearly defined management pathways, based on national guidance, attending professionals will be best placed to improve safety and the quality of the labour process for both mother and baby.

The auditing and monitoring of standards and outcomes are vital to the organization and improvement of maternity services. The recent introduction of Clinical Dashboards (Appendix A) promises to be a major advance by facilitating the monitoring through traffic light recording of performance and governance (including clinical activity, workforce, outcomes risk incidents, complaints/ women's feedback about care) against locally or nationally agreed benchmarked standards.

This book contains the most up-to-date references and evidence base, including from the Guidelines and Standards of the Royal College of Obstetricians and Gynaecolgists (www.rcog.org.uk) and the National Institute for Health and Clinical Excellence (www.nice.org.uk). We believe that this textbook will be of great value for all midwives and doctors overseeing and managing childbirth.

Richard Warren
Sir Sabaratnam Arulkumaran

Acknowledgements

The editors would like to acknowledge the help of each and every author who has given their time generously to contribute the chapters and Mrs Sue Cunningham of St George's University of London who helped with the invitation and organization of the chapters. We are indebted to Nick Danton, Katie James and Dawn Preston of Cambridge University Press for their invaluable help in publishing this book and helping us all keep to time.

We are greatly indebted to our families Jane, Pippa and Joffy Warren and Gayatri, Shankari, Nishkantha and Kailash Arulkumaran for their tolerance and understanding of the time away from them during our own careers and in editing this book.

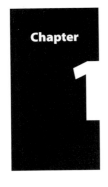

Chapter

1

Pelvic and fetal cranial anatomy and mechanism of labour

Louay S. Louis and Richard Warren

Introduction

Labour is the series of events whereby the contents of the gravid uterus, the fetus, amniotic fluid, placenta and membranes, are expelled from the pregnant woman. This process usually occurs approximately 280 days from conception.

In order for labour to be successful there needs to be a combination of efficient uterine contractions (power), an adequate roomy pelvis (passage) and an appropriate fetal size (passenger).

The female pelvis

The human being has an unusual pelvis; the distinctive shape of the hominid pelvis is probably as a result of an adaptation to bipedal gait [1].

The pelvis is comprised of two hip (innominate) bones that are joined anteriorly via the symphysis pubis (3.5 cm long), and posteriorly they articulate with the sacrum (12 cm long) at the sacro-iliac joint. Each hip bone is composed of three bones that are joined together at the acetabulum; these bones are the pubis, ischium and ilium (Figure 1.1).

The female pelvis is tilted forwards relative to the spine. The angle of inclination is variable between different individuals and between different races; in adult Caucasian females, the pelvis is usually about 55° to the horizontal plane. Pelvic 'tilt', or inclination, is position-dependent and increases with growth into adulthood [2].

The 'true' pelvis is bounded anteriorly by the symphysis pubis, the iliopectineal line laterally, and the sacrum posteriorly. It is composed of an inlet, a cavity and an outlet (Figure 1.2).

The female pelvis can be classified into four basic shapes [3]; gynaecoid (which is the classical female pelvis and the most common), android (heart-shaped inlet, a funnel-shaped cavity and a narrow outlet), anthropoid (the inlet is oval with the widest diameter being antero-posterior, the cavity is long and narrow) and platypoid (flattened inlet with the antero-posterior diameter at the inlet shorter than a gynaecoid pelvis and the transverse diameter wider) (Figure 1.3). The final shape of the female pelvis seems to be determined by culture and environment, as well as by genetics, with a suggestion that the age of acquisition of erect posture might play a vital role [4].

The pelvic inlet of an adequately sized gynaecoid pelvis is usually more than 12 cm antero-posteriorly, and 13.5 cm in the transverse diameter. The inlet is bounded anteriorly by the pubic crest, posteriorly by the promontory of the sacrum, and laterally by the ilio-pectineal line. The antero-posterior diameter of the pelvic inlet is also known as the true conjugate. However, clinically the most important diameter is the obstetric conjugate, which is the line between the promontory of the sacrum and the innermost part of the symphysis pubis – it is usually more than 10 cm (Figure 1.2). The line between the sacral promontory and the lowermost point of the symphysis is termed the diagonal conjugate. The mid cavity is spacious yet shallow, with both antero-posterior and transverse diameters usually approximately 12.5 cm. The birth canal narrows down inferiorly in the transverse section at the level of the ischial spines, but still measures more than 10 cm. In an ideal pelvis the ischial spines do not indent prominently into the pelvic cavity. The pelvic outlet is bounded by the inferior aspect of the pubic arch anteriorly, the tip of the coccyx posteriorly, and the ischial tuberosities and the surrounding ligaments laterally, with diameters of 12.5 cm antero-posteriorly and 11 cm transversely.

Best Practice in Labour and Delivery, ed. R. Warren and S. Arulkumaran. Published by Cambridge University Press.
© Cambridge University Press 2009.

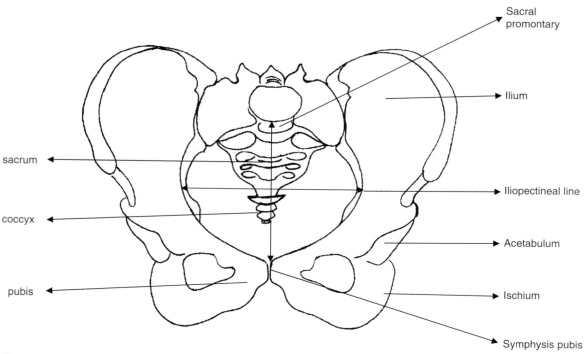

Figure 1.1 The female pelvis. The anterior–posterior diameter of the pelvic inlet is 12 cm and the transverse diameter is 13.5 cm

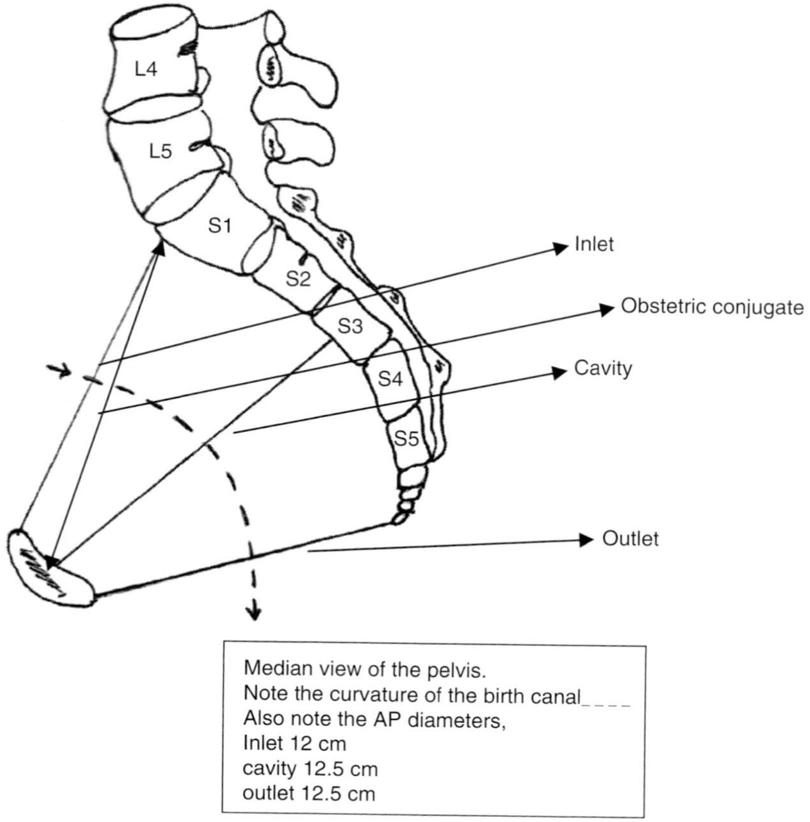

Figure 1.2 Vertical section of the pelvis

Median view of the pelvis.
Note the curvature of the birth canal____
Also note the AP diameters,
Inlet 12 cm
cavity 12.5 cm
outlet 12.5 cm

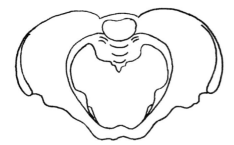

Gynaecoid, most common, 55%, inlet transverse diameter is wider than the antero-posterior diameter

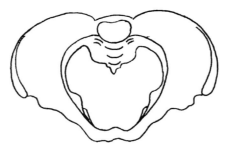

Android, 20% of women, heart-shaped inlet, funnel-shaped cavity, narrow outlet

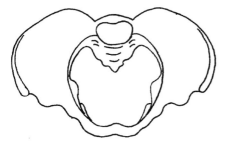

Anthropoid, 20% of women, oval-shaped inlet, maximum diameter AP with a long and narrow cavity

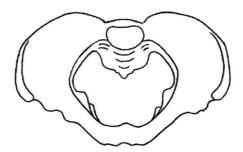

Platypoid, 5% of women, flattened transversely oval, shallow cavity and spacious outlet

Figure 1.3 Basic shapes of the female pelvis

It is through these various curves and bony canal that the fetus has to pass in order to achieve a successful vaginal delivery.

The fetal skull

Compared to the adult skull, the fetal skull is made of the large cranium and a relatively small face. The fetal cranium is composed of nine bones (occipital, two parietal, two frontal, two temporal, sphenoid and ethmoid). The first five are of clinical importance during birth. These bones are held together by membranes, also called sutures, which permit their movement and overlap during labour. The junction between the two parietal bones is called the sagittal suture, between the two frontal bones it is called the frontal suture, between the two frontal and two parietal bones the suture is called the coronal suture, and the suture between the two parietal bones and the occipital bone is called the lambdoid suture. The diamond-shaped junction where the two coronal sutures meet with the frontal and sagittal sutures is

called the anterior fontanelle, whilst the triangular junction between the sagittal suture and the two lambdoid sutures is called the posterior fontanelle (Figure 1.4).

Moulding is the process whereby the anatomical relationship between the cranial bones is changed as a response to external pressures/forces. Moulding occurs in labour to a varying degree as the fetal head descends in the birth canal, allowing the fetal head to accommodate to the geometry of the birth canal. Moulding is often more marked when there is a partially contracted pelvis, as moulding reduces the diameter of the presenting part of the fetal head and helps descent and progress towards a vaginal delivery. Classically, it was thought that moulding is due to overlapping of the parietal bones over other cranial bones. Some authors, however, argue that the actual mechanism is due partially to unbending and straightening of the parietal bones that allow moulding, with a locking mechanism occurring in protracted labours when the free edges of the cranial bones are forced into one another [5,6].

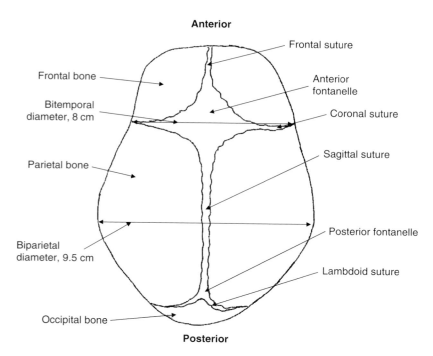

Anterior

Frontal suture

Frontal bone

Anterior fontanelle

Bitemporal diameter, 8 cm

Coronal suture

Sagittal suture

Parietal bone

Biparietal diameter, 9.5 cm

Posterior fontanelle

Lambdoid suture

Occipital bone

Posterior

Figure 1.4 The sutures and fontanelles of the fetal skull

For descriptive purposes, the fetal head has been divided into regions that aid in defining the lower-most presenting part on vaginal examination during labour. The vertex is the area between the anterior and posterior fontanelle and extends to the parietal eminences on each side. The occiput is the area behind the posterior fontanelle. The area of the anterior fontanelle is called the bregma and the area in front of the anterior fontanelle to the root of the nose is known as the brow. The area between the root of the nose and the chin is the face (Figure 1.5).

The degree of flexion of the fetal head during labour determines which region of the fetal skull is presenting, and hence it is customary to describe lines that correspond to the diameter of the presenting region of the head (Figure 1.6). The suboccipito-bregmatic (fully flexed vertex) and the submento-bregmatic (face) are the narrowest diameters at 9.5 cm each. The widest diameter is 13.5 cm which is the mento-vertical of a brow presentation and the other diameters are suboccipito-frontal (10.5 cm) and occipito-frontal (11.5 cm); both the latter are seen with deflexed vertex presentations.

Caput succedaneum is the term that refers to the subcutaneous sero-haematic extravasation that usually, but not always, occurs in a labour that is especially protracted and when the vertex is the presenting part. It is a boggy and soft swelling that may extend over the suture line. It usually resolves within a few days after birth, although extremely rarely it may result in alopecia [7]. Preterm prelabour rupture of the membranes seems to be a predisposing factor for in-utero formation of caput succedaneum [8]. The presence of severe caput succedaneum can make defining the position of the fetus in the second stage of labour difficult [9]; however, it seems to have only minimal influence on the pH of blood obtained from the scalp during fetal blood sampling [10].

Parturition, initiation of labour and myometrial contractility

Uterine activity in pregnancy, or 'phenotype', can be described in four different stages during the parturition process. Uterine myometrial activity is quiescent during 95% of pregnancy (phase 0); it is believed that this is mainly due to the action of progesterone. Activation corresponds to phase 1 and is affected predominantly by mechanical influence, but also by uterotrophins such as oestrogen and through increased expression of contraction-associated proteins. Stimulation corresponds to phase 2, when endogenous uterotronins,

Figure 1.5 The regions of the fetal skull

1. Suboccipito-bregmatic, 9.5 cm
2. Suboccipito-frontal, 10.5 cm
3. Occipito-frontal, 11.5 cm
4. Mento-vertical, 13.5 cm
5. Submento-bregmatic, 9.5 cm

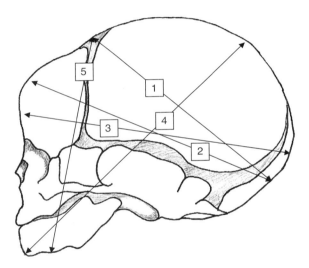

Figure 1.6 The diameters of the fetal skull

including prostaglandins and oxytocin, act on the activated myometrium. Postpartum involution corresponds to phase 3. In this sequence of events, the initiation of parturition corresponds to the transition from phase 0 to phase 1 [11].

The mechanisms that instigate parturition in humans have been elusive to discovery [12]. Unlike animals, the fetal hypothalamic–pituitary–adrenal (HPA) axis has a supportive, rather than an essential, role [13]. During pregnancy the uterus grows under the action of oestrogen; growth ceases towards the end of pregnancy, and at the same time an increasing tension of the uterus may herald the signal of the onset of labour. Relaxation of the uterine myometrium appears to be regulated by progesterone [12]. Progesterone levels do not fall with the onset of labour per se, but it is believed that there is a change in the expression of progesterone receptors from type B to types A and C, constituting a 'functional' progesterone withdrawal [12,14,15].

As pregnancy advances, there is an increased production of placental corticotrophin-releasing hormone (CRH). Maternal levels of CRH increase, peaking at the time of delivery. As a result, the adrenals release cortisol and dehydroepiandrosterone sulphate (DHEAS). The latter is rapidly metabolized by the placenta into oestrogen. Increased cortisol stimulates further production of CRH, generating a positive feed-forward reaction. CRH acts on multiple sites in the mother and the fetus to initiate the changes associated with parturition. Cortisol production by the fetus induces maturation of the lungs via surfactants and phospholipids. The latter enter the amniotic fluid and result in increased levels of cyclooxygenase-2 (COX-2) and prostaglandin E_2. Prostaglandins mediate the release of the metalloproteases that weaken the placental membranes, leading to rupture of membranes [12,16]. Prostaglandins mediate cervical ripening, directly stimulate uterine contractions, and indirectly increase fundally dominant myometrial contractility by up-regulation of oxytocin receptors and, thereby, allow synchronization of contractions [17].

The microanatomy of the term-pregnant human uterus is that of clearly defined structural elements [18]. In labour, a group of proteins called contraction-associated proteins (CAPs) act on the relaxed uterus to initiate powerful rhythmic contractions that push the fetus down the birth canal. There are three types of CAPs: those that cause myocyte contraction, those that increase myocyte excitability, and those that promote intercellular connectivity [12]. This has led to the suggestion of a functional partitioning of the myometrium during pregnancy, whereby the lower segment displays a contractile phenotype throughout gestation but changing to a relaxatory phenotype at labour, whereas the upper uterine segment maintains a relaxatory phenotype throughout most of gestation to accommodate the growing fetus and adopts a contractile phenotype during labour [19]. Myometrial contraction itself is a function of actin and myocin; this is aided by myocin light-chain kinase, calmodulin, calcium and connexin-43. The electrochemical potential of the myocytes' plasma membrane is intracellularly negative, due to the action of the sodium–potassium pump. This changes at the time of labour, with a low-intensity stimulus only required for depolarization and thereby contraction. Connections between myocytes in labour are formed by paracrine release of prostaglandins $F_{2\alpha}$. The end result is extensive depolarization waves over large areas of the uterus. This activity is fundally dominant, synchronized, (with periods of relaxation in between contractions to allow increased blood flow to the fetus), and leads to expulsion of the fetus [12].

Labour and its mechanism

In order to achieve a safe and successful vaginal delivery and to minimize the risks of complications to the mother and baby, the fetal lie, presentation and position should be determined at the beginning of the first stage of labour.

Lie

This describes the relationship of the fetal longitudinal axis to that of the uterus. It is either longitudinal (which is the case in over 99% of singleton term babies), transverse (0.3%) or oblique. Oblique lies usually change during the course of labour into either longitudinal or transverse.

The main causes for persistent transverse lie in pregnancy include prematurity, multiparity, multiple pregnancy, placenta praevia, a fundal placenta, polyhydramnios, uterine fibromatas, congenital uterine anomalies, intrauterine fetal death and extrauterine masses obstructing the birth canal, e.g. a large ovarian cyst.

Compared to those babies presenting with a longitudinal lie at the onset of labour, babies who are in transverse lie have been found to have a lower absolute pH, more frequent chance of developing severe acidosis, lower birth weight, and are more likely to sustain birth trauma and long-term residual effects [20].

Presentation

The presenting part of the fetus is the lowermost part of the fetal body within the birth canal that can be felt during a vaginal examination. At term most babies present by the vertex. The degree of flexion of the fetal head will determine the presentation, and whereby, for example, a deflexed head may result in a brow or face presentation.

In transverse or oblique lies, the presenting part is usually the shoulder or, rarely, the umbilical cord.

In breech presentation, the description of the presenting part depends on the relationship of the lower extremities to the fetal hips. With extended (frank) breech, both thighs are flexed and both knees are extended, this being the most common (65%). Flexed (complete) breech is when both the thighs and the knees are flexed (25%). Least common is the footling (incomplete) breech, when one hip is flexed whilst the other is extended (10%).

Finally, compound presentations refer to more than one part of the fetal body presenting together, e.g. a hand and vertex.

Position

The fetal position refers to the relation of a reference point that is an easily definable point on the periphery of the presentation, usually a bony prominence, to fixed points of the maternal pelvis. The 'denominator' for the vertex is the occiput (O). For the face, the denominator is the chin (mentum) (M); for the shoulder, the acromion (A), although for practical reasons the back is taken as reference; and for the breech it is the sacrum (S).

Since, at term, the presentation of most fetuses is cephalic, the occiput is used in this text for descriptive purposes. A left-sided (L) occiput is more common than a right (R) occiput. Either side, the occiput can be placed anteriorly (A), transversely (T) or posteriorly (P), resulting in eight possible different positions. The same principles apply to each of the other three presentations when describing their denominator's relationship to the maternal pelvis.

Asynclitism

Asynclitism describes the relationship of the sagittal plane of the fetal head to that of the coronal planes of the symphysis pubis and the sacral promontory. Usually the planes are not parallel and a slight degree of asynclitism is the norm. Significant asynclitism occurs with relative cephalo-disproportion, as the fetal head rocks on entering the pelvis in an attempt to make progress, the infra-supra parietal diameter (8.5 cm) usually being nearly 1 cm shorter than the biparietal. If the tilt of the sagittal plane is directed towards the symphysis pubis, then more of the posterior aspect of the fetus's head is felt vaginally during examination; this is called posterior asynclitism. Anterior asynclitism occurs if more of the anterior part of the fetal head is felt on examination.

Attitude

This refers to the characteristic posture that the fetus adopts during the last weeks of pregnancy. Attitude describes the relation of the various fetal parts to other parts of the body, e.g. arms folded over the chest or parallel by the sides. During the latter months of pregnancy, with the fetal head, trunk and limbs all flexed, the universal attitude is that of flexion.

Abdominal and pelvic examination during pregnancy and labour

Abdominal examination

The uterus may be palpated through the maternal abdomen from 12 weeks gestation and the uterine fundus reaches the level of the xiphisternum by 36 weeks.

In addition to the usual standard methods of clinical assessment of inspection, palpation, percussion and auscultation, there are specific palpation methods used in pregnancy; these include the assessment of the symphyseal–fundal height (SFH) and the Leopold manoeuvres.

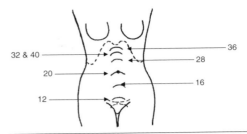

The abdominal markings of uterine growth related to the number of weeks of pregnancy. At 12 weeks the uterus is just palpable abdominally, by 20 weeks the uterine fundus is at the level of the umbilicus. Maximum fundal height is achieved at 36 weeks gestation.

Figure 1.7 The SFH at different stages in pregnancy

SFH may be used as a screening tool to assess fetal growth; it can be achieved either by hand or by using a tape measure. When a tape measure is used, the measurement is made by identifying the variable point, the fundus, and then measuring to the fixed point of the top of the symphysis pubis, with the option of centimetre values being hidden from the examiner [21].

Alternatively, without a measure, approximately every two finger breadths between the symphysis pubis and the umbilicus equals 2 weeks gestation added to the 12 weeks mark suprapubically; therefore, the uterus is about 20 weeks size when it is at the level of the umbilicus. Above the umbilicus every single finger breadth equals approximately 2 weeks gestation (see Figure 1.7).

In the nineteenth century, Christian G. Leopold described the manoeuvres which came to bear his name. The aim of these manoeuvres is to check fetal lie, presentation, position, station and attitude (see Figure 1.8). Leopold's manoeuvres are undertaken with the patient, having emptied her bladder, in a reclining position, preferably with a left-sided tilt.

First manoeuvre

The uterine fundal area is palpated in order to determine what part of the fetus is occupying the fundus (Figure 1.8a), usually the breech or head; the head is round and ballottable, while the breech is softer.

Second manoeuvre

The lateral walls of the uterus are felt to determine on which side is the fetal back, which is large and firm. The fetal abdomen is soft and extremities are soft and mobile (Figure 1.8b).

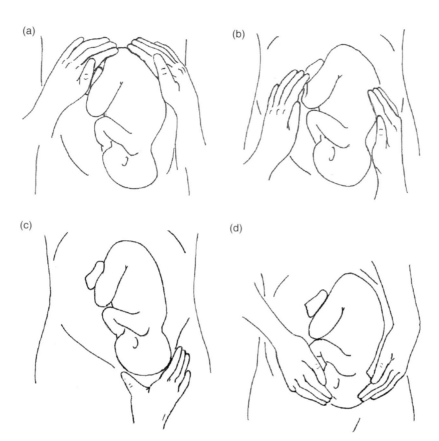

(a)   (b)   (c)   (d)

Figure 1.8 The Leopold Manoeuvres

Third manoeuvre

Also called the Pawlik's manoeuvre. A gentle grip with thumb and fingers placed on the area over the symphysis pubis to determine what part of the fetal head is lying over the pelvic inlet and the amount of that presenting part that is palpable abdominally (Figure 1.8c). The same principles apply in differentiating a cephalic from a breech presentation. Pawlik's manoeuvre may be uncomfortable for the pregnant woman and, if examination is performed in this way, it must be undertaken gently. Alternatively, and in preference, the necessary clinical information may be obtained through the fourth manoeuvre.

Fourth manoeuvre

The examiner turns towards the patient's feet and places his/her hands on the lower part of the uterus to confirm the presentation and on which side is the prominence of the presenting part (Figure 1.8d).

When used by experienced clinicians, the above manoeuvres can be used as a screening tool for fetal malpresentation with a high sensitivity (88%) and specificity (94%) [22].

Whichever technique is used, it is customary to describe the amount of the fetal head that is palpable outside of the pelvis in fifths (Figure 1.9). Traditionally, the fifths are described based on the number of fingers needed to cover the fetal head above the pelvic brim. When all of the fetal head is palpable above the pelvis it is described as 5/5 (five-fifths palpable). When the fetal head is engaged, it is usually 2/5th palpable, and when it is deeply engaged it is 0/5th palpable.

On completion of a clinical examination it is usual to describe, in order, the sympyseal–fundal height, fetal lie, presentation and engagement. The fetal heart should be auscultated.

Pelvic examination

This is divided into two types: speculum examination and digital vaginal examination.

A sterile **speculum examination**, allowing visual inspection, is indicated in cases of preterm labour,

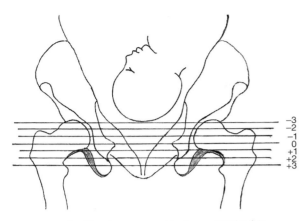

−3
−2
−1
0
+1
+2
+3

Figure 1.9 Fetal head engagement in the maternal pelvis

Table 1.1 Bishop score for status of the cervix.

Score	0	1	2	3
Dilatation (cm)	0	1–2	3–4	5+
Length of cervix (cm)	3	2	1	0
Station	−3	−2	−1, 0	+1, +2
Consistency	Firm	Medium	Soft	
Position	Posterior	Mid	Anterior	

Note: Score each component and add scores.

vaginal bleeding and suspected rupture of membranes. It must be avoided when there is any suspicion of placenta praevia.

During examination the following should be described and noted: inspection of vulva and vagina to ascertain/establish the presence or absence of any liquor, blood or discharge, and inspection of the cervix to establish its length, thickness and position (anterior, mid-position or posterior).

The features assessed during sterile **digital vaginal examination** change during the course of labour. Throughout prelabour, during assessment for induction of labour, and during the initial stages of labour, it is customary to start with an assessment of the cervical length (effacement), dilatation, consistency, position, and the presentation and station of the presenting part relative to the ischial spines. These features make up the Bishop score (see Table 1.1). Cervical dilatation is a better predictor of the likelihood of successful induction of labour and vaginal delivery than the Bishop score or any other Bishop score component characteristic [23]. In the active stage of labour, the clinician assesses the progress of cervical dilatation, the shortening of the length of the cervix (effacement), the station and position of the presenting part, and whether there is any caput succedaneum, asynclitism and/or moulding.

Cervical effacement

The normal prelabour cervical length is 3–4 cm. The cervix is said to be 50% effaced when it shortens to approximately 2 cm, and fully effaced when there is no length and it is as thin as the adjacent lower segment of the uterus. Effacement is determined by assessing the length of the cervix from the external to the internal os. Complete cervical effacement is associated with a characteristic and profound alteration in the gene expression profile of cervical cells. The majority of these genes encode cytokines, transcription factors and cell-matrix-associated proteins [24].

The process of cervical effacement and dilatation differs between primigravida and multiparous patients. In the latter, effacement and dilatation are occurring simultaneously, whilst in the case of primigravidae, effacement precedes dilatation.

Cervical position describes the location of the cervix in relation to the maternal pelvis. During labour, the position progresses from posterior to mid-position and then to anterior.

Cervical consistency ranges from firm to soft. Cervical softening during pregnancy is a unique phase of the tissue remodelling process characterized by increased collagen solubility, maintenance of tissue strength, and up-regulation of genes involved in mucosal protection [25]. During this process, the junction between the fetal membranes and the deciduas breaks down, and an adhesive protein – fetal fibronectin – enters vaginal fluids. This is a clinically useful predictor of imminent delivery [12].

Identifying the **position of the presenting part** is accomplished by identifying the bony sutures of the fetal head, following the suture until it leads to a fontanelle and then identifying the sutures radiating from it. Provided the head is low and the patient has good pain relief, it may also be possible to locate the ear of the fetus and to assess to which side it faces. The nose and mouth can usually be identified in a face presentation, whilst the sacrum, genitalia and anus should be identifiable with a breech presentation.

The **station** of the presenting part describes the distance of the leading bony part of the fetal head relative to the ischial spines. The usual method is to measure the distance above and below the spines in centimetres, with the areas above being given a minus sign and those below the spines being given a positive sign. For example, −2 indicates that the lowest part of the fetal head is 2 cm above the level of the ischial spines, whilst +1 indicates that the head is 1 cm below the level of the spines (Figure 1.9).

Stages of labour, its mechanism and cardinal movements

Labour is divided into three stages, with the first stage of labour beginning with the onset of painful regular contractions resulting in cervical changes. The first stage ends when the cervix is fully dilated at 10 cm. The second stage of labour then starts, ending with the delivery of the fetus. The third stage begins from the birth of the baby and lasts until the uterus is emptied with the expulsion of placenta and membranes.

The **first stage of labour** is divided into a latent phase and an active phase. The **latent phase** is defined as the period of time, not necessarily continuous, when there may be painful contractions as well as cervical change, including cervical effacement and with cervical dilatation up to 4 cm. The established, **active phase of labour** begins when there are regular painful contractions and there is progressive cervical dilatation from full effacement and 4 cm dilatation onwards. The length of the active first stage of labour varies between women; first labours last on average 8 h and are unlikely to last over 18 h. Second and subsequent labours last on average 5 h and are unlikely to last over 12 h [26] [27].

Mechanism of labour

The mechanism of labour, or its cardinal movements, describes the series of changes in the position of the fetal head with its passage through the birth canal (Figures 1.10 and 1.11). These are as follows.

Engagement

This is the mechanism whereby the biparietal diameter of the fetal head enters the 'true' pelvis. The fetal head is engaged when its maximum diameters (suboccipito-bregmatic and biparietal, when the head is well flexed) have passed the pelvic inlet. On engagement, the biparietal diameter lies at the level of the true conjugate and the vertex is 1 cm above the ischial spines. In nulliparous women, engagement usually takes place from the middle of the third trimester onwards, but in some of these women, and in most multiparous women, engagement may not take place until the onset of labour. Studies that have looked at post-term nulliparous patients (defined after 41 weeks gestation) with an unengaged vertex concluded that they are 12.4-times more likely to be delivered by caesarean section than those with an engaged fetal head.

Descent

This is the downward movement of the fetal head in the pelvis. Descent is usually described by the number of fifths of the presenting part still palpable above the pelvis, and by the station (the relative position of the presenting part to the ischial spines). In nulliparous women, descent may not take place until the second stage of labour. Descent is usually brought about by uterine contractions and is aided in the second stage of labour by maternal effort.

Flexion

Uterine contractions will usually cause flexion of the fetal head forwards as it is pressed against the lower segment of the uterus, the pelvic side walls and pelvic floor. This results in the fetal chin coming into contact with the fetal chest and the smallest diameter (suboccipito-bregmatic diameter, in the case of a fully flexed head) continues to pass through the birth canal.

Internal rotation

This is the gradual turning of the fetal head (which usually enters the pelvis with the sagittal suture in the transverse) so that the occiput turns to be behind the symphysis pubis (occipito-anterior). In preterm labour and with small babies, labour may progress without internal rotation of the fetal vertex.

Extension

As the fetal head descends to the level of the pelvic outlet, the base of the occiput will come into contact with the inferior margin of the symphysis pubis where the birth canal curves upward and forward. The head is delivered through the maternal vaginal introitus by extension from the flexed position. First to deliver is the occiput, then with further extension the vertex, bregma, forehead, nose, mouth and finally the chin.

Figure 1.10 The Bishop Score

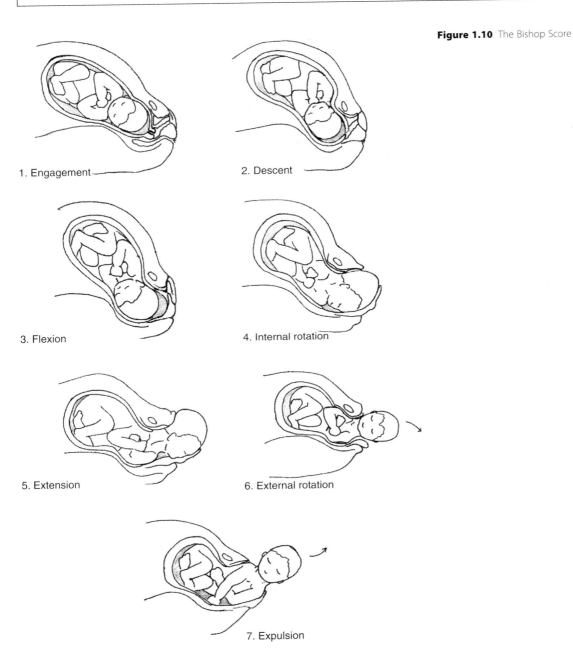

1. Engagement

2. Descent

3. Flexion

4. Internal rotation

5. Extension

6. External rotation

7. Expulsion

External rotation (restitution)

Having delivered with the sagittal suture vertical and the occiput anterior, the delivered fetal head returns to the position it occupied in the vagina. For example, if the position was left occipito anterior (LOA), the head will 'restitute' to the left. This is followed by complete rotation of the sagittal suture to the transverse position so that the shoulders align in the antero-posterior diameter of the pelvic outlet, so facilitating their passage (i.e. one shoulder will lie behind the symphysis pubis, the other will be posterior, in front of the sacral promontory).

Expulsion

The rest of the fetal body is delivered. Birth of the baby is completed by delivery of the anterior shoulder first then, by lateral flexion, the posterior shoulder and finally the remainder of the torso.

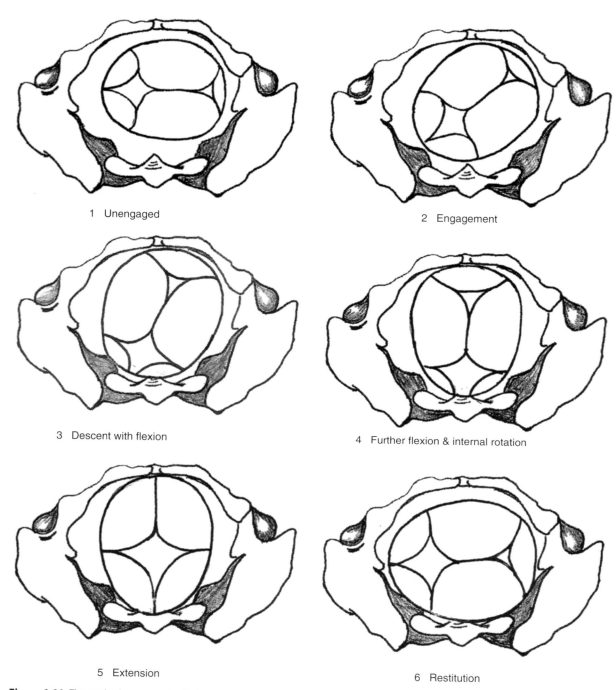

1   Unengaged

2   Engagement

3   Descent with flexion

4   Further flexion & internal rotation

5   Extension

6   Restitution

Figure 1.11 The cardinal movements of labour

Management of the third stage of labour. (See Chapter 14.)

References

1. Stewart D B. The pelvis as a passageway. I. Evolution and adaptations. *Br J Obstet Gynaecol* 1984; **91**: 611–7.

2. Mac-Thiong J M, Berthonnaud E, Dimar J R II, Bets R R, Labelle H. Sagittal alignment of the spine and pelvis during growth. *Spine* 2004; **29**: 1642–7.

3. Caldwell W E, Moloy H C. Anatomical variation in the female pelvis and their effect in labor with a suggested classification. *Am J Obstet Gynecol* 1933; **26**: 479–505.

4. Abitbol M M. The shapes of the female pelvis. Contributing factors. *J Reprod Med* 1996; **41**: 242–50.

5. Lapeer R J, Prager R W. Fetal head moulding: finite element analysis of a fetal skull subjected to uterine pressures during the first stage of labour. *J Biomech* 2001; **34**: 1125–33.

6. Carlan S J, Wyble L, Lense J, Mastrogiannis D S, Parsons M T. Fetal head moulding. Diagnosis by ultrasound and a review of the literature. *J Perinatol* 1991; **11**: 105–11.

7. Lykoudis E G, Spyropoulou G A, Lavasidis L G, Paschopoulos M E, Paraskevaidis E A. Alopecia associated with birth injury. *Obstet Gynecol* 2007; **110**: 487–90.

8. Bats A S, Senat M V, Mohlo M, Ville Y. Discovery of caput succedaneum after premature rupture of membranes at 28 weeks gestation. *J Gynecol Obstet Biol Reprod (Paris)* 2003; **32**: 179–82.

9. Dupuis O, Ruimark S, Corrine D, Simone T, André D, René-Charles R. Fetal head position during the second stage of labor: comparison of digital vaginal examination and transabdominal ultrasonographic examination. *Eur J Obstet Gynecol Reprod Biol* 2005; **123**: 193–7.

10. Boenisch H, Saling E. The reliability of pH-values in fetal blood samples – a study of the second stage. *J Perinat Med* 1976; **4**: 45–50.

11. Norwitz E R, Robinson J N, Challis J R. The control of labor. *N Eng J Med* 1999; **341**: 660–6.

12. Smith R. Parturition. *N Eng J Med* 2007; **356**: 271–83.

13. Bernal A L. Overview of current research in parturition. *Exp Physiol* 2001; **86**: 213–22.

14. Smith R, Mesiano S, McGrath S. Hormone trajectories leading to human birth. *Regul Pept* 2002; **108**: 159–64.

15. Zakar T, Hertelendy F. Progesterone withdrawal: key to parturition. *Am J Obstet Gynecol* 2007; **196**: 289–96.

16. Majzoub J A, McGregor J A, Lockwood C J, *et al.* A central theory of preterm and term labor: putative role for corticotrophin-releasing hormone. *Am J Obstet Gynecol* 1999; **180**: 232–41.

17. Slater D, Dennes W, Sawdy R, Allport V, Bennett P. Expression of cyclo-oxygenase type-1 and -2 in human fetal membranes throughout pregnancy. *J Mol Endocrinol* 1999; **22**: 125–30.

18. Young R C, Hession R O. Three-dimensional structure of the smooth muscle in the term-pregnant human uterus. *Obstet Gynecol* 1999; **93**: 94–9.

19. Grigsby P L, Sooranna S R, Adu-Amankwa B, *et al.* Regional expression of prostaglandin E2 and F2 alpha receptors in human myometrium, amnion, and choriodecidua with advancing gestation and labor. *Biol Reprod* 2006; **75**: 297–305.

20. Hankins G D, Hammond T L, Snyder R R, Gilstrap L C III. Transverse lie. *Am J Perinatol* 1990; **7**: 66–70.

21. *The Investigation and Management of the Small-For-gestational-age Fetus.* Royal College of Obstetricians and Gynaecologists. Green-top guidelines No. 31. London: RCOG, 2002.

22. Lydon-Rochelle M, Albers L, Gorwoda J, Craig E, Qualls C. Accuracy of Leopold maneuvers in screening for malpresentation: a prospective study. *Birth* 1993; **20**: 132–5.

23. Williams M C, Krammer J, O'Brien W F. The value of the cervical score in predicting successful outcome of labor induction. *Obstet Gynecol* 1997; **91**: 315–6.

24. Huber A, Hudelist G, Czerwenka K, *et al.* Gene expression profiling of cervical tissue during physiological cervical effacement. *Obstet Gynecol* 2005; **105**: 91–8.

25. Read C P, Word R A, Ruscheinsky M A, Timmons B C, Mahendroo M S. Cervical remodeling during pregnancy and parturition: molecular characterization of the softening phase in mice. *Reproduction* 2007; **134**: 327–40.

26. National Institute for Health and Clinical Excellence. *Intrapartum Care: Care of Healthy Women and their Babies during Childbirth.* London: NICEM; 2007 Sep. CG55.

27. Shin K S, Brubaker K L, Ackerson L M. Risk of cesarean delivery in nulliparous women at greater than 41 weeks' gestational age with an unengaged vertex. *Am J Obstet Gynecol* 2004; **190**: 129–34.

The first stage of labour

Sambit Mukhopadhyay and David Fraser

The management of spontaneous labour remains an important issue. The perils of prolonged and often neglected labour are well known. In the developing world where there is a lack of appropriate health care both in terms of provision and access, the morbidity and mortality from prolonged and neglected labour is alarming. The causes of death and morbidity include obstructed labour, sepsis, rupture of the uterus and postpartum haemorrhage. In the developed world this is extremely rare, but rising caesarean section (CS) rate without significant benefit to maternal and neonatal outcomes is a matter of concern. The increasing CS rate for dystocia or difficult labour contributes at least a third to the overall CS rate, and almost 70% of those women who have a CS in their first labour will request an elective CS in subsequent pregnancies [1]. CS leads to increased maternal morbidity as well as mortality, especially when it is performed as an emergency procedure [2,3]. Furthermore, long-term risks of caesarean section have been reported, including an increased risk of placenta praevia and ectopic pregnancy [4]. Maternal and fetal morbidity and mortality due to prolonged labour and CS for dystocia may be reduced by the proper management of poor progress in labour – especially the first labour.

Normal labour

The precise definition of normal labour is the spontaneous onset of regular, painful uterine contractions associated with the effacement and progressive dilatation of the cervix and descent of the presenting part – with or without a 'show' or ruptured membranes. This process culminates in the birth of a healthy baby followed by expulsion of the placenta and membranes. In most cases, the outcome can be predicted prospectively by observing the progress of cervical dilatation and descent of the presenting part. Although labour is a dynamic, continuous process, it is normally divided into three functional stages for the purpose of management: the first, second and third stages of labour.

The basis for the scientific study of the progress of labour was developed by Friedman. He described the labour progress of 100 consecutive primigravid women in spontaneous labour at term. The progress was presented graphically by plotting the rate of cervical dilatation against time. The resulting graph of cervical dilatation forms the basis of the modern partogram – a pictorial representation of the key events in labour presented chronologically on a single page. The maternal and fetal parameters recorded include cervical dilatation, the level of the presenting part (in fifths of the fetal head palpable above the pelvic brim, rather than the station which relates the level of the head to the ischial spines and is measured in cm above or below), the fetal heart rate (FHR), the frequency and duration of uterine contractions, and the colour and quantity of amniotic fluid. Other maternal parameters include temperature, pulse and blood pressure, and drugs used. This pictorial documentation of labour facilitates the early recognition of poor progress. Plotting of the cervical dilatation at regular intervals also enables prediction of the time of onset of the second stage of labour.

Nomograms of cervical dilatation

The rate of cervical dilatation in labour has been studied in various ethnic groups in different countries [5–8]. The nomograms derived show similar rates of cervical dilatation in the different ethnic groups, and comparative studies have confirmed that ethnicity has little influence on the rate of cervical dilatation [9], or on uterine activity in spontaneous normal labour [10].

Best Practice in Labour and Delivery, ed. R. Warren and S. Arulkumaran. Published by Cambridge University Press.
© Cambridge University Press 2009.

Observations during the first stage of labour (defined from the time of admission to the labour ward to full dilatation of the cervix) show that the rate of cervical dilatation is composed of two phases. Following a slow 'latent' phase of labour, during which the cervix shortens from 3 to less than 0.5 cm long (effacement) and dilates to 4 cm, there is a faster 'active phase', when the cervix dilates from 4 cm to full dilatation (conventionally taken as 10 cm, although in reality it refers to a situation when no cervix is palpable). In order to identify women at risk of prolonged labour, a line of acceptable progress is drawn on the partogram, i.e. the alert line. If the rate of cervical dilatation falls to the right of this line, progress is deemed unsatisfactory. Conventionally, the line of acceptable progress has been based on the slowest tenth percentile rate of cervical dilatation observed in women who progress without intervention and deliver normally; in other words, 1 cm per hour. However, a certain grace period is given before intervention and is based on a line drawn parallel and one to four hours to the right of this – the action line. Accordingly, the proportion of labours deemed to have unsatisfactory progress can vary from 5 to 50%. WHO [11] and, more recently, NICE recommend the use of 4 h action line [12]. In the presence of good contractions (at least >2 in 10 min, lasting >40 s), the latent phase may last for up to 8 h in nulliparas and up to 6 h in multiparas. During the peak of the active phase of labour, the cervix dilates at a rate of 1 cm per hour in both in nulliparas and multiparas. Multiparas appear to dilate faster because they have shorter labours overall; not only do they have a shorter latent phase resulting in a more advanced cervical dilatation on admission, they have an increased rate of progress as full dilatation approaches. Construction of nomograms of anticipated normal progress or 'alert' lines, with the addition of 'action' lines to the right of this, reduces the likelihood of prolonged labour being overlooked, and is of considerable diagnostic and educational value (Figure 2.1). Studies looking at the efficacy of the use of the partogram, and comparison of a partogram with action line and one without, should be carried out [12].

Diagnosis of labour

The accurate diagnosis of labour at term may be difficult – and can be even more difficult in those labouring in the preterm period. If the contractions are painful and regular and if the cervix is >4 cm dilated (in other words, in the active phase), there is little difficulty in diagnosing labour. However, if the patient is in the latent phase of labour, it may be necessary to perform two examinations at least 2 h apart (and preferably done by the same examiner) in order to detect any progressive cervical change and diagnose labour. Uterine contractions without effacement and dilatation of the cervix occur in the third trimester. They are usually termed Braxton-Hicks contractions and are painless. These contractions may become more frequent and painful without affecting cervical changes of effacement and dilatation and may abate spontaneously. Differentiating points between false and true labour are shown in Table 2.1.

Management of first stage of labour

Good antecedents for 'natural' or 'physiological' labour and childbirth are antepartum education that eliminates fears and anxieties about labour, regular exercise to promote relaxation, muscle control and breathing without hyperventilation throughout labour. In addition, the importance of the 1:1 attention of a skilled professional attendant throughout labour to comfort the mother and give her constant reassurance has been shown to promote normal labour and good outcome.

The general principles of management are:

1. initial assessment,
2. observation and intervention if labour becomes abnormal,
3. close monitoring of the fetal and maternal condition,
4. adequate pain relief,
5. emotional support, and
6. adequate hydration.

Initial assessment

On admission, an initial assessment should be done by eliciting a detailed history and listening to the woman, by clinical examination and basic investigation. The aim is to identify high-risk pregnancies: a proportion being identified as high-risk before the onset of labour and others being identified as at-risk only during labour.

General examination

This should include the general condition of the woman, whether she has pallor or jaundice, the state of hydration, her blood pressure, pulse, temperature

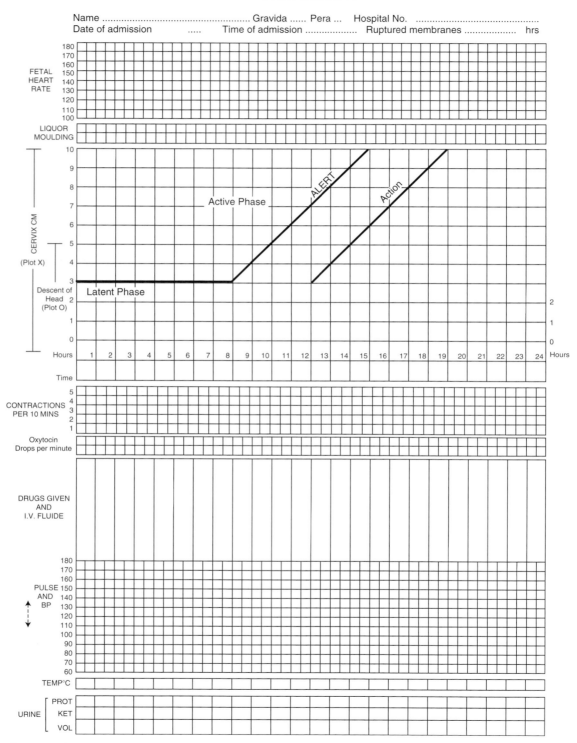

Figure 2.1 The WHO partograph

Table 2.1 Differences between true and false labour.

True labour	False labour
1. Contractions occur at regular intervals	Contractions occur at irregular intervals
2. Interval gradually shortens	Interval remains irregular
3. Intensity of pain gradually increases	Intensity of pain remains the same
4. Duration of contractions increases	Duration of contractions varies and tends to become less
5. There is progressive cervical effacement and dilatation	There is no progress in cervical effacement and dilatation
6. Progress of labour not stopped by sedation	Usually painful contractions are relieved by sedation and there is no progress in labour

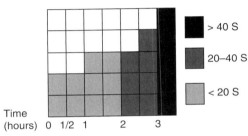

Figure 2.2 Quantification of uterine contractions by clinical palpation. Frequency per 10 min is recorded by shading the equivalent number of boxes. The type of shading indicates the duration of each contraction

and breathing should be checked. The cardiovascular status should be assessed and any oedema noted. The frequency of bladder emptying and urinary output should be noted.

Abdominal examination

Uterine contractions should be assessed by palpation, with relevance to their frequency and duration (every 30 min) and is assessed over a 10-minute period (Figure 2.2). The fundal height should be measured to identify babies felt to be significantly above or below the average birthweight, and the level of the presenting part should be noted. The level of the head should be estimated in 'fifths' (Figure 2.3) – clinical estimation of descent of the head in fifths excludes variation due to excessive caput and moulding and that produced by different depths of pelvis. It is easily reproducible. The fetal heart rate should be auscultated after a contraction for a minimum period of 1 min, and at least every 15 min in the first stage of labour and every 5 min in the second stage [13].

Vaginal examination

It is important to ensure consent, privacy, dignity and comfort before vaginal examination is undertaken. The following points should be noted during vaginal examination:

- any abnormal discharge from the vagina;
- the colour and quantity of any amniotic fluid and whether it is clear, blood-stained or contains meconium;
- the consistency, position, effacement and dilatation of the cervix;
- the presenting part in relation to the ischial spines, caput and moulding of the head; and
- the bony pelvis should be assessed with regard to its adequacy for childbirth.

Investigations

The urine should be examined for protein, ketones and sugar. Commercial dip 'stix' will also test for leukocytes, nitrites and blood – their presence may signify a urinary tract infection.

Oral intake is often restricted in labour to reduce the risk of gastric aspiration and Mendelson's syndrome should general anaesthesia be required. The details of nutrition and hydration in labour is discussed in Chapter 7.

When rehydration is necessary in labour, it is best to give normal saline or Hartman's solution, to maintain a more physiological fluid and electrolyte balance. This may also help to avoid water intoxication if intravenous oxytocin is used over a long period in high doses.

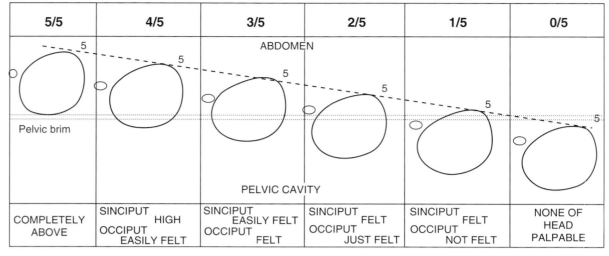

5/5	4/5	3/5	2/5	1/5	0/5
COMPLETELY ABOVE	SINCIPUT HIGH OCCIPUT EASILY FELT	SINCIPUT EASILY FELT OCCIPUT FELT	SINCIPUT FELT OCCIPUT JUST FELT	SINCIPUT FELT OCCIPUT NOT FELT	NONE OF HEAD PALPABLE

Figure 2.3 Clinical estimation of descent of head in fifths palpable above the pelvic brim

Mobility and posture in labour

It is preferable not to confine the mother to bed in early labour. She may prefer ambulation or sitting in a chair. The upright posture may increase the pelvic diameters and assist in the descent of the fetal head. Although many women prefer to be ambulatory early in labour, few remain upright for long, and they may wish to sit or adopt a reclining, lateral recumbent position or lie down as labour progresses. The dorsal position may cause aorta–caval compression and should be discouraged. The actual position the mother chooses does not appear to influence labour outcomes, and hence the mothers should be encouraged and helped to adopt whatever positions they find most comfortable throughout labour [12].

Use of analgesia and anaesthesia

Women should be offered support and encouraged to ask for analgesia at any point during labour. Non-pharmacological measures like labouring in water, supporting women's use of breathing/relaxation techniques, massage and music should be considered. In the UK, the four most widely used forms of pain relief for labour are transcutaneous electrical nerve stimulation (TENS), nitrous oxide (Entonox), intramuscular narcotics (e.g. Pethidine) and epidural analgesia. TENS may not be effective in women in well-established labour [12].

A more detailed discussion of analgesia in labour is found in Chapter 3.

Meconium

Between 15 and 20% of term pregnancies are associated with meconium staining of the amniotic fluid (MSAF), which is not a cause for concern in the vast majority of labours. Meconium may be demonstrated in the fetal gut in the first trimester, but in utero passage is rare before 34 weeks. Meconium reflects fetal gut maturity.

However, the passage of meconium in labour may have a more sinister explanation. An association between meconium passage in utero and poor neonatal outcome has been recorded by Aristotle. Meconium aspiration can occur with intrauterine gasping or when the baby takes its first breath, and accounts for 2% of perinatal deaths.

The appearance of fresh meconium in labour should prompt evaluation of fetal well-being. Continuous electronic fetal monitoring should be instituted. Fetal scalp blood sampling should be considered in the presence of fetal heart rate abnormalities. This is particularly true for thick meconium, since this implies that there is little liquor to dilute the meconium, and this itself may indicate placental problems before the onset of labour. Thin meconium, on the other hand, is thin because it has been diluted with an adequate volume of liquor.

In the presence of a normal fetal heart rate, MSAF is not an indication for immediate delivery or fetal blood sampling, especially if it is thin staining. However, if the heart rate becomes abnormal in association with thick fresh meconium, early delivery should be considered, particularly in high-risk pregnancies.

Diagnosis of poor progress of labour

Progress in labour is confirmed by observing the progressive effacement and dilatation of the cervix and the descent of the presenting part.

The use of a partogram for the management of labour facilitates the early detection of abnormal labour progress and identifies those women most likely to require intervention. This can be used at all levels of obstetric care by basic care providers who have been trained to assess cervical dilatation. When used properly, it helps to detect abnormal labour progress promptly, allowing timely intervention. In a WHO multicentre trial in southeast Asia involving over 35,000 women, the introduction of the partograph as part of an agreed labour management protocol was associated with a reduction in prolonged labour from 6.4 to 3.4%, and the proportion of labours requiring augmentation reduced from 20.7 to 9.1%. The caesarean section rates also fell from 9.9 to 8.3% and intrapartum stillbirths from 0.5 to 0.3%. There were also improvements in fetal and maternal mortality and morbidity in both nulliparous and multiparous women [11].

The term 'dystocia' or difficult labour refers to poor progress of labour and is diagnosed when the rate of cervical dilatation is slower than anticipated. When a woman is admitted in the active phase of labour, the cervical dilatation can be plotted on the partogram and an expected progress or alert line can be constructed, usually corresponding to 1 cm per hour. Another line, the action line, can be added 4 h to the right of the alert line, and parallel to it [11,12].

The outcome of spontaneous labours has been studied and three distinct patterns of abnormal progress described [14–16]. These are:

(a) prolonged latent phase,
(b) primary dysfunctional labour, and
(c) secondary arrest of cervical dilatation.

The duration of latent phase is difficult to define. It is considered prolonged if it is greater than 15 h in a nullipara. The latent phase in parous patients has not been studied in detail [12], therefore no such figure exists for multiparas. Once established in the active phase of labour, primary dysfunctional labour is diagnosed when the progress falls to the right of the nomogram. If labour progresses normally in the early active phase but the cervix fails to dilate or dilates slowly thereafter, secondary arrest of cervical dilatation is diagnosed (Figure 2.4). More than one of these abnormal labour patterns may occur in the same patient, since they frequently share a common aetiology.

The use of the partogram with the anticipated progress line for an individual patient annotated allows the prompt recognition of abnormal cervical progress. The descent of the presenting part as the proportion of the presenting part (expressed as fifths) palpable abdominally is also an integral component of the partogram, and it too is plotted at each review. A poor rate of descent may also be an indication of developing mechanical problems in the labour. Poor progress has conventionally been related to the three 'P's namely:

(a) powers – adequacy of the uterine contractions;
(b) passages – resistance of the birth canal;
(c) passenger – relating to the size, position, degree of flexion, etc., of the baby.

To these can be added a fourth 'P': poor practice.

Poor progress in labour does not identify the specific cause (that is, fault with the powers, passage or passenger), since these are frequently interrelated.

Primary dysfunctional labour (PDL) is the commonest abnormality of the first stage of labour, occurring in up to 25% of spontaneous primigravid labours [15] and 8% of multiparas [16]. The commonest cause is inadequate uterine activity. Secondary arrest of cervical dilatation (SACD) is much less common than the above, said to affect 6% of nulliparas and only 2% of multiparas.

Although the commonest cause of SACD (especially in nulliparas) is still inefficient uterine activity, relative disproportion is far more likely to be the explanation than with PDL. Secondary arrest does not always indicate genuine cephalo-pelvic disproportion, as inadequate uterine contractions can be corrected, resulting in spontaneous vaginal delivery [17]. However, a diagnosis of secondary arrest (especially in a multiparous woman) should prompt a search for obvious problems in the passenger (for example, hydrocephalus, brow presentation, undiagnosed shoulder presentation, large baby, malposition) and the passages (for example, a congenitally small pelvis, a deformed pelvis due to fracture following an accident, or masses in the pelvis). Unfavourable pelvic diameters

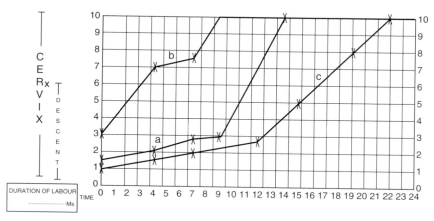

Figure 2.4 Various forms of dysfunctional labour: (a) prolonged latent phase, (b) secondary arrest of labour, (c) prolonged latent phase and primary dysfunctional labour

are rarely a cause of cephalo-pelvic disproportion in the developed world. The fetus is more commonly the cause of relative disproportion by presenting a larger diameter of the vertex due to a malposition or deflexion, or both. In such cases, the dystocia may be overcome if the flexion and rotation to an occipito-anterior position can be encouraged by efficient uterine contractions.

Management options

Augmentation

Indications

Prolonged labour is associated with high rates of maternal infection, obstructed labour, uterine rupture and postpartum haemorrhage, which may end in maternal morbidity and rarely in mortality.

In many areas of the developing world it remains a common axiom 'not to allow the sun to set twice on a woman in labour', in order to prevent such tragic outcomes. In the early 1970s, Philpott and Castle in Harare, Zimbabwe, O'Driscoll and his colleagues in Dublin and Studd in the UK all advocated and popularized the concept of one-to-one midwifery care, use of partogram and augmentation of labour with poor progress to reduce the incidence of prolonged labour.

The active management of labour was based on the principle of anticipating and identifying that there may be a problem and then taking action. Increasing the uterine power, which was the common problem, is one of the many components of the policy of active management. It also helped to overcome any

Table 2.2 The key components of active management of labour.

- Special antenatal classes to prepare women for labour
- Strict criteria for diagnosing labour
- Routine 2-hourly vaginal examination
- Early amniotomy
- Early recourse to oxytocin
- A designated midwife in constant attendance and continuous one-to-one support during labour
- A guarantee that labour would last no longer than 12 h

borderline disproportion by promoting flexion, rotation and moulding in vertex presentation. Each component of the active management, i.e. one-to-one midwifery care, reassurance, pain relief, hydration and fetomaternal surveillance, is essential to prevent prolonged labour in the nulliparae and to reduce the CS rate.

However, randomized control studies suggest that active management of labour shortens the length of labour but does not affect the rate of caesarean section or maternal or fetal morbidity [18–20]. There was no assessment of pain perceived by women or neonatal outcomes. Companionship in labour and continuity of care during pregnancy and childbirth is highly recommended. The entire package of active management of labour need not be offered routinely [12].

The decision to augment labour should be governed by the rate of cervical dilatation based on the partogram, after the exclusion of gross disproportion or malpresentation. Minor degrees of disproportion due to malposition and poor flexion of the head may be overcome by oxytocin infusion. More forceful uterine contractions cause flexion at the atlanto-occipital joint and reduce the presenting diameter. This allows rotation of the occiput from a posterior to an anterior position. The increased force of contraction helps **moulding**, i.e. the overlapping of skull bones over the suture lines, which helps to reduce the presenting diameter of the head. It may increase the pelvic dimensions due to the descending head distending the pelvis and widening the sacro-iliac and symphysis pubic joints. The parietal, occipital and frontal bones of the skull first come together (moulding +), followed by one parietal bone going under the other. The occipital and frontal bones traverse below the parietal bones. If gentle digital pressure is adequate to reduce the overlapping of the bones, it is recorded as moulding ++, and when digital pressure does not restore the overlapping bones to their original position, it is recorded as moulding +++. Caput is the soft tissue swelling caused by the oedema of the scalp that develops as the fetal head descends in the pelvis. The degree of caput increases in prolonged labour, although it is a less reliable sign of mechanical disproportion compared to moulding.

When to augment labour

The mechanical 'efficiency' of uterine contractions should be defined in terms of their clinical effect (that is, the progress of cervical dilatation and descent of the head) and not in relation to the magnitude of uterine contractions, because normal labour progress is observed with a wide range of uterine activity in both nulliparas and multiparas. The more rapid the rate of progress for a given level of uterine activity, the more 'efficient' the contractions. It is also important to recognize the difference between inefficient uterine activity and 'incoordinate' contractions. *Inefficiency* is the failure of the uterus to work in such a way that the labour progress is normal. It can be demonstrated when cervimetric progress is abnormal in the absence of disproportion (although both of these often co-exist). *In-coordinate* uterine action is a descriptive term for the tocographic tracings (Figures 2.5 and 2.6). Most records of uterine contractions will show some degree of

irregularity, but they need not necessarily be associated with abnormal labour progress. Therefore the decision to augment labour should be governed primarily by the dynamic effects of the uterine activity – that is, by the rate of cervical dilatation after disproportion and malpresentation have been excluded. The issue of whether oxytocin augmentation is appropriate in the presence of slow progress but apparently normal contractions as demonstrated by intrauterine pressure measurement needs further elucidation.

Further research is required to assess the cervical contribution to abnormal labour progress. Traditionally, the active management of labour has sought to improve the outcome by enhancing the uterine contractions with oxytocin. However, a significant proportion of labours augmented for abnormal progress still result in caesarean section, implying that other factors are important. A recent in vivo study suggested that cervical smooth muscle activity contributed to the duration of the latent phase [21]. Other researchers have drawn attention to the importance of the head-to-cervix relationship, linking this to the intrauterine pressures developed during labour [22,23]. Further research on this important topic is obviously essential.

Practical aspects of labour management

The diagnosis of active labour is dependent on a careful cervical assessment to define dilatation, effacement, consistency, position and station of the head. These are more important than 'soft' indicators, such as regular contractions, a show, or even amniotic membrane rupture.

On admission, the cervical dilatation should be plotted on the partogram, provided the diagnosis of labour has been made. An alert line is drawn at 1 cm/h once the active phase of labour has been reached, and an action line is then drawn parallel and to the right of this. There is no consensus as to the 'correct' placement of the action line. Recent NICE guidelines on intrapartum care recommend the action line to be drawn 4 h to the right of the alert line. Modifying factors include the level of nursing and medical care available for the supervision of labour once oxytocin has been commenced, the risk of complications associated with prolonged labour (likely to be higher in the more disadvantaged communities), and social factors.

The actual presence of the action line on the partogram is more important than the precise time

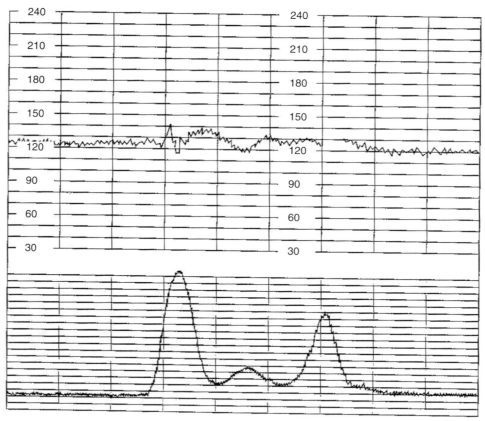

Figure 2.5 Mild degree of in-coordination of uterine contractions

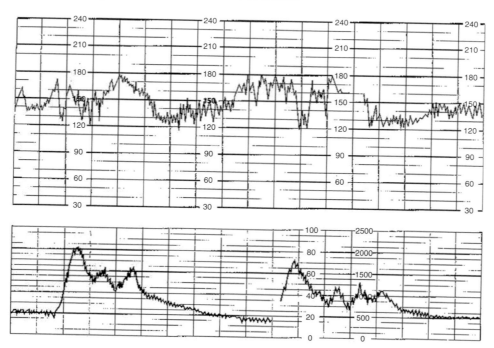

Figure 2.6 Severe degree of in-coordination of uterine contractions

interval between it and the alert line – its presence indicates that action will be necessary if labour progress falls to the right of that projected. When action is needed, amniotomy alone may suffice to correct slow progress in some cases (see below), although oxytocin will be necessary if there is poor progress after amniotomy.

Augmentation in the latent phase of labour

The duration of the latent phase of labour varies widely and is a period when the diagnosis of labour can be very difficult. Appreciable proportions of women have painful contractions for long periods in the latent phase with little cervical change. The management of the latent phase, once maternal and fetal well-being has been confirmed, consists of explanation, reassurance, hydration, nutrition and ambulation. The mainstay of management of a prolonged latent phase is to avoid unnecessary intervention. The decision to augment in the latent phase should be based on clear medical or obstetric indications, since augmentation with an unfavourable cervix is associated with a high risk of caesarean section. However, when the woman has been experiencing frequent, painful but apparently fruitless contractions for a long time, some action has to be taken. In these circumstances, augmentation may be appropriate.

Augmentation in the active phase of labour

Most patients are admitted in the active phase with cervical dilatation >3 cm. The expected progress line or 'alert line' can be drawn at 1 cm/h on the partogram. Proponents of active management of labour augment labour when the progress is to the right of this alert line, whereas most advocate augmentation only when the progress has deviated to the right of the 'action line' drawn 1–4 h parallel to the alert line. By allowing a 'period of grace', fewer patients will require augmentation: 55% of nulliparas with no period of grace [6] compared to 19% of women given a 2 h period of grace [17]. Both methods of management yield comparable results, although prompt intervention does decrease the duration of labour and may be more appropriate when labour ward staffing is inadequate and/or number of beds are limited. However, 'natural childbirth' should be encouraged, and hoping to avoid intervention, the action line may be drawn 4 h to the right of the alert line, since the obstetric outcomes are similar. The WHO study with the action line drawn 4 h to the right of the alert line

showed a reduction in prolonged labour and CS rates [11]. Recent NICE guidelines on intrapartum care also support the use of the 4 h action line [12].

The role of artificial rupture of the membranes (ARM)

The artificial rupture of the membranes need not be performed as a routine. Once the active phase has started, i.e. when the cervix is more than 3 cm dilated, the membranes may be ruptured, and such a policy of early amniotomy leads to a reduction, on average, of between 1 and 2 h in the duration of labour, and also to a reduction in the incidence of dystocia [24]. However, it does not lower the rate of CS or operative vaginal deliveries, and a policy of routine amniotomy is not normally recommended [25]. When ARM is not routinely performed, there are some occasions when it is indicated:

(a) to enhance the strength of contractions when labour progress is abnormal;
(b) to assess the volume and nature of the liquor in a high-risk labour, especially if the fetal heart rate pattern is abnormal; and
(c) to attach a fetal scalp electrode or to insert an intrauterine pressure catheter.

ARM does have some drawbacks. When the presenting part is high there is a chance of cord prolapse, and if labour becomes unduly prolonged the risk of intrauterine infection is increased. Furthermore, there is also an increased rate of fetal heart abnormalities.

Oxytocin dosage and time increment schedules

Oxytocin receptors in the uterus increase during pregnancy and labour, so that the uterus may be sensitive to very small doses of administered oxytocin. The drug is best titrated in an arithmetical or geometric manner starting from a low dose. Oxytocin should not be administered by gravity-fed drips, because they are unreliable and potentially unsafe. Overdosage may lead to uterine hyperstimulation and fetal distress, while a suboptimal dose may lead to failure to progress in labour, resulting in unnecessary intervention. The dangers of uncontrolled infusions include severe fetal hypoxia and uterine rupture. Ideally, intravenous oxytocin should be administered using a peristaltic infusion pump.

Published protocols vary widely in terms of the oxytocin dilution. A more detailed discussion of oxytocin administration for augmenting labour may be found in Chapter 18 relating to induction and augmentation of labour.

Achievement of optimal uterine activity

There remains a dearth of literature regarding the level of uterine activity that should be produced by oxytocin titration to produce a good obstetric outcome. It has been suggested that the use of intrauterine pressure catheters may identify those who are most likely to need a caesarean section for failure to progress. It is known that active contraction area measurements using an intrauterine pressure catheter correlate better with the rate of cervical dilatation than do the individuals of frequency or amplitude of contractions. Despite this, there is little evidence that using an intrauterine pressure catheter to measure uterine activity or using oxytocin titration to achieve a preset active contraction area profile is associated with a better obstetric outcome in augmented labours, compared with an oxytocin infusion titrated against the frequency of contractions [26].

In most centres, facilities to monitor the uterine activity with pressure catheters are not available. The uterine activity has to be judged clinically, on the basis of the frequency and duration of the palpated contractions. As a guide, 3 contractions in 10 min is an appropriate target uterine activity with oxytocin titration, but if there is no progress with this frequency of contractions, the oxytocin dose may be increased to achieve a frequency of 4 or 5 in 10 min, provided the fetal heart is normal.

The measurement of uterine contractions

The frequency of contractions can be assessed by either external or internal tocography. Some centres use intrauterine pressure catheters when oxytocin is administered because they feel that hyperstimulation of the uterus can be identified early and the oxytocin infusion rate adjusted accordingly, in the hope that this will improve the neonatal outcome. However, excessively frequent contractions can also be identified by external tocography. Internal tocography for augmented labour does not give rise to a better obstetric outcome when compared with external tocography. Therefore, in a busy clinical practice, it is far easier, less invasive, cheaper and perfectly appropriate to assess uterine contractions using external tocography. On the other hand, in certain high-risk cases (such as pregnancies complicated by intrauterine growth restriction, or in those practices where medico-legal concerns

are important) there are theoretical advantages to using intrauterine pressure catheters. In addition, internal tocography can be valuable in very obese women, where external tocography is less reliable. The use of intrauterine pressure catheters has also been recommended in women with a previous caesarean section who are being augmented for poor labour progress. A sudden decline in uterine activity may precede any clinical signs of scar rupture, such as scar pain, vaginal bleeding or maternal collapse. Overall, there is only a limited place for intrauterine pressure measurement outside a research setting.

Duration of augmentation

There is general agreement that the use of the partogram and oxytocin augmentation for the management of abnormal labour progress is valuable. However, there is far less consensus regarding how long augmentation should continue before performing a caesarean section for 'failure to progress'.

A period of 8 h of augmentation with adequate monitoring in the absence of gross disproportion should result in the majority of nulliparous and multiparous women delivering vaginally with little risk of intrauterine hypoxia or birth injury. It is doubtful whether more than 8 h of augmentation in the presence of poor progress will result in a greater number of vaginal deliveries without compromise to the fetus. Fetal and maternal surveillance and monitoring of the progress of labour is important to avoid iatrogenic fetal morbidity.

Labour is a natural physiological phenomenon leading to childbirth. Many women have the rewarding experience of a safe vaginal birth of a healthy baby, while a small proportion continue to suffer from the complications of prolonged labour and its sequelae. In an attempt to minimize the risks of adverse outcomes, obstetric interventions in labour have become more common. However, a perception of the widespread use of what are seen as unnecessary interventions has caused a healthy degree of scepticism among patients and some clinicians. These concerns, expressed by the general public in recent years, are perfectly valid and will continue to increase if obstetric practice is not continually scrutinized and subjected to rigorous scientific evaluation wherever possible.

This is one of the many challenges currently faced by those with an interest in the welfare of pregnant and labouring women and their babies.

References

1. Thomas J, Paranjothy S. Royal College of Obstetricians and Gynaecologists. Clinical Effectiveness Support Unit. *The National Sentinel Caesarean Section Audit Report*. London: RCOG Press, 2001.

2. Bewley S, Cockburn J I. The unfacts of 'request' caesarean section. *Br J Obstet Gynaecol* 2002; **109**: 597–605.

3. Villar J, Carroli G, Zavaleta N, *et al*. Maternal and neonatal individual risks and benefits associated with caesarean delivery: multicentre prospective *Br Med J* 2007; **335**: 1025.

4. Hemminki E, Merilainen L. Long term effects of cesarean section: ectopic pregnancies and placental problems. *Am J Obstet Gynecol* 1996; **174**: 1569–74.

5. Philpott R H. Graphic records in labour. *Br Med J* 1972; **iv**: 163–5.

6. O'Driscoll K, Stronge J M, Minogue M. Active management of labour. *Br Med J* 1973; **iii**: 135–8.

7. Studd J W W. Partograms and nomograms in the management of primigravid labour. *Br Med J* 1973; **iv**: 451–5.

8. Ilancheran A, Lim S M, Ratnam S S. Nomograms of cervical dilatation in labour. *Sing J Obstet Gynecol* 1977; **8**: 69–73.

9. Duignan N M, Studd J W W, Hughes A O. Characteristics of labour in different racial groups. *Br J Obstet Gynaecol* 1975; **82**: 593–601.

10. Arulkumaran S, Gibb D M F, Chau S, Piara Singh, Ratnam S S. Ethnic influences on uterine activity in spontaneous labour. *Br J Obstet Gynaecol* 1989; **96**: 1203–6.

11. World Health Organization Maternal Health and Safe Motherhood Programme. World Health Organization partograph in management of labour. *Lancet* 1994; **343**: 1399–404.

12. NICE Intrapartum Care. *Care of Healthy Women and their Babies during Childbirth*. Clinical guideline 55. London: RCOG Press, 2007.

13. RCOG Clinical Effectiveness Support Unit. *The Use of Electronic Fetal Monitoring*. Evidence-based clinical guideline number 8. London: RCOG Press, 2001.

14. Studd J, Clegg D R, Saunders R R, Hughes A O. Identification of high risk labours by labour nomogram. *Br Med J* 1975; **ii**: 545–7.

15. Cardozo L D, Gibb D M F, Studd J W W, Vasant R V, Cooper D J. Predictive value of cervimetric labour patterns in primigravidae. *Br J Obstet Gynaecol* 1982; **89**: 33–8.

16. Gibb D M F, Cardozo L D, Studd J W W, Magos A L, Cooper D J. Outcome of spontaneous labour in multigravidae. *Br J Obstet Gnaecol* 1982; **89**: 708–11.

17. Arulkumaran S, Koh C H, Ingemarsson I, Ratnam S S. Augmentation of labour. Mode of delivery related to cervimetric progress. *Aust NZ J Obstet Gynecol* 1987; **27**: 304–8.

18. Lopez-Zeno J A, Peaceman A M, Adashek J A, Socol M L. A controlled trial of a program for the active management of labor. *N Eng J Med* 1992; **326**: 450–4.

19. Frigoletto F D, Lieberman E, Lang J M, *et al*. A clinical trial of active management of labor. *N Eng J Med* 1995; **333**: 745–50.

20. Sadler L C, Davison T, McCowan L M E. A randomised controlled trial and meta-analysis of active management of labour. *Br J Obstet Gynaecol* 2000; **107**: 909–15.

21. Pajntar M, Leskosek B, Rudel D, Verdenik I. Contribution of cervical smooth muscle activity to the duration of latent and active phases of labour. *Br J Obstet Gynaecol* 2001; **108**: 533–8.

22. Gough G W, Randall N J, Genevier E S, Sutherland I A, Steer P J. Head to cervix pressure and their relationship to the outcome of labour. *Obstet Gynecol* 1990; **75**: 613–8.

23. Allman A C J, Genevier E S G, Johnson M R, Steer P J. Head-to-cervix force: an important physiological variable in labour. *Br J Obstet Gynaecol* 1996; **103**: 763–8.

24. Fraser W D, Krauss I, Brisson-Carrol G, Thornton J, Breart G. Amniotomy for shortening spontaneous labour. *The Cochrane Library* 2002; **2**.

25. The UK Amniotomy Group. A multicentre randomised trial of amniotomy in spontaneous first labour at term. *Br J Obstet Gynaecol* 1994; **101**: 307–9.

26. Arulkumaran S, Yang M, Ingemarsson I, Piara S, Ratnam S S. Augmentation of labour. Does oxytocin titration to achieve preset active contraction area values produce better obstetric outcome? *Asia Oceania J Obstet Gynecol* 1989; **15**: 333–7.

Chapter 3

Analgesia and anaesthesia in labour

Jason Scott and Geraldine O'Sullivan

Introduction

Women vary in their needs and desire for pain relief during labour, with some aiming for a natural childbirth with no pain relief and others wishing to employ more-invasive techniques, such as neuraxial analgesia. It must be appreciated, and this fact needs to be emphasized to women, that most non-neuraxial methods of analgesia will never provide complete pain relief during labour, but represent at best techniques that allow a woman 'to cope' with her labour pain. It should also be noted that the complete removal of pain does not necessarily mean a more satisfying birth experience for a woman [1].

Women's views and experiences of pain and pain relief in childbirth

Hodnett, in a systematic review, specifically addressed the issue of women's views on the experience of childbirth in relation to their intrapartum analgesia [1]. Women in labour, with no medical or obstetric complications, were studied. Analysis of the evidence from all the reviewed papers led to the conclusion that four factors – personal expectations, amount of support from caregivers, quality of the caregiver–patient relationship, and involvement in decision-making were critical to women's experience of childbirth.

Simple analgesic techniques

a. Support during labour

A Cochrane review has specifically addressed the effect of continuous support for women during childbirth [2] [3]. The conclusion of the review was that women who had continuous one-to-one support during labour were

(1) more likely to have a spontaneous vaginal birth,
(2) less likely to require analgesia, and
(3) less likely to report dissatisfaction with their childbirth experience.

b. Hydrotherapy

All maternity units should provide women with the option to labour and deliver in water. Election manifesto, Labour Party, 2005, UK.

There has been one major systematic review on the effects of immersion in water during labour [4]. The review included eight trials and showed that the use of water in the first stage of labour reduced the use of regional analgesia. There was no difference in the duration of the first and second stages of labour or the caesarean section rate. Ideally, therefore, hospitals and birthing centres should provide facilities for women to spend part or even all of their labour in a suitable bath/pool. If hydrotherapy is used there should be local protocols that address issues such as the temperature of the water, the use of concomitant analgesia, fetal monitoring, and evacuation from the pool in the event of an emergency.

Complementary and alternative therapies

a. Acupuncture

Acupuncture is not in widespread use in China as a means of relieving pain in childbirth, and perhaps significantly no acupuncture points are described in traditional Chinese literature for pain relief in labour!

Several randomized controlled trials (RCT) have tried to evaluate the use of acupuncture as an analgesic in labour. Some of these RCTs suggested that

Best Practice in Labour and Delivery, ed. R. Warren and S. Arulkumaran. Published by Cambridge University Press.
© Cambridge University Press 2009.

acupuncture improved pain scores and reduced the use of both parenteral opioids and epidural analgesia. However, some of these RCTs had serious flaws; for example, in some of the studies [5], the midwife performing the acupuncture was also clinically responsible for the patient and the patient only received other analgesics if 'thought appropriate by the midwife'.

Current evidence suggests that, in most women, acupuncture does not provide adequate analgesia throughout labour, although some women do appreciate the technique. However, before a definite conclusion on the place of acupuncture as an analgesic in labour can be reached, further RCTs, which should include the use of sham acupuncture, should be undertaken.

b. Transcutaneous electrical nerve stimulation (TENS)

TENS is a technique whereby low-voltage electrical impulses are administered through electrodes that, for the relief of labour pain, are usually sited in the lower lumbar area. A systematic review on the efficacy of TENS was conducted in 1997: it included 10 studies and involved 877 women – 436 women received active TENS and 441 women acted as controls (sham TENS or no treatment). There was no difference in pain intensity, pain relief or the need for additional analgesia between TENS and controls [6].

There is no evidence that TENS has any beneficial effect on labour pain, but on the plus side its use is associated with no side effects. Whilst the use of TENS during active labour should not be encouraged, it may help with backache during the latent phase of labour.

Pharmacological analgesia in labour
a. Inhalational analgesia

Inhalational analgesia is provided by inhaling sub-anaesthetic concentrations of volatile anaesthetic gases, the aim being that the mother should remain conscious with preservation of her laryngeal reflexes. The technique first achieved fame and later gained widespread acceptance when John Snow administered chloroform to Queen Victoria for the birth of her eighth and ninth children in 1853 and 1857. However, the only agent that has really survived the test of time is nitrous oxide, which is most commonly administered as Entonox (a 50:50 oxygen : nitrous oxide mixture).

Nitrous oxide

Nitrous oxide (N_2O) is usually administered via a demand valve connected to a face mask or mouthpiece. This demand valve only opens when the user applies negative pressure by inspiring through a mouthpiece or a properly applied face mask.

A systematic review on the efficacy of N_2O was published in 2002 [7]. Seven studies described significant analgesia with N_2O and, interestingly, in two studies women continued to use N_2O even after the study period was over. Nausea and vomiting was reported as ranging from 5 to 36%. Neonatal Apgar scores were reported in four studies and no differences were shown.

Therefore, there is a moderate level of evidence to support the use of N_2O in labour, in that N_2O is effective for some women with no apparent adverse outcomes for either mother or baby.

b. Systemic opioid analgesia
Pethidine

Systemic opioids are the commonest mode of analgesia used during labour, probably because they are readily available, cheap and easy to administer. Since its introduction into obstetrics during the 1940s, without any trials, pethidine has been the main opioid used during labour. Its perceived analgesic efficacy probably owes as much to its sedative as to its analgesic effects. It was initially believed that pethidine caused little respiratory depression and that the effect on the fetus was minimal. Later studies demonstrated that the effect on the fetus was significant [8]. A double-blind RCT, conducted in Hong Kong, compared intramuscular (IM) pethidine with an IM placebo [9]. Ethical considerations demanded that the initial study period (after which rescue analgesia would be available) would be limited to 30 min to minimize the period during which patients would be exposed to a placebo. A significant reduction in pain scores was observed in the women who received pethidine ($N=25$) compared to those who had received placebo ($N=25$) (Figure 3.1). Thirty minutes after drug administration, the women were also asked to rate on a five-point scale how satisfied they were with their analgesia (1 = totally dissatisfied, 5 = totally satisfied). Scores were significantly higher for women in the pethidine group, although neither had very high scores (the median was 2 in the pethidine group and 1 in the placebo group). Eight per cent of women

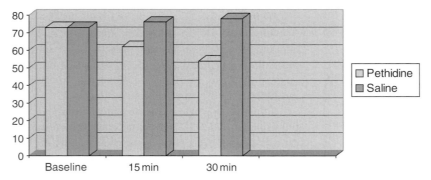

Figure 3.1 Pethidine vs saline for analgesia in labour. At 30 min the median visual analogue pain score (VAS) was lower in the pethidine compared with the saline group (0 = no pain, 100 = worst pain imaginable). (See colour plate section.)

in the pethidine group were totally dissatisfied with the pain relief received, compared with 60% in the control group.

This and other studies using opioids to relieve pain in labour suggest that opioids reduce pain intensity by an average of 25–35%, but will only provide pain relief in less than 30% of women [10]. It has been shown that unless visual analogue pain scores (VAS) fall below 40 (on a VAS scale of 0–100), a patient will request further analgesia. Therefore the poor efficacy of systemic opioids during labour combined with their effects on the neonate suggests that women should not be encouraged to use these agents during labour.

Remifentanil

Neuraxial analgesia is contra-indicated in some women and not desired by others, and thus remifentanil, a short-acting μ-opioid agonist, could be the opioid of choice for such women. It has a rapid onset of action and undergoes hydrolysis by non-specific tissue and blood esterases to almost completely inactive metabolites, which are eliminated in the urine. The context specific half-life is only 3 min. The pharmacokinetics of remifentanil has been investigated in babies under two months and the half-life is similar to that found in adults.

Studies are currently ongoing to assess the efficacy and optimum dose of remifentanil during labour. Some of these studies indicate that remifentanil may cause significant respiratory depression [11], and thus currently its use mandates one-to-one nursing and monitoring with maternal pulse oximetry and fetal CTG. Further large-scale RCTs are required before remifentanil can be routinely used as an analgesic in labour.

Regional analgesia in labour

A Cochrane review of epidural analgesia in labour concluded that epidural analgesia provides significantly better pain relief than non-epidural techniques.

Pain is conducted from the uterine body by Aδ and C fibres which travel with the sympathetic fibres through the hypogastric plexus and enter the spinal cord at the 11th and 12th thoracic roots. There is also some overlap into the 10th thoracic and first lumbar roots (Figure 3.2). Labour pain is therefore felt in the lower abdominal and lumbar areas. Pain during the second stage of labour is conducted through the pudendal nerve (S 2,3,4). Branches of the ilioinguinal nerve, genito-femoral nerve, and the long cutaneous nerve of the thigh also innervate the vagina and perineum. This means that a pudendal block alone cannot provide complete anaesthesia of the perineum for an episotomy. The pudendal block must be supplemented with local infiltration to achieve effective analgesia.

The indications for regional analgesia in labour could include:

- maternal request,
- hypertensive disorders of pregnancy,
- pre-existing medical disease,
- multiple pregnancy,
- previous caesarean section,
- prolonged labour, and
- deterioration in fetal well-being.

Contra-indications to regional analgesia include:

- maternal refusal,
- coagulopathy and thrombocytopenia,
- local or systemic infection, and
- inadequate staffing or facilities.

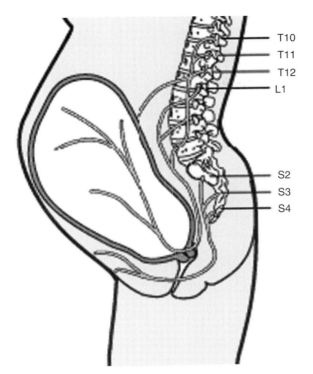

Figure 3.2 Nerve supply of the uterus. The perineum also receives innervation from the ilioinguinal nerve, the genito-femoral nerve and the long cutaneous nerve of the thigh

In current obstetric practice the aim of regional analgesia in labour is to produce a selective sensory block from T10 to L1, whilst at the same time sparing the motor supply to the lower limbs, L2–L5, the 'Mobile Epidural'. This sparing of motor fibres has been achieved by decreasing the concentration of local anaesthetic used by the addition of opioid, most commonly fentanyl. Solutions of bupivacaine ranging in concentration from 0.0625 to 0.1% with fentanyl 2 µg/ml are the most commonly used agents for epidural analgesia in the UK. The synergistic effect of local anaesthetics and opioids achieves excellent intrapartum analgesia whilst at the same time minimizing the unwanted side effects of both groups of drugs.

a. Establishing regional analgesia in labour

An initial loading dose of 10–15 ml of bupivacaine 0.1% with fentanyl 2 µg/ml is commonly used to establish epidural analgesia in labour. Analgesia is usually established in 10–15 min (i.e. 2–3 contractions).

Women who are in severe pain at the time of the request for regional analgesia will often benefit from a rapid onset of analgesia. This can be best achieved by the intrathecal administration of local anaesthetic and opioid, either as a single-shot spinal or as a combined spinal epidural (CSE) technique. In the latter technique, a long spinal needle is passed through the previously sited epidural needle and into the subarachnoid space, where local anaesthetic and opioid (e.g. 2.5 mg bupivacaine with 15–20 µg fentanyl) is then administered. The spinal needle is then withdrawn and a catheter is then passed through the epidural needle into the epidural space (Figure 3.3).

NICE guidelines recommend that continuous electronic fetal monitoring should be employed during the establishment of epidural analgesia.

b. Maintenance of regional analgesia during labour

This can be achieved by:

- regular top-ups, usually administered by a midwife,
- an epidural infusion, or
- patient-controlled epidural analgesia (PCEA).

Although more expensive, as it requires a dedicated machine, PCEA is being used in an increasing number of units (Figure 3.4). Analgesia is established as described above, whilst subsequent doses are self-administered by the woman. Evidence shows that, when compared to techniques using continuous infusions, less local anaesthetic and opioid are used with PCEA, and in addition the woman has more control over her level of analgesia.

Complications and side effects of regional analgesia
Hypotension

Local anaesthetics block the preganglionic autonomic fibres, which results in vasodilatation, a reduction in venous return, cardiac output and systemic vascular resistance, and a consequent fall in blood pressure. This maternal hypotension may also cause fetal heart rate abnormalities. With the advent of low-dose local anaesthetic and opioid solutions, this complication is now rare.

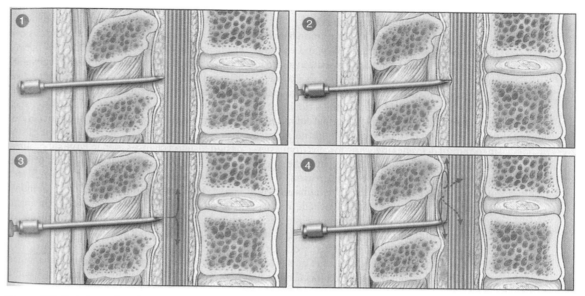

Figure 3.3 Technique of combined spinal epidural (CSE) analgesia/anaesthesia.
1. Tuohy needle in epidural space.
2. Long spinal needle passing through Tuohy needle and piercing the dura mater.
3. Injecting drugs through the spinal needle and into the cerebrospinal fluid (CSF).
4. Spinal needle now withdrawn and epidural catheter is passed through the Tuohy needle into the epidural space.

Accidental dural puncture and postdural puncture headache

If the epidural needle is inadvertently allowed to advance beyond the epidural space, thereby puncturing the dura mater and causing a leak of cerebrospinal fluid (CSF), a low-pressure headache may develop. Classically, the headache, which can be very severe, occurs 24–72 h after the dural puncture and is postural in nature, in that it is relieved by lying down. The definitive treatment of a postdural puncture headache is an epidural blood patch, which should be performed without delay once the headache is diagnosed. Caffeine has also been shown to have a minimal effect in the treatment of postdural puncture headache.

Backache

Several excellent prospective studies have shown that epidural analgesia in labour does **not** result in post-partum backache. Short-term (5–7 days) local tenderness at the site of the needle puncture occurs in about 50% of mothers.

Bladder dysfunction

If a low-dose local anaesthetic with opioid is used to achieve analgesia in labour, the mother should be able to walk for a few hours after the epidural has been sited. Thereafter she can use a bed pan. However, in some mothers, epidural analgesia can result in difficulty in passing urine. Bladder distension must not be allowed to occur during labour, and the insertion of a urinary catheter should be considered for mothers who are having difficulty passing urine or whose epidural analgesia has been in progress for greater than 6 h.

Effect of regional analgesia on the progress and outcome of labour

The recently published NICE Guidelines on Intrapartum Care [12] indicate that epidural analgesia:

- is **not** associated with a longer first stage of labour or an increased risk of a caesarean birth, but
- is associated with a longer second stage of labour and an instrumental birth.

However, the most important factors determining labour outcome are anaesthetic and obstetric management. Therefore:

- low concentrations of local anaesthetics should be used to minimize motor block;
- oxytocin should be used to augment labour when required; and

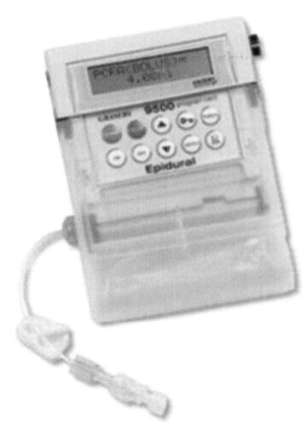

Figure 3.4 Apparatus for patient-controlled epidural analgesia (PCEA)

- maternal pushing in the second stage of labour should be delayed, if possible, until the presenting part is visible, or until 1 h after reaching full cervical dilatation.

Education is an important part of preparing for labour and delivery. Therefore all women should be provided with written information on the types of analgesia available in the local maternity unit. Ideally, anaesthetists should provide input into local childbirth preparation classes.

Anaesthesia for caesarean section

a. Introduction

The developments of asepsis and anaesthesia in the nineteenth century paved the way for the introduction of caesarean section. The evolution of anaesthesia for this procedure was initially slow – ether and chloroform were the only two agents available until the

addition of cyclopropane. Regional anaesthesia was not available until 1900 [13].

Anaesthetic-related maternal mortality has decreased remarkably over the last 50 years as evidenced by the Confidential Enquiry into Maternal and Child Health (CEMACH) [14]. (Figure 3.5) This shows that anaesthesia (spinal, epidural and general) is much safer than it was in the years after the confidential enquiries were first published.

Reductions in anaesthetic risk have been achieved by:

- the increased use of regional anaesthesia;
- improvements in training and better understanding of anaesthetic techniques; and
- the use of H_2 blockers coupled with sodium citrate.

b. Pre-operative considerations
Selection of anaesthetic technique

The increased risks of aspiration and of encountering a 'difficult airway' (i.e. failure to intubate and/or ventilate) have made regional anaesthesia a more attractive option for most caesarean sections. Regional anaesthesia for caesarean section has also become increasingly popular over the past couple of decades as more experience has been gained, and initial fears that epidural and spinal anaesthesia would affect fetal well-being were allayed. However, the indication for caesarean section, the urgency, the medical conditions of both mother and fetus, and also the mother's wishes, will all have a bearing on the anaesthetist's choice.

For most elective or urgent caesarean sections in patients without a pre-existing epidural, a spinal technique seems to offer the best risk–benefit ratio. Blood loss at caesarean section may be less with a regional technique, although studies in support of this finding have been criticized, as patients in whom excessive blood loss is predicted are more likely to be selected for general anaesthesia [15]. However, the avoidance of volatile anaesthetic agents will certainly aid in uterine contraction post delivery.

Postoperative opioid requirements are much lower in those who receive neuraxial opioids than in patients who receive a general anaesthetic. As a result, postoperative recovery is also better, with the mother more mobile the next day, able to breastfeed and care for her baby. Fewer postop complications are likely to develop, such as pyrexia and chest infections, and the

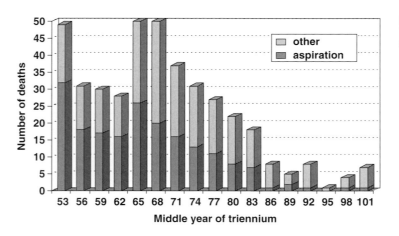

Figure 3.5 Maternal deaths due to anaesthesia 1952–2005. Deaths in the darker shading were due to pulmonary aspiration of gastric contents

result of all these effects is that there is less depression in mothers both immediately and at one week. If there are indications that the surgery may be prolonged, for example a tertiary caesarean section, a combined spinal epidural (CSE) technique may be most appropriate.

In patients with a pre-existing epidural, the block can usually be extended for caesarean section. Epidurals may also provide an advantage when trying to prevent maternal hypotension, or when trying to avoid motor blockade of the thoracic segments and intercostal muscles in cases of respiratory comprom-ise, as the dose can be titrated to the desired sensory/motor level.

In cases of fetal distress, the anaesthetist and obstetrician must together weigh the severity of the fetal compromise against the maternal risks of general anaesthesia. General anaesthesia may sometimes be indicated for a Category 1 caesarean section where every minute counts. However, clinical studies have shown that fetal outcome is not affected by the deci-sion to administer regional anaesthesia in cases of moderate fetal distress.

In cases of parturients presenting with medical illness, the nature and severity of the condition will influence the choice of anaesthesia. Patients with a significant coagulopathy are at increased risk for epi-dural haematoma after a regional technique. General anaesthesia is usually considered best in cases of severe maternal haemorrhage. However, it is accept-able to use regional anaesthesia in cases of placenta praevia with no evidence of hypovolaemia – recent studies do not support the idea that blood loss is increased in these cases when regional anaesthesia is employed [16].

Premedication

Aspiration of gastric contents during general anaes-thesia used to be a major cause of maternal morbidity and mortality (Figure 3.5). In 1986, a large Swedish study reported an aspiration incidence of 1 in 661 cases of general anaesthesia for caesarean section: four times higher than the incidence for non-obstetric surgery. However, in the last two triennial reports on maternal death from the UK, there was only one case of aspiration and this was in a woman with multi-organ failure in intensive care. Other western countries have seen a similar decline in morbidity and mortality from this cause. This success has been a result of the implementation of several measures.

First, a good pre-anaesthetic assessment identifies the patients at greatest risk of difficult intubation and therefore aspiration. A simple test often used to esti-mate those at risk of difficult intubation is the Mal-lampati score. Whilst sitting upright and looking straight ahead the patient is asked to open their mouth wide and stick out their tongue. The view is then graded I to IV: patients with a Grade III or IV view could be difficult to intubate (Figure 3.6). The most effective way to minimize the risk of aspiration is to use regional anaesthesia and maintain a patient' airway with intact reflexes. If regional anaesthesia is contra-indicated, awake fibre optic intubation should be considered in the patient with a difficult airway. Application of cricoid pressure, with a rapid sequence induction, and intubation with a cuffed endotracheal tube should be performed when a difficult airway is not predicted.

Pharmacological prophylaxis against acid pul-monary aspiration includes measures to increase gas-tric pH and decrease gastric volume. A total of 30 ml

Class I   Class II   Class III   Class IV

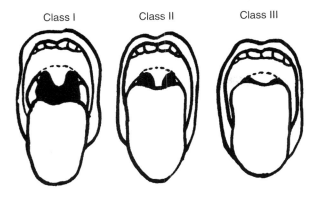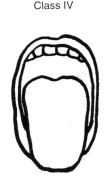

Figure 3.6 Mallampati Score. The patient, sitting upright, is asked to open their mouth as widely as possible and the view is assessed and scored. Classes III and IV are potentially difficult intubations

of 0.3 M sodium citrate will raise the gastric fluid pH above 2.5. However, it must be given in theatre immediately before induction of general anaesthesia, as the duration of action of sodium citrate can be relatively short. Sodium citrate has no effect on gastric volume. Non-particulate antacids such as sodium citrate are preferred, as particulate antacid aspiration results in pulmonary damage similar to that caused by acid aspiration.

H₂-receptor antagonists such as ranitidine will significantly reduce gastric acid secretion, reducing pH and, to a lesser degree, gastric volume. They have no effect on the volume or acidity of the gastric contents already present. Ranitidine 150 mg administered orally will take 40–60 min to exert an effect, and has a duration of action of 6–8 h. The recommended regimen is an oral dose at bedtime and in the morning for patients undergoing elective caesarean section. The intravenous administration of ranitidine 50 mg with oral administration of sodium citrate 30 ml results in a greater increase in gastric pH than when sodium citrate was used alone, providing 30 min has elapsed from the dose of ranitidine to intubation. Ranitidine can also be administered at 8-hourly intervals during labour to those mothers 'at risk' of requiring an emergency caesarean section.

Metoclopramide, a dopamine antagonist, promotes gastric emptying in the pregnant woman even during labour, raises the lower oesophageal tone, and has anti-emetic properties. In cases where urgent general anaesthesia is planned, the administration of sodium citrate with intravenous metoclopramide and an H₂-receptor antagonist is highly recommended.

Maternal position

Aortocaval compression, also known as maternal supine hypotensive syndrome, occurs when the pregnant woman lies supine. The aetiology is probably multifactorial. The gravid uterus compresses the inferior vena cava and the aorta against the bodies of the lumbar vertebrae. The decreased venous return may result in decreased maternal cardiac output and blood pressure. Compression of uterine venous drainage results in an increased uterine venous pressure and therefore a reduced uterine perfusion pressure. Compression of the aorta or common iliac arteries also results in a reduced uterine artery perfusion pressure. For these reasons, left uterine displacement must be maintained during caesarean section. This can be effected by placing a wedge underneath the right buttock or tilting the operating table to the left by 15 degrees. This practice results in a similar incidence of maternal hypotension and fetal bradycardia as that seen if anaesthesia is performed in the lateral decubitus position. Adequacy of tilt can also be assessed by palpation of the left femoral artery whilst displacing the uterus to the left: if the position is adequate there should be no significant decrease in pulse quality.

Regional anaesthesia for caesarean section

a. General considerations

A bilateral sensory block to T4 including sacral roots accompanied by motor block is generally accepted as necessary for caesarean section. Zones of differential blockade exist at the upper and lower edges of a regional block. Loss of sensation to cold is two dermatomes higher than loss of sensation to pinprick, which is in turn two dermatomes higher than loss of sensation to light touch. Loss of sensation to light touch from S1 to at least T6, with corresponding loss of sensation to cold to T4 and a dense motor block of

33

hips and ankles, are good signs that anaesthesia is adequate. The sensation of cold can be measured with ice or ethyl chloride spray, pin prick with a neurological pin, and light touch with a nylon filament (Von Frey hair) or tissue. Measuring with these techniques is highly anaesthetist-dependant, and consistency of technique is important.

After delivery and cord clamping, IV oxytocin 5 iu should be administered to the mother to aid uterine involution and reduce blood loss. An infusion of 40 iu could be administered over the next 2–4 h if there is concern about continued blood loss.

Many methods for preventing hypotension during spinal anaesthesia have been investigated, including fluids administered as preloads or coloads, and vasopressors administered as infusions and/or boluses. A combination of fluid coloading administered with a phenylephrine infusion appears particularly effective [17].

b. Spinal anaesthesia

Spinal anaesthesia is popular because of its relative simplicity, fast onset time, reliability and 'density' of block.

Technique

Patient position for administration of spinal blockade can influence the rate of onset and spread of the drug. The sitting position is often used, as many anaesthetists can perform dural tap more easily in this position, but spread of anaesthesia may be slower. The sitting position is particularly suitable for the obese parturient where identification of the midline can be difficult. The right or left lateral decubitus position is preferable in obstetric anaesthesia, as it avoids the problems associated with vena-caval occlusion.

Lumbar puncture is performed at the L2–L3 or L3–L4 interspace. Smaller (25–27 G), atraumatic pencilpoint needles such as Sprotte or Whittacre result in headache rates of less than 1%.

Doses of bupivacaine required for spinal anaesthesia during pregnancy are about 25% less than those required in non-pregnant women. Vena-caval obstruction resulting in engorged epidural veins and therefore decreased epidural and CSF volume probably contributes to this effect, and is even more pronounced with multiple pregnancies. The dose of bupivacaine used ranges from 7.5 to 12.5 mg. Opioids such as diamorphine or fentanyl should be added to the local

anaesthetic solution as intrathecal opioids enhance intraoperative anaesthesia and reduce the postoperative analgesia requirement.

c. Epidural anaesthesia

Most caesarean sections performed under epidural blockade are urgent or emergent cases where the epidural catheter is in-situ, having been used for labour analgesia. However, there remain some indications for the establishment de novo of epidural anaesthesia for caesarean section.

Technique

Epidural catheters are usually placed at L2–L3 or L3–L4. Infiltration of the skin and subcutaneous tissues with 2% lidocaine helps allow easy and painfree insertion of the Tuohy needle, and helps the mother to remain still during epidural insertion.

The midline approach is used by most anaesthetists, with the paramedian approach being used by some practitioners in difficult patients. With the midline approach, the epidural needle passes through skin, subcutaneous fat, supraspinous ligament, interspinous ligament, and finally the ligamentum flavum before entering the epidural space. The epidural space is located using a loss of resistance technique. Either saline or air can be used. Saline has been advocated as having a lower incidence of accidental dural puncture. Evidence suggests that approximately 5 cm of catheter should be advanced into the epidural space [18].

Having inserted the epidural catheter, the catheter should be aspirated observing for blood or fluid, and then a test dose of the local anaesthetic solution should be administered. The local anaesthetic dose should be equivalent to the intrathecal dose used for caesarean section (e.g. bupivacaine 7.5–10 mg or lidocaine 45–60 mg) to detect intrathecal administration. No technique for detecting intrathecal administration is completely reliable, and it should be remembered that catheters can migrate to a different space at any time, so vigilance should be maintained whenever a drug is bolused through the epidural catheter.

Dosing

At 3–5 min after the test dose there should be no evidence of motor blockade or dense sensory blockade or haemodynamic disturbances. If this is the case the therapeutic dose can then be administered. The pregnant woman requires approximately 1 ml of local anaesthetic solution for each level of anaesthetic blockade. Therefore a block to T4 will require 18 segments and usually 15–20 ml of local anaesthetic.

The choice of anaesthetic agent depends on the desired speed of onset and the duration of action. Lidocaine 2%, levo-bupivacaine 0.5%, and ropivacaine 0.75% have durations of action which should be sufficient for caesarean section (75–100 min for lidocaine, and 120–180 min for levo-bupivacaine and ropivacaine). Lidocaine has a faster onset of action, about half that of levo-bupivacaine. Lidocaine has been associated with a higher incidence of inadequate block. The addition of epinephrine to the local anaesthetic to achieve a concentration of 1 in 200,000 or 1 in 400,000 (1 ml or 0.5 ml of 1 in 1000 epinephrine) may decrease vascular absorption of the local anaesthetic and improve the quality and duration of the block; and is particularly efficacious when used with lidocaine [19].

Topping up a labour epidural for emergency caesarean section means that a large dose of local anaesthetic may have to be given quickly as there may not be time to dose incrementally. Unless there has been a recent top-up during labour, 15–20 ml of local anaesthetic is required. Topping up in the delivery room is controversial and should be avoided whenever possible. Once the top-up has been given it is imperative to stay with the mother and have a means of measuring her blood pressure. Appropriate vasopressors must be readily available. If epidural analgesia has not been effective during labour, the epidural should be abandoned and spinal or general anaesthesia performed depending on the degree of urgency.

Combined spinal epidural anaesthesia

The combined spinal epidural (CSE) technique is useful as it both increases the reliability of the epidural and allows for prolongation of the block in cases of potential prolonged caesarean section, such as caesarean section after previous pelvic or abdominal surgery, or caesarean section and tubal ligation.

The sequential block

Ten minutes after a spinal injection, 10 ml of epidural saline can produce a more cephalad spread of the block. This has been confirmed by myelography to be a volume effect, a squeezing of the dural sac resulting in a decrease in CSF volume [9] (Figure 3.3). Extension

of a low-dose subarachnoid block in this way with epidural local anaesthetic can help facilitate cardiovascular stability in the sicker patient.

General anaesthesia for caesarean section

Neither general anaesthesia nor regional anaesthesia (which is always accompanied by the risk of having to institute general anaesthesia) should be considered in the absence of a minimum equipment requirement.

a. Pre-oxygenation

At term there is an increase in oxygen consumption of 20%, a further increase of 20% during labour, and an increase of up to 100% over non-pregnant controls during the second stage of labour. Consequently, desaturation occurs much more rapidly in pregnant women. Therefore the parturient must be pre-oxygenated prior to inducing general anaesthesia for a caesarean section. If the mask is not tightly fitted, room air can entrain, decreasing the efficacy of denitrogenation. Normal tidal volume breaths for 3 min will decrease alveolar nitrogen to 1%, four vital capacity breaths decreases alveolar nitrogen to 5%. The tidal volume method buys about 15 s more time.

b. Rapid sequence induction

Cricoid pressure was first described by Sellick in 1961, and is often referred to as Sellick's manoeuvre. It is employed to reduce the risk of reflux of gastric contents into the pharynx, and therefore the risk of aspiration, prior to securing the airway with a cuffed endotracheal tube. He described a two-handed technique. The thumb and middle finger of one hand are placed either side of the cricoid and backward pressure compresses the oesophagus on the vertebral column at C6, thus occluding it. The other hand is placed behind the neck and forward pressure is applied, placing the head in the sniffing position and making the oesophagus easier to occlude. In practice when only one assistant is present, the second hand of the assistant is more usefully employed in reaching for additional equipment and one-handed cricoid pressure is most commonly used. If cricoid pressure is incorrectly applied it may make intubation more difficult.

c. The failed intubation

Careful positioning of the mother is important to optimize the chances of a successful intubation. This includes adjusting the table height to one most

Difficult Airway Algorithm

1. Assess the likelihood and clinical impact of basic management problems.
   A. Difficult ventilation
   B. Difficult intubation
   C. Difficulty with patient cooperation or consent
   D. Difficult tracheostomy

2. Actively pursue opportunities to deliver supplemental oxygen throughout the process of difficult airway management.

3. Consider the relative merits and feasibility of basic management choices:

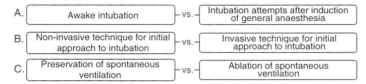

4. Develop primary and alternative strategies.

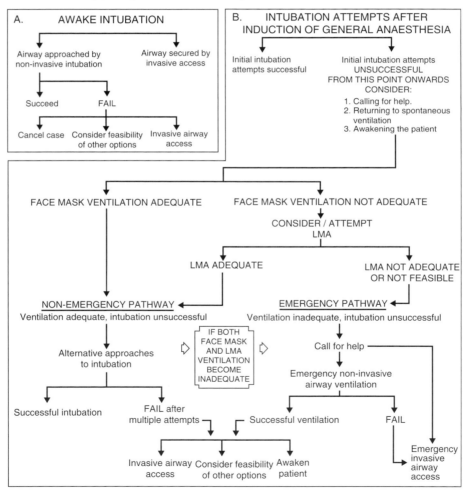

Figure 3.7 Algorithm for a potential difficult intubation

comfortable for the anaesthetist, placing pillows under the mother's head to provide support, good head extension on the neck, and ensuring that the mother's arms are not resting on her chest, as this may exacerbate difficulty in inserting the laryngoscope blade.

If a failed intubation is encountered it is important to have a plan of action: failed intubation algorithms can be useful for this (Figure 3.7). Failure to intubate the mother will cause no harm as long as oxygenation can be maintained and passive regurgitation prevented. If intubation has failed, a second dose of the muscle relaxant suxamethonium should not be given. Repeated attempts at intubation will increase the chance of aspiration, and in the presence of hypoxaemia the second dose may produce profound maternal bradycardia.

If it remains possible to maintain oxygenation and ventilation via a laryngeal mask or face mask, then a decision needs to be made regarding whether or not to wake the mother up. This will be based on an evaluation of the mother and fetus, and the reliability of the airway. If the mother's life depends on completion of the surgery, as in massive haemorrhage or cardiac arrest, then surgery should continue. In the case of sudden and severe fetal distress with no recovery between contractions, for example with placental abruption or prolapsed cord, and where the airway is manageable, then to save the life of the fetus it is reasonable to continue with anaesthesia. The depth of anaesthesia should be increased in the spontaneously breathing patient as light anaesthesia may precipitate coughing, vomiting and breath-holding. If the mother's life is deemed to be at risk from continued anaesthesia, she should be woken. In all other cases the safest course of action is to wake the mother and form an alternative plan. This will be regional anaesthesia or an awake fibre optic intubation.

References

1. Hodnett E D. Pain and women's satisfaction with the experience of childbirth: a systematic review. *Am J Obstet Gynecol* 2002; **186**: S160–72.

2. Hodnett E D, Gates S, Hofmeyr G J, Sakala C. Continuous support for women during childbirth. *Cochrane Database Syst Rev* 2003; **3**: CD003766.

3. Smith C A, Collins C T, Cyna A M, Crowther C A. Complementary and alternative therapies for pain management in labour. *Cochrane Database Syst Rev* 2005; **2**:

4. Cluett E R, Nikodem V C, McCandlish R E, Burns E E. Immersion in water in pregnancy, labour and birth. *The Cochrane Library* 2004; CD000111.

5. Nesheim B-I, Kinge R, Berg B, *et al.* Acupuncture during labor can reduce the use of meperidine: a controlled clinical study. *Clin J Pain* 2003; **19**: 187–91.

6. Carroll D, Moore R A, Tramer M R, McQuay H J. Transcutaneous electrical nerve stimulation does not relieve labor pain: updated systematic review. *Contemp Rev Obstet Gynaecol* 1997; **9**: 205.

7. Rosen M A. Nitrous oxide for relief of labor pain: a systematic review. *Am J Obstet Gynecol* 2002; **186**: S110–26.

8. Kuhnert B R, Linn P L, Kennard M J, *et al.* Effect of low doses of meperidine on neonatal behaviour. *Anesth Analg* 1985; **64**: 335–42.

9. Tsui M H Y, Ngan Kee W D, Ng F F, *et al.* A double blind randomised placebo-controlled study of intramuscular Pethidine for pain relief in the first stage of labour. *Br J Obstet Gynaecol* 2004; **111**: 648.

10. Nelson K E, Eisenach J C. Intravenous butorphanol, meperidine, and their combination relieve pain and distress in women in labor. *Anesthesiology* 2005; **102**: 1008–13.

11. Blair J M, Dobson G T, Hill D A, *et al.* Patient controlled analgesia for labour: a comparison of remifentanil with pethidine. *Anaesthesia* 2005; **60**: 22–7.

12. MCE. *Intrapartum Care. Care of Healthy Women and their Babies during Childbirth.* NICE guideline 55. London: NICE

13. Drife J. The start of life: a history of obstetrics. *Postgrad Med J* 2002; **78**: 311–5.

14. Lewis G (ed.). The Confidential Enquiry into Maternal and Child Health (CEMACH). Saving mothers' lives: reviewing maternal deaths to make motherhood safer 2003–2005. *The Seventh Report on Confidential Enquiries into Maternal Death in the United Kingdom.* London: CEMACH, 2007.

15. T, Halpern S H, Crosby E T, Huh C. Uterine incision and maternal blood loss in preterm caesarean section. *Arch Gynecol Obstet* 1993; **252**: 113–7.

16. MacCallum N S, Cox M. Anaesthesia for caesarean section complicated by placenta praevia. *Hosp Med* 2002; **63**: 636.

17. Ngan Kee W D, Khaw K S, Ng F F. Prevention of hypotension during spinal anaesthesia for cesarean delivery: an effective technique using combination phenylephrine infusion and crystalloid cohydration. *Anesthesiology* 2005; **103**: 744–50.

18. Reynolds F. Dural puncture and headache. *Br Med J* 1993; **306**: 874–6.

19. Lucas D N, Ciccone G K, Yentis S M. Extending low-dose epidural analgesia for emergency Caesarean section. A comparison of three solutions. *Anaesthesia* 1999; **54**: 1173–7.

Intrapartum fetal surveillance

Rohan D'Souza and Sabaratnam Arulkumaran

With the onset of labour, the fetus embarks upon a most perilous journey – a journey fraught with risks of asphyxia, trauma, intervention and even death. Yet, this journey must be made, as the odds today still favour a vaginal birth. Although it is unlikely that scientific advances will be able to make this journey any easier, there certainly have been attempts at making this journey safer for both mother and baby. To this end, the concept of 'intrapartum fetal surveillance' was introduced decades ago. What began with the listening to the fetal heart beat using a Pinard stethoscope has now become a sophisticated discipline, incorporating the ever-increasing knowledge of the science of obstetrics and the latest technology.

The aim of fetal surveillance during labour is to identify the fetus at risk of an adverse outcome based on our ability to understand how the fetus reacts to stress before it becomes compromised. Sadly, no single method is foolproof, and even in the developed world, intrapartum asphyxia with resultant mortality or severe morbidity continues to be a cause for concern. The most recent Perinatal Mortality report for England and Wales [1] reveals that 256 stillbirths and 165 neonatal deaths in the year 2006 were a direct result of intrapartum causes. The fear of litigation remains the obstetrician's worst nightmare, and ensuring a good outcome with minimum intervention his greatest challenge.

When electronic fetal monitoring (EFM) was introduced in the 1960s, a drastic reduction in perinatal morbidity and mortality was anticipated. However, the only consistently proven and clinically significant benefit from the routine use of continuous EFM compared with intermittent auscultation has been found to be the reduction of neonatal seizures, with an increase in caesarean section (CS) and

operative vaginal deliveries [2]. The widespread implementation of EFM does not appear to have brought about a reduction in cerebral palsy [3]. Despite its subjective nature, the frequency of falsely non-reassuring patterns and persistent questions regarding efficacy, EFM remains the predominant method of intrapartum fetal surveillance in the developed world. The search for a 'worthy accomplice' continues, with newer methods constantly being tried and tested. While some of these have been all but abandoned, some others have stuck around. A few of these have, however, shown practical potential and are being subjected to further scrutiny. These will be discussed in further detail.

Intermittent fetal monitoring

Intermittent surveillance of the fetal heart rate (FHR) during labour involves either intermittent auscultation (IA) or intermittent EFM at predetermined intervals during labour.

Intermittent auscultation

The auscultation of the fetal heart using a Pinard stethoscope or a hand-held Doppler is common practice in low-risk pregnancies. However, there is emerging evidence that there may be a role for IA in some high-risk pregnancies as well. A study in post-caesarean section pregnancies has suggested that intermittent auscultation may also be a safe mode of fetal surveillance as long as close monitoring is ensured [4].

A systematic review of recent trials comparing EFM with IA in low-risk pregnancies [5] has shown that women with continuous EFM were more likely to have CS and instrumental vaginal birth for abnormal FHR pattern compared with those with IA. There was also evidence that women having continuous EFM were less likely to have babies with neonatal seizures and more likely to have babies admitted to neonatal units compared with those having IA, with no evidence of difference in perinatal mortality. The findings were similar even when both low- and high-risk pregnancies were included in the analysis. IA is also a less expensive option than EFM because of the higher cost of equipment and increased rate of CS with the latter [6].

The use of the Pinard stethoscope has been compared with the hand-held Doppler, and it was found that although women monitored using a hand-held Doppler device had less spontaneous vaginal births and more CS, there was evidence that women monitored by Doppler were less likely to have babies with admissions to neonatal units, neonatal seizures, and hypoxic encephalopathy than those monitored using a Pinard stethoscope. There was no evidence of differences in perinatal mortality or low Apgar scores (Apgar score less than 6 at 5 min) [7].

Intermittent EFM

Intermittent use of EFM in the first stage of labour has been compared with continuous EFM in one RCT [8]. Here the use of intermittent EFM for 15–30 min every second hour with IA in between during the first stage was compared with the use of continuous EFM in the first stage of labour. Both groups had continuous EFM in the second stage of labour. Intermittent EFM (with stethoscope auscultation in between) was as effective as continuous EFM in low-risk labours.

Based on recent evidence, the National Institute for Clinical Excellence (NICE) [9] has made the following recommendations with regard to intermittent fetal surveillance in labour.

1. IA of the FHR may be used for low-risk women in established labour in any birth setting.
2. Initial auscultation of the fetal heart should be done at first contact in early labour and at each further assessment undertaken, to determine whether labour has become established.
3. Once a woman is in established labour, IA of FHR after a contraction be continued every 15 min during the first stage and every 5 min during the second stage for 60 s immediately after a contraction.
4. The 'moderate-level evidence' suggesting the superiority of the hand-held Doppler over the Pinard stethoscope was not robust enough to

differentiate between the two techniques and therefore either technique may be used for the purpose of IA.

5. Pregnancies being monitored by IA should be converted to continuous EFM following:

- meconium-stained liquor – significant or light;
- abnormal FHR detected by IA (less than 110 beats per minute (bpm); greater than 160 bpm; any decelerations after a contraction);
- maternal pyrexia (defined as 38.0°C once or 37.5°C on two occasions 2 h apart);
- fresh bleeding developing in labour;
- oxytocin use for augmentation;
- the woman's request.

The admission cardiotocograph (CTG)

Many units use a 20-minute CTG on admission to the delivery suite as a screening test to identify the fetus at risk of intrapartum hypoxia. This has not been shown to improve neonatal outcome, although operative delivery rates remain unchanged [10]. A systematic review including 3 RCTs and 11 observational studies, and assessing the prognostic value of the admission CTG and its effectiveness compared with auscultation alone, has been published recently [11]. This showed that women with admission CTG were more likely to have epidural analgesia, continuous EFM and fetal blood sampling (FBS). There was also borderline evidence that women with continuous EFM were more likely to have an instrumental birth and CS compared with the auscultation group, although there was no evidence of differences in augmentation, perinatal mortality or other neonatal morbidities. Therefore, the routine use of the admission CTG is not recommended.

Continuous electronic fetal monitoring (EFM)

Continuous EFM involves the use of a Doppler ultrasound transducer placed on the maternal abdomen or a scalp electrode to monitor the baby's heart rate and a pressure gauge transducer placed on the abdomen between the uterine fundus and the umbilicus to monitor uterine contractions. The CTG is a continuous recording of the fetal heart rate combined with a recording of uterine activity. This is the most widely

39

used method of intrapartum fetal surveillance in high-risk labour.

In view of the dubious performance of the CTG in RCTs and the poor specificity of CTG patterns to correlate with subsequent injury in a specific way, the continued reliance on CTG by the medical profession is being lambasted on both medical and legal grounds [12]. However, since this is the most widely studied and accepted modality of fetal surveillance at the moment, and since there is insufficient evidence to allow the exclusive use of other techniques, the CTG remains indispensable. The proper understanding of the precepts, use and interpretation of the CTG trace therefore becomes vital to the practice of obstetrics and midwifery.

Acceptable indications for the use of continuous EFM are given in Table 4.1 [13].

The highly litigious environment we live in would require that attention be given to the minutest detail and this must commence even prior to the commencement of the recording. Good practice would demand that the following measures be ensured.

1. The patient's name, hospital number, date of birth, the date and time of the recording, pulse rate and temperature should always be checked and recorded before starting the actual recording.

2. The time is automatically recorded on new CTG machines, but the clock on these machines must always be checked. The time at the end of the trace must also be recorded.

3. If monitoring extends beyond one pack of paper, the packs should be labelled Part 1, 2, 3, etc. The timing and order of events is often crucial in Court and commonly disputed areas in cases of fetal compromise are the timing of intervention and what is an acceptable time delay from the time of decision-making to delivery.

4. The FHR should be auscultated by a Pinard's stethoscope or a Doppler device before commencing EFM to avoid the maternal pulse being recorded by the fetal monitor. A sudden, significant shift of baseline FHR during the course of the recording should prompt an immediate review of the CTG and a correlation between the recorded FHR and maternal pulse. Persistent signal loss should be investigated and should prompt the changing of the transducer, electrodes, connections and machine, if necessary. If these actions do not rectify the problem, intermittent auscultation should be performed and this should

Table 4.1 Acceptable indications for continuous EFM in labour.

Labour abnormalities
- Induced labour
- Augmented labour
- Prolonged labour
- Prolonged rupture of membranes
- Regional analgesia
- Previous caesarean section
- Abnormal uterine activity

Suspected fetal distress in labour
- Meconium staining of amniotic fluid
- Suspicious fetal heart trace on auscultation
- Abnormal FHR on admission CTG
- Vaginal bleeding in labour
- Intrauterine infection

Fetal problems
- Multiple pregnancies (all fetuses)
- Small fetus
- Preterm fetus
- Breech presentation
- Oligohydramnios
- Post-term pregnancy
- Rhesus isoimmunisation

Maternal medical disease
- Hypertension
- Diabetes
- Cardiac disease (especially cyanotic)
- Haemoglobinopathy
- Severe anaemia
- Hyperthyroidism
- Collagen disease
- Renal disease

be documented in the medical records. The Courts will view an un-interpretable CTG with utmost suspicion and such a recording might jeopardize a successful defence.

5. All intrapartum events, e.g. vaginal examination, FBS, siting of an epidural or an epidural top-up, must be noted on the CTG.

6. Any member of staff who is asked to provide an opinion on a trace should note their findings on both the trace and the woman's medical records along with the date, time and signature.

7. Following birth, the healthcare professional should sign and note the date, time and mode of birth on the FHR trace.

8. Ideally both tocograph and cardiograph tracings should be clearly recorded in a continuous manner. FHR pattern recognition should be in relationship to the uterine contractions.

9. A review of litigation cases found that around 30% of traces were missing and that another 20% could not be interpreted [14]. It has also been recommended that CTG should be kept for a minimum of 25 years. Electronic storage systems provide a robust system of storage and facilitate easy retrieval, research and audit. CTG tracings can be downloaded and stored online in powerful central servers. Other systems make use of write-once-read-many-times (WORM) optical disks that can archive 4000 cases, with an average of 8 h of trace, along with the clinical data.

Pitfalls surrounding the interpretation of the CTG resulting in adverse outcomes have been highlighted repeatedly in the Confidential Enquiries [15]. Correct interpretation requires the complete understanding of the basic features of CTG. The four main features are the baseline heart rate, baseline variability, accelerations and decelerations.

Baseline heart rate

This refers to the mean FHR when this is stable, excluding accelerations and decelerations, determined over a period of 5–10 min and expressed in beats per minute (bpm) [8]. This baseline rate should be considered to be within a narrow range, perhaps 5 bpm at best [16]. A baseline rate between 110 and 160 bpm is regarded as 'normal'. Earlier studies have shown that uncomplicated bradycardia (defined as an FHR between 90 and 119 bpm) and tachycardia (160–179 bpm) had a poor predictive value for an umbilical artery cord pH of less than 7.20, although the predictive value increased with the duration and the degree of the baseline abnormality [17,18]. While these definitions help in identifying a fetus at risk in most instances, defining fetal bradycardia and tachycardia using arbitrary limits violates fundamental physiological principles by not using the fetus as its own control. It has been argued that it is far more appropriate to use the relative rise or fall of the baseline [16]. In the light of current research, it has been suggested that in the absence of infection, a baseline FHR of 160–179 bpm (moderate tachycardia) and 100–109 bpm (moderate bradycardia) are probably not associated with adverse neonatal outcome, although in the presence of other non-reassuring FHR features or if there has been a rise in the baseline FHR, this needs further investigation [9].

Baseline variability (BLV)

The abrupt and usually chaotic changes of the interval between consecutive heart beats in the normal fetus gives rise to a pseudo-random pattern of changes that can be characterized as 'baseline variability'. This has been defined as the minor fluctuations in baseline FHR occurring at 3–5 cycles per minute [9]. It is important to note that the appearance of variability will depend on physiological factors such as the fetal sleep cycle, interventions and administration of certain medications and on technical factors including whether the tracing is obtained from an internal or external transducer. Reduced BLV (<5 bpm) may be seen for up to 40 min and may represent a fetal sleep cycle. Although some studies show that this may last up to 90 min [19], most guidelines would recommend a review of the whole case and appropriate intervention by this point.

A cut-off of 5 bpm for amplitude and 5 cycles per minute for frequency maximizes the sensitivity for detection of neonatal acidosis (cord artery pH<7.20) or 5-min Apgar score of less than 7 [20]. Reduced BLV is associated with an increased risk of cerebral palsy [21,22].

Although most attention has been paid to the abnormalities associated with decreased variability, it is important to emphasize that increased BLV is no more 'normal' than decreased BLV. Here again, the pattern and the evolution are important [16].

Accelerations

Defined as abrupt increases in the baseline FHR of more than 15 bpm and lasting over 15 s, the presence of accelerations is generally considered a good indicator of good perinatal outcome. CTGs with more than two accelerations in a 20 min window are called reactive traces and have a sensitivity of 97% for an Apgar score greater than 7 at 5 min [23,24]. Accelerations are a very reassuring feature, so much so that neurological injuries seen with a reactive intrapartum FHR pattern are deemed to have occurred either in early pregnancy, as a consequence of birth trauma or after birth [16].

With regard to accelerations, it is important to note that their incidence may be lower prior to

41

30 weeks, steadily increasing to term. Also, their size may be less than 15 bpm in the early preterm period.

Cycling

CTG with reactive segments with good variability (active sleep period) alternates with segments of reduced variability and no or occasional accelerations (quiet sleep). Alternating segments of active and quiet epochs are termed cycling and are indicative of a fetus with a normal behavioural status.

Decelerations

Five types of decelerations have been described as follows.

Early decelerations

Uniform, repetitive, periodic slowing of FHR with onset early in the contraction and return to baseline at the end of contraction. They generally do not drop to more than 40 beats from the baseline heart rate. These decelerations have been attributed to head compression and are not associated with metabolic acidosis or a low Apgar score [25–27].

Late decelerations

Uniform, repetitive, periodic slowing of FHR with onset mid to end of contraction, nadir >20 s after the peak of the contraction and ending after the contraction. In the presence of a non-accelerative trace with baseline variability <5 bpm, the definition should include decelerations of <15 bpm [9]. These represent a transient fall in partial pressure of oxygen (hypoxaemia) below a certain threshold. There is an association between late decelerations and reduced Apgar scores at 5 min [28,29], metabolic acidosis [27,30] and marked increase in the odds of cerebral palsy, the risk of which is higher if both late decelerations and reduced variability are present [31]. Late decelerations have a high sensitivity for predicting subsequent abnormal neurological examinations at 2, 4, 6, 9 and 12 months [32]. When accompanied by reduced BLV and the absence of accelerations, recurrent late decelerations are found to be associated with a low pH (<7.1) in >50% of cases [33].

Variable decelerations – uncomplicated

These refer to the variable, intermittent, periodic slowing of FHR with rapid onset and recovery. Time relationships with contraction cycles are variable and they may occur in isolation. They have a pre-shouldering followed by a sudden decline and quick recovery to the baseline, followed by another shouldering of the FHR. They are generally believed to be due to cord compression and may be relieved by repositioning of the mother or by amnioinfusion. Uncomplicated variable decelerations are not consistently shown to be associated with reduced 5 min Apgar scores, metabolic acidosis or poor neonatal outcome [34–38].

Variable decelerations – complicated or 'atypical'

Variable decelerations with the following additional features represent transient hypoxaemia and are associated with poor adverse neonatal outcome when compared with FHR tracings with no decelerations or simple variable decelerations.

- Loss of primary or secondary rise in baseline rate.
- Slow return to baseline FHR after the end of the contraction (late recovery).
- Prolonged increase of secondary rise in baseline (rebound tachycardia).
- Biphasic or 'combined' decelerations – variable followed by late component.
- Loss of variability during deceleration.
- Continuation of baseline heart rate at lower level.
- Decelerations with depth >60 beats and duration >60 s.

Prolonged decelerations

Prolonged decelerations ('bradycardia') of less than 80 beats for less than 3 min are categorized as suspicious, and for more than 3 min as abnormal [9] The decline in pH is rapid in the presence of a prolonged deceleration of less than 80 bpm. Prolonged decelerations arising from a previously normal FHR pattern are only occasionally associated with fetal acidosis if the deceleration stabilizes at 80 bpm or above for a short duration, especially if variability is maintained [39]. Immediate delivery should be undertaken in the presence of abruption, scar rupture and cord prolapse. Measures such as altering position, stopping oxytocin and tocolysis should be considered in other cases, and failure of the FHR to show signs of recovery within the next 6–9 min is an indication for immediate delivery.

The interpretation of decelerations

The interpretation of decelerations is a rather complex topic and cannot be viewed in isolation. It is crucial to the understanding of CTG patterns that in the presence of uterine contractions, fetal hypoxia will be reflected by the appearance of decelerations before a rise in the baseline rate or a decrease in variability [40]. With continued mild-to-moderate hypoxia, the decelerations continue accompanied by a rising baseline heart rate and a diminution in baseline variability [40], eventually leading to a fixed elevated rate. The previously normal fetus will not fail to respond to significant hypoxia with a change in baseline rate and variability. As the fetus approaches death, the baseline falls and becomes unstable; decelerations might be less obvious and less easily separable into type, i.e. late or variable. Alternatively, the initial response to severe or profound hypoxia might be a prolonged deceleration (bradycardia).

CTGs permit discrimination between the mechanisms of hypoxia according to the pattern of deceleration:

- hypoxia related primarily to decreased availability of oxygen (hypoxaemic hypoxia); and
- hypoxia related primarily to interference with blood flow and the regional interference with oxygen availability (ischaemic hypoxia).

Those changes associated with late decelerations appear to be hypoxaemic, whereas those associated with variable or prolonged decelerations of sudden onset are ischaemic [41–46]. The distinction, readily supported by the literature, is important because of the different ways the fetus responds to such limitations of oxygen, in the speed of deterioration, and in the relationship to subsequent injury. Late decelerations associated with a rising baseline rate and decreasing variability are associated with a slow decrease in oxygen availability and cerebral blood flow, and might be tolerated for 60–90 min or more but the condition of the fetus is better checked by FBS [44].

Sinusoidal trace

A sinusoidal pattern is defined as a regular oscillation of the baseline rate with markedly reduced baseline variability resembling a sine wave. This smooth, undulating pattern, lasting at least 10 min, usually has a relatively fixed period of 3–5 cycles per minute and amplitude of 5–15 bpm above and below the baseline. Fetal anaemia has been reported previously as an associated risk factor for sinusoidal FHR patterns with poor neonatal outcome [47]. However,

segments of sinusoidal patterns can be seen in uncompromised babies and are not necessarily associated with adverse neonatal outcome. However, the occurrence of this pattern should be viewed with suspicion and a feto-maternal haemorrhage must be excluded.

A fetus that has a reactive CTG after the segment of sinusoidal pattern is unlikely to be anaemic. Continuation of the trace for 90 min or stimulation of the fetus (to look for accelerations) will help to identify the sinusoidal trace that has a physiological basis such as thumb-sucking without anaemia.

Categorization of FHR features [9]

Feature	Baseline (bpm)	Variability (bpm)	Decelerations	Accelerations
Reassuring	110–160	≥5	None	Present
Non-reassuring	100–109 161–180	<5 for 40–90 min	Typical variable decelerations with over 50% of contractions, occurring for over 90 min	The absence of accelerations with otherwise normal trace is of uncertain significance.
			Single prolonged deceleration for up to 3 min	
Abnormal	<100 >180 Sinusoidal pattern ≥10 min	<5 for 90 min	Either atypical variable decelerations with over 50% of contractions or late decelerations, both for over 30 min	
			Single prolonged deceleration for more than 3 min	

Categorization of FHR traces – definition of normal, suspicious and pathological FHR traces [9]

Category	Definition
Normal:	An FHR trace in which all four features are classified as reassuring

Suspicious: An FHR trace with one feature classified as non-reassuring and the remaining features classified as reassuring

Pathological: An FHR trace with two or more features classified as non-reassuring or one or more classified as abnormal

However, in addition to the correct interpretation of CTG, the importance of adequate communication of the findings, timely clinical response for a suspicious or pathological trace and the consideration of the clinical picture cannot be overemphasized. The Confidential Enquiry into Stillbirths and Deaths in Infancy [48] found that 50% of intrapartum deaths of babies over 1500 g with no chromosomal or congenital malformations could have been avoided and were due to non-recognition of abnormal CTG patterns, poor communication and delay in taking appropriate action. These findings were one of the many factors that prompted the need for national guidelines for EFM.

Acting on a suspicious or pathological CTG

Inaction is a common feature in many claims. A pathological CTG is considered to indicate a risk of fetal hypoxia; it is indefensible to take no action and, indeed, it is not acceptable practice.

An appropriate action might include a decision to 'wait and see' for a limited period while taking remedial actions such as repositioning the mother, stopping the oxytocin infusion, using tocolysis in the presence of hyperstimulation or improving placental perfusion by maternal hydration. FBS might be obtained if the cervix is sufficiently dilated. Based on the clinical situation, immediate delivery might be the only option. The time of observation and the action taken including a decision to 'wait and see' should be recorded in the notes. Initialling the CTG is not enough, and if a decision that has been taken is not clearly documented in the notes it will appear in retrospect that the CTG abnormality was simply ignored.

Time is of the essence in cases of prolonged FHR deceleration because hypoxia and acidosis can develop rapidly. In such cases, especially if the bradycardia is due to placental abruption, cord prolapse or scar dehiscence, an immediate delivery needs to be performed, ideally within 15 min and certainly no longer than 30 min. There is a strong correlation between poor neonatal outcome and a delayed decision to delivery interval.

NICE has devised a practice algorithm to guide the clinicians in management of suspicious and pathological traces [9]. They recommend that:

- in cases where the CTG falls into the suspicious category, conservative measures should be used;
- in cases where the CTG falls into the pathological category, conservative measures should be used and fetal blood sampling performed where appropriate/feasible; and
- in situations where fetal blood sampling is not possible or appropriate, delivery should be expedited.

Interpretation of CTG – education and training

Interpretation of the CTG is subject to intra- and interobserver differences. The best way to achieve competence in CTG interpretation is probably through a combination of education and training strategies rather than a single approach. The following have been recommended by various authorities [49].

- A regular and structured programme of compulsory training on the interpretation of CTGs for all midwives and doctors.
- Mandatory introductory training whenever an individual takes up a new post.
- Regular rolling 'CTG study days' every 6 months 'protected from clinical work' to maximize attendance.
- Weekly case review meetings, as this is the best way of reinforcing knowledge.
- Self-directed learning should be encouraged. Units should provide learning resources such as books, interactive CD-ROMs or access to websites.

Interpretation of CTG – expert vs. computer interpretation

A new review of the use of computerized FHR interpretation including six studies concluded that computerized systems have not been demonstrated to be superior to expert interpretation of the FHR trace and that further study investigating computerized expert systems should be undertaken [9].

Incorporating the clinical picture

The clinical picture should always have a major influence on the action planned in the face of a disquieting CTG. It must always be borne in mind that the CTG is only an investigation and that monitoring labour using only a single parameter is never sufficient. With any given CTG, the clinical actions and decisions will vary depending on the clinical picture. When there is abruption, cord prolapse or possible scar rupture, a suboptimal CTG needs immediate intervention because these traces can suddenly change for the worse, resulting in a poor outcome [50]. Fetal hypoxia and acidosis may develop faster with an abnormal trace when there is scanty thick meconium, intrauterine growth restriction, intrauterine infection with pyrexia and/or pre- or post-term labour [49]. In preterm fetuses (especially <34 weeks), hypoxia and acidosis can increase the likelihood of respiratory distress syndrome [51] and may contribute to intraventricular haemorrhage [52], warranting an early intervention in the presence of an abnormal trace. Hypoxia can be made worse by oxytocin, epidural analgesia and difficult operative deliveries [53]. Abnormal patterns may represent the effects of drugs, fetal anomaly, fetal injury or infection – not only hypoxia [50].

Intrapartum fetal scalp stimulation tests

Scalp stimulation tests include fetal scalp puncture that is incidental to performing an FBS and digital stimulation of the fetal scalp, which is performed by gentle digital stroking of the fetal scalp. For any of the methods of scalp stimulation, a reassuring response is defined as acceleration in the FHR. A meta-analysis of available data revealed that there is observational evidence that response to digital stimulation of the fetal scalp is a good predictive test and response to fetal scalp puncture during FBS is a moderately predictive test for fetal acidaemia [54]. Based on the above findings, it has been recommended that digital stimulation of the fetal scalp by the healthcare professional during a vaginal examination be considered as an adjunct to continuous EFM [9].

Fetal scalp blood sampling for pH and lactate measurements

Fetal scalp blood sampling (FBS) during the first stage of labour was introduced by Saling in 1962 and was based on pH analysis [55]. The technique involves the introduction of an illuminated plastic endoscopic cone into the vagina and through the cervical os, so that it rests against the fetal presenting part. After drying and appropriate preparation of the part, the fetal scalp is punctured with a micro-scalpel and blood is collected by capillary action in a heparinized capillary tube and transported on ice to the laboratory for analysis.

Empirically, based on some 80 cases, Saling suggested pH cut-off values and consequently recommended interventional guidelines. These guidelines are still by-and-large regarded as the 'gold standard' with respect to the diagnosis of intrapartum fetal distress.

Fetal blood sample result (pH) Interpretation of the results [9]	
≥7.25	Normal FBS result
7.21–7.24	Borderline FBS result
≤7.20	Abnormal FBS result

These results should be interpreted taking into account the previous pH measurement, the rate of progress in labour and the clinical features of the woman and baby.

After an abnormal FBS result, consultant obstetric advice should be sought.

After a normal FBS result, sampling should be repeated no more than 1 h later if the FHR trace remains pathological, or sooner if there are further abnormalities.

After a borderline FBS result, sampling should be repeated no more than 30 min later if the FHR trace remains pathological or sooner if there are further abnormalities.

The time taken to take a fetal blood sample needs to be considered when planning repeat samples.

If the FHR trace remains unchanged and the FBS result is stable after the second test, a third/further sample may be deferred unless additional abnormalities develop on the trace.

Where a third FBS is considered necessary, consultant obstetric opinion should be sought.

It has now been shown that respiratory acidaemia (CO_2 accumulation) is harmless to the fetus, whereas metabolic acidaemia (lactic acid accumulation) is associated with neonatal morbidity [56–58]. Most delivery units would therefore have guidelines requiring

45

the full analysis of acid–base status at FBS, to be able to discriminate between the two. The relationship between fetal asphyxia and brain damage is complex and may be influenced by a number of factors including fetal maturity, degree, duration and nature of asphyxia, and the fetal cardiovascular response [59]. Our understanding of this relationship has been based on studies in research laboratories and a direct extrapolation to the clinical context may not be totally appropriate. A thorough analysis of current evidence suggests that there is no correlation between scalp blood pH and improved longer-term outcomes, and limited correlation between fetal base deficit and longer-term outcomes [9].

Metabolic acidaemia (pH<7.00) is said to be moderate when the base deficit (BD) is >8 mmol/l, and severe when BD>12 mmol/l [60]. Umbilical artery blood-measure of metabolic acidosis is a good indicator of tissue oxygen debt experienced by the fetus. Recent studies suggest that an increased risk to the fetus begins when umbilical artery BD exceeds the mean [61]. Moderate and severe newborn complications have only been shown to occur in fetuses with an umbilical artery BD>12 mmol/l and the incidence was 10% with BD 12–16 mmol/l [62]. These umbilical artery BD values are often applied to FBS but have not been evaluated in clinical trials. Besides, no cut-off values are derived from FBS blood to fit with the higher pH values (<7.20) [63].

There is a good correlation between lag-time ST event on fetal ECG and scalp pH [64]. For want of a more suitable and clinically tested method of surveillance, FBS for pH is still recommended on the premise that 'although the research evidence does not support the use of FBS because of the lack of direct comparison, clinical experience and evidence from indirect comparisons suggests that FBS avoids some instrumental births and CS' [9].

The other problems associated with FBS include the following.

- The procedural and technical difficulties in collecting a sufficient quantity of blood for analysis and the need to repeatedly perform this invasive procedure make it rather unattractive for clinicians and women in labour.
- Although acid–base machines have improved over the years, analysis can be compromised by air bubbles or clots in the blood sample; the machine might also be busy with its automatic calibrating system at the time for analysis. pH blood sampling or analysis has been reported to fail in 20% of cases [65]. On average, the procedure takes 18 min to perform and therefore cannot be used in cases of acute fetal compromise [66].
- Optimal interpretation requires a paired sample from both umbilical artery and vein, and the accuracy of calculated measures of metabolic acidosis is dependant upon the quality of pH and pCO_2 estimations [59].
- It has also been recommended that the use of FBS be avoided in bleeding disorders such as haemophilia A and in women with certain maternal viral infections such as HIV, Hepatitis B and Herpes simplex. In the presence of abnormal FHR patterns in preterm labour (<34 weeks' gestation) the use of FBS may be associated with an increase in adverse neonatal outcome and an early delivery is advised [9].

Lactate measurements

While the interest in scalp blood pH is in decline, the measurement of scalp blood lactate might still hold some promise. It has recently been shown that lactate in arterial umbilical cord blood might be a more direct and correct indicator of fetal asphyxia at delivery than pH [67].

Lactate measurements have been evaluated in intrapartum fetal surveillance for over three decades, and the launch of reliable, hand-held, microvolume devices in the 1990s has made the measurement of scalp blood lactate a clinical option. Maternal and fetal lactate concentrations increase with the duration of active bearing-down. It is estimated that fetal lactate increases by 1 mmol/l for every 30 min of pushing; the corresponding value for the woman is 2 mmol/l per 30 min [68]. A lactate concentration of 4.8 mmol/l has been recommended as the cut-off value for intervention and the following guidelines (table) have been published [69].

Clinical guidelines for fetal scalp blood pH and lactate (using Lactate Pro™) [55,69].

An RCT [65] comparing these two measurements found lactate to be more favourable in clinical practice in terms of less sampling failure and reduced time from the decision to do a fetal scalp blood sample to

	pH	Lactate (mmol/l) using Lactate Pro™
Normal	>7.25	<4.2
Pre-acidaemia/ pre-lactaemia	7.20–7.25	4.2–4.8
Acidaemia/ lactaemia	<7.20	>4.8

the clinician receiving the result. Although this RCT was too small to allow analysis of severe neonatal outcome, there is a lot of retrospective data on fetal scalp blood pH and lactate analyses (Lactate Pro™), in selected normal cases as well as in cases with fetal distress [69,70]. A good correlation between lactate obtained at FBS close to delivery and from cord arterial blood immediately after delivery has been found [71].

Another advantage of scalp lactate measurement is that a much smaller quantity of blood suffices (5 µl) as compared to pH measurements that require approximately 35 µl [65]. There is also a suggestion that caput formation does not significantly alter the correlation between values obtained at FBS and values in the central fetal circulation [63].

At present, a large multicentre RCT is in progress in Sweden to compare lactate and pH measurement for the clinical management of suspected fetal compromise. The main end-points of this study are metabolic acidaemia or pH<7.00 in cord arterial blood at delivery and the results are awaited.

Fetal electrocardiogram (ECG)

Fetal electrocardiographic surveillance includes ST segment analysis and PR–RR interval analysis which are computerized methods to analyse the ST and PR–RR segments of fetal ECG, respectively.

ST segment analysis

The ST waveform of the fetal ECG provides continuous information on the ability of the fetal heart muscle to respond to the stress of labour. An elevation of the ST segment and T wave, quantified by the ratio between the T wave and QRS amplitudes (T/QRS), identifies fetal heart muscle responding to hypoxia by a surge of stress hormones (catecholamines), which leads to utilization of glycogen stored in the heart (an extra source of energy). ST segment depression can

indicate a situation where the heart is not fully able to respond. The basis for ST waveform interpretation is given in Figure 4.1 [72].

A special fetal monitoring device, STAN®, has been developed to allow detailed assessment of both fetal heart rate and ST waveform during labour after a standard fetal scalp electrode has been applied. The ST waveform changes are identified automatically, and clinical action should be taken strictly according to the guidelines, which are based on extensive research.

Summary of the pathophysiology of the ST waveform changes

From key experimental studies, the following conclusions can be drawn [72].

- During acute hypoxaemia, a mature fetus reacts with an elevation of the ST segment and a progressive increase in T wave height quantified by the ratio between the amplitude of the T wave and the QRS complex.
- This pattern emerges in parallel to a surge of adrenaline and is linked to the activation of myocardial beta-adrenoceptors.
- An increase in T/QRS emerges as a sign of functional adaptation of the myocardium to the hypoxic stress with myocardial glycogenolysis and enhanced myocardial performance and workload.
- In fetuses suffering from infections, hypotension and anaemia, persistently elevated ST waveforms were noted to precede intrauterine death.
- This functional response to hypoxia appears well in advance of any signs of failing function of the CNS. The integrity of the CNS is maintained as long as there is adequate cerebral blood perfusion.
- ST depression with negative T waves appears to provide information on a myocardium not fully responding to the hypoxic stress. Such a situation might emerge during the initial phase of hypoxia, but also as the dominant pattern seen in fetuses exposed to long-term reduction of oxygen and nutritional supply, and exposed to acute hypoxia. Endotoxin seems to play a role as well.
- The electrophysiological mechanism behind this is a situation of uncoordinated repolarization

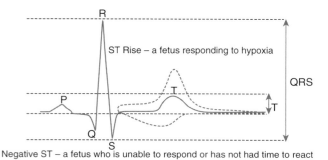

Negative ST – a fetus who is unable to respond or has not had time to react

Table 4.2 STAN clinical guidelines: ST changes indicating clinical intervention if CTG is intermediary or abnormal [72].

ST	CTG		
	Intermediary	Abnormal	Pre-terminal
Episodic T/QRS rise	Increase >0.15 from baseline	Increase >0.10 from baseline	Immediate delivery regardless of ST changes
Baseline T/QRS rise	Increase >0.10 from baseline	Increase >0.05 from baseline	Delivery regardless of ST changes
Biphasic ST: a component of the ST segment below the baseline	Continuous >5 min or >two episodes of coupled biphasic ST type 2 or 3	Continuous >2 min or >one episode of coupled biphasic ST type 2 or 3	

within the myocardial wall with prolonged repolarization in the endocardium.

The most recent meta-analysis [9] that includes a recently published RCT [73] as well as a systematic review of ST analysis [74] showed evidence that ST analysis significantly reduced the rate of instrumental vaginal birth and the need for FBS. There was no evidence of a difference in the CS rate and fetal acid–base status. There is evidence that ST analysis reduced the number of babies who developed neonatal encephalopathy and the number of babies with cord blood acidosis (pH less than 7.05, base excess less than −12 mmol/l), although there was no evidence of differences in other neonatal outcomes, i.e. perinatal deaths, Apgar score less than 7 at 5 min and admission to neonatal unit. When perinatal deaths and neonatal encephalopathy are combined, there is no evidence of difference.

In the light of current evidence, it was concluded [9] that ST analysis seems to add value to the use of EFM and reduces intervention, but it is recommended that another RCT to consolidate these findings be undertaken. The limitations identified were as follows.

1. Added cost.
2. The use of fetal scalp electrodes.
3. Additional staff training.
4. If used when fetal heart rate abnormalities are already present, it may be necessary to perform FBS before using ST analysis.

Fetal pulse-oxymetry (FPO)

FPO made its formal debut in the late 1980s, when investigators in the UK independently reported their initial experiences in measuring fetal oxygen saturation ($FSpO_2$) using cannibalized components of adult oxymeters [75–77]. During the 1990s, large volumes of data were published regarding feasibility, physiology and clinical application of this technology [78–84].

One of the most important questions addressed was the 'critical threshold' of $FSpO_2$ – the level of fetal arterial oxygen saturation above which acidaemia does not occur. Clinical observations of thousands of cases, and published studies, suggest that a critical threshold of 30% would be appropriate for human clinical use, a threshold used in the American RCT and subsequently approved by the US Food and Drug Administration (FDA) [85–88].

The American multicentre RCT was the first large-scale study to assess clinical utility of this new technology and remains the only RCT published to date [89]. The study concluded that although the CS rate for non-reassuring EFM was reduced by more than 50%, the overall CS rate was unchanged between the control and the test group, secondary to an increased incidence of CS for dystocia in the FPO group. The failure to reduce the overall caesarean rate led many to question whether there was any clear benefit to FPO monitoring, despite improved prediction of fetal condition using FPO. In September 2001, the American College of Obstetricians and Gynaecologists (ACOG) released a Committee Opinion [90] on FPO, stating that the adoption of this device in clinical practice could not be endorsed because of concerns that its introduction would escalate the cost of medical care without necessarily improving clinical outcome. This was followed by a similar directive by the Society of Obstetricians and Gynaecologists of Canada in March 2002 [91,92].

Although neither of these publications has recommended that FPO should not be used by clinicians, they resulted in a significant reversal in enthusiasm for the technology. The NICHHD MFM Units Network is currently conducting an RCT involving 10,000 nulliparous women in labour and is aiming to study the impact of FPO as an adjunct to EFM on the CS rate. The study was initiated in 2002 and results are awaited.

Although there have been a few recent publications on FPO [93,94], the future of FPO will depend largely on the findings of the above-mentioned RCT. As of now, what is known about FPO is that although FPO improves the prediction of the fetal acid–base condition as an adjunct to EFM and also reduces the CS rate for non-reassuring EFM patterns, as currently used, it does not decrease the overall CS rate and therefore cannot be recommended for routine use.

Conclusion

Despite the recent developments in the discipline of intrapartum fetal surveillance and the incorporation of a number of newer devices to the existing armamentarium, the search for the 'perfect tool' continues. While intermittent auscultation, electronic fetal monitoring and fetal blood sampling have established themselves as the best available tools, the interest in ST-segment analysis (fetal ECG) and fetal pulse-oxymetry continues to grow. Although more than two decades have passed since its introduction, Near Infra-Red Spectroscopy (NIRS) remains very much a developmental technique, while the current research in intrapartum fetal Doppler studies and fetal PR–RR intervals do not warrant their routine usage in clinical practice. Until a perfect method is devised to detect intrapartum hypoxia, the importance of the judicious use and the meticulous interpretation of the CTG will continue to dominate the science of fetal surveillance. A reminder of the following 'Clinical Pearls' [50] would go a long way in avoiding litigation, while simultaneously ensuring an optimal obstetric outcome.

1. Accelerations and normal baseline variability are hallmarks of fetal health.
2. Periods of decreased variability may represent fetal sleep.
3. Hypoxic fetuses may have a normal baseline FHR of 110–150 bpm with no accelerations and baseline variability of <5 bpm for >40 min.
4. In the presence of baseline variability <5 bpm, even shallow decelerations <15 bpm are ominous in a non-reactive trace.
5. Abruption, cord prolapse and scar rupture can give rise to acute hypoxia and should be suspected clinically.
6. Hypoxia and acidosis may develop faster with an abnormal trace in patients with scanty thick meconium, intrauterine growth restriction (IUGR), intrauterine infection with pyrexia, and those who are pre- or post-term.
7. In preterm fetuses (especially <34 weeks), hypoxia and acidosis can aggravate respiratory distress syndrome (RDS) and may contribute to intraventricular haemorrhage and sequelae warranting early action in the presence of an abnormal trace.
8. Hypoxia can be worsened by oxytocin, epidural analgesia and difficult operative deliveries.
9. During labour, if decelerations are absent, asphyxia is unlikely.
10. Abnormal patterns may represent effects of drugs, fetal anomaly, infection – not only hypoxia.

References

1. Confidential Enquiry into Maternal and Child Health (CEMACH). *Perinatal Mortality 2006: England, Wales and Northern Ireland*. London: CEMACH, 2008.

2. Thacker S B, Stroup D, Chang M. Continuous electronic heart rate monitoring for fetal assessment during labor. *Cochrane Database Syst Rev. (Online)* 2001; **2**: CD000063.

3. Clark S L, Hankins G D. Temporal and demographic trends in cerebral palsy – fact and fiction. *Am J Obstet Gynecol* 2003; **188**: 628–33.

4. Madaan M, Trivedi S S. Intrapartum electronic fetal monitoring vs. intermittent auscultation in postcesarean pregnancies. *Int J Gynaecol Obstet* 2006; **94**: 123–5.

5. Alfirevic Z, Devane D, Gyte G M. Continuous cardiotocography (CTG) as a form of electronic fetal monitoring (EFM) for fetal assessment during labour. *Cochrane Database Syst Rev. (Online)*. 2006; **3**: CD006066.

6. Mugford M. The costs of continuous electronic fetal monitoring in low risk labour. In: Spencer J A D, Ward R H T, eds. *Intrapartum Fetal Surveillance*. London: RCOG Press, 1993; 241–52.

7. Mahomed K, Nyoni R, Mulambo T, Kasule J, Jacobus E. Randomised controlled trial of intrapartum fetal heart rate monitoring. *BMJ* 1994; **308**: 497–500.

8. Herbst A, Ingemarsson I. Intermittent versus continuous electronic monitoring in labour: a randomised study. *Br J Obstet Gynaecol* 1994; **101**: 663–8.

9. RCOG. *Intrapartum Care: Care of Healthy Women and their Babies during Childbirth*. London: RCOG Press, 2007.

10. Impey L, Reynolds M, MacQuillan K, *et al.* Admission cardiotocography: a randomised controlled trial. *Lancet* 2003; **361**: 465–70.

11. Bix E, Reiner L M, Klovning A, Oian P. Prognostic value of the labour admission test and its effectiveness compared with auscultation only: a systematic review. *Br J Obstet Gynaecol* 2005; **112**: 1595–604.

12. Lent M. The medical and legal risks of the electronic fetal monitor. *Stanford Law Rev* 1999; **51**: 807–37.

13. Steer P J D. Fetal distress in labour. In: James D K, Steer P J, Weiner C P, Gonik B, eds. *High Risk Pregnancy: Management Options*, 2nd ed. Philadelphia: W B Saunders, 1999; 1121–49.

14. Ennis M, Vincent C A. Obstetric accidents: a review of 64 cases. *BMJ* 1990; **300**: 1365–7.

15. Lewis G. The Confidential Enquiry into Maternal and Child Health (CEMACH). Saving mothers' lives: reviewing maternal deaths to make motherhood safer – 2003–2005. *The Seventh Report on Confidential Enquiries into Maternal Deaths in the United Kingdom*. London: CEMACH, 2007.

16. Schifrin B S. The CTG and the timing and mechanism of fetal neurological injuries. *Best Pract Res* 2004; **18**: 437–56.

17. Gilstrap L C, 3rd, Hauth J C, Hankins G D, Beck A W. Second-stage fetal heart rate abnormalities and type of neonatal acidemia. *Obstet Gynecol* 1987; **70**: 191–5.

18. Gilstrap L C, 3rd, Hauth J C, Toussaint S. Second stage fetal heart rate abnormalities and neonatal acidosis. *Obstet Gynecol* 1984; **63**: 209–13.

19. Spencer J A, Johnson P. Fetal heart rate variability changes and fetal behavioural cycles during labour. *Br J Obstet Gynaecol* 1986; **93**: 314–21.

20. Samueloff A, Langer O, Berkus M, *et al.* Is fetal heart rate variability a good predictor of fetal outcome? *Acta Obstet Gynecol Scand* 1994; **73**: 39–44.

21. Schifrin B S, Hamilton-Rubinstein T, Shields J R. Fetal heart rate patterns and the timing of fetal injury. *J Perinatol* 1994; **14**: 174–81.

22. Shields J R, Schifrin B S. Perinatal antecedents of cerebral palsy. *Obstet Gynecol* 1988; **71**: 899–905.

23. Krebs H B, Petres R E, Dunn L J, Smith P J. Intrapartum fetal heart rate monitoring. VI. Prognostic significance of accelerations. *Am J Obstet Gynecol* 1982; **142**: 297–305.

24. Powell O H, Melville A, MacKenna J. Fetal heart rate acceleration in labor: excellent prognostic indicator. *Am J Obstet Gynecol* 1979; **134**: 36–8.

25. Cibils L A. Clinical significance of fetal heart rate patterns during labor. VI. Early decelerations. *Am J Obstet Gynecol* 1980; **136**: 392–8.

26. Krebs H B, Petres R E, Dunn L J, Jordaan H V, Segreti A. Intrapartum fetal heart rate monitoring. I. Classification and prognosis of fetal heart rate patterns. *Am J Obstet Gynecol* 1979; **133**: 762–72.

27. Low J A, Victory R, Derrick E J. Predictive value of electronic fetal monitoring for intrapartum fetal asphyxia with metabolic acidosis. *Obstet Gynecol* 1999; **93**: 285–91.

28. Cibils L A. Clinical significance of fetal heart rate patterns during labor. II. Late decelerations. *Am J Obstet Gynecol* 1975; **123**: 473–94.

29. Ellison P H, Foster M, Sheridan-Pereira M, MacDonald D. Electronic fetal heart monitoring, auscultation, and neonatal outcome. *Am J Obstet Gynecol* 1991; **164**: 1281–9.

30. Low J A, Cox M J, Karchmar E J, *et al.* The prediction of intrapartum fetal metabolic acidosis by fetal heart

rate monitoring. *Am J Obstet Gynecol* 1981; **139**: 299–305.

31. Nelson K B, Dambrosia J M, Ting T Y, Grether J K. Uncertain value of electronic fetal monitoring in predicting cerebral palsy. *N Engl J Med* 1996; **334**: 613–8.

32. Painter M J, Depp R, O'Donoghue P D. Fetal heart rate patterns and development in the first year of life. *Am J Obstet Gynecol* 1978; **132**: 271–7.

33. Sameshima H, Ikenoue T. Predictive value of late decelerations for fetal acidemia in unselective low-risk pregnancies. *American J Perinatol* 2005; **22**: 19–23.

34. Cibils L A. Clinical significance of fetal heart rate patterns during labor. V. Variable decelerations. *Am J Obstet Gynecol* 1978; **132**: 791–805.

35. Gaziano E P. A study of variable decelerations in association with other heart rate patterns during monitored labor. *Am J Obstet Gynecol* 1979; **135**: 360–3.

36. Krebs H B, Petres R E, Dunn L J. Intrapartum fetal heart rate monitoring. VIII. Atypical variable decelerations. *Am J Obstet Gynecol* 1983; **145**: 297–305.

37. Ozden S, Demirci F. Significance for fetal outcome of poor prognostic features in fetal heart rate traces with variable decelerations. *Arch Gynecol Obstet* 1999; **262**: 141–9.

38. Tortosa M N, Acien P. Evaluation of variable decelerations of fetal heart rate with the deceleration index: influence of associated abnormal parameters and their relation to the state and evolution of the newborn. *Eur J Obstet Gynecol Reprod Biol* 1990; **34**: 235–45.

39. Parer J T, Livingston E G. What is fetal distress? *Am J Obstet Gynecol* 1990; **162**: 1421–5; discussion 5–7.

40. Murata Y, Martin C B, Jr, Ikenoue T, *et al.* Fetal heart rate accelerations and late decelerations during the course of intrauterine death in chronically catheterized rhesus monkeys. *Am J Obstet Gynecol* 1982; **144**: 218–23.

41. Aldrich C J, D'Antona D, Spencer J A, *et al.* Fetal heart rate changes and cerebral oxygenation measured by near-infrared spectroscopy during the first stage of labour. *Eur J Obstet Gynecol Reprod Biol* 1996; **64**: 189–95.

42. Aldrich C J, D'Antona D, Spencer J A, *et al.* Late fetal heart decelerations and changes in cerebral oxygenation during the first stage of labour. *Br J Obstet Gynaecol* 1995; **102**: 9–13.

43. Ball R H, Parer J T. The physiologic mechanisms of variable decelerations. *Am J Obstet Gynecol* 1992; **166**: 1683–8; discussion 8–9.

44. Fleischer A, Schulman H, Jagani N, Mitchell J, Randolph G. The development of fetal acidosis in

the presence of an abnormal fetal heart rate tracing. I. The average for gestational age fetus. *Am J Obstet Gynecol* 1982; **144**: 55–60.

45. Harris J L, Krueger T R, Parer J T. Mechanisms of late decelerations of the fetal heart rate during hypoxia. *Am J Obstet Gynecol* 1982; **144**: 491–6.

46. Itskovitz J, LaGamma E F, Rudolph A M. Heart rate and blood pressure responses to umbilical cord compression in fetal lambs with special reference to the mechanism of variable deceleration. *Am J Obstet Gynecol* 1983; **147**: 451–7.

47. Modanlou H D, Freeman R K. Sinusoidal fetal heart rate pattern: its definition and clinical significance. *Am J Obstet Gynecol* 1982; **142**: 1033–8.

48. *The Confidential Enquiry into Stillbirths and Deaths in Infancy. The Fourth Annual Report.* London: Maternal and Child Health Consortium, 1997.

49. Williams B, Arulkumaran S. Cardiotocography and medicolegal issues. *Best Pract Res* 2004; **18**: 457–66.

50. Gibb D, Arulkumaran S, eds. *Fetal Monitoring in Practice*, 3rd ed. Edinburgh: Churchill Livingstone, 2008.

51. Krasomski G, Broniarczyk D. [The influence of perinatal asphyxia on the occurrence of respiratory distress syndrome in preterm labor.] *Ginekol Pol* 1994; **65**: 547–52.

52. Lavrijsen S W, Uiterwaal C S, Stigter R H, *et al.* Severe umbilical cord acidemia and neurological outcome in preterm and full-term neonates. *Biol Neonate* 2005; **88**: 27–34.

53. Okosun H A S. Intrapartum fetal surveillance. *Curr Obstet Gynaecol* 2005; **15**: 18–24.

54. Skupski D W, Rosenberg C R, Eglinton G S. Intrapartum fetal stimulation tests: a meta-analysis. *Obstet Gynecol* 2002; **99**: 129–34.

55. Bretscher J, Saling E. pH values in the human fetus during labor. *Am J Obstet Gynecol* 1967; **97**: 906–11.

56. Andres R L, Saade G, Gilstrap L C, *et al.* Association between umbilical blood gas parameters and neonatal morbidity and death in neonates with pathologic fetal acidemia. *Am J Obstet Gynecol* 1999; **181**: 867–71.

57. Goldaber K G, Gilstrap L C, 3rd, Leveno K J, Dax J S, McIntire D D. Pathologic fetal acidemia. *Obstet Gynecol* 1991; **78**: 1103–7.

58. Low J A, Panagiotopoulos C, Derrick E J. Newborn complications after intrapartum asphyxia with metabolic acidosis in the term fetus. *Am J Obstet Gynecol* 1994; **170**: 1081–7.

59. Low J A. Fetal monitoring during labour. In: Edmonds D K, ed. *Dewhurst's Textbook of Obstetrics & Gynaecology*. Oxford: Blackwell Publishing, 2007; 56–62.

60. Herbst A, Thorngren-Jerneck K, Wu L, Ingemarsson I. Different types of acid–base changes at birth, fetal heart rate patterns, and infant outcome at 4 years of age. *Acta Obstet Gynecol Scand* 1997; **76**: 953–8.

61. Victory R, Penava D, Da Silva O, Natale R, Richardson B. Umbilical cord pH and base excess values in relation to adverse outcome events for infants delivering at term. *Am J Obstet Gynecol* 2004; **191**: 2021–8.

62. Low J A, Lindsay B G, Derrick E J. Threshold of metabolic acidosis associated with newborn complications. *Am J Obstet Gynecol* 1997; **177**: 1391–4.

63. Nordstrom L. Fetal scalp and cord blood lactate. *Best Pract Res* 2004; **18**: 467–76.

64. Luttkus A K, Noren H, Stupin J H, *et al*. Fetal scalp pH and ST analysis of the fetal ECG as an adjunct to CTG. A multi-center, observational study. *J Perinatal Med* 2004; **32**: 486–94.

65. Westgren M, Kruger K, Ek S, *et al*. Lactate compared with pH analysis at fetal scalp blood sampling: a prospective randomised study. *Br J Obstet Gynaecol* 1998; **105**: 29–33.

66. Tuffnell D, Haw W L, Wilkinson K. How long does a fetal scalp blood sample take? *Br J Obstet Gynaecol* 2006; **113**: 332–4.

67. Gjerris A C, Staer-Jensen J, Jorgensen J S, Bergholt T, Nickelsen C. Umbilical cord blood lactate: a valuable tool in the assessment of fetal metabolic acidosis. *Eur J Obstet Gynecol Reprod Biol* 2008; **139**: 16–20.

68. Nordstrom L, Achanna S, Naka K, Arulkumaran S. Fetal and maternal lactate increase during active second stage of labour. *Br J Obstet Gynaecol* 2001; **108**: 263–8.

69. Kruger K, Hallberg B, Blennow M, Kublickas M, Westgren M. Predictive value of fetal scalp blood lactate concentration and pH as markers of neurologic disability. *Am J Obstet Gynecol* 1999; **181**: 1072–8.

70. Nordstrom L, Ingemarsson I, Kublickas M, *et al*. Scalp blood lactate: a new test strip method for monitoring fetal wellbeing in labour. *Br J Obstet Gynaecol* 1995; **102**: 894–9.

71. Kruger K, Kublickas M, Westgren M. Lactate in scalp and cord blood from fetuses with ominous fetal heart rate patterns. *Obstet Gynecol* 1998; **92**: 918–22.

72. Rosen K G, Amer-Wahlin I, Luzietti R, Noren H. Fetal ECG waveform analysis. *Best Pract Res* 2004; **18**: 485–514.

73. Ojala K, Vaarasmaki M, Makikallio K, Valkama M, Tekay A. A comparison of intrapartum automated fetal electrocardiography and conventional cardiotocography – a randomised controlled study. *Br J Obstet Gynaecol* 2006; **113**: 419–23.

74. Neilson J. Fetal electrocardiogram (ECG) for fetal monitoring during labour. *Cochrane Database Syst Rev*. 2006; **3**.

75. Gardosi J, Carter M, Becket T. Continuous intrapartum monitoring of fetal oxygen saturation. *Lancet* 1989; **2**: 692–3.

76. Johnson N, Johnson V A, Bannister J, Lilford R J. Measurement of fetal peripheral perfusion with a pulse oximeter. *Lancet* 1989; **1**: 898.

77. Peat S, Booker M, Lanigan C, Ponte J. Continuous intrapartum measurement of fetal oxygen saturation. *Lancet* 1988; **2**: 213.

78. Carbonne B, Audibert F, Segard L, *et al*. Fetal pulse oximetry: correlation between changes in oxygen saturation and neonatal outcome. Preliminary report on 39 cases. *Eur J Obstet Gynecol Reprod Biol* 1994; **57**: 73–7.

79. Dildy G A, Clark S L, Loucks C A. Preliminary experience with intrapartum fetal pulse oximetry in humans. *Obstet Gynecol* 1993; **81**: 630–5.

80. Dildy G A, Clark S L, Loucks C A. Intrapartum fetal pulse oximetry: past, present, and future. *Am J Obstet Gynecol* 1996; **175**: 1–9.

81. East C E, Colditz P B. Women's evaluations of their experience with fetal intrapartum oxygen saturation monitoring and participation in a research project. *Midwifery* 1996; **12**: 93–7.

82. Luttkus A, Fengler T W, Friedmann W, Dudenhausen J W. Continuous monitoring of fetal oxygen saturation by pulse oximetry. *Obstet Gynecol* 1995; **85**: 183–6.

83. Yam J, Chua S, Arulkumaran S. Intrapartum fetal pulse oximetry. Part I: Principles and technical issues. *Obstet Gynecol Surv* 2000; **55**: 163–72.

84. Yam J, Chua S, Arulkumaran S. Intrapartum fetal pulse oximetry. Part 2: Clinical application. *Obstet Gynecol Surv* 2000; **55**: 173–83.

85. Dildy G A, Thorp J A, Yeast J D, Clark S L. The relationship between oxygen saturation and pH in umbilical blood: implications for intrapartum fetal oxygen saturation monitoring. *Am J Obstet Gynecol* 1996; **175**: 682–7.

86. Kuhnert M, Seelbach-Goebel B, Butterwegge M. Predictive agreement between the fetal arterial oxygen saturation and fetal scalp pH: results of the German multicenter study. *Am J Obstet Gynecol* 1998; **178**: 330–5.

87. Richardson B S, Carmichael L, Homan J, Patrick J E. Electrocortical activity, electroocular activity, and breathing movements in fetal sheep with prolonged and graded hypoxemia. *Am J Obstet Gynecol* 1992; **167**: 553–8.

88. Seelbach-Gobel B, Heupel M, Kuhnert M, Butterwegge M. The prediction of fetal acidosis by means of

intrapartum fetal pulse oximetry. *Am J Obstet Gynecol* 1999; **180**: 73–81.

89. Garite T J, Dildy G A, McNamara H, *et al.* A multicenter controlled trial of fetal pulse oximetry in the intrapartum management of nonreassuring fetal heart rate patterns. *Am J Obstet Gynecol* 2000; **183**: 1049–58.

90. ACOG Committee Opinion. Number 258, September 2001. Fetal pulse oximetry. *Obstet Gynecol*. 2001; **98**: 523–4.

91. Liston R, Crane J, Hamilton E, *et al.* Fetal health surveillance in labour. *J Obstet Gynaecol Can* 2002; **24**: 250–76; quiz 77–80.

92. Liston R, Crane J, Hughes O, *et al.* Fetal health surveillance in labour. *J Obstet Gynaecol Can* 2002; **24**: 342–55.

93. Hajek Z, Srp B, Haddad el R, *et al.* [Analysis of present diagnostic methods of intrapartum fetal hypoxia.] *Ceska Gynekol* 2005; **70**: 22–6.

94. Sobotkova D, Kucerova I, Dittrichova J, Velebil P. [Psychomotor development of children with signs of intrapartum hypoxia and monitored by intrapartum fetal pulse oxymetry.] *Ceska Gynekol* 2004; **69**: 114–20.

53

Uterine contractions

Vivek Nama and Sabaratnam Arulkumaran

Introduction

Uterine contractions are a prerequisite for vaginal delivery. Unless there are mechanical difficulties such as disproportion or malposition, efficient contractions and the expulsive efforts of the mother should result in unassisted vaginal delivery. In most centres, uterine contractions are assessed by external palpation at regular intervals, and the clinical outcome with such practice is generally satisfactory. Dysfunctional labour has been estimated to affect up to 21% of primigravid labours [1]. It is the commonest cause of emergency caesarean sections and hence a significant health and economic issue [2]. Much research has been devoted to the identification of better methods of measuring uterine activity, but the appropriate use of this technology is difficult to define. This chapter discusses the molecular mechanisms involved in uterine contractions, methods used to measure uterine contractions, their reliability and uterine activity in normal, augmented and induced labour and in women with a caesarean scar.

Electric and physical basis of uterine contractions

Myometrium is predominantly a phasic muscle, although it can exhibit tonic contractions when exposed to high concentration of contractants [3]. Uterine contractions are a direct consequence of the underlying electrical activity in the myometrial cells. The action potentials in uterine smooth muscle result from voltage and time-dependent changes in membrane ionic permeability [4]. Phosphorylation of Serine-19 on the light chain of myosin brings about a significant interaction between myosin and actin in the uterus. This phosphorylation is by myosin light chain kinase activated by calcium channels binding to calmodulin. The frequency, amplitude and duration of contractions are mainly determined by the frequency of occurrence of the uterine electrical bursts, the total number of cells that are simultaneously active during the bursts, and the duration of the uterine electrical bursts, respectively [5].

Is there a need to measure uterine contractions?

Myometrial contractions initiated too early in pregnancy lead to preterm deliveries. Contractions at term that are too frequent will cause fetal hypoxia and distress; while if contractions are too weak or infrequent, the labour may be dysfunctional and require an emergency caesarean section. Uterine contractions temporarily impede replenishment of the retroplacental pool of blood necessary for oxygen transfer or compress the umbilical cord and cause compromise in fetuses with low reserves. Since the abnormal progress of spontaneous labour cannot be predicted prospectively, and the deleterious effect of uterine contraction on the fetal heart rate is interpreted in relation to uterine contractions, measurement of uterine activity is of value.

Measurement of uterine contractions is of importance to decide the interval between prostaglandin administered for induction of labour, and in induced labour to titrate the dose of syntocinon. Different contraction parameters are explained in Table 5.1.

Methods of measurement
Maternal perception

Mothers may be asked to time their contractions to assess their frequency and duration, but the reliance is

Table 5.1 Definition of contraction parameters.

Parameter	Definition
Relaxation time	Time in seconds between the end of one contraction and the beginning of the next contraction
Contraction duration	Time in seconds between onset and offset of a contraction
Contraction amplitude	Maximum uterine pressure above basal tone, mmHg
Contraction surface	Surface underneath the contraction, compared with the basal tone, between onset and offset of the contraction, mmHg seconds
Contraction frequency	Number of contractions in a 10-min period

on the woman's perception. An intrauterine pressure of 15 mmHg from the baseline pressure is effective in producing cervical changes and is experienced as pain. However, the threshold of pain varies from woman to woman and may be influenced by parity and maternal weight; obese and nulliparous women have difficulty in perceiving contractions [6].

Manual palpation

In many centres, uterine contractions are assessed by external palpation performed at regular intervals. The reliability of measurement is dependent on the experience of the obstetrician or midwife. Since the first and the last part of the contractions may not be palpable, the duration estimated may be less than the actual duration of the contraction [7]. Manual palpation of contractions is not influenced by a woman's position in labour, her parity, or the gestational age. The only parameter that can be correctly assessed by manual palpation is the contraction frequency. However, the clinical outcome with such practice is satisfactory.

External tocography

External tocography is performed using a tocodynamometer which has a centrally located, pressure-sensitive button (guard-ring type) or a diaphragm. Placed on the fundus, it detects myometrial contractility by a change in antero-posterior diameter of the abdomen resulting from uterine contractions. An on-line graphical record using such devices provides information

on the duration and frequency and an approximation of the strength of contractions.

The advantage of external tocography is that it is non-invasive. It provides a continuous record (trace) and does not require constant attendance of labour ward staff. External tocography is influenced by changes in position and abdominal wall musculature contractions, such as coughing and vomiting. The intensity is dependent on the tightness of the belt and thickness of the abdominal wall [8]. The quality of the recording in obese and restless women is poor. During the second stage of labour where the fetus is most at risk, the recording of uterine contractions is often inadequate.

External tocography provides adequate information of contraction frequency [9] and is suitable for use in an antenatal patient to predict preterm labour and in a parturient with normally progressing, spontaneous labour. Information on baseline tone, duration and intensity of contractions recorded by internal tocography is more accurate [10] compared with external tocography.

Internal tocography

Internal tocography is unaffected by maternal position. It is more comfortable for the patient, allows for amnioinfusion, and gives quantitative information on uterine activity such as baseline tone, contraction frequency, duration and amplitude [11]. Intrauterine pressure measurements in labour using transducer-tipped catheters inserted in the extra-amniotic space may not provide comparable information to a similar catheter inserted intra-amniotically when membranes are ruptured [12]. Internal tocography is invasive and carries certain risks. Since the rupture of membranes is a requirement, it has an increased risk of infection. There have been reports of occasional uterine perforation, fetal haemorrhage due to puncture of a fetal vessel, and placental abruption [13,14].

There are two varieties of intrauterine pressure catheters: fluid-filled or transducer-tipped. Both provide similar mean baseline uterine tone, contraction interval and duration. Fluid-filled catheters require more frequent readjustment and have an increased tendency for artefact due to air bubbles, kinked cables and catheter occlusion by meconium, blood, or fetal parts [15]. The transducer-tipped catheter is a bridge strain gauge deposited on a thin metal pressure-sensing surface. It is mounted on the end of a 90-cm

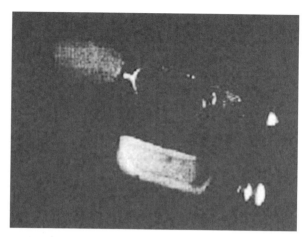

Figure 5.1 The tip of a fibre optic catheter with a smooth dome and distal fenestration housing the mirror arrangement is shown alongside the tip of the Gaeltec catheter with a recessed area behind the rounded tip

catheter, with a sensing area which is recessed, thus minimizing accidental damage and enabling lateral pressure measurements without impact of head or end-on pressure (Figure 5.1). The introduction of flexible fibre optic catheters has decreased the incidence of placental or fetal injury and these catheters can be kept in the uterus during the second stage of labour [16]. A dual-channel, multifunctional uterine probe and balloon probe has the advantage of accurate electronic monitoring of the fetal heart rate whilst also recording uterine activity [17].

There are variations in intrauterine pressure measurements from contraction to contraction when two intrauterine catheters are used in utero. The reasons for the individual variations from contraction to contraction remain obscure, but may be due to mechanical (direct force) rather than fluid pressure acting on the transducer. However, cumulative active pressure measurements recorded by each catheter were only 5% different, and hence have very little bearing on the management of labour [18,19].

External tocography correlates well with internal tocography with respect to frequency and may be the case even in the moderately obese [9]. If there is a fetal heart rate (FHR) abnormality in labour, the accuracy of contraction monitoring may be of benefit. In abnormal labour, when compared to external tocography, internal tocography has not been shown to change the obstetric outcome. Randomization of 250 pregnant women with slow progress and augmented labour into either intrauterine pressure transducer or external monitoring did not show any differences in neonatal outcome or reduction in caesarean section rates [20]. Similarly, uterine monitoring by external or internal tocography in women with induced labour did not show any difference in duration of labour, caesarean section rates and neonatal outcome [21]. Women who are obese, and/or restless, and those with poor progress in labour despite high doses of oxytocin infusion, may benefit from intrauterine monitoring.

Uterine electromyography (EMG)

A typical uterine EMG system includes abdominal surface electrodes, electrical filters/amplifiers and acquisition and analysis hardware/software. The EMG waves can be analysed by a number of sophisticated mathematical methods in order to determine the extent of the electrochemical preparedness of the myometrium for labour and subsequent delivery [4]. It is possible to detect, by non-invasive abdominal recordings, a risk of preterm birth as early as the 27th week of pregnancy [22]. EMG measurement may be used to measure the synchronization and concordance of contractions [23]. The uterine electromyogram is the result of electrical activity generated at the microscopic level. Measurements of uterine activity by transabdominal electromyography are comparable to intrauterine pressure catheters for measuring the strength of uterine contractions [24].

Given the current state of the art in monitoring uterine contractions, intrauterine pressure catheters are limited by their invasiveness and the need for ruptured membranes; at present, external uterine monitors are uncomfortable, often inaccurate, and depend on the subjectivity of the examiner. Neither of these methods directly measures properties that control both the function and state of the uterus or cervix during pregnancy. The frequency and duration of contractions appear to be of greater importance in terms of adequate placental perfusion and the avoidance of fetal compromise than amplitude alone. As both of these parameters can be assessed externally, this has remained the mainstay of uterine activity assessment [17].

Quantification of uterine activity

The necessity to quantify uterine contractions is of importance to understand and interpret the tocogram. The elements of uterine contractions which relate to efficiency are frequency, active pressure, duration and co-ordination (Figures 5.2 and 5.3). Duration is the time between onset and offset of the contractions in seconds. It may be difficult to measure if the contractions are overlapping or coupling. The amplitude is the difference between the maximum intrauterine pressure and the resting intrauterine pressure. Basal intrauterine pressure is the pressure at the lowest point of the tracing between

contractions, due to atmospheric pressure, hydrostatic pressure, and elastic recoil of the uterus and surrounding tissues [8]. This pressure should be excluded from quantitative measures because they are affected by variables which are not related to uterine activity. The baseline tone is important to recognize there is a rise in the baseline tone secondary to placental abruption [25] or excessive oxytocin stimulation [26]. The shape of the contraction appears to be important in patients with dysfunctional labour. The shape is measured by the F : R ratio, where the F (fall) is the time for a contraction to return to baseline from its peak and the R (rise) is the time for a contraction to rise to its peak [27]. An increased F : R ratio is associated with a higher need for caesarean delivery, although the evidence is not robust [28]. The total amount of uterine activity per unit time can be described in different ways (Table 5.2).

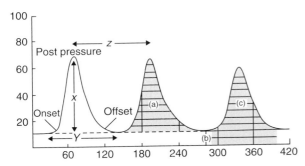

Figure 5.2 Elements and terminology of uterine contractions. X: active pressure or amplitude, Y: duration, Z: contraction interval related to frequency, (a) active contraction area, (b) basal tone, (c) total contraction area

Uterine activity units

Many authors have described the total amount of uterine activity per unit of time in different ways.

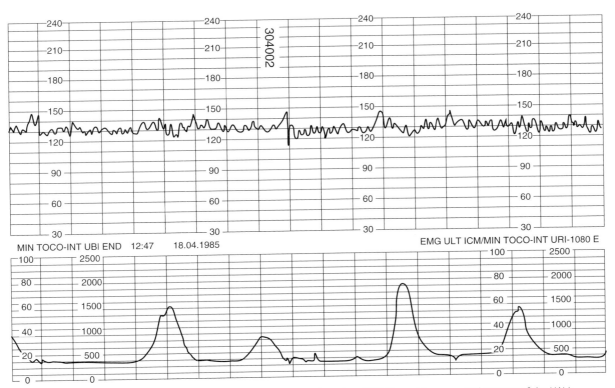

Figure 5.3 Recording of UAI as a short dark line against a vertical axis from 0 to 2500 kPa and the numerical printout of the UAI in addition to mode of recording, paper speed and time

Table 5.2 Measurements of uterine activity per unit of time by different methods.

Units	Measurements	Disadvantages
Montvideo unit [29]	Mean amplitude × mean frequency over 10 min (initially described as intensity × frequency)	Ignores any contribution from the duration of contractions and shape of the contractions
Alexandria unit [30]	Montvideo unit × mean duration over 10 min	No contributions taken from the shape. Incorporating the duration showed that longer contractions decreased the duration of labour
Uterine activity unit (UAU) [31]	Area under the pressure curve (Torr-min) over 1 min – 1UAU = 1 Torr min	Includes the contraction frequency, duration and amplitude, but also includes the baseline tone and hence is not widely adopted
Uterine activity integral (UAI) or active contraction area [32]	Active area under the pressure curve over 15 min (intrauterine pressure minus the baseline pressure) (Figure 5.3)	Measures active pressure including maternal efforts, especially in the second stage
Mean active pressure (MAP) [33]	UAI divided by 900 (kPa), measuring over 1 s (15 min – 900 s)	Independent of the duration of the integration period
Mean contraction active pressure (MCAP) [33]	UAI/total duration of contraction	When the integration period is with respect to one contraction

The quantification techniques of uterine activity still do not consider the shape of contractions. Low-amplitude, high-frequency contraction (tachysystole) may cause fetal compromise and still be within normal limits of current quantification methods. Hence it is necessary to record frequency and duration even if defined activity units are used to quantify uterine contractions [17]. Although an increase in baseline tone is not measured by many quantification methods, it is usually associated with an increase in the frequency of contractions, or an excessive active contraction area. Uterine activity monitoring is quintessential in labours, but quantification may not be required unless high doses of oxytocin are being used, because quantification has not led to improvement in spontaneous deliveries or fetal outcome in augmented or induced labours [34,35].

Uterine activity in normal labour

Characteristically, uterine activity at the end of first stage of labour has an amplitude of more than 50 mmHg, a duration of approximately 60 s and a frequency of 3–5 contractions in a 10-min period. Achieving a contraction frequency of 4–5 per 10 min and each lasting for at least 40 s is desirable to overcome dysfunctional labour [36], with a relaxation time of 51 s in the first stage and 36 s in the second

stage [37]. An increase in the contraction frequency and a decrease in relaxation time are associated with lower umbilical artery pH. The ideal contraction interval, in which fetal cerebral oxygen saturation remains stable or even increases, is 2–3 min or longer [38].

Uterine contractions and parity

A uterus has to perform a given quantum of activity in labour to effect delivery (Figure 5.6). The total uterine activity is a reflection of the cervical and pelvic tissue resistance. If the expected total uterine activity for the given parity and cervical score is exceeded, and there is little progress, it may suggest cephalopelvic disproportion or failed induction. However, there is a wide range of uterine activity associated with normal progress of labour in primigravid women [32,39,40]. As there is a wide range of uterine activity in labour, it is difficult to predict the progress of labour prospectively, and hence uterine activity quantification is unlikely to provide additional information if partographic progress is normal (Figure 5.4). The parous uterus needs to expend significantly less effort to effect normal vaginal delivery than its nulliparous counterpart until the late first stage, suggesting that parity may have a greater influence on the resistance offered by the cervix than the pelvic tissues [41].

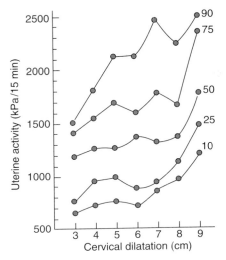

Figure 5.4 Cervical dilatation specific uterine activity in KPa/15 min in nulliparous spontaneous normal labour

Maternal characteristics that affect uterine contractions

Obesity or raised BMI is associated with dysfunctional labour due to poor uterine contractility [42]. In-vitro findings relating to cholesterol manipulation suggest that elevated cholesterol in obese women may disrupt the signalling mechanisms, impairing contractions and producing dysfunctional labours [43]. Intracellular acidification decreases and alkalization increases contractility [44]. Myometrial hypoxia can lead to myometrial lactic acidosis and dysfunctional labour [45].

Uterine contractions and previous caesarean section (CS)

Women with a caesarean scar, who had a previous vaginal delivery, are able to deliver with lower uterine activity than if they had had no vaginal delivery [46]. If they had no previous vaginal delivery, the caesarean was done electively, or in the latent phase of labour, the uterine activity needed to deliver is higher compared to those who had CS in the active phase of labour. Those women who are likely to deliver vaginally show satisfactory progress in the first few hours of labour. A satisfactory outcome can be achieved in most women with a caesarean scar, even if they need augmentation, by careful selection and a limited period of augmentation [47,48].

Quantification of uterine activity and internal tocography may help in the identification of scar dehiscence in some cases, but cannot predict impending rupture. There is conflicting evidence as to whether intrauterine pressure catheters are useful in diagnosing uterine rupture [49,50]. A breach in the scar affects the uterine wall tension and reduces the build-up of intrauterine pressure. The decline in the amplitude or absence of recording contractions may indicate scar dehiscence [51]. The reduction of intrauterine pressure does not become apparent if the catheter is placed posteriorly and is localized in an isolated pool of amniotic fluid. Since there is no loss of contractions, such localization will still demonstrate uterine contractions of good amplitude. Scar dehiscence with intact peritoneum may show no loss of intrauterine pressure, but the contractions may stretch the dehisced scar, causing poor cervical dilatation [52]. A reduction of uterine activity seen using internal tocography is more reliable than external tocography, as a sudden reduction with external tocography may be attributed to loosening of the belt or alteration in the patient's position.

Uterine contractions and induced labour

Induction of labour is common in modern obstetric practice and rates can be as high as 30%. Uterine activity in induced labour is higher than that in normal labour [53]. Induced labours also have a higher incidence of tachysystoles or polysystoles (>5 contractions in 10 min). Induction with oxytocin reduces the intercontraction interval and increases the contraction regularity, and can be used as a predictor for likely progress of labour [54]. Oxytocin in augmented labour first increases the frequency of contractions followed by an increase in their amplitude, after which a stable phase is achieved [55]. Any further increase in oxytocin will increase the baseline tone and frequency of contractions, with a reduction in their amplitude causing hyperstimulation. This led to the belief that monitoring of the uterine contraction area would lead to a decrease in the number of cases of inadequate stimulation. However, titration of oxytocin to achieve 4–5 contractions in 10 min, or the 75th centile of uterine activity expected in normal labour according to parity, using automated pumps, did not offer any advantage in induced labour [56].

Quantification of uterine activity has been shown to detect true active phase arrest [57], but its use in clinical settings is not proven.

The incidence of uterine contraction abnormalities are dependent on the dose, route of administration and the type of drug used [58]. Misoprostol is associated with a greater incidence of tachysystoles and dinoprostone with hyperstimulation. Contraction abnormalities increase with repeated doses [58]. In cases of uterine hyperstimulation, combining the use of terbutaline and stopping syntocinon significantly reduces the time taken for reduction in uterine activity [59].

Abnormal contraction patterns (in-coordinate uterine contractions)

Abnormalities of contraction shape, frequency and tone are seen as polysystole (merging of contractions), paired contractions and tachysystole (more than 5 contractions in 10 min), and hypertonia (increase in baseline pressure). In-coordinate uterine contractions can be associated with normal labour [60], and are not an indication for oxytocin unless they are inefficient in producing the expected cervical dilatation. The use of oxytocin in dysfunctional labours may improve the efficiency, but may also increase the in-coordinate nature of uterine contractions. Various degrees of in-coordinate uterine activity are shown in Figures 5.5 and 5.6.

Polysystole (Figure 5.7) is one with contraction frequency > 7 in 10 mins but may appear as a single contraction with more than one peak and the tone in between the peaks not falling to the baseline [27]. Paired contractions have a relaxation time of less than 60 s in between successive contractions. Contractions which merge to form a sustained contraction lasting for >3 min are defined as tetanic contractions. They are not generally seen in natural labour and are due to oxytocins (Figure 5.8). When contractions do not merge but the baseline pressure is elevated by more than 20 mmHg for more than 3 min, they are called hypertonic contractions (Figure 5.9). Tetanic contractions will cut off perfusion to the retroplacental pool of blood, while hypertonic activity will reduce perfusion. Spiral arterioles are completely compressed with an intrauterine pressure of 30 mmHg. Intrauterine pressure reaches up to 60 mmHg in normal labour, with relaxation in between to replenish the intervillous space. Sustained elevation of the baseline tone causes compromise to uteroplacental perfusion and fetal oxygenation.

Conclusion

When oxytocin is used, the incidence of tachysystoles reaches 57% of cases in the first stage of labour and 27% in the second stage [17]. The latter might be lower because of poor recording of uterine contractions during the second stage. Of labours requiring fetal

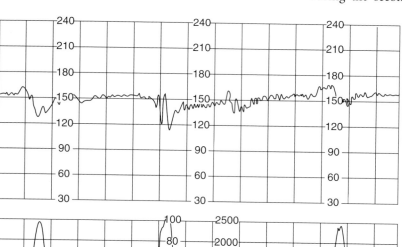

Figure 5.5 Moderate degree of in-coordinate contractions

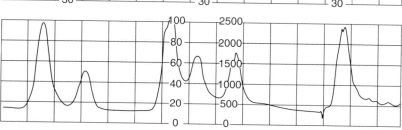

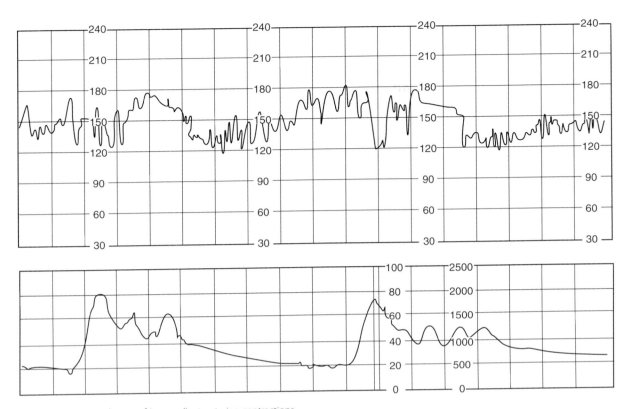

Figure 5.6 Severe degree of in-coordinate uterine contractions

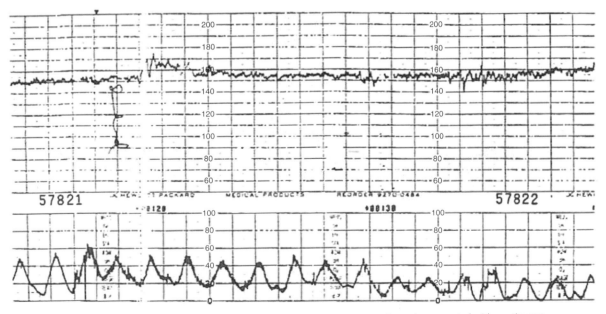

Figure 5.7 Polysystolic contractions of low amplitude due to abruptio placenta in a patient who presented with continuous abdominal pain and bleeding per vaginum with the cervix 1 cm dilated. There is associated fetal tachycardia

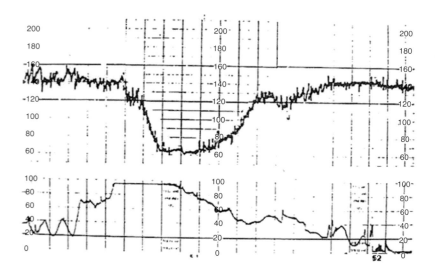

Figure 5.8 Tetanic contractions caused by accidental bolus infusion of oxytocin when the infusion was run fast to check whether the intravenous line was patent

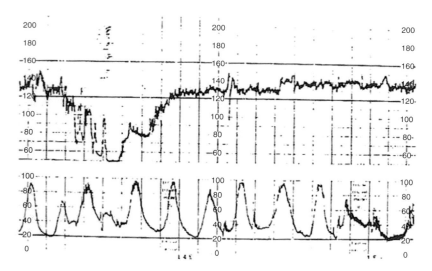

Figure 5.9 Hypertonic uterine contractions, showing the elevation of the baseline pressure, which has caused a transient bradycardia

scalp blood sampling, 50% had a poor tocography for a quarter of the total monitoring time, indicating that more satisfactory recording is required. Medico-legal issues are commonly due to inadequate uterine contraction monitoring, cessation of monitoring of FHR, or uterine contractions much earlier than the time of delivery, failure to recognize that the uterus is contracting more than 5 times in 10 min, and pathological FHR patterns caused by uterine hyper-stimulation. Hence, monitoring of uterine contractions is indispensable, especially with the use of oxytocin infusion. FIGO has provided guidelines on methods of uterine activity monitoring [61] and their interpretation. Computer-assisted automated analysis of uterine activity along with FHR interpretation may aid the improvement of reporting criteria and clinical management of cases [62].

References

1. Selin L, Wallin G, Berg M. Dystocia in labour – risk factors, management and outcome: a retrospective observational study in a Swedish setting. *Acta Obstet Gynecol Scand* 2008; **87**: 216–21.

2. Thomas J, Callwood A, Paranjothy S. National Sentinel Caesarean Section Audit: update. *Pract Midwife* 2000; **3**(11): 20.

3. Sanborn B M. Cell and molecular biology of myometrial smooth muscle function. *Semin Cell Dev Biol* 2007; **18**: 287–8.

4. Garfield R E, Maner W L. Physiology and electrical activity of uterine contractions. *Semin Cell Dev Biol* 2007; **18**: 289–95.

5. Marshall J M. Regulation of activity in uterine smooth muscle. *Physiol Rev Suppl* 1962; **5**: 213–27.

6. Cottrill H M, Barton J R, O'Brien J M, Rhea D L, Milligan D A. Factors influencing maternal perception of uterine contractions. *Am J Obstet Gynecol* 2004; **190**: 1455–7.

7. Gibb D. *Uterine Activity in Labour*. Turnbridge Wells, Kent: Castle House Publications, 1989.

8. Steer P J. Standards in fetal monitoring – practical requirements for uterine activity measurement and recording. *Br J Obstet Gynaecol* 1993; **100** (Suppl 9): 32–6.

9. Miles A M, Monga M, Richeson K S. Correlation of external and internal monitoring of uterine activity in a cohort of term patients. *Am J Perinatol* 2001; **18**(3): 137–40.

10. LaCroix G E. Monitoring labor by an external tokodynamometer. *Am J Obstet Gynecol* 1968; **101**: 111–9.

11. Nageotte M. *Uterine Contraction Monitoring*. 3rd ed. Philadelphia: Lippincott Williams and Wilkins, 2003.

12. Chua S, Arulkumaran S, Yang M, Steer P J, Ratnam S S. Intrauterine pressure: comparison of extra vs. intra amniotic methods using a transducer tipped catheter. *Asia Oceania J Obstet Gynaecol* 1994; **20**: 35–8.

13. Chan W H, Paul R H, Toews J. Intrapartum fetal monitoring. Maternal and fetal morbidity and perinatal mortality. *Obstet Gynecol* 1973; **41**: 7–13.

14. Nuttall I D. Perforation of a placental fetal vessel by an intrauterine pressure catheter. *Br J Obstet Gynaecol* 1978; **85**: 573–4.

15. Devoe L D, Gardner P, Dear C, Searle N. Monitoring intrauterine pressure during active labor. A prospective comparison of two methods. *J Reprod Med* 1989; **34**: 811–4.

16. Svenningsen L, Jensen O. Application of fiberoptics to the clinical measurement of intra-uterine pressure in labor. *Acta Obstet Gynecol Scand* 1986; **65**: 551–5.

17. Vanner T, Gardosi J. Intrapartum assessment of uterine activity. *Baillieres Clin Obstet Gynaecol* 1996; **10**: 243–57.

18. Arulkumaran S, Yang M, Tien C Y, Ratnam S S. Reliability of intrauterine pressure measurements. *Obstet Gynecol* 1991; **78**: 800–2.

19. Chua S, Arulkumaran S, Yang M, Ratnam S S, Steer P J. The accuracy of catheter-tip pressure transducers for the measurement of intrauterine pressure in labour. *Br J Obstet Gynaecol* 1992; **99**: 186–9.

20. Chua S, Kurup A, Arulkumaran S, Ratnam S S. Augmentation of labor: does internal tocography result in better obstetric outcome than external tocography? *Obstet Gynecol* 1990; **76**: 164–7.

21. Chia Y T, Arulkumaran S, Soon S B, Norshida S, Ratnam S S. Induction of labour: does internal tocography result in better obstetric outcome than external tocography. *Aust NZ J Obstet Gynaecol* 1993; **33**: 159–61.

22. Marque C K, Terrien J, Rihana S, Germain G. Preterm labour detection by use of a biophysical marker: the uterine electrical activity. *BMC Pregnancy Childbirth* 2007; **7**: S5.

23. Jiang W, Li G, Lin L. Uterine electromyogram topography to represent synchronization of uterine contractions. *Int J Gynaecol Obstet* 2007; **97**: 120–4.

24. Maul H, Maner W L, Olson G, Saade G R, Garfield R E. Non-invasive transabdominal uterine electromyography correlates with the strength of intrauterine pressure and is predictive of labor and delivery. *J Matern Fetal Neonatal Med* 2004; **15**: 297–301.

25. Odendaal H J, Brink S, Steytler J G. Clinical and haematological problems associated with severe abruptio placentae. *S Afr Med J* 1978; **54**: 476–80.

26. Woolfson J, Steer P J, Bashford C C, Randall N J. The measurement of uterine activity in induced labour. *Br J Obstet Gynaecol* 1976; **83**: 934–7.

27. Bakker P C, van Geijn H P. Uterine activity: implications for the condition of the fetus. *J Perinat Med* 2008; **36**: 30–7.

28. Althaus J E, Petersen S, Driggers R, *et al.* Cephalopelvic disproportion is associated with an altered uterine contraction shape in the active phase of labor. *Am J Obstet Gynecol* 2006; **195**: 739–42.

29. Caldeyro-Barcia R, Sica-Blanco Y, Poseiro J J, *et al.* A quantitative study of the action of synthetic oxytocin on the pregnant human uterus. *J Pharmacol Exp Ther* 1957; **121**: 18–31.

30. el-Sahwi S, Gaafar A A, Toppozada H K. A new unit for evaluation of uterine activity. *Am J Obstet Gynecol* 1967; **98**: 900–3.

31. Miller F C, Yeh S Y, Schifrin B S, Paul R H, Hon E H. Quantitation of uterine activity in 100 primiparous patients. *Am J Obstet Gynecol* 1976; **124**: 398–405.

32. Steer P J, Carter M C, Beard R W. Normal levels of active contraction area in spontaneous labour. *Br J Obstet Gynaecol* 1984; **91**: 211–9.

33. Phillips G F, Calder A A. Units for the evaluation of uterine contractility. *Br J Obstet Gynaecol* 1987; **94**: 236–41.

34. Arulkumaran S, Yang M, Ingemarsson I, Singh P, Ratnam S S. Augmentation of labour: does oxytocin titration to achieve preset active contraction area values produce better obstetric outcome? *Asia Oceania J Obstet Gynaecol* 1989; **15**: 333–7.

35. Gibb D M, Arulkumaran S, Ratnam S S. A comparative study of methods of oxytocin administration for induction of labour. *Br J Obstet Gynaecol* 1985; **92**: 688–92.

36. Arulkumaran S, Chua S, Chua T M, *et al.* Uterine activity in dysfunctional labour and target uterine activity to be aimed with oxytocin titration. *Asia Oceania J Obstet Gynaecol* 1991; **17**: 101–6.

37. Bakker P C, Kurver P H, Kuik D J, Van Geijn H P. Elevated uterine activity increases the risk of fetal acidosis at birth. *Am J Obstet Gynecol* 2007; **196**: 313 e311–6.

38. Peebles D M, Spencer J A, Edwards A D, *et al.* Relation between frequency of uterine contractions and human fetal cerebral oxygen saturation studied during labour by near infrared spectroscopy. *Br J Obstet Gynaecol* 1994; **101**: 44–8.

39. Cowan D B, van Middelkoop A, Philpott R H. Intrauterine-pressure studies in African nulliparae: normal labour progress. *Br J Obstet Gynaecol* 1982; **89**: 364–9.

40. Fairlie F M, Phillips G F, Andrews B J, Calder A A. An analysis of uterine activity in spontaneous labour using a microcomputer. *Br J Obstet Gynaecol* 1988; **95**: 57–64.

41. Arulkumaran S, Gibb D M, Lun K C, Heng S H, Ratnam S S. The effect of parity on uterine activity in labour. *Br J Obstet Gynaecol* 1984; **91**: 843–8.

42. Zhang J, Bricker L, Wray S, Quenby S. Poor uterine contractility in obese women. *Br J Obstet Gynaecol* 2007; **114**: 343–8.

43. Wray S. Insights into the uterus. *Exp Physiol* 2007; **92**: 621–31.

44. Parratt J R, Taggart M J, Wray S. Changes in intracellular pH close to term and their possible significance to labour. *Pflugers Arch* 1995; **430**: 1012–4.

45. Quenby S, Pierce S J, Brigham S, Wray S. Dysfunctional labor and myometrial lactic acidosis. *Obstet Gynecol* 2004; **103**: 718–23.

46. Arulkumaran S, Gibb D M, Ingemarsson I, Kitchener H C, Ratnam S S. Uterine activity during spontaneous labour after previous lower-segment caesarean section. *Br J Obstet Gynaecol* 1989; **96**: 933–8.

47. Chua S, Arulkumaran S, Singh P, Ratnam S S. Trial of labour after previous caesarean section: obstetric outcome. *Aust NZ J Obstet Gynaecol* 1989; **29**: 12–7.

48. Arulkumaran S, Ingemarsson I, Ratnam S S. Oxytocin augmentation in dysfunctional labour after previous caesarean section. *Br J Obstet Gynaecol* 1989; **96**: 939–41.

49. Arulkumaran S, Chua S, Ratnam S S. Symptoms and signs with scar rupture – value of uterine activity measurements. *Aust NZ J Obstet Gynaecol* 1992; **32**: 208–12.

50. Beckley S, Gee H, Newton J R. Scar rupture in labour after previous lower uterine segment caesarean section: the role of uterine activity measurement. *Br J Obstet Gynaecol* 1991; **98**: 265–9.

51. Gee H, Taylor E W, Hancox R. A model for the generation of intrauterine pressure in the human parturient uterus which demonstrates the critical role of the cervix. *J Theor Biol* 1988; **133**: 281–91.

52. Paul R H, Phelan J P, Yeh S Y. Trial of labor in the patient with a prior cesarean birth. *Am J Obstet Gynecol* 1985; **151**: 297–304.

53. Arulkumaran S, Gibb D M, Ratnam S S, Heng S H, Lun K C. Uterine activity in oxytocin induced labour. *Asia Oceania J Obstet Gynaecol* 1986; **12**: 533–40.

54. Oppenheimer L W, Bland E S, Dabrowski A, *et al.* Uterine contraction pattern as a predictor of the mode of delivery. *J Perinatol* 2002; **22**: 149–53.

55. Steer P J, Carter M C, Beard R W. The effect of oxytocin infusion on uterine activity levels in slow labour. *Br J Obstet Gynaecol* 1985; **92**: 1120–6.

56. Arulkumaran S, Ingemarsson I, Ratnam S S. Oxytocin titration to achieve preset active contraction area values does not improve the outcome of induced labour. *Br J Obstet Gynaecol* 1987; **94**: 242–8.

57. Hauth J C, Hankins G D, Gilstrap L C, III. Uterine contraction pressures achieved in parturients with active phase arrest. *Obstet Gynecol* 1991; **78**: 344–7.

58. Crane J M, Young D C, Butt K D, Bennett K A, Hutchens D. Excessive uterine activity accompanying induced labor. *Obstet Gynecol* 2001; **97**: 926–31.

59. Pacheco L D, Rosen M P, Gei A F, Saade G R, Hankins G D. Management of uterine hyperstimulation with concomitant use of oxytocin and terbutaline. *Am J Perinatol* 2006; **23**: 377–80.

60. Gibb D M, Arulkumaran S, Lun K C, Ratnam S S. Characteristics of uterine activity in nulliparous labour. *Br J Obstet Gynaecol* 1984; **91**: 220–7.

61. FIGO Study Group on the Assessment of New Technology. International Federation of Gynecology and Obstetrics. Intrapartum surveillance: recommendations on current practice and overview of new developments. *Int J Gynaecol Obstet* 1995; **49**: 213–21.

62. Ayres-de Campos D, Bernardes J, Garrido A, Marques-de-Sa J, Pereira-Leite L. SisPorto 2.0: a program for automated analysis of cardiotocograms. *J Matern Fetal Med* 2000; **9**: 311–8.

The management of intrapartum 'fetal distress'

Bryony Strachan

Introduction

The aim of good obstetric care is to reduce the number of infants that die or are damaged from birth asphyxia. Permanent brain damage or death resulting from asphyxia around the time of birth is a major tragedy for any family. The challenge is to find the fetus at risk of asphyxia without causing harm from unnecessary intervention for the mother or fetus.

Fetal asphyxia and 'fetal distress' in labour – definitions

The term 'asphyxia' is derived from the Greek and means 'without pulse'. Its current usage in obstetrics is to describe fetal distress before or during labour. Fetal distress or fetal asphyxia are poorly defined terms, but have been widely used in a number of different meanings to describe a range of pathological conditions. Asphyxia is defined experimentally as impaired respiratory gas exchange accompanied by the development of metabolic acidosis. It is usually reserved for experimental situations in which these changes can be accurately established. In the clinical context, fetal asphyxia is progressive hypoxaemia and hypercapnia with a significant metabolic acidaemia. Fetal distress is a commonly used but poorly defined term. Its common usage is to describe concern about a fetal condition that pre-empts a caesarean section or instrumental delivery. It is not a diagnosis as such, but a concern or indication for delivery. Presumed fetal distress was the indication for 22% of caesarean births in the UK [1]. The underlying 'cause' (for example, hyperstimulation, placental insufficiency, cord compression or abruption) is often not known, even after delivery.

Perinatal mortality and morbidity

Labour has been described as the most dangerous journey of our lives, and remains so in many parts of the world. Perinatal mortality has declined considerably over the last 50 years in developed countries as a result of greatly improved antenatal and intrapartum care. In 1960, the perinatal mortality rate in England and Wales was 33 per 1000 births, with a third of these deaths caused by intrapartum asphyxia [2]. In 2005, the combined stillbirth and neonatal mortality rate had fallen to 8 per 1000 births, with less than a tenth of these deaths caused by intrapartum events. This still corresponds to the death of 471 babies in England and Wales per year [3].

By contrast, in the less and least developed countries of the world, the perinatal mortality rate is over six times greater than that of the UK, at rates of 47 and 60 per 1000 births, respectively. Intrapartum deaths still account for one-third of these deaths. The World Health Organization argues that intrapartum deaths are largely avoidable with skilled care. In developing countries, just over 40% of births will occur in a healthcare facility, and little more than one in two will have the assistance of a doctor, nurse or midwife [4]. Intrapartum asphyxia still accounts for significant perinatal morbidity. The incidence of hypoxic ischaemic encephalopathy is 2–5 per 1000 live births, with around half being severely affected. Intrapartum asphyxia will account for nearly a third of these cases [5].

The consequences of intervention for fetal distress

Interventions for presumed fetal distress are common. Although caesarean sections are becoming safer, they still have 2–4 times the mortality and 5–10 times the morbidity of a spontaneous vaginal birth for the mother. Similarly, operative intervention for presumed fetal distress in the form of forceps delivery or vacuum extraction is not without risk to mother and to fetus. The risks of haemorrhage, urinary and bowel symptoms, perineal trauma and pain and post-traumatic syndrome to the mother are greater with an instrumental delivery. Operative delivery for the fetus is also not without risk. Delivering a fetus by a forceps or vacuum delivery increases the chance of a cephalohaematoma, facial nerve injury, retinal haemorrhage, life-threatening intracranial haemorrhage or skull fracture [1,6].

Ideally, therefore, fetal monitoring should identify the fetus at risk without causing undue harm to the mother or fetus from unnecessary intervention. The challenge is to accurately identify those babies that are coping well with the 'stress' of labour from those which are getting 'distressed' with enough time to expedite delivery before asphyxia occurs.

Management of 'fetal distress' – decision-making

For the obstetrician there are three key 'decision-makers' in managing presumed fetal distress in labour:

- the fetal reserve,
- the likely cause, and
- the potential response to resuscitation.

The fetal reserve

The first 'decision-maker' is to assess the reserve of the fetus for the stress of labour by reviewing the antenatal history (Table 6.1). The effect of antenatal factors on the development of fetal hypoxia in labour is complex. In the Western Australia series, antenatal factors were common findings in the infants that developed neonatal encephalopathy [5]. These included

Table 6.1 Antenatal factors affecting fetal reserve.

Factors affecting the fetal reserve
Presumed fetal growth restriction
Pre-eclampsia
Intrapartum bleeding
Infection, e.g. chorioamnionitis
Postmaturity
Antepartum haemorrhage

intrauterine growth restriction, postmaturity and pre-eclampsia. These conditions affect placental function and transfer, making hypoxia in labour more likely. If fetal growth is impaired, glycogen stores in the fetal liver are depleted, which reduces the ability of the fetus to cope with a hypoxic insult. Growth restriction or placental insufficiency makes the fetus more likely to be delivered for presumed fetal distress. However, routine antenatal care including abdominal palpation and symphyseal fundal height will only detect a third of 'small for gestational age' babies before birth. Using a customized growth centile chart where maternal characteristics such as height, weight, ethnicity and parity are considered, the sensitivity increases to 48% [7]. Therefore, half of growth-restricted babies will not be recognized before labour.

In the presence of infection, the fetus will increase its metabolic and oxygen requirement, making the fetus more likely to become hypoxic. Inflammatory cytokines compound the effects of hypoxia on cell damage.

Assessment of fetal reserve – preparation before labour

An anaesthetist will assess the risk of a patient before an anaesthetic according to a standardized grading. In a similar way, an obstetrician could assess the fetus before labour (Table 6.2). For example, a normal healthy fetus will have a low risk for developing fetal distress in labour; the aim is to reduce unnecessary intervention by using intermittent auscultation. For a fetus known to be growth-restricted or postmature, the risk of developing fetal distress is higher, warranting a careful plan for the type and frequency of monitoring and the intervention required. Some babies are at such a high perceived risk of developing fetal distress and asphyxia that a prelabour caesarean section may be recommended. Other babies will have a very poor outcome after birth because of severe congenital problems or extreme prematurity. A careful and sensitive discussion is needed to make a plan for appropriate monitoring in labour taking into account parental wishes and the neonatal plan for assessment and resuscitation at birth. For a stillbirth, although there is no need for fetal monitoring, a plan for monitoring maternal vital signs should be made, particularly in the presence of a uterine scar.

The cause of fetal distress in labour

The second key 'decision-maker' for the obstetrician is to consider the underlying cause of the fetal

67

Table 6.2 Comparison of grading systems for anaesthesia and fetal reserve for labour.

ASA grading before anaesthesia [8]		Fetal reserve before labour	
P1	Normal healthy patient	F1	Normal healthy term infant
P2	Mild systemic disease	F2	Mild systemic disease, e.g. mild to moderate pre-eclampsia, minor antepartum haemorrhage, postmaturity, mild IUGR, 34–36 weeks gestation
P3	Severe systemic disease	F3	Severe systemic disease, e.g. severe IUGR or 27–33 weeks gestation
P4	Severe systemic disease that is a constant threat to life	F4	Severe systemic disease that is an imminent threat to life, e.g. severe IUGR with abnormal CTG Suspected severe chorioamnionitis with abnormal CTG in preterm infant
P5	Moribund patient	F5	Fetus with lethal congenital malformations or unlikely to survive because of extreme prematurity
P6	Brain-dead patient	F6	Stillbirth

distress. This will determine the likely response to intrauterine resuscitation and the likelihood of continuing with the labour or expediting delivery.

Contractions

The fetus is at risk during labour because the supply of oxygen from the mother may be interrupted by contractions of the uterus affecting placental exchange, and compressing the cord. The exchange of oxygen and carbon dioxide with the maternal circulation is compromised by uterine contractions. This was demonstrated by Borell *et al.* in 1965 [9]. They used arteriographic techniques on three women in labour, who were carrying congenitally lethal fetuses. Injecting radio opaque dye during and after a contraction demonstrated that during a contraction the dye entering the villous spaces was considerably delayed, reducing placental perfusion and thus the gaseous exchange during normal labour. The Ferguson reflex, at full dilatation of the cervix, releases further oxytocin, increasing the strength of contractions, and may cause further compromise to gaseous exchange during second stage. The start of maternal pushing (the active phase of the second stage) increases the risk of acidaemia with higher levels of lactic acid and carbon dioxide and increasing acidosis. No changes were seen with the passive second stage [10]. Thus the two parts of the second stage of labour actually differ in their potential to stimulate fetal acidosis. There is no evidence to suggest that a Valsalva manoeuvre has an additive effect to this.

Hyperstimulation will increase the risk of fetal hypoxia by reducing the time the uterus spends at rest with optimum placental perfusion. A diseased placenta will be more susceptible to the effects of uterine activity on the reduction of gaseous exchange.

Cord compression

The delivery of oxygenated blood to the fetus is via the umbilical cord. This is prone to compression against the fetal part during contractions. The presence of Wharton's jelly in the cord is usually protective of severe compression. Infants with intrauterine growth restriction (IUGR) have a reduction of Wharton's jelly, and both the total and lumen vein areas are reduced [11]. Thus a growth-restricted infant is more susceptible to cord compression. A normally grown fetus is protected from the effects of cord compression except in the extremes of cord prolapse or severe entanglement.

Failure to progress or dystocia

In study and audit data, reasons for performing an emergency caesarean are categorized to aid analysis, but often there is a combination of fetal distress and failure to progress in labour rather than one or the other. In reality, these definitions overlap. A prolonged or obstructed labour will eventually exhaust the fetus. Therefore an accurate assessment of the progress of labour is important in considering the causes of fetal distress.

Maternal positioning

As early as the eighteenth century, obstetricians favoured mothers delivering in the left lateral position. Most historical pictures of birth are in the upright position. Aortocaval compression by the term-gravid uterus can exacerbate any fetal compromise.

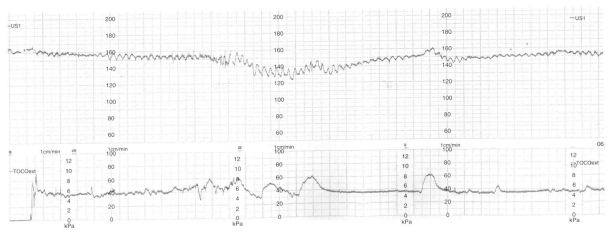

Figure 6.1 Sinusoidal pattern seen after ruptured membranes associated with anaemia from vasa praevia

Aortocaval compression from the gravid uterus reduces the uterine artery flow and reduces the pre-load to the mother's heart, reducing cardiac output. Aortocaval compression can be measured using toe phlesmography, where changes in blood pressure in the toe can reflect poor perfusion to the lower limbs associated with aortocaval compression. Using this technique, aortocaval compression was seen in about half of the women in labour. The left or right lateral positions abolished this. Aortocaval compression was seen most commonly in the supine position, and less frequently in the standing and semi-recumbent positions. An occipito-posterior position in labour increased the likelihood. Ten percent of women will have a 'revealed' aortocaval compression syndrome with hypotension in the supine position. But in about a third of women, this aortocaval compression is concealed with no apparent drop in blood pressure as measured in the upper arm. Fetal heart deceler-ations were not seen in all cases of aortocaval com-pression, presumably because of the collaterals from the ovarian arteries and placental reserve. Pelvic tilt alone was not good enough to relieve aortocaval compression. A lateral tilt of 15 degrees is recom-mended; however, angle of tilt is often overestimated, and even at 15 degrees, both left and right pelvic tilt failed to reverse the decreased blood flow in the leg associated with the supine position [12].

Sudden dramatic events

Most 'fetal distress' is of an insidious onset as the strength of the contractions increase and the head descends in the pelvis. However, sudden events such as a cord prolapse, abruption, or vasa praevia can cause profound dramatic distress.

Vasa praevia

Vasa praevia is rare and must be considered to be diagnosed. The blood loss is from the fetal side and this carries high mortality. The diagnosis should be considered with any bleed after a spontaneous or artificial rupture of membranes accompanied by acute fetal distress. Alerting the attending neonatolo-gist to the possibility of vasa praevia is vital to ensure the provision of blood for transfusion of the fetus. The characteristic sinusoidal pattern of the cardio-tocograph with anaemia can be present (Figure 6.1). Prolonged decelerations of the fetal heart rate coin-ciding with membrane rupture can be another pattern.

Cord prolapse

The diagnosis of cord prolapse is made on vaginal examination. The management is to deliver the fetus promptly. Elevation of the presenting part above the pelvic brim will relieve cord compression. This can be achieved by digital displacement, keeping the hand in the vagina until delivery. Alternatively a knee elbow position or an exaggerated Sims' position can be used. Bladder filling with 500 ml of saline using a Foley catheter can also be useful. Tocolysis will help reduce compression of the cord from contractions. If the fetal heart rate recovers with these measures then a rapid sequence spinal block can be used in favour of a general anaesthetic.

Table 6.3 Potential response to intrauterine resuscitation.

Yes	Maybe	No
Hyperstimulation	Cord compression	Placental abruption
Supine hypotension	Placental insufficiency	Uterine rupture
Dehydration	Infection	Vasa praevia
Hypotension following regional anaesthetic	Cord prolapse	

Abruption

The presence of continued pain between contractions with or without bleeding may suggest an intrapartum abruption as a cause of the fetal distress. This is unlikely to respond to resuscitation.

Uterine rupture

Fetal distress may be the first sign of impending uterine rupture. The presence of pain between contractions, vaginal bleeding, sudden cessation of contractions, or a rise of the presenting part should alert the obstetrician to the possibility of uterine rupture, particularly in a woman at risk. Again, this will not respond to resuscitation.

Fetal distress caused by sudden dramatic labour events will not be reversed with intrauterine resuscitation. However, intrauterine resuscitation is rarely contra-indicated, even when immediate delivery is planned, as it will optimize fetal oxygenation during preparation for delivery. Table 6.3 summarizes the potential response to intrauterine resuscitation.

Intrauterine resuscitation

Maternal positioning in left lateral

An upright or left lateral position reduces the risk of fetal heart decelerations. It makes sense to prevent the effects of aortocaval compression by discouraging the use of supine or tilt positions in favour of the lateral or upright position. If fetal distress is suspected then using the lateral position is good practice to correct any revealed or concealed aortocaval compression.

Stopping the contractions

Maternal blood flow to the placental villous space is reduced or altered during a contraction. Increasing the frequency of contractions above 4 in 10 min will reduce gaseous exchange across the placenta.

Recognizing hyperstimulation is the first step in preventing this. Commonly, this is missed. In the Swedish survey of malpractice claims, 71% had injudicious use of oxytocin, with greater than 6 in 10 contractions observed [13]. With hyperstimulation, the oxytocin infusion must be stopped for a short period of time before recommencing at a lower rate once the fetus has recovered. Oxytocin has a half-life of 15 min; therefore, reducing the rate of the infusion will reduce the serum levels quickly. An infusion should be stopped for at least 15 min before recommencing. Tocolytics should be considered in addition to stopping oxytocin.

Tocolysis

Acute tocolysis or uterine relaxation can be a valuable tool in the management of fetal distress. By correcting the hyperstimulation causing the fetal distress, it may be possible to continue with the labour or convert an immediate category one caesarean to a less-urgent category two.

Terbutaline, a betasympathomimetic, is the tocolytic with most published data. The NICE guidance recommends a dose of 250 μg given subcutaneously [14]. The effect of abolishing contractions can be seen in Figure 6.2. Fears regarding risk of postpartum haemorrhage are largely unfounded in practice. If this does occur, the action can be reversed with 1 mg propanolol i.v.

Atosiban, an oxytocin antagonist, developed for the treatment of preterm labour, has the potential for use as an acute tocolytic as it has a favourable side effect profile and is currently being evaluated. Nitroglycerin as a sublingual preparation (400 μg) has been shown to be useful for acute tocolysis. Its very short duration of action (2–3 min) makes it ideal for use at caesarean section to aid delivery – for example in a transverse lie with no liquor – but not so good for tocolysis in labour, as the dose has to be repeated every 2 min. Side effects such as hypotension, nausea and headache are common.

Intravenous fluids

Maternal hypovolaemia and hypotension can decrease the uteroplacental blood supply. For this reason, the NICE guidance recommends assessing the mother for signs of dehydration and/or hypotension when assessing a suspicious cardiotocograph (CTG) in

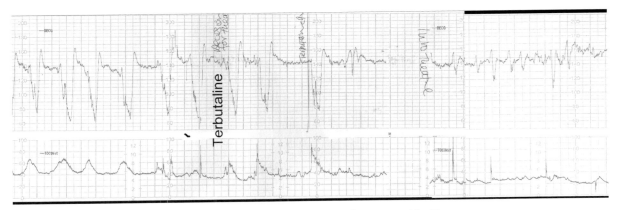

Figure 6.2 Cardiotocograph showing the effect of terbutaline on contraction frequency and fetal heart rate

labour and treatment with a bolus of 500 ml crystalloid is recommended [14]. There are no randomized trials looking at the use of an intravenous fluid bolus for the management of fetal distress, and caution must be used in the presence of pre-eclampsia because of the risk of pulmonary oedema. However, it does seem sensible to correct dehydration and hypotension if present. Intravenous fluid boluses of glucose-containing solutions should be avoided because of potentially detrimental effects on fetal status, including increased fetal lactate and decreased fetal pH.

Amnioinfusion

Amnioinfusion has been used as a treatment for fetal distress. One potential use is in the case of meconium staining of the liquor to dilute the meconium and therefore make the incidence of meconium aspiration less likely. Unfortunately, trials have not shown the benefit of this [14]. It is likely that the meconium has already been inhaled in utero down to the alveoli levels. Therefore adding in more fluid once thick meconium has been seen is unlikely to be of significant benefit.

The other potential use is in the presence of variable decelerations thought to be due to cord compression. The addition of fluid would cushion the cord compression occurring during a contraction. A meta-analysis did show a modest reduction in fetal heart rate abnormalities and a reduction in low Apgars and low arterial pH at birth. However, the trials included were too small to address rare but serious maternal side effects of amnioinfusion [15].

Therefore, there is no current role for amnioinfusion in the acute management of intrapartum fetal distress.

Oxygen

The use of oxygen in the management of acute fetal distress is controversial. Oxygen administration has been shown to increase fetal oxygenation as measured by pulse oximetry, and some studies have shown improvements in fetal heart rate patterns. There is limited evidence on its use in the acute setting. One study found deterioration in cord blood gas values with routine oxygen administration in the second stage of labour. In the non-acute setting of managing intrauterine growth restriction, its use is potentially harmful. In the acute resuscitation of the newborn infant, high concentrations of oxygen may have ill effects. In newborn life support, air is used for initial ventilation if required. At present, routine oxygen administration cannot be recommended for intrauterine resuscitation for the fetus [14]. However, pre-oxygenation is important for the mother if a general anaesthetic is being considered.

Delivering the fetus

Having considered the fetal reserve, the nature of the insult and the potential or actual response to resuscitation, the decision is whether to expedite delivery.

There is only one randomized trial comparing delivery for fetal distress to a conservative approach published in 1959 from South Africa. Women were randomized to intervention (delivery by caesarean, symphysiotomy or forceps), or a conservative approach to fetal distress as picked up by fetal heart rate abnormalities on intermittent auscultation or the presence of meconium staining of the liquor. There was a high perinatal mortality rate in both arms of the study with significant number of deaths in the intervention group due to trauma. The study was underpowered for differences in perinatal mortality. There are no trials within contemporary practice. The Cochrane reviewers concluded that there was too little evidence to show whether operative management is more beneficial than treating factors which may be causing the baby's distress, and that further research is needed. Such a trial will be difficult to perform [16].

Caesarean section or operative delivery

Once the decision has been made to expedite delivery, then the decision is how to deliver. During preparation for delivery, resuscitation methods can continue. In the first stage of labour the only available option for delivery is caesarean section. In only rare circumstances (for example, rapid progress in a multiparous patient or a second twin) would a vaginal delivery at less than 9 cm be contemplated.

The classification of urgency is useful in determining good communication with the anaesthetist. The choice of anaesthesia has to be made between the anaesthetist and the mother. Increasingly, regional analgesia is favoured in preference to a general anaesthesia. With the use of a 'rapid sequence' spinal anaesthetic, a decision interval can be less than the gold standard of 30 min [1].

The instances of poor fetal outcome with instrumental vaginal births relate to inappropriate application and/or excessive traction, particularly at mid cavity and rotational deliveries in the presence of fetal distress.

A prospective cohort study of 393 women experiencing operative delivery in the second stage of labour reported an increased risk of neonatal trauma and admission to the special care baby unit (SCBU) following excessive pulls (more than three pulls) and sequential use of instruments. The risk was further increased where delivery was completed by caesarean section following a protracted attempt at operative vaginal delivery [17].

The bulk of malpractice litigation results from failure to abandon the procedure at the appropriate time, particularly the failure to eschew prolonged, repeated or excessive traction efforts in the presence of poor progress. The choice of instrument will depend on the skill and expertise of the operator and the assessment of the ease and difficulty of the planned delivery. Mid cavity and rotational deliveries will have a higher complexity (and thus higher morbidity) than low cavity and non-rotational deliveries. Opting for caesarean section is not always the safest way for mother or baby, and considerable morbidity can occur to either. The wise obstetrician in the presence of fetal distress will choose the instrument that will have the best chance of delivering the baby the safest and quickest way with the least risk of failure or use of multiple instruments.

Forceps or vacuum delivery

Forceps and vacuum extraction are associated with different benefits and risks. The options available for rotational delivery include Kielland forceps, manual rotation followed by direct traction forceps, or rotational vacuum extraction. There is an increasing trend for opting for a manual rotation, despite this being the least assessed by research. Rotational deliveries should be performed by experienced operators, the choice depending upon the expertise of the individual operator.

Decision to deliver by caesarean section in the presence of fetal distress is between 30 and 40 min on average. Delivery by instrumental birth is, on average, between 20 and 30 min [14]. There appears to be no advantage of forceps over a vacuum delivery in the presence of fetal distress, and the decision to delivery intervals are similar between these instruments. Delivery in theatre compared to the room will result in a longer decision to delivery interval, but this must be balanced against the risk of failure in the room causing increased morbidity [18].

Managing fetal distress – non-technical skills

In a recent survey of malpractice cases in Sweden, the most common events were neglecting to supervise fetal well-being in 173 cases (98%), neglecting signs of fetal asphyxia in 126 cases (71%), including incautious use of oxytocin in 126 cases (71%), and choosing a non-optimal mode of delivery in 92 cases (52%). The authors conclude that there is a great need and a challenge to improve cooperation and to create security barriers within our labour units. Similar findings are seen in the UK Confidential Enquiries, which found substandard care in 75% of intrapartum-related deaths, related to failure to recognize a problem, failure to act appropriately or to communicate. A long delay has been highlighted as a major contribution to

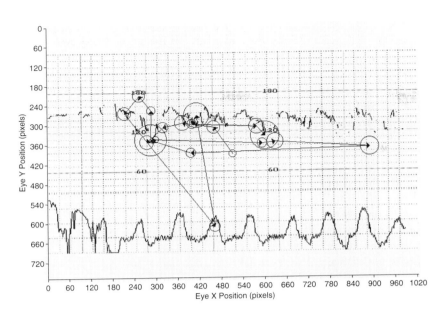

Figure 6.3 Eye tracking chart of a cardiotocograph showing that over 90% of the time is spent looking at the fetal heart rate. The circles represent the fixation point, with the larger circles indicating a longer fixation time. The arrows indicate the saccadic movements of the eye

intrapartum deaths. This suggests that there is often a window of opportunity where intervention could make a difference. Midwives and obstetricians need to improve their shared understanding of how to act in cases of imminent fetal asphyxia and how to choose a timely and optimal mode of delivery [13,19].

The complexity of patient care in modern obstetrics demands a wide range of skills and attributes. Conventional training has placed great emphasis on acquisition of the necessary knowledge and practical skills to ensure competent practice. However, good outcomes will only be realized if appropriate plans can be put in place effectively. This requires both technical and non-technical skills, such as communication, team-working, planning, resource management and decision-making. Such skills are not new in obstetrics; good practitioners have always demonstrated these competencies, but they have not featured explicitly in formal training programmes. These skills are sometimes referred to under the general heading of 'human factors'. There are several teamwork dimensions, based on commercial and military aviation models, which have been applied in medical settings [20]. There are barriers to teamwork, particularly in labour wards with a complexity of hierarchy, communication and decision-making.

How do we make the 'right' decisions?

Most work on medical decision-making is 'low-velocity'; i.e. time constraints are modest, and there is a cool-off period for adjustment and reconsideration. 'High-velocity' decision-making in the busy labour ward is different.

The nature of high-velocity decision-making

In the heat of an emergency situation, a decision needs to be made within huge time pressure, and the impact of the decision (delivery or not) may have major implications.

In this situation, the human mind works in a different way. Understanding this enables the clinician to improve their decision-making. In simple terms, the human brain filters visual and auditory information under stressful conditions. This prevents 'information overload'. Visually, data are concentrated on the focal field with reduced input from the periphery. When reading the two lines of data such as on a CTG, the focal field cannot take in both the heart rate and the contractions, and only a small part of the time looking at the CTG is spent looking at contractions (Figure 6.3).

Auditory information is also filtered to the task concerned. For example, when an obstetrician is concentrating on an examination or the start of a difficult delivery, fetal bradycardia may not be heard by them although clearly audible to all others in the room. Understanding this allows the clinician to make concerted efforts to gain the vital information and to rely on their 'wing men', the fellow members of the team, to alert them to danger.

73

Filtering of information is crucial

A good decision-maker is able to filter the correct information, and compute the information correctly. Not being able to filter the information leads to information overload and an inability to make a timely decision. Filtering the wrong information and concentration of the minutia leads to the wrong decision.

Conclusions

Fetal distress is an imprecise term for a fetus at risk of intrapartum asphyxia.

Losing a baby from intrapartum asphyxia is now uncommon in the developed world. We are still dealing with an imperfect tool to monitor the baby, namely the CTG. An obstetrician needs to balance the risk of unnecessary intervention with the need to correctly identify babies that are distressed. Normal labour involves challenges to the normal gaseous exchange of the fetus for which a normal healthy baby will almost certainly cope. Good decision-making involves assessing the fetal reserve to identify the fetus at risk of distress in labour, the likely cause of the fetal distress, and the likely response to resuscitation. Starting intrauterine resuscitation is rarely contra-indicated and should be commenced even when immediate delivery is planned. This should include positioning in left lateral, stopping the contractions and giving intravenous fluids. Understanding how we make decisions in the acute setting will help develop our decision-making skills. Good communication and team-working on the labour ward is vital.

Summary of management options

1. Make a decision – assess:
   - the fetal reserve,
   - the likely cause of distress,
   - the likely response to resuscitation.
2. Resuscitate the fetus:
   - place mother in left lateral,
   - stop the contractions by stopping oxytocin and give tocolysis,
   - give intravenous fluids.
3. Communicate clearly with the team.

References

1. National Collaborating Centre for Women's and Children's Health. *Caesarean Section. Clinical Guideline*. London: RCOG Press, 2004.

2. Fryer J G, Ashford J R. Trends in perinatal and neonatal mortality in England and Wales 1960–69. *Br J Prev Soc Med* 1972; **26**: 1–9.

3. Confidential Enquiry into Maternal and Child Health. *Perinatal Mortality 2005: England, Wales and Northern Ireland*. London: CEMACH, 2007.

4. World Health Organization. *Neonatal and Perinatal Mortality: Country, Regional and Global Estimates in 2004*. Geneva: WHO Maternal Health and Safe Motherhood Programme, 2007.

5. Badawi N, Kurinczuk J J, Keogh J M, *et al*. Antepartum risk factors for newborn encephalopathy: the Western Australian case-control study. *Br Med J* 1998; **317**: 1549–53.

6. Towner D, Castro M A, Eby-Wilkens E, Gilbert W M. Effect of mode of delivery in nulliparous women on neonatal intracranial injury. *New Engl J Med* 1999; **341**: 1709–14.

7. RCOG. *The Investigation of the Small for Gestational Age Fetus*. Green top guideline No. 31. London: RCOG Press, 2002.

8. American Society of Anesthesiologists. *ASA Physical Status Classification System*. Available online at: http://www.asahq.org/clinical/physicalstatus.htm (accessed 22 November 2005).

9. Borell U, Fernstrom I, Ohlsen L, Wiqvist N. Influence of uterine contractions on the uteroplacental blood flow at term. *Am J Obstet Gynecol* 1965; **93**: 44–57.

10. Piquard F, Schaefer A, Hsiung R, Dellenbach P, Haberey P. Are there two biological parts in the second stage of labor? *Acta Obstet Gynecol Scand* 1989; **68**: 713–8.

11. Gill P, Jarjoura D. Wharton's jelly in the umbilical cord. A study of its quantitative variations and clinical correlates. *J Reprod Med* 1993; **38**: 611–4.

12. Kinsella S M, Lee A, Spencer J A. Maternal and fetal effects of the supine and pelvic tilt positions in late pregnancy. *Eur J Obstet Gynecol Reprod Biol* 1990; **36**: 11–7.

13. Berglund S, Grunewald C, Pettersson H, Cnattingius S. Severe asphyxia due to delivery-related malpractice in Sweden 1990–2005. *Br J Obstet Gynaecol* 2008; **115**: 316–23.

14. National Collaborating Centre for Women's and Children's Health. *Intrapartum Care of Healthy Women and their Babies during Childbirth*. London: RCOG Press, 2007.

15. Hofmeyr G J. Amnioinfusion for potential or suspected umbilical cord compression in labour. *Cochrane Database Syst Rev.* 1996, 2. Art. No.: CD000013. DOI: 10.1002/14651858.CD000013.

16. Hofmeyr G J, Kulier R. Operative versus conservative management for 'fetal distress' in labour. *Cochrane Database Syst Rev.* 1998, 2. Art. No.: CD001065. DOI: 10.1002/14651858.CD001065.

17. Murphy D J, Liebling R E, Patel R, Verity L, Swingler R. Cohort study of operative delivery in the second stage of labour and standard of obstetric care. *Br J Obstet Gynaecol.* 2003; **110**: 610–5.

18. Murphy D J, Koh D K. Cohort study of the decision to delivery interval and neonatal outcome for emergency operative vaginal delivery. *Am J Obstet Gynecol* 2007; **196**: 145.e1–7.

19. Maternal and Child Health Research Consortium. *Confidential Enquiry into Stillbirths and Deaths in Infancy: 4th Annual Report.* London: Department of Health, 1997.

20. Fletcher G, Flin R, McGeorge P, *et al.* Anaesthetists' Non-Technical Skills (ANTS): evaluation of a behavioural marker system. *Br J Anaesth* 2003; **90**: 580–8.

Nutrition and hydration in labour

David Fraser and Sambit Mukhopadhyay

Whenever lay people, midwives, obstetricians and anaesthetists sit down to discuss the optimum management of the labouring patient, few topics seem to excite as much comment as that of nutrition and hydration in labour. Views quickly appear polarized, with little room for consensus, and these opposing views of the subject appear to have been permitted to fill the vacuum left by a paucity of good-quality evidence with which to guide clinical practice. Given the interest in so many other aspects of perinatal physiology, such a lack of reliable evidence on which to base clinical practice remains a matter of some regret.

Introduction

In December 1945, at a meeting of the New York Obstetrical Society, Curtis Mendelson first described his studies on aspiration of stomach contents associated with general anaesthesia in pregnant women – these findings were published the following year [1]. Mendelson had noted 66 cases of aspiration of stomach contents into the lungs in over 44,000 pregnancies at the New York Lying-In Hospital from 1932 to 1945, an incidence of 1.5 per 1000 deliveries. In 45 of these cases, the aspirated material was recorded; 40 mothers aspirated liquid and 5 aspirated solid food. Only two of the mothers actually died, both dying on the delivery table as a result of suffocation, having ingested solid material. The surviving women went on to develop an aspiration pneumonitis, thought to be due to the aspiration of gastric acid. So the risks of gastric aspiration were noted to be twofold: the aspiration of solid particles sufficiently large to obstruct the airway, and the pneumonitis secondary to acidic gastric contents.

The significance of this seminal paper lies not only in the description of this eponymous condition for the first time, but also on the profound effect it had on the subsequent management of labouring women. Nil-by-mouth (NBM) policies were introduced into many Western labour wards in the 1940s and 1950s in the belief that this would reduce the incidence of pulmonary aspiration of acidic gastric contents should general anaesthesia be required.

Pulmonary aspiration is increasingly rare, and in the years 1994–2005 only one maternal death from the aspiration of gastric contents under general anaesthesia has been recorded in the United Kingdom, a 12-year period when approximately 8 million women delivered [2–5].

Despite the fact that maternal death from pulmonary aspiration of gastric contents has virtually disappeared, the practice of restricted oral intake in normal labour appears to persist. Indeed, as recently as October 2006, the American Society of Anesthesiologists recommended that 'solid foods should be avoided in labouring patients' [6].

Practical obstetric considerations

A number of anatomical and physiological changes occur in pregnancy and labour which increase the risk of pulmonary aspiration, if general anaesthetic is required.

The anatomical changes that can increase the difficulty of obstetric intubation include the raised body mass index (an increasing problem) and enlarged breasts. These can make laryngoscopy more difficult, particularly if the situation is exacerbated by the laryngeal oedema that may complicate obstetric conditions such as pre-eclampsia.

These considerations may also jeopardize effective airway protection by making it more difficult to apply cricoid pressure correctly. These are particular concerns

Best Practice in Labour and Delivery, ed. R. Warren and S. Arulkumaran. Published by Cambridge University Press.
© Cambridge University Press 2009.

in the emergency situation, when rapid sequence induction is required.

In pregnancy, symptomatic gastroesophageal reflux is much more likely to occur. This occurs due to a combination of rising intra-abdominal pressure caused by the gravid uterus, and the steady decline in lower oesophageal sphincter tone as a result of high progesterone levels. The tone of the sphincter is also reduced by general anaesthesia – increasing the likelihood of reflux of gastric contents into the oropharynx, and their subsequent pulmonary aspiration.

Labour also causes significant depression of gastric motility and delays in gastric emptying in proportion to its duration [7]. Following a standard 'meal' of 750 ml of water containing a dye, the volume of fluid remaining in the stomach after 30 min was compared in 3 groups of women: non-pregnant, late pregnancy (pregnancy of at least 34 weeks gestation), and labouring. The mean volume remaining during labour was significantly higher than in non-pregnant women and pregnancy women before labour. The authors proposed that these results might be attributed to the pain and emotional disturbances which accompany labour.

Finally, narcotic analgesics exacerbate the problem of delayed gastric emptying in labour, and women who have received intramuscular narcotic analgesics such as pethidine or diamorphine in labour are more likely to vomit or to have increased volumes of gastric residuals at delivery [8].

A recent postal survey of UK obstetric practice found that the use of such intramuscular opioids is still widespread, at least in consultant-led maternity units. A total of 234 consultant-led obstetric units in the UK were questioned about their use of intramuscular opioids, and of units responding to the survey questionnaire over 84% were using pethidine and 34% used diamorphine [9].

Changes in obstetric anaesthetic practice

A number of profound changes in obstetric anaesthetic practice have occurred in over 60 years since Mendelson's paper was published, which have contributed to the extremely low rates of maternal mortality and morbidity witnessed today.

Diminishing rates of general anaesthesia

Although the rates of obstetric interventions, including caesarean section, are increasing, the proportion of women receiving a general anaesthetic (GA) as a result of a complication of labour is low. At the Norfolk and Norwich University Hospital, for example, only 3.1% of women required GA in the 5461 births in 2006. The indications for the GA are given in Table 7.1.

The majority of these GAs (131/172) were administered for an emergency caesarean section (2.4% overall) and, in particular, those obstetric emergencies where concern for maternal – or, more usually, fetal – well-being was such that attempts were made to deliver the baby within 30 min or less of taking the decision to perform a CS. This group of obstetric patients accounts for approximately three-quarters of all CS performed in 2006, and for 2% of all GAs performed in 2006. Many of these CS were undertaken on women who did not fall into recognizably 'high-risk' obstetric groups.

Nevertheless, these figures indicate that the substantial majority of labouring women in the hospital did *not* require a GA. Unfortunately, those women who will ultimately need a GA cannot, to a large extent, be predicted.

Table 7.1 Norfolk and Norwich University Hospital figures for obstetric GAs in 2006.

Total number of deliveries	5461
Total number of GAs	172 (3.1% of all deliveries)
Indications for GA:	
1. Emergency CS	
Category A CS (DDI less than 20 min)	81
Category B CS (DDI less than 30 min)	29
Category C CS (DDI less than 75 min)	15
Category D CS (DDI less than 360 min)	6
2. Elective CS	14
3. Other	
Examination under anaesthesia	7
Perineal repair	3
Assisted vaginal delivery	3
Manual removal of retained placenta	5
Unknown	9
DDI = decision-delivery interval	

(*Source:* Dr L. Rowe, personal communication.)

Furthermore, it must be recognized that some obstetric patients will *choose* to have a GA for their delivery.

One approach to this difficulty is to assume that all women in normal labour are at equal risk of requiring a GA (and, therefore, of pulmonary aspiration of gastric contents) and offering everyone routine prophylactic drugs. However, a recent review of the limited number of randomized controlled trials of such an approach found no evidence that either H2-receptor antagonists or antacids in labour reduced the incidence of gastric aspiration, and recommended that they should not be routinely given to low-risk women in normal labour [10].

Increasing rates of epidural anaesthesia

The proportion of women who opt to have regional anaesthesia for pain relief in labour and/or caesarean section continues to rise; for example, in our own obstetric unit, 23% of all patients had an epidural anaesthetic in labour. In addition, the majority of women who have a caesarean section – either as an elective procedure or as an emergency – have their surgery carried out with some form of regional anaesthetic technique, rather than GA. Overall, 97.3% of the elective caesareans and 82.7% of the emergency caesareans performed in 2006 employed an epidural anaesthetic (Dr L. Rowe, personal communication).

In spite of the increase in epidural rates, there does not appear to have been a commensurate decrease in the use of systemic opioids in consultant-led maternity units [9]. Furthermore, many of the standard solutions used for epidural anaesthesia contain not only a local anaesthetic agent but also an opioid, typically fentanyl. The addition of one of the opioids to the solution permits a lower dose of the local anaesthetic to be used without compromising analgesia. As expected, systemic fentanyl inhibits gastrointestinal motility in a dose-dependent manner, but there is also some data on other routes of fentanyl administration. For example, the influence of epidural-administered fentanyl on gastric emptying was the subject of a randomized controlled study of 55 women published in 1997 [11]. Women were randomly allocated to receive bupivacaine 0.125% alone or bupivacaine 0.0625% with fentanyl 2.5 µg/ml at an infusion rate of 10–12 ml/h. Gastric emptying in the fentanyl group was delayed only after it had been infused for mean time of 4.5 h, when women had received over 100 µg. It seems likely, therefore, that any delay in gastric emptying in women with an epidural will be directly related to the duration of their labour and the dose of epidural fentanyl. Lower doses of epidural opioids are used currently; the standard epidural solution used in the Norfolk and Norwich University Hospital consists of bupivicaine 0.1% with fentanyl 2 µg/ml, administered as bolus doses.

These delays in gastric emptying are over and above those associated with labour and although the delay is less than witnessed with systemic opioids, it is present nevertheless.

Despite the increase in the rates of regional anaesthesia for operative obstetrics, approximately 3% of labouring women in the Norfolk and Norwich Hospital will still require a GA, the majority for an emergency caesarean section. Many of these could not have been anticipated, but all remain at risk of pulmonary aspiration of gastric contents.

Other changes in obstetric anaesthetic practice

The dramatic decline in maternal deaths from aspiration of gastric contents cannot all be explained by the starvation policies introduced after Mendelson's paper, or the changes in practice described above.

A number of other clinical recommendations that changed obstetric anaesthetic practice may have also contributed to this fall [12]. The suggested changes include:

- intubation and rapid sequence induction,
- antacids and H2-receptor antagonists, and
- increased training and education of obstetric anaesthesiologists.

Oral intake in labour

The evidence relating to the benefits (or otherwise) of eating and drinking in labour has recently been summarized by the authors of the national guidance on intrapartum care, published in September 2007 [13].

Labour is a metabolically challenging time for mother and fetus. Non-diabetic women in late pregnancy have been shown to exhibit a state of 'accelerated starvation' if denied food and drink [14]. This results in the increased production of ketones – in particular β-hydroxybutyrate and aceto-acetic acid – and the non-esterified fatty acids from which they are derived, and significant reductions in plasma glucose and insulin levels. The changes seem to occur equally in lean and obese women. These physiological changes are exacerbated by the metabolic changes of labour, and the authors cautioned against the common practice of skipping breakfast in pregnant women.

The production of ketones is a normal physiological adaptation to generate an alternative energy supply when glucose supply is limited. Despite this, concerns about the detrimental effects of maternal starvation and subsequent ketosis in labour in the 1960s and 1970s led to the intrapartum administration of high-dose intravenous dextrose solutions as a preventative measure. However, it is now clear that ketones are not so detrimental to the mother and fetus as once thought. In addition, it quickly became apparent that while strategies employing high-dose intravenous dextrose throughout labour could swiftly correct maternal ketosis, the practice was associated with adverse consequences for the mother and fetus, so the practice was abandoned [15].

Attention subsequently switched to intrapartum measures that might attenuate the metabolic consequences of eating and drinking in labour. These have been evaluated in a number of randomized controlled studies.

Light diet

In 1999, Scrutton et al. published the results of a prospective study examining the effect of light diet on the metabolic profile, outcome of labour, and the risk of aspiration [16]. Women presenting in early labour (cervical dilatation less than 5 cm) were randomly allocated to one of two groups; those in the eating group were permitted to eat a low-residue diet throughout their labour, whereas those in the starved group received water only. By the end of labour, plasma β-hydroxybutyrate and non-esterified fatty acids were significantly lower in the eating group. Conversely, the plasma glucose and insulin levels were higher in the eating group. However, those women who ate had significantly higher gastric volumes within an hour of delivery, and were twice as likely to vomit at or around delivery. The volumes vomited by women in the eating group were also significantly larger than volumes vomited by women in the starved group (309 ml vs. 104 ml). The vomit contained a considerable amount of solid and semi-solid residue.

There were no significant differences between groups with respect to duration of labour, mode of delivery or neonatal outcome. These results suggest that those women allowed a light diet in labour are at reduced risk of developing ketosis without any discernible benefit to the labour progress or outcome for mother or fetus. However, the residual gastric volume around the time of birth is significantly higher in the eating group, who are almost certainly at greater risk of pulmonary aspiration should they require an emergency GA.

Isotonic 'sport drinks'

Sport drinks have become very popular in the last decade. Most contain mixtures of carbohydrates (such as glucose and dextrose), sodium, potassium and calcium, together with flavouring to make them more palatable.

The results of a study of the effect of one such sport drink on the outcome of labour were published by Kubli et al. in 2002 [17]. Sixty women in early labour (cervical dilatation less than 5 cm) were randomly allocated to receive either isotonic sport drink or water only. In this case, the oral sport drink used was Lucozade Sport™. Women in the sport drink group were permitted to consume up to 500 ml in the first hour and then a further 500 ml every 3–4 h. By the end of labour, plasma β-hydroxybutyrate and non-esterified fatty acids were significantly increased and the plasma glucose significantly decreased in the water-only group. There were no significant differences between the groups in gastric volume measured within 45 min of delivery, or in the volume vomited or number of vomiting episodes within 1 h of birth or throughout labour. The mean calorific intake in the sport drink group was 47 kcal/h – it was zero in the water-only group. There was no difference between the two groups in duration of labour, mode of delivery or neonatal outcome.

Thus, isotonic sport drinks appear to prevent the ketosis of labour without the increase in gastric volumes and tendency to vomit seen in women who eat during labour.

Carbohydrate solutions

Three randomized controlled trials evaluating the effects of carbohydrate versus placebo have been published by the same group of researchers in the Netherlands.

In the first study, 201 consecutive nulliparous women in early labour (cervical dilatation 2–4 cm at entry) were allowed to drink at will [18]. One group of women were randomized to the placebo arm of the study and received flavoured water. The other group received an isotonic solution containing 12.6 g carbohydrate per 100 ml. Both solutions had an identical taste and colour.

A high proportion of women recruited to this study had high-risk pregnancies (80% of the carbohydrate and 82% for the placebo – not statistically significant), presumably because in the Netherlands women considered at low risk are delivered by independent midwives. The median total intake of the study solution was 300 ml in the placebo group and 400 ml in the carbohydrate group (P value 0.04). The median total caloric intake during the study was 0 kJ in the placebo group and 802 kJ in the carbohydrate group (P value <0.001). There was no statistically significant difference in the percentage of those women who required augmentation or pain relief. Although there was no significant difference between the carbohydrate and placebo groups for spontaneous births or for instrumental vaginal delivery, the caesarean section rate for the carbohydrate group (21%) was significantly higher than that noted in the placebo group (7%).

The reasons for the caesarean sections performed were as listed on Table 7.2.

The low rate of caesarean section in the placebo arm of the study is particularly surprising given that 82% of the women allocated to this treatment arm were regarded as 'high-risk'. The authors postulated that the increase in caesarean section for non-progress in the carbohydrate group was due to a redistribution of blood in favour of the gastrointestinal tract at the expense of the myometrium. This, in turn, might lead to less energy for uterine contractions.

There were no significant differences in neonatal outcome between the carbohydrate and placebo groups.

Table 7.2 Reasons for performing caesarean section.

	Carbohydrate group	Placebo group[18]
Non-progressing labour	12	3
Fetal distress	4	2
Combination of factors	5	2

In a second study conducted by the same group, 202 nulliparous women were recruited just before the start of the second stage of labour (cervical dilatation 8–10 cm at entry) [19]. The women were then randomized to receive bottles containing 200 ml of either the same carbohydrate solution as used above, or placebo. Once again, the bottles were identical and the solutions used had identical appearances and taste.

The proportion of women considered to have a high-risk pregnancy was, again, high: 73% in the carbohydrate group and 70% in the placebo group.

The median total intake of the study solution was 200 ml in the placebo group and 200 ml in the carbohydrate group (P value 0.42). In contrast to the first study, there were no significant differences in changes in glucose, lactate or plasma β-hydroxybutyrate when the two treatment groups were compared, but the plasma free fatty acid levels were lower in the carbohydrate group (P value 0.09). Similarly, there were no significant differences in spontaneous birth or instrumental vaginal delivery. However, the figures with respect to delivery by caesarean section are in marked contrast to those reported above; only eight caesarean sections in total were performed, seven in the placebo group and one in the carbohydrate group. This difference was not significant, and the authors were unable to find a logical explanation for these differences in results. There were also no significant differences in neonatal outcome.

The third study, a smaller one, focused on the fetal effects of carbohydrate use in labour and used similar methodology to that described above [20]. A total of 100 nulliparous women considered to be of medium to high risk were randomized when the cervical dilatation was 8–10 cm. Half received bottles containing 200 ml of carbohydrate solution, the other half comparable bottles containing placebo. A higher proportion of the carbohydrate group delivered spontaneously and the only caesarean section reported occurred in the placebo group. However, the numbers reported are too small for meaningful comparisons. The arterial umbilical cord pH, pCO_2, pO_2, HCO_3- and base excess was comparable in both groups, although no statistical analysis was presented. The venous umbilical cord blood results were also similar.

No information regarding incidence of vomiting, or volumes vomited, was reported in any of these three papers.

Patient choice

There is a paucity of high-quality data exploring women's preferences with respect to eating and drinking in labour.

In a study published in 1997, a multidisciplinary team comprising a research midwife, a consultant anaesthetist and a consultant obstetrician formulated a written policy in favour of oral intake in labour with an uncomplicated pregnancy [21]. A subsequent audit of 250 women reported that 40% said they felt hungry at some point in labour, and 92% felt thirsty. Approximately 68% of women questioned drank water only while in labour in hospital and many stated this was all they wanted, although the actual number was not reported. The same study reported that a 'considerable number' of women questioned did not eat while they were in labour in hospital, usually because they did not feel like eating. However, many appreciated the option of eating and drinking, even if few chose to do so.

In a Scottish study published in 2000, 149 postnatal women were invited to complete an audit questionnaire within 36 h of delivery which incorporated questions on their oral intake in labour [22]. Only a minority of women questioned (30%) said that they would wish to eat during their labour, generally in the early stages. When the 'food' and 'no food' groups were compared, there were no statistical differences in the duration of labour, choice of analgesia or mode of delivery.

In the study of sport drink in labour quoted earlier, a progressive decrease in the desire to drink the sport drink was noted towards the end of labour after consuming 750–1000 ml [16]. Similarly, in the studies of carbohydrate solutions in labour, the volumes consumed in labour were modest: a median volume of 400 ml when women were recruited in early labour [17], and 200 ml when recruitment took place just before the start of the second stage [18].

So while a desire to eat in early labour may be common, on the basis of what little information is currently available, it would appear that the majority of women do not usually wish to eat – or even drink – once they are in the active phase of labour, and it may be inappropriate to encourage them do so.

Summary

The policy of starvation in labour was introduced over 50 years ago in an order to prevent maternal morbidity and mortality from pulmonary aspiration of gastric contents (Mendelson's syndrome) in those labouring women who required a general anaesthetic.

The proportion of women who require a GA for a complication of labour has fallen dramatically since Mendelson's original paper – it currently stands at approximately 3%. The majority of the obstetric GAs administered at this institute are undertaken for an emergency CS where the clinician has indicated a desire to deliver the baby within 30 min of taking this decision. Many of these deliveries were performed on patients who had been regarded as 'low-risk' prior to this.

The maternal mortality and morbidity due to the pulmonary aspiration of gastric contents is now so rare in Western practice as to make the 'nil-by-mouth' policy largely unsustainable for low-risk women in normal labour.

Unfortunately, relatively little evidence exists on which to base modern obstetric practice regarding eating and drinking in labour. The randomized controlled studies that have been published have recruited relatively few patients to draw meaningful conclusions. Randomized controlled trials to evaluate this specific intervention in labour need large numbers.

Metabolic changes in late pregnancy predispose to a ketotic state, and these changes are exacerbated by the physical demands of labour and delivery. These metabolic changes, once considered detrimental, are now regarded with more equanimity. Nevertheless, a number of intrapartum strategies to attenuate these changes have been evaluated.

There is limited evidence that light diet in labour significantly reduces plasma markers of 'starvation', while significantly increasing plasma glucose. However, eating causes a significant increase in volumes vomited and the residual gastric volume around the time of delivery. There were no significant differences in maternal or neonatal outcomes.

Isotonic sports drinks containing calories consumed in labour also appear to reduce markers of 'starvation' in labour, while preventing the significant fall in plasma glucose levels seen in the water-only group. Gastric volumes, incidence and volume of vomiting were comparable to the water-only group, and there were no significant differences between the groups in maternal or neonatal outcomes.

The use of carbohydrate solutions in labour appears to have little effect on neonatal outcome when compared to placebo-treated women. Similarly, there appears to be no difference in rates of spontaneous birth and instrumental vaginal delivery rates. There appear to be conflicting evidence about the effect of drinking carbohydrate solutions in labour on the risk of subsequently requiring a caesarean section. However, these differences could be due to the heterogeneity of the women recruited and/or the fact the trials were underpowered – only 403 women were recruited to the two relevant studies.

There is no compelling evidence that maternal outcomes such as duration of labour, type of analgesia required or mode of delivery is affected by any of the interventions tested thus far, although the trials conducted to date may be statistically underpowered.

Finally, there is some evidence that even when given the choice, only a minority of labouring women actually wish to eat in labour, particularly near to delivery.

Conclusions

While the subject cries out for a randomized controlled trial of the maternal and neonatal benefits, or otherwise, of a more liberal policy with respect to eating and drinking in normal labour with sufficient statistical power to provide meaningful results, this is unlikely to take place. Given the rarity of pulmonary aspiration of gastric contents in United Kingdom obstetric practice, this study would have to be of intimidating size.

Low-risk women in normal labour may eat a light diet, but should be advised that this appears to increase the risk of vomiting.

Low-risk women in normal labour may drink freely throughout the labour, and there is some evidence that isotonic sport drinks containing some calories may be more beneficial than water.

Low-risk women who receive systemic opioids or develop other risk factors that make general anaesthesia more likely should be advised to refrain from eating. It would also be appropriate to consider prescribing either a regular H2-receptor antagonist or antacid for such women.

For those women at high risk of obstetric intervention, solids and semi-solids should be avoided and patients should probably be advised to restrict their intake to isotonic drinks.

Ultimately, the matter of what to drink and eat in labour must be a matter of patient choice. Information should be made widely available to allow women to make an informed choice.

References

1. Mendelson C L. The aspiration of stomach contents into the lungs during obstetric anesthesia. *Am J Obstet Gynecol* 1946; **52**: 191–205.

2. Department of Health, Welsh Office, Scottish Office Department of Health, and Department of Health and Social Services, Northern Ireland. *Why Mothers Die. Report on Confidential Enquiries into Maternal Deaths in the United Kingdom, 1994–1996*. London: The Stationary Office, 1998.

3. Department of Health, Welsh Office, Scottish Office Department of Health, and Department of Health and Social Services, Northern Ireland. *Why Mothers Die. Report on Confidential Enquiries into Maternal Deaths in the United Kingdom, 1997–1999*. London: RCOG Press, 2001.

4. Lewis, G. (ed.). The Confidential Enquiry into Maternal and Child Health (CEMACH). Why mothers die 2000–2002. *The Sixth Report on Confidential Enquiries into Maternal Deaths in the United Kingdom.* London: RCOG Press, 2004.

5. Lewis, G (ed.). The Confidential Enquiry into Maternal and Child Health (CEMACH). Saving mothers' lives: reviewing maternal deaths to make motherhood safer – 2003–2005. *The Seventh Report on Confidential Enquiries into Maternal Deaths in the United Kingdom.* London: CEMACH, 2007.

6. American Society of Anesthesiologists' practice guidelines for obstetric anesthesia: Update 2006. *Int J Obstet Anesth* 2006; **16**: 103–5.

7. Davison J S, Davison M C, Hay D M. Gastric emptying time in late pregnancy and labour. *J Obstet Gynaecol Br Commonw* 1970; **77**: 37–41.

8. Nimmo W S, Wilson J, Prescott L F. Narcotic analgesics and delayed gastric emptying during labour. *Lancet* 1975; **i**: 890–3.

9. Tuckey J P, Prout R E, Wee M Y. Prescribing intramuscular opioids for labour analgesia in consultant-led maternity units: a survey of UK practice. *Int J Obstet Anesth* 2007; **17**: 3–8.

10. Gyte G M L, Richens Y. Routine prophylactic drugs in normal labour for reducing gastric aspiration and its effects. *Cochrane Database Syst Rev.* 2006, **3**. Art. No.: CD005298. DOI: 10.1002/14651858. CD005298.pub2.

11. Porter J S, Bonello E, Reynolds F. The influence of epidural administration of fentanyl infusion on gastric emptying in labour. *Anesthesia* 1997; **52**: 1151–6.

12. O'Sullivan G, Scrutton M. NPO during labor – is there any scientific validation? *Anesthesiology Clin N Am* 2003; **21**: 87–98.

13. National Collaborating Centre for Women's and Children's Health. *Intrapartum Care: Care of Healthy Women and their Babies during Childbirth*. London: RCOG Press, 2007.

14. Metzger B E, Ravnikar V, Vileisis R A, Freinkel N. 'Accelerated starvation' and the skipped breakfast in late normal pregnancy. *Lancet* 1982; **i**: 588–92.

15. Lawrence G F, Brown V A, Parsons R J, Cooke I D. Feto-maternal consequences of high-dose glucose infusion during labour. *Br J Obstet Gynaecol* 1982; **89**: 27–32.

16. Scrutton M J, Metcalfe G A, Lowy C, Seed P T, O'Sullivan G. Eating in labour: a randomised controlled trial assessing risks and benefits. *Anaesthesia* 1999; **54**: 329–34.

17. Kubli M, Scrutton M J, Seed P T. An evaluation of isotonic 'sport drinks' during labour. *Anesth Analg* 2002; **94**: 404–8.

18. Scheepers H C J, Thans M C J, de Jong P A, *et al*. A double-blind, randomised, placebo controlled study on the influence of carbohydrate solution intake during labour. *Br J Obstet Gynaecol* 2002; **109**: 178–81.

19. Scheepers H C J, de Jong P A, Essed G G M, Kanhai H H H. Carbohydrate solution intake during labour just before the start of the second stage: a double-blind study on metabolic effects and clinical outcome. *Br J Obstet Gynaecol* 2004; **111**: 1382–7.

20. Scheepers H C J, Thans M C J, de Jong P A, Essed G G M, Kanhai H H H. The effects of oral carbohydrate administration on fetal acid base balance. *J Perinat Med* 2002; **30**: 400–4.

21. Newton C, Champion P. Oral intake in labour: Nottingham's policy formulated and audited. *Br J Midwif* 1997; **5**: 418–22.

22. Armstrong T S H, Johnston I G. Which women want food during labour? Results of an audit in a Scottish DGH. *Health Bulletin* 2000; **58**: 141–4.

8 Prolonged second stage of labour including difficult decision-making on operative vaginal delivery and caesarean section

Hajeera Butt and Deirdre J. Murphy

Introduction

The second stage of labour is an important component of the natural phenomenon of childbirth. From the perspective of the mother and the midwife it is often seen as the climax of the birth process, and from the perspective of the obstetrician it is the period of increased risk. The second stage begins with full dilatation of the cervix and ends with the birth of the baby. It is difficult to ascertain exactly when full dilatation of the cervix occurs as it is an event in the continuum of the labour process. It is diagnosed by either routine vaginal examination during labour or when the patient reports experiencing the sensation to bear down.

The second stage of labour has two phases.

- A passive phase that begins with full dilatation of the cervix and ends when bearing down efforts begin.

- An expulsive phase when the mother feels the sensation of bearing down due to pressure of the presenting part on the rectum and active maternal pushing occurs.

The primary outcome following effective management of the second stage of labour is safe delivery of a healthy infant to a mother who has had a rewarding experience retaining both physical and psychological well-being. The ideal management of the second stage of labour is where spontaneous vaginal birth is facilitated without use of instruments or additional procedures. This should be possible in most cases. There are, however, difficult decisions to be made in cases that deviate from normal. The optimal approach in these circumstances is one where the midwife and obstetrician work together (with the anaesthetist and neonatal specialist if required) in supporting a woman through appropriate intervention or operative birth.

Duration of the second stage of labour

It is perhaps surprising that there is no single accepted definition of an appropriate duration for the second stage of labour. The approach in recent years has been to allow the woman as long as possible to achieve a vaginal birth, particularly with epidural anaesthesia. The American College of Obstetricians and Gynaecologists (ACOG) define the limits for the second stage of labour as 2 h for nulliparous women and 1 h for multiparous women without regional anaesthesia [1]. When a woman is given regional anaesthesia, an extra hour is added in both cases. Both the ACOG practice bulletin and 'green-top' guideline of the Royal College of Obstetricians and Gynaecologists (RCOG)[2] describe a prolonged second stage as lack of continuous progress for 3 h with regional anaesthesia or 2 h without regional anaesthesia in nulliparous women. In multiparous women, prolonged second stage is no progress for 2 h with or 1 h without regional anaesthesia[1,2]. The RCOG guidelines emphasize that the durations stated are a combined total of both active and passive phases of the second stage. The recently developed National Institute for Health and Clinical Excellence (NICE) guideline on intrapartum care allows longer intervals of active second stage to achieve spontaneous vaginal birth as follows [3].

- Nulliparous women:

  - birth would be expected to take place within 3 h of the start of the active second stage in most women;
  - a diagnosis of delay in the active second stage should be made when it has lasted 2 h and women should be referred to a healthcare

professional trained to undertake an operative vaginal birth if birth is not imminent.

- Parous women:
  - birth would be expected to take place within 2 h of the start of the active second stage in most women;
  - a diagnosis of delay in the active second stage should be made when it has lasted 1 h and women should be referred to a healthcare professional trained to undertake an operative vaginal birth if birth is not imminent.

With the above criteria it would be considered acceptable for the second stage of labour to last 5 h for a nulliparous woman with an epidural where up to 2 h are allowed for passive descent and 3 h for the active phase. Intervention in the second stage of labour because an arbitrary time limit has been exceeded must be balanced with the risks of an adverse outcome for the mother or her baby as a result of a prolonged second stage of labour.

Outcomes of prolonged second stage of labour

Undue prolongation of the second stage of labour can potentially result in maternal and/or fetal compromise, although the published data are far from consistent. A large US cross-sectional study ($n=15,759$) investigated the relationship between prolonged duration of the second stage (defined as more than 4 h) and pre-specified outcomes in nulliparous women [4]. Logistic regression analyses, controlling for various confounders, showed that there was evidence of an association between a prolonged second stage and chorioamnionitis (OR 1.79 [95% CI 1.44–2.22]), third- or fourth-degree lacerations (OR 1.33 [95% CI 1.07–1.67]), caesarean section (OR 5.65 [95% CI 4.46–7.16], operative vaginal birth (OR 2.83 [95% CI 2.38–3.36]) and low Apgar score (<7 at 5 min OR 0.45 [95% CI 0.25–0.84]). The reduced incidence of low Apgar scores suggests that intervention occurred without delay in the context of suspected fetal compromise. There was no evidence of an association between prolonged second stage of labour and endomyometritis (OR 0.79 [95% CI 0.49–1.26]), postpartum haemorrhage (PPH) (OR 1.05 [95% CI 0.84–1.31]), meconium-stained liquor (OR 1.11

[95% CI 0.93–1.33]), or admission to the neonatal unit (OR 0.59 [95% CI 0.35–1.03]). In a study of 5158 women, the same authors concluded that multiparous women with a second stage of 3 h or greater have an increased risk of operative delivery, peripartum morbidity, five minute Apgar score less than 7, fetal acidosis (umbilical artery pH<7.0, base excess (BE) < −12), presence of meconium-stained amniotic fluid and admission to neonatal intensive care unit [5].

A German cross-sectional study ($n=1200$) investigated prolonged second stage of labour (more than 2 h) and intrapartum outcomes [6]. The results showed evidence of an association of prolonged second stage with a low Apgar score at 1 min, PPH, perineal tears and postpartum fever, although the analyses did not control for confounding factors. A large UK cross-sectional study ($n=25,069$) investigated prolonged second stage of labour and perinatal outcomes [7]. Logistic regression analysis showed that there was evidence of an association between a longer duration and a higher rate of PPH (durations: 120–179 min OR 1.6 [95% CI 1.3–1.9]; 180–239 min OR 1.7 [95% CI 1.3–2.3]; 240+ min OR 1.9 [95% CI 1.2–2.8]), but there was no evidence of an association with postpartum infection or an Apgar score less than 7 at 5 min.

There is no clear consensus on the optimal duration of the second stage of labour, and the research addressing this question is currently limited. The question of 'how long is too long' needs to be addressed by prospective randomized studies with long-term outcomes. The ACOG practice bulletin and the RCOG guideline emphasize the need to individualize care for the specific circumstances, stating that 'the length of the second stage of labour is not in itself an absolute or even strong indication for operative termination of labour' [1], and that 'the question of when to intervene should involve balancing the risks and benefits of continuing pushing as against operative delivery' [2]. However, the potential for maternal or neonatal adverse outcomes is reflected in the NICE guideline recommendation that 'following initial obstetric assessment for women with delay in the second stage of labour, ongoing obstetric review should be maintained every 15–30 minutes' [3]. The practical implications for an obstetrician of being available for regular reviews at close intervals needs to be considered in the context of busy maternity units.

85

Causes of prolonged second stage of labour

At a basic level, prolonged second stage of labour can be considered in terms of deviations from normal of the powers, passages or passenger, or a combination of these factors. The powers reflect maternal uterine activity and maternal effort when actively pushing. Various factors influence the powers, including support and encouragement, rate, rhythm, duration and strength of contractions, maternal position when pushing, and degree of motor and sensory blockage with analgesia or anaesthesia. The bony pelvis (passages) is limited in terms of actual dimensions; however, repositioning of the mother may optimize the available diameters at the pelvic inlet and outlet. Occasionally the passages may be obstructed by a cervical fibroid or ovarian cyst, although this is usually apparent long before the second stage of labour.

The passenger (the baby) may be large for the mother or may descend into the pelvis in an abnormal presentation (brow or face), abnormal position (occipito-posterior or occipito-transverse), or may fail to rotate and flex, resulting in asynclitism and deflexion. Most fetuses with a cephalic presentation present by the vertex because of the pelvic shape. In labour, 80–90% of vertex presentations are occipito-anterior position. Of the remaining 10–20%, almost 90% will become occipito-anterior with progress of labour [8]. Persistent occipito-posterior position (POP) can occur in 2–5% of cases. This results in a larger head diameter being presented, resulting in poor progress in both first and second stages of labour – on average, 38% of these can deliver vaginally. Any presentation other than vertex is defined as malpresentation. The various types are breech, face, brow, and shoulder presentation. If the umbilical cord presents at the cervix and the membranes are intact, it is a cord presentation. This should be delivered by caesarean section, otherwise cord prolapse will occur after rupture of the membranes. A deflexed head causes a brow presentation. If the head becomes flexed due to the mechanics of labour, a brow presentation can become vertex. On the other hand, if further deflexion occurs, brow presentation becomes a face presentation. Persistent brow needs to be delivered by caesarean section. Face presentation is diagnosed by palpation of the orbital ridges, nose, mouth and chin. A mento-anterior position can deliver vaginally due to smaller presenting diameters. If the face is in a mento-posterior position, the presenting diameter will be larger than the pelvis and vaginal delivery is not possible. The safe option in this case is caesarean section.

In general terms, assessment of progress should include maternal behaviour, effectiveness of pushing and fetal well-being, taking into account the fetal position and station at the onset of the second stage. These factors will assist in deciding the timing of further vaginal examinations and the need for obstetric review.

Epidural anaesthesia and prolonged second stage of labour

Epidural anaesthesia may contribute to the likelihood of a prolonged second stage of labour and subsequent intervention, but equally it may have a role to play in the successful management of prolonged second stage of labour.

A Cochrane systematic review of epidural anaesthesia in labour concluded that epidural anaesthesia provides significantly better, safer and effective pain relief than non-epidural techniques [9]. It is the method of choice for many women. A systematic review of the effects of epidural analgesia on labour, maternal and neonatal outcomes was performed with a meta-analysis of 14 randomized controlled trials. The following observations were made.

- Mothers receiving an epidural had lower pain scores and were more satisfied with their analgesia than those on parenteral opioids or no analgesia.
- Length of first stage did not differ between the epidural and parenteral opioid groups.
- Epidural is associated with prolongation of second stage, more frequent oxytocin augmentation. The duration of second stage was increased by an average of 15 min in the epidural group.
- The total operative vaginal delivery rate was higher for epidural (12 trials; $n=3653$; OR 2.08 [95% CI 1.48–2.93]), but the incidence of operative vaginal delivery for dystocia was not.
- The incidence of caesarean section for any indication did not differ between patients randomized to receive parenteral opioids (7.7%) and patients randomized to receive epidural analgesia (8.0%).

Certain side effects are specifically associated with epidural anaesthesia. Common side effects are itching, shivering, maternal pyrexia >38°C, and urinary retention. Less common side effects include hypotension, headache due to accidental dural puncture, and respiratory arrest. Some interventions can be avoided if the woman does not have an epidural – these include intravenous lines, intravenous fluids, bladder catheterization and continuous electronic fetal monitoring.

However, the corollary is that epidural anaesthesia provides safe and effective anaesthesia in the second stage of labour for interventions such as labour augmentation, episiotomy, operative vaginal delivery and emergency caesarean section. The NICE Intrapartum Care guideline specifically recommends effective anaesthesia in these circumstances [3].

- Consideration should be given to the use of oxytocin, with the offer of regional analgesia, for nulliparous women if contractions are inadequate at the onset of the second stage.
- Tested effective analgesia should be provided prior to carrying out an episiotomy, except in an emergency due to acute fetal compromise.
- Instrumental birth is an operative procedure that should be undertaken with tested effective anaesthesia.

When effective epidural analgesia has been achieved it should not be discontinued. There is insufficient evidence to support the hypothesis that discontinuing epidural analgesia reduces the incidence of operative vaginal delivery (23% vs. 28%; RR 0.84 [95% CI 0.61–1.15]), but there is evidence that it increases women's pain (22% vs. 6%; RR 3.68 [95% CI 1.99–6.80]) [9].

How to avoid prolonged second stage of labour

There are several approaches that may help a woman achieve a spontaneous vaginal birth within the limits set for a normal duration for the second stage of labour and thereby avoid operative delivery. At a simple level, if pushing is ineffective or if requested by the woman, strategies to assist birth can be used, such as support, change of position, emptying of the bladder and encouragement.

Support in labour

There is evidence to show that continuous support for women during childbirth can reduce the incidence of operative vaginal delivery, particularly when the carer is not a member of staff (14 trials; $n=12,757$; RR 0.89 [95% CI 0.83–0.96]) [10]. All women should be encouraged to have continuous support during labour.

Women's position in the second stage of labour

The position or positions a woman adopts in the second stage of labour may have an important impact on the duration of the second stage and the need for operative intervention. The NICE Intrapartum Care guideline and the RCOG guideline reflect this in the following recommendation.

- Women should be discouraged from lying supine or semi-supine in the second stage of labour and should be encouraged to adopt any other position that they find most comfortable.

A systematic review has been updated recently which assesses the benefits and risks of the use of different positions during the second stage of labour [11]. The review included 19 trials involving 5764 women. The use of any upright or lateral position compared with supine or lithotomy was associated with reduced duration of second stage of labour: weighted mean reduction in duration 16.9 min [95% CI 14.3–19.5 min]; a reduction in assisted births: RR 0.84 [95% CI 0.73–0.98] and a reduction in episiotomies RR 0.84 [95% CI 0.79–0.91].

Pushing in the second stage of labour

When and how a woman is encouraged to push requires consideration and is summarized in the following NICE recommendations.

- Women should be informed that in the second stage they should be guided by their own urge to push.
- If full dilatation of the cervix has been diagnosed in a woman without epidural analgesia, but she does not get an urge to push, further assessment should take place after 1 h.

A recent meta-analysis demonstrated that nulliparous women with epidurals were likely to have fewer rotational or mid cavity operative interventions when pushing was delayed for 1–2 h or until they had a strong urge to push [12]. Allowing passive descent and rotation is recommended where the fetal status is satisfactory.

Two US randomized controlled trials (RCTs) of good quality have compared coached with uncoached pushing in the second stage of labour [13,14]. The mean duration of the second stage of labour was significantly shorter for women in the coached group compared with the uncoached group (46 min vs. 59 min, $p=0.014$) [13]. There were no differences noted in any other maternal or neonatal outcomes in either trial. There is therefore no high-level evidence that directed pushing affects outcomes.

Oxytocin augmentation

Consideration should be given to the use of oxytocin, with the offer of regional analgesia, for nulliparous women if contractions are inadequate at the onset of the second stage [3]. However, caution is required, particularly for multiparous women. While it may be possible to augment the uterine contractions with the use of oxytocin, clearly this should not be contemplated where uterine activity is already effective and if disproportion or obstructed labour is suspected.

Role of episiotomy in prolonged second stage of labour

Episiotomy can be used to facilitate delivery if there is a clinical need, such as for operative vaginal delivery or suspected fetal compromise (e.g. fetal bradycardia). However, it should be limited to specific clinical indications and not employed routinely. This is reflected in guideline recommendations [3].

- A routine episiotomy should not be carried out during spontaneous vaginal birth.
- An episiotomy should be performed if there is a clinical need, such as instrumental birth or suspected fetal compromise.
- Where an episiotomy is performed, the recommended technique is a mediolateral episiotomy originating at the vaginal fourchette and usually directed to the right side. The angle to the vertical axis should be between 45 and 60 degrees at the time of the episiotomy.
- Tested effective analgesia should be provided prior to carrying out an episiotomy, except in an emergency due to acute fetal compromise.

A Cochrane review of six randomized trials involving 4850 women found that as compared to routine use (73%), restrictive episiotomy use (28%) was more beneficial as it was associated with less posterior perineal trauma, less need for suturing and fewer healing complications [15]. On the other hand, it caused more anterior perineal trauma and there was no difference in severe vaginal or perineal trauma, dyspareunia, urinary incontinence or severe pain. The evidence overall was in favour of a restrictive approach to episiotomy.

A prospective observational study involving 241 women giving birth for the first time aimed to identify risk factors associated with third- and fourth-degree tears following childbirth [16]. Episiotomies angled closer to the midline were significantly associated with anal sphincter injuries (26 vs. 37 degrees, $p=0.01$). The authors recommended that the angle to the vertical axis should be between 45 and 60 degrees at the time of the episiotomy.

Assessment prior to operative delivery

The vast majority of avoidable maternal and neonatal morbidity at operative vaginal delivery relates to inappropriate application of the instrument and operator inexperience [17]. Therefore an essential prerequisite for operative vaginal delivery is a skilled operator. The obstetrician must be able to assess the bony pelvis and unequivocally determine the fetal position and station, as well as any degree of flexion, caput, moulding and asynclitism. The instrument must then be correctly placed and an appropriate amount of traction applied in the right direction. In such circumstances, successful operative vaginal delivery rates are high and morbidity low. However, these skills are not easy to acquire, and certainly cannot be self-taught. In addition, the trainee obstetrician must know when to ask for help. Predictors of failed operative vaginal delivery include occipito-posterior position, high presenting part (station spines $+0$), inadequate analgesia and birthweight >4000 g, and these criteria should alert the obstetrician to be cautious and seek senior support [18,19].

The RCOG has recommended that obstetricians be confident and competent in the use of both vacuum and forceps, and that operators should choose the instrument most appropriate to the clinical circumstances and their level of skill [2]. Clear and detailed guidelines are available and should be adapted within local practice-based protocols and followed up with regular audit and multidisciplinary review of adverse incidents. A UK study demonstrated substantial differences between consultant assessment regarding fetal position and station compared with specialist registrars, and that the consultant was more likely to reverse a decision for caesarean section and safely conduct an operative vaginal delivery [20]. A review of failed vacuum extractions reported suboptimal application in 40% of cases [21]. Clearly, appropriate supervision and the availability of skilled obstetricians on the labour ward at all times will be an essential component of training initiatives.

The following prerequisites must be fulfilled when assessing a woman before attempting an operative vaginal delivery.

- No more than one-fifth of the head should be palpable on abdominal palpation.
- Cervix fully dilated and membranes ruptured.
- Station at level of ischial spines or below.
- Exact position of fetal head should be determined.
- Excessive caput or moulding should not be present.
- There should be noticeable descent of head with uterine contraction and bearing down efforts.

Operative delivery in the second stage of labour

Vacuum vs. forceps

There is ongoing debate on the relative merits and hazards of vacuum and forceps delivery. A systematic review of several RCTs reported that use of the vacuum extractor was associated with significantly less maternal trauma (OR 0.41, 95% CI 0.33–0.50) and with more completed deliveries (OR 1.69, 95% CI 1.31–2.19) than forceps delivery [22]. However, this is potentially misleading, as attempted vacuum delivery has a higher failure rate than forceps as a first line instrument, with failed vacuum deliveries frequently completed by forceps. Vacuum failure rates of between 20 and 30% have been reported in two recent RCTs, with higher failure rates for the hand-held vacuum device [23,24]. Failure of vacuum delivery is three to four times more likely with a fetal malposition and is associated with an increased risk of postpartum haemorrhage [25,26]. In a prospective cohort study of women transferred to theatre for arrested progress in the second stage of labour, attempted forceps was more likely to result in completed vaginal delivery than attempted vacuum (63% vs. 48%, $p<0.01$) [18].

Operative vaginal delivery is associated with increased pelvic floor morbidity, but comparisons between vacuum and forceps remain controversial. Forceps delivery incurred a higher risk of third-degree laceration than vacuum in two population-based studies (OR 1.94, 95% CI 1.30–2.89 and OR 3.33, 95% CI 2.97–3.74, respectively) [27,28]. In a recent randomized trial assessing anal sphincter function, symptoms of altered faecal continence were significantly more common following forceps delivery compared to vacuum [29]. More reassuringly, there was no difference in rates of urinary and bowel dysfunction at five-year follow-up of a previous randomized controlled study comparing forceps and vacuum delivery [30]. However, in the prospective cohort study of operative delivery in the second stage of labour, there was a threefold increased risk of urinary incontinence at one and three years following operative vaginal delivery compared to second stage caesarean section [31,32].

The neonatal outcome is critical to the debate on the role of operative vaginal delivery in modern obstetric practice. The operator's expertise may ultimately determine the preferred mode of delivery, but each obstetrician should have the necessary skills to deliver the baby by the swiftest and safest means according to the individual circumstances. The neonatal morbidity related to operative delivery needs to be evaluated where operative vaginal delivery is successfully achieved, where caesarean section is undertaken following failed attempt at operative vaginal delivery, and where delivery is by immediate caesarean section. In a systematic review of trials comparing vacuum extraction with forceps delivery, Johanson and Menon reported that use of the vacuum extractor was associated with an increase in neonatal cephalhaematoma and retinal haemorrhages [22]. Despite this finding, the vacuum extractor has become the instrument of choice in the interest of minimizing maternal morbidity. If speed is of the essence, particularly in the presence of suspected fetal hypoxia, then there is a higher chance of completed operative vaginal delivery with forceps than vacuum. However, operative vaginal delivery is likely to incur an increased risk of birth trauma (usually transient) that may be avoided by immediate recourse to caesarean section, and a back-up plan needs to be in place in the event of abandoning an attempted operative vaginal delivery.

In situations where the baby is born in poor condition, fears about early morbidity are quickly replaced by concerns about survival and long-term neurological disability. Badawi *et al.* have reported an increased risk of neonatal encephalopathy following both operative vaginal delivery and emergency caesarean section in a large Australian population-based study (OR 2.3, 95% CI 1.2–4.7) and (OR 2.2, 95% CI 1.0–4.6, respectively) [33]. Moderate and severe neonatal encephalopathy are strongly associated with cerebral palsy and death. The use of sequential instruments particularly vacuum and forceps has been associated with scalp trauma, intracranial haemorrhage and neonatal death [34]. Reassuringly, a five-year follow-up of the second stage prospective cohort study reported low overall rates of neuro-developmental morbidity with comparable outcomes for each mode of delivery [35].

Deciding between operative vaginal delivery and caesarean section

Rotational delivery and mid cavity arrest in the second stage of labour present the obstetrician with a choice between a potentially difficult operative vaginal delivery and caesarean section at full dilatation, each with inherent risks. In a prospective cohort study of women transferred to theatre for second stage arrest, caesarean section was associated with an increased risk of major haemorrhage (adjusted OR 2.8, 95% CI 1.1–7.6) and prolonged hospital stay (OR 3.5, 95% CI 1.6–7.6) [18]. However, caesarean delivery (OR 0.63, 95% CI 0.38–1.00) and major haemorrhage were less likely with an experienced obstetrician (OR 0.5, 95% CI 0.3–0.9). High rates of third- and fourth-degree tears are reported following operative vaginal delivery. The comparable morbidity at caesarean section relates to extension of the uterine incision into the cervix, vagina or broad ligaments. Extension of the uterine incision at full dilatation has been reported in up to 35% of cases and has been associated with an increased risk of caesarean hysterectomy and febrile morbidity [36]. Long-term follow-up will determine whether this results in subsequent difficult deliveries or an increased risk of uterine rupture.

To date, there has been inconsistency in the reported early neonatal morbidity when comparing operative vaginal delivery with caesarean section for mid cavity arrest. Older retrospective studies found little difference in short-term neonatal morbidity, and, reassuringly, the study by Revah *et al.* [37] found no increase in neonatal morbidity among women who had a failed operative vaginal delivery in a setting where caesarean section could follow promptly. In a prospective cohort study of women transferred to theatre in the second stage of labour, delivery by caesarean section was associated with an increased risk of admission to the special care baby unit (SCBU) compared to operative vaginal delivery (OR 2.6, 95% CI 1.2–6.0) [18]. Of note, there were equal rates of ominous fetal heart rate tracings in the two groups. The greater risk of admission to SCBU following caesarean section did not appear to be the result of a selective decision based on pre-existing fetal compromise but may reflect the decision to delivery interval, which is frequently longer for a caesarean section. However, neonatal trauma was significantly less common following caesarean delivery compared to operative vaginal delivery (OR 0.4, 95% CI 0.2–0.7). In the majority of cases this represented facial and scalp bruising, but there was one facial laceration in each group, and a fractured clavicle and six cases of brachial plexus injury in the operative vaginal delivery group. A low umbilical artery pH was more frequently recorded following failed operative vaginal delivery, but there was no increase in admissions to SCBU. Trauma was significantly more likely following failed operative vaginal delivery than immediate caesarean section ($p=0.03$), but was still less common than following completed operative vaginal delivery [17]. In a large North American population-based study, the sequential use of vacuum and forceps was associated with an increased need for mechanical ventilation in the infant [38]. These findings suggest that neonatal complications could be reduced, with careful selection of cases for attempted operative vaginal delivery and a judicious choice of instrument.

A previous delivery experience can have important implications for future pregnancies, not least whether a woman would contemplate another pregnancy. Fear of childbirth has been reported in up to 26% of women at five years following either operative vaginal delivery or caesarean section compared with 10% following spontaneous vaginal delivery [39]. In the second stage prospective cohort study, women were far more likely to aim for a future vaginal delivery (79% vs. 39%) and to achieve a subsequent vaginal delivery (78% vs. 31%) following operative vaginal delivery than caesarean section, although fear of childbirth was a frequently reported reason for avoiding a further pregnancy in both groups [40,41]. Women who have experienced a previous caesarean section at full dilatation generate anxiety in subsequent labours relating to the risk of further emergency caesarean section and potential uterine rupture. Mid cavity and rotational operative vaginal deliveries have become unpopular in the US and are increasingly abandoned in favour of caesarean section. This may be a short-sighted view, however, if one fails to consider the outcome of future deliveries in the assessment of overall morbidity. In a follow-up study of primigravidae who required mid cavity operative vaginal delivery, more than 75% achieved a spontaneous vaginal delivery with heavier babies in the second pregnancy and very low overall rates of birth trauma or asphyxia [39].

Clearly, choice of operative delivery in the second stage of labour presents a difficult risk/benefit dilemma in terms of short- and long-term maternal and infant well-being. Caesarean section at full dilatation with anhydramnios and an engaged fetal head is a difficult procedure. This is reflected in high rates of major obstetric haemorrhage, extension of the uterine incision and prolonged hospital admission. These risks must be balanced with the potential for pelvic floor trauma and neonatal injury following operative vaginal delivery.

Conclusion

Decisions regarding the most appropriate management of prolonged second stage of labour will continue to be subjective. Individual clinical circumstances, maternal preferences and the skill of the obstetrician will influence the approach taken. A balance needs to be achieved between avoiding unnecessary intervention and preventing avoidable morbidity. Every woman has a right to expect high-quality care in labour, and in the event of a prolonged second stage she should be assessed carefully and advised on a course of action that will result in a safe and timely delivery. Most women who have reached the second stage of labour will prefer an operative vaginal delivery to a caesarean section if this can be safely achieved with a minimum of morbidity. In such circumstances women should be encouraged that the probability of a spontaneous vaginal birth in a subsequent pregnancy is very high.

References

1. American College of Obstetricians and Gynecologists. Operative vaginal delivery use of forceps and vacuum extractors for operative vaginal delivery. *ACOG Practice Bulletin* 2000; **17**: 1–6.
2. Royal College of Obstetricians and Gynaecologists. *Operative Vaginal Delivery*. Green-top Guideline No. 26. London: RCOG, 2005.
3. NICE. *Intrapartum Care; Care of Healthy Women and their Babies during Childbirth*. NICE clinical guideline. London: NICE, 2007.
4. Cheng Y W, Hopkins L M, Caughey A B. How long is too long: does a prolonged second stage of labor in nulliparous women affect maternal and neonatal outcomes? *Am J Obstet Gynecol* 2004; **194**: 933–8.
5. Cheng Y W, Hopkins L M, Laros R K Jr, Caughey A B. Duration of the second stage of labour in multiparous women: Maternal and neonatal outcomes. *Am J Obstet Gynecol* 2007; **196**: 585.e1–e6.
6. Janni W, Schlessl B, Poschers U, *et al*. The prognostic impact of a prolonged second stage of labor on maternal and fetal outcome. *Acta Obstet Gynecol Scand* 2002; **81**: 214–21.
7. Saunders N S, Pearson C M, Wadsworth J. Neonatal and maternal morbidity in relation to the length of the second stage of labour. *Br J Obstet Gynaecol* 1992; **99**: 381–5.
8. Ponkey S E, Cohen A P, Heffner L J, Liberman E. Persistent fetal occiput posterior position: obstetric outcome. *Obstet Gynecol* 2003; **101**: 915–20.
9. Howell C W. Epidural versus non-epidural analgesia for pain relief in labour (Cochrane Review). In: *The Cochrane Library*, Issue 3, Oxford; 2000.
10. Hodnett E D, Gates S, Hofmeyr G J, Sakala C. Continuous support for women during childbirth. *Cochrane Database Syst Rev.* 2003; **3**: CD003766. Review.
11. Gupta J K, Hofmeyr G J. Position for women during second stage of labour. *Cochrane Database Syst Rev.* 2003; **3**. Art. No.: CD002006.pub2. DOI: 10.1002/14651858.CD002006.pub2.
12. Roberts C L, Torvaldsen S, Cameron C A, Olive E. Delayed versus early pushing in women with epidural analgesia: a systematic review and meta-analysis. *Br J Obstet Gynaecol* 2004; **111**: 1333–40.
13. Bloom S L, Casey B M, Schaffer J I, *et al*. A randomized trial of coached versus uncoached maternal pushing during the second stage of labor. *Am J Obstet Gynecol* 2006; **194**: 10–3.
14. Schaffer J I, Bloom S L, Casey B M, *et al*. A randomized trial of coached versus uncoached maternal pushing during the second stage of labor on postpartum pelvic floor structure and function. *Am J Obstet Gynecol* 2005; **192**: 1692–6.

15. Carroli G, Belizan J. Episiotomy for vaginal birth. *Cochrane Database Syst Rev.* 2003; **1**: CD000081(1).

16. Andrews V, Sultan A H, Thakar R, *et al.* Risk factors for obstetric anal sphincter injury: a prospective study. *Birth* 2006; **33**: 117–22.

17. Murphy D J, Liebling R E, Patel R, Verity L, Swingler R. Cohort study of operative delivery in the second stage of labour and standard of obstetric care. *Br J Obstet Gynaecol* 2003; **110**: 610–5.

18. Murphy D J, Liebling R E, Verity L, Swingler R, Patel R. Cohort study of the early maternal and neonatal morbidity associated with operative delivery in the second stage of labour. *Lancet* 2001; **358**: 1203–7.

19. Ben-Haroush A, Melamed N, Kaplan B, Yogev Y. Predictors of failed operative vaginal delivery: a single-center experience. *Am J Obstet Gynecol* 2007; **197**: 308.e5–47.

20. Olah K S. Reversal of the decision for Caesarean section in the second stage of labour on the basis of consultant vaginal assessment. *J Obstet Gynecol* 2005; **25**: 115–6.

21. Sau A, Sau M, Ahmed H, Brown R. Vacuum extraction: is there any need to improve the current training in the UK? *Acta Obstet Gynecol Scand* 2004; **83**: 466–70.

22. Johanson R B, Menon B K. Vacuum extraction versus forceps for assisted vaginal delivery. *Cochrane Database Syst Rev* 2000; **2**: CD000224.

23. Attilakos G, Sibanda T, Winter C, Johnson N, Draycott T. A randomised controlled trial of a new handheld vacuum extraction device. *Br J Obstet Gynaecol* 2005; **112**: 1510–5.

24. Groom K M, Jones B A, Miller N, Paterson-Brown S. A prospective randomised controlled trial of the Kiwi Omnicup versus conventional ventouse cups for vacuum-assisted vaginal delivery. *Br J Obstet Gynaecol* 2006; **113**: 183–9.

25. Bhide A, Guven M, Prefumo F, *et al.* Maternal and neonatal outcome after failed ventouse delivery: comparison of forceps versus cesarean section. *J Matern Fetal Neonatal Med* 2007; **20**: 541–5.

26. Damron D P, Capeless E L. Operative vaginal delivery: a comparison of forceps and vacuum for success rate and risk of rectal sphincter injury. *Am J Obstet Gynecol* 2004; **191**: 907–10.

27. MacArthur C, Glazener C M A, Wilson P D, *et al.* Obstetric practice and faecal incontinence three months after delivery. *Br J Obstet Gynaecol* 2001; **108**: 678–83.

28. De Leeuw J W, Struijk P C, Vierhout M E, Wallenburg H C S. Risk factors for third degree perineal ruptures during delivery. *Br J Obstet Gynaecol* 2001; **108**: 383–7.

29. Fitzpatrick M, Behan M, O'Connell P R, O'Herlihy C. Randomised clinical trial to assess anal sphincter function following forceps or vacuum assisted vaginal delivery. *Br J Obstet Gynaecol* 2003; **110**: 424–9.

30. Johanson R B, Heycock E, Carter J, *et al.* Maternal and child health after assisted vaginal delivery: five-year follow up of a randomised controlled study comparing forceps and ventouse. *Br J Obstet Gynaecol* 1999; **106**: 544–9.

31. Liebling R E, Swingler R, Patel R R, *et al.* Pelvic floor morbidity up to one year after difficult instrumental delivery and cesarean section in the second stage of labor: a cohort study. *Am J Obstet Gynecol* 2004; **191**: 4–10.

32. Bahl R, Strachan B, Murphy D J. Pelvic floor morbidity at three years after instrumental delivery and caesarean section in the second stage of labor and the impact of a subsequent delivery. *Am J Obstet Gynecol* 2005; **192**: 789–94.

33. Badawi N, Kurinczuk J J, Keogh J M, *et al.* Intrapartum risk factors for newborn encephalopathy: the Western Australian case-control study. *Br Med J* 1998; **317**: 1554–8.

34. Towner D, Castro M A, Eby-Wilkens E, Gilbert W M. Effect of mode of delivery in nulliparous women on neonatal intracranial injury. *N Engl J Med* 1999; **341**: 1709–14.

35. Bahl R, Patel R R, Swingler R, Ellis N, Murphy D J. Neurodevelopmental outcome at 5 years after operative delivery in the second stage of labor: a cohort study. *Am J Obstet Gynecol* 2007; **197**: 147e1–6.

36. Rodriguez A I, Porter K B, O'Brien W F. Blunt versus sharp expansion of the uterine incision in low-segment transverse cesarean section. *Am J Obstet Gynecol* 1994; **171**: 1022–5.

37. Revah A, Ezra Y, Farine D, Ritchie K. Failed trial of vacuum or forceps – maternal and fetal outcome. *Am J Obstet Gynecol* 1997; **176**: 200–4.

38. Demissie K, Rhoads G G, Smulian J C, *et al.* Operative vaginal delivery and neonatal and infant adverse outcomes: population based retrospective analysis. *Br Med J* 2004; **329**: 24–9.

39. Jolly J, Walker J, Bhabra K. Subsequent obstetric performance related to primary mode of delivery. *Br J Obstet Gynaecol* 1999; **106**: 227–32.

40. Murphy D J, Liebling R. Cohort study of maternal views on future mode of delivery following operative delivery in the second stage of labour. *Am J Obstet Gynecol* 2003; **188**: 542–8.

41. Bahl R, Strachan B, Murphy D J. Outcome of subsequent pregnancy three years after previous operative delivery in the second stage of labour – cohort study. *Br Med J* 2004; **328**: 311–4.

Operative vaginal deliveries: indications, techniques and complications

Stergios K. Doumouchtsis and Sabaratnam Arulkumaran

Introduction

Operative vaginal delivery involves the use of the ventouse (vacuum extractor) or obstetric forceps to facilitate descent of the fetal head along the pelvic curve and delivery of the fetus. Ventouse delivery is performed by traction of the fetal scalp with a suction cup. Forceps cradle the parietal and malar bones of the fetal skull and apply traction, as well as laterally displace maternal tissues.

The incidence of operative vaginal delivery in different countries varies between 10 and 15% [1,2]. Although the incidence has remained unchanged, ventouse has become more popular than forceps. Over the past two decades, in the United Kingdom, the use of forceps has decreased by 50% in favour of vacuum extraction or caesarean section [3]. In the USA, the rate of vacuum delivery exceeded the rate of forceps delivery in 1992 [2,4]. In Canada, forceps delivery has decreased in the last decade from 11.2% in 1991 to 6.8% in 2001 [5].

Although ventouse delivery is associated with a significant reduction of maternal morbidity compared to the use of forceps [6], it has higher failure rates (RR 1.7) [7,8], which is a concern in the light of the risks of sequential instrumentation for delivery [9].

Operative vaginal deliveries are classified by the station of the leading bony point of the fetal head and the degree of rotation of the sagittal suture from the midline. According to the ACOG classification, operative deliveries are classified as *outlet* if the fetal scalp is visible without separating the labia, the sagittal suture is in an antero-posterior diameter or right or left occipito-anterior or posterior position (rotation does not exceed 45°) and the fetal head is at or on the perineum. *Low cavity* deliveries include those where the leading point of the skull is at station $\geq$+2 cm and not on the pelvic floor. This type is further subdivided if the rotation is $\leq$45° or $>$45°. *Mid cavity* deliveries are those with an engaged fetal head but the leading point of the skull is above +2 cm station [10].

Indications

The most common indication is prolonged second stage of labour, which is usually associated with inadequate uterine contractions, poor expulsive maternal efforts and minor disproportion or malposition of the fetal head. The occipito-posterior (OP) and occipito-transverse positions (OT) occur frequently with regional anaesthesia. The tone of the musculature of the pelvic floor is reduced, preventing rotation of the fetal head to the optimal occipito-anterior (OA) position. Regional anaesthesia has also been associated with a longer second stage of labour, increased use of oxytocin and compromised maternal forces resulting in an increased incidence of operative vaginal deliveries [11]. This occurs because the increase in endogenous oxytocin, which occurs as the presenting part descends onto the pelvic floor (Ferguson's reflex), is reduced with epidural anaesthesia, thereby reducing the natural increase of uterine activity in the second stage. Fetal distress or presumed fetal compromise is also a common indication for operative delivery. It may result in hypoxic brain damage or fetal death if no intervention is undertaken.

Maternal indications are most commonly maternal distress or maternal exhaustion. Medically significant conditions are less common indications. These include cardiac disease, cerebral vascular disease, pre-eclampsia, etc. Vaginal birth after previous caesarean section may be a relative indication to minimize the risk of scar rupture if the second stage is likely to be prolonged.

Best Practice in Labour and Delivery, ed. R. Warren and S. Arulkumaran. Published by Cambridge University Press.
© Cambridge University Press 2009.

Contra-indications

Operative vaginal delivery is contra-indicated in fetal malpresentation (e.g. brow, face mento-posterior), unengaged fetal head (fetal head is above the ischial spines or more than one-fifth of the head is palpable abdominally), cephalopelvic disproportion, fetal coagulopathy or bone demineralization disorder. Operative vaginal delivery should not be attempted when the cervix is not fully dilated. Possible exceptions include vacuum delivery (not forceps) for cord prolapse at 9 cm in a multiparous woman or a second twin [1] and situations where the benefits significantly outweigh the risks and there is no viable alternative [5].

The most common relative contra-indications are high presenting part and fetal prematurity. Among premature newborns delivered by vacuum extraction, 14.29% exhibit scalp oedema, 21.43% bone fracture and 21.43% cephalhematoma [12]. The Royal College of Obstetricians and Gynaecologists (RCOG) recommends avoiding the use of ventouse below 34 weeks because of the susceptibility of the preterm fetus to trauma [1].

Forceps may only be applied in vertex presentation, face presentation if the fetal position is mento-anterior and in breech presentation for the delivery of the after-coming head. Unknown position of the fetal head is a contra-indication for both vacuum and forceps delivery due to the increased risks of failure and fetal trauma [13,14]. Vaginal examination during operative delivery fails to identify the correct fetal head position in 25% [15] to 65% [16] of cases. Intrapartum ultrasound may provide objective information on the fetal head station, position, and progress of labour [17], and hence some authors recommend routine performance of abdominal and translabial ultrasound scanning in the labour room [18].

Techniques
Prerequisites

Prior to performing an operative vaginal delivery, the condition of the mother and the fetus and the clinical situation should be thoroughly reviewed. Assessment should be undertaken with the presence of a chaperone. The findings and the procedure that is to follow should be explained to the parturient and her partner. Verbal or written consent should be obtained and documented after detailed counselling about the indication, advantages and disadvantages.

General examination includes condition of the mother, analgesia and hydration. Pudendal block and local perineal infiltration of 1% lignocaine may be adequate for low forceps or ventouse deliveries. For mid cavity operative deliveries and for a trial of operative delivery, epidural or spinal anaesthesia may be more suitable. The condition of the fetus should be evaluated. In cases of cord prolapse, antepartum bleeding or prolonged deceleration, delivery should be expedited and actions should be undertaken without delay.

Abdominal examination is important to assess the size of the fetus, the uterine contractions and the descent of the fetal head in 'fifths' above the pelvic brim. Oxytocin infusion should be considered if the contractions are inadequate (less than 4 in 10 min each lasting >40 s) in the absence of signs of fetal compromise. The bladder should be empty and therefore not abdominally palpable. Otherwise, it should be emptied by catheterization. If the fetus appears large, extra caution should be taken to avoid prolonged traction and to be prepared for possible shoulder dystocia.

Vaginal examination should confirm full dilatation of the cervix and absent membranes. The colour and quantity of amniotic fluid should be noted. The presentation should be vertex. Excess caput (soft tissue swelling) or moulding may be suggestive of cephalopelvic disproportion. The fetal head should be below the ischial spines. Descent of the head with contraction and bearing down effort should be ascertained during vaginal examination. The degree of descent of the leading bony part of the fetal head in relation to the ischial spines can be misleading with vaginal examination alone because of the possible presence of caput and moulding. The accurate assessment of the true descent of the fetal head requires both abdominal and vaginal examination. The vaginal assessment of the exact position of the head and of any degree of asynclitism is also critical and decisive for the correct application of any instrument. When there is synclitism, the parietal eminences are at the same level and indicated by the sagittal suture placed centrally in the pelvis and equal portions of the skull are felt on either side. Other prerequisites include adequate facilities and personnel, antiseptic and aseptic conditions, skilled and experienced operator in the use of the instruments and the management of possible complications and an alternative plan in case of difficulty in delivery, failure to deliver, or any adverse event. The fetal heart rate is continuously monitored during an operative vaginal delivery. Conditions where difficulty or failure are anticipated include one-fifth or more of head palpable abdominally, presenting part at the level of the spines, occipito-posterior position, excessive moulding of the fetal head, fetal macrosomia, dysfunctional or prolonged labour and body mass index >30 [19]. In those cases, a trial of operative vaginal delivery should be performed in the operating theatre under effective epidural or spinal anaesthesia with facilities and personnel available for caesarean section.

Vacuum-assisted deliveries

The vacuum extractor is a device with a suction cup attached with tubing to a vacuum source and a handle, which is used to apply traction to the cup. Traction is applied to the fetal head along the axis of the birth canal. Malmström devised the stainless steel vacuum cup in the 1950s. It has rounded edges and a diameter of 60 mm, with the vacuum tubing and the traction chain attached on the centre of the upper surface of the cup. Bird modified the Malmström vacuum extractor by attaching the vacuum tubing and the traction chain on the side of the cup. This allows the placement of the cup close and anterior to the occiput in occipito-posterior and lateral positions. Kobayashi introduced a single unit silastic cup with a diameter of 65 mm and a stainless steel valve that allows the release of suction between contractions without loss of application of the cup to the head. Kiwi Omnicup (Clinical Innovations Inc., Murray, Utah, USA) is a disposable vacuum extractor with a rigid flat plastic cup and a hand pump-traction system directly applied to the vacuum cup (Figure 9.1). The accurate development of negative pressure can be monitored via an indication gauge on the traction handle. Randomized studies [20] suggest that rigid cups are more likely to result in vaginal birth than soft cups, but they are more likely to cause scalp trauma.

The parturient should be in lithotomy position with adequate analgesia. Prior to cup placement, the fetal presentation, the amount of fetal head in 'fifths' palpable abdominally above the symphysis pubis, the position of the fetal head, and the station should be confirmed. Correct placement of the cup is a major determinant of the outcome. The 'flexion point' is the site on the fetal scalp over which the centre of

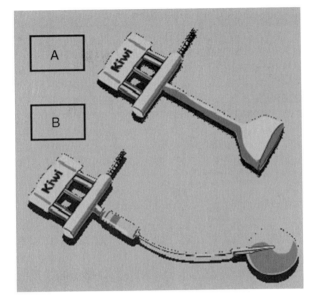

Figure 9.1 Kiwi™ vacuum cup. A: anterior cup (Procup). B: posterior cup (Omnicup)

the vacuum cup should be placed to achieve a flexing median application. This point is on the sagittal suture 3 cm anteriorly to the posterior fontanelle (Figure 9.2). Application of the vacuum cup on this point promotes synclitism and flexion of the fetal head, presenting the optimal diameter of the fetal head (sub-occipito-bregmatic, 9.5 cm) to the maternal pelvis. By incorrect application of the vacuum cup (deflexing and paramedian, Figure 9.3), the fetal head will present with a larger diameter which will increase the difficulty and risk of failure or fetal injury [21,22]. In occipito-lateral or posterior positions, a vacuum cup with the tubing emerging from the lateral aspect (posterior metal cup) or through a groove in the cup (posterior rigid plastic cup – Omnicup) should be used, as it can be inserted between the vaginal wall and the head to reach the flexion point. Soft silk, plastic or anterior metal cups, where the tubing is attached in the centre of the cup, are not suitable for occipito-posterior or lateral positions as the lateral vaginal wall would not permit a cup with the central stem or suction tubing on the dorsum to be shifted to the flexion point. These cups are suitable for occipito-anterior positions as the flexion point is directly accessible.

After the application of the cup to the fetal head and before inducing negative pressure, any maternal tissue entrapment between the cup and the fetal head

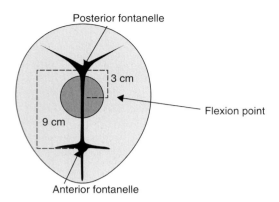

Figure 9.2 The flexion point about 3 cm anterior to the posterior fontanelle along the sagittal suture

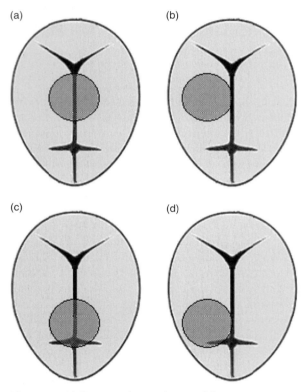

Figure 9.3 (a) Flexing median application of the vacuum cup (correct application). (b–d) Various malapplications of the vacuum cup. (b) Flexing paramedian. (c) Deflexing median. (d) Deflexing paramedian

should be excluded. Apart from causing significant vaginal or cervical trauma and maternal haemorrhage, entrapment of maternal tissue may cause detachment of the cup and failure of the procedure.

Detachment of the cup is associated with increased incidence of cranial fractures (9.58%; RR 2.11) cephalhaematoma (18.56%; RR 1.86) and scalp oedema (26.34%; RR 1.41) [12].

Suction is developed by gradual increments of negative pressure and the fetal scalp is sucked into the hollow of the cup creating an artificial caput (chignon). Effective traction usually requires a negative pressure of at least 0.6 kg/cm^2 (440 mmHg) and usually 0.8 kg/cm^2 (588 mmHg). Higher pressures are associated with increased risk of fetal head injury. The traction force indicators of the vacuum devices should be checked throughout the delivery as attention to the force and duration may help to reduce the incidence of fetal injuries [23]. Traction should be in line with the axis of the pelvis, perpendicularly to the plane of the vacuum cup and co-ordinated with maternal expulsive efforts. Descent must be observed with the initial traction effort. If the cup is dislodged, the reason for the 'pop-off' should be evaluated, and if there are no contra-indications it can be reapplied after careful inspection of the fetal scalp for injury. There is no consensus on the maximum number of traction attempts, the duration of a vacuum application, or the number of 'pop-offs' that should be allowed. Vacca suggests that the traction force should not exceed 11.5 kg, the duration of the procedure should be restricted to 15 min and the number of pulls limited to three for the descent phase and three for the perineal phase [24]. A traction force exceeding 13.5 kg is associated with an increased risk of fetal scalp injury [24]. Higher levels of traction force and a greater number of pulls may, however, be required during the outlet phase of the vacuum delivery as resistance is greatest at this stage. For this reason, additional time and pulls should be allowed for the perineum to stretch over the head, especially if the birth is managed without episiotomy [24].

The traction force is less when the head descends with the cup during traction compared with a situation when the head does not descend with traction. Hence additional pulls with descent are less likely to be harmful compared with traction on a head that does not descend with three pulls. The RCOG guidelines recommend that 'operative vaginal delivery should be abandoned where there is no evidence of progressive descent with each pull or where delivery is not imminent following three pulls of a correctly applied instrument by an experienced operator' [1]. The SOGC guidelines advise that if delivery has not occurred after four contractions the intended method of delivery should be reassessed [5]. With efficient uterine contractions and good maternal expulsive efforts almost all vacuum-assisted deliveries should be completed within 15 min. If a 20-min limit is exceeded, the procedure should be abandoned unless delivery is imminent [13]. The procedure should also be abandoned if there is evidence of fetal scalp trauma.

Forceps deliveries

Forceps are a paired instrument with a handle, shank, lock and blade. The blades have a cephalic and a pelvic curve between the heel and toes (at the distal end) and are attached to each other by a lock on the shank. There are over 700 different types of forceps. They are grouped in two major categories: classical and special. Classical forceps were originally designed by Sir James Y. Simpson (1848) and George Elliot (1858). This group includes the Simpson, Luikart–Simpson, Elliot, Neville–Barnes, Chamberlain, DeLee, Anderson, Tucker–McLane, Wrigley and Naegle forceps. Simpson forceps have a spread shank and a long cephalic curve. Elliot forceps have overlapping shanks and a shorter cephalic curve. In Luikart–Simpson forceps the blade is pseudofenestrated and in Tucker–McLane forceps it is solid.

The special forceps include the Kielland's forceps designed for correction of malposition and asynclitism and for rotational deliveries; the Barton forceps for transverse arrest in a flat pelvis; and the Piper forceps for the delivery of the after-coming head in breech presentations.

The mechanism of action of forceps includes correction of deflexion, asynclitism, or positional abnormalities of the fetal head, extraction by assisting or replacing the maternal expulsive forces, reduction of the friction between the fetal head and the birth canal, and transient reduction of the resistance of the outlet by enlargement of the soft tissue of the birth canal. The cephalic curve grasps the fetal head over the maxilla or malar eminences while the length of the blade grasps the sides of the head from the malar area along the side of the head in front of the ear and the parietal bones in front of the occiput. This bimalar–biparietal application exerts uniform pressure on the head. In this position the shank is over the flexion point, allowing the correct direction of traction. The pelvic curve fits the pelvis and is minimal in those forceps used for rotation, e.g. Kielland's forceps.

The choice of the type of forceps depends on the indication and the clinical situation, the preferences of the obstetrician and the availability of instruments. For occipito-anterior positions in the mid or low cavity or low direct occipito-posterior positions, the Neville–Barnes with or without axis traction handle or the Simpson's forceps can be used. Wrigley's forceps is ideal for outlet deliveries. If the position is occipito-lateral or posterior Kielland's forceps can achieve rotation without inflicting trauma to the fetus or the maternal passages. Non-fenestrated blades are indicated in cases with oedematous soft maternal tissues to minimize risk of tearing. Face presentation with mento-anterior position can be delivered using Kielland's or Simpson forceps.

Proper application of the forceps to the fetal head is extremely important for a safe procedure with a successful outcome. The exact location of the sagittal suture and posterior fontanelle should be ascertained. The arrangement of the blades should be rehearsed prior to insertion. The forceps blades should be applied gently between contractions. The left blade is applied first to the left side of the maternal pelvis using the left hand, whilst the right hand guides and protects the head and the vagina. The right blade is applied to the right side of the maternal pelvis using the right hand. No force should be required. If there is resistance the blade should be removed and reapplied. The blades are correctly placed when they are situated in the spaces between the fetal orbits and ears and this will be reflected by the shanks and handles being horizontal and there is easy locking of the blades. When the blades are locked and prior to applying traction the obstetrician should confirm correct application by ensuring that the forceps have not inadvertently penetrated the lateral vaginal walls, the sagittal suture is symmetrically and perpendicularly in the midline between the two shanks, the occiput is 3–4 cm above the shanks (so that the traction line is along the flexion point, thus promoting flexion and exposing the minimal diameter) and the space between the heel of the blade and the head does not admit more than a finger breadth (ensures synclitism).

Once the forceps have been applied and the position of the blades checked, traction should be co-ordinated with maternal contractions. The axis of the traction forces should follow the pelvic curve (curve of Carus). The traction is initially downward and as the head descends in the birth canal, the angle moves forward and upward at the outlet. The Pajot manoeuvre involves the combined exertion of outward and downward forces, which produce a vector that follows the pelvic curve. Traction should be released between contractions in order to reduce the intracranial pressure and the associated vagally induced bradycardia. An episiotomy is usually indicated when the head is crowning at the perineum.

Delivery in malposition of the fetal head

Occipito-transverse (OT) position of the fetal head results in a deep transverse arrest and cephalopelvic disproportion. The delivery options include digital or manual rotation, autorotation with traction using a ventouse, rotation with forceps or caesarean section. In a digital rotation the index and middle fingers are placed onto the part of the anterior parietal bone that overlaps the occipital bone in the area of the posterior fontanelle and gentle pressure is applied with the tips of the fingers to rotate the posterior fontanelle upward and toward the symphysis pubis. In a manual rotation, rotational pressure is applied by the hand under the posterior parietal bone and the thumb on the anterior parietal bone. When a ventouse is used, rotation should only be achieved by traction and not by twisting or rotational motions of the vacuum cup. By applying traction in the correct direction, flexion and asynclitism of the head can be corrected and autorotation occurs as the head descends by virtue of the anatomy of the pelvis. The use of a rotational motion should be avoided as the shearing forces on the fetal head may result in scalp injury especially with the use of a metal cup. Rotation of the fetal head can be attempted using special rotational forceps (Kielland's). Before Kielland's forceps are used, it is essential to identify abdominally the side of the baby's back and the occiput on vaginal examination. The forceps are applied with the 'knobs' facing towards the baby's occiput. The anterior or posterior blade may be applied first directly depending on the preference of the obstetrician. The anterior blade can be positioned by direct, reverse, or classical and wandering method. In the wandering method the anterior blade is placed over the face and then moved to lie on the side of the fetal head. The posterior blade can be applied directly. The blades are locked and asynclitism corrected by sliding the shanks on each other until the sliding locks come to the same level. If there is no asynclitism the sagittal suture of the fetus will lie

equidistant from the two blades of the forceps. If the blades cannot be locked easily, their position should be checked and they should be removed and reinserted.

An abnormal position (e.g. occipito-transverse) is corrected by rotating the handles of the forceps blades and directing the fetal occiput to the anterior position to emerge underneath the symphysis pubis. The risk of injury can be minimized by avoiding excessive torsion during rotation, rotation in the wrong direction, forceful rotation or combined rotation with traction. In a rotational delivery the movements of traction and rotation should always be separate unless rotation occurs spontaneously with traction. Rotation should be avoided during a uterine contraction [25].

Complications
Maternal injuries

Maternal complications of operative vaginal deliveries are usually those of soft tissue trauma. Although operative delivery has been associated with a higher incidence of maternal injuries compared to spontaneous vaginal deliveries, most of the complications of an operative vaginal delivery can occur after a spontaneous vaginal delivery. Vaginal, cervical, labial, periurethral lacerations, pelvic haematomas, perineal injuries, episiotomy extension and the associated haemorrhage are the most common complications. Severe maternal morbidity is increased after operative vaginal deliveries [26] and maternal deaths from traumatic operative delivery have been reported [14].

Maternal injury is less frequent and less extensive with the use of vacuum compared to forceps [8,27,28]. Maternal complications of vacuum delivery include cervical lacerations, severe vaginal lacerations, periurethral lacerations, vaginal haematomas, and third- and fourth-degree tears [8]. The use of forceps has been associated with a higher rate of episiotomies and third- and fourth-degree perineal and vaginal tears [29].

The most common vaginal lacerations are the posterior midline tears or the anterior periurethral tears. Inadvertent entrapment of the cervix or the vaginal wall with consequent lacerations can occur during an operative delivery. Posterior tears should be repaired if they involve more than the vaginal mucosa. Anterior labial and periurethral tears do not usually require repair unless they are bleeding. Injury to the bladder or the urethra may cause urinary retention secondary to oedema or haematoma and late fistula formation. Insertion of a Foley's catheter is advisable if the tear is close to the urethra. Vaginal lacerations may extend into the ischiorectal fossae.

A third- or fourth-degree perineal tear with anal sphincter injury is a potentially severe complication of vaginal delivery, which may result in anal incontinence and rectovaginal fistula formation. A third-degree perineal tear and altered faecal continence occurs more frequently after forceps than vacuum deliveries [30] and in occipito-posterior positions [31,32]. The incidence of third- or fourth-degree perineal tears with forceps-assisted delivery can be as high as 31% and 17% with the use of vacuum, respectively. This rate is significantly higher than at an unassisted delivery [28]. However, normal vaginal delivery without evidence of sphincter injury is also associated with significant effect on anal sphincter function [33]. Anal incontinence can occur regardless of the mode of delivery [34].

Trauma to the pelvic floor musculature and its innervation as a result of forceps and vacuum delivery may contribute to the occurrence of urinary incontinence [35]. Arya et al. found that in primiparous women, urinary incontinence after forceps delivery is more likely to persist compared with spontaneous vaginal or vacuum delivery [36]. Liebling et al. studied the symptoms of pelvic floor morbidity after difficult operative vaginal deliveries and caesarean sections during the second stage of labour, and concluded that although a caesarean section does not completely protect women from pelvic floor morbidity, operative vaginal delivery was associated with a greater prevalence of urinary symptoms and dyspareunia for up to a year after delivery [37].

Psychological morbidity is also important. Operative vaginal delivery can be associated with fear of subsequent childbirth which may be as severe as a post-traumatic stress type syndrome termed 'tokophobia'.

Fetal injuries
Scalp bruises and lacerations

Fetal scalp injuries occur in most operative vaginal deliveries. They are usually transient and of no clinical significance. The more significant injuries are related to wrong application of the instrument, excessive or incorrectly directed traction, or cephalopelvic disproportion.

During application of the vacuum cup on the fetal head a collection of interstitial fluid and microhaemorrhages (chignon) fill the internal diameter of the vacuum cup in a 'key-in-lock' fashion. This is less pronounced when using soft cups, and resolves within 12–18 h. The incidence of scalp abrasions and lacerations after vacuum extraction is 10%. The incidence of scalp abrasions is higher in infants delivered by Kiwi Omnicup vacuum (Clinical Innovations Inc., Murray, Utah, USA) or metal cup devices compared to those delivered by silastic cup [38]. Correct cup placement and traction, and avoidance of cup detachments ('pop-offs') reduces the risk of scalp injuries [13].

Cephalhaematoma

Cephalhaematoma is secondary to rupture of blood vessels between the skull and the periosteum. It is delineated by the suture lines and thus can be differentiated from subgaleal haemorrhage. As the capacity of the subperiosteal space is limited, these haematomas are small. Cephalhaematoma occurs in 1–2% of spontaneous vaginal deliveries, in 6–10% of vacuum extractions (range 1–26%) [8,12,20,21] and in 4% of forceps deliveries [8]. Vacuum extraction therefore has a stronger association with cephalhaematoma compared with forceps (odds ratio: 2.38) [8]. Metal cups are more likely to cause cephalhaematoma than silastic cups or the Omnicup [39]. Vacuum extractions at mid or low station are associated with a higher incidence of cephalhaematoma (13.11% and 13.56%) when compared with vacuum applied at the outlet (6.81%; RR 1.92; RR 1.99) [12].

Subgaleal haemorrhage and cranial trauma

Subgaleal, also known as subaponeurotic, haemorrhage develops between the skull periosteum and the galea aponeurotica. This space has a capacity of up to 260 ml in term infants. The pathogenesis includes avulsion of the aponeurosis from the cranium and haemorrhage caused by traction forces during operative delivery, skull fracture or rupture of an interosseous synchondrosis. Subgaleal haemorrhage with a loss of 20–40% of the circulating blood volume will result in hypovolaemic shock, disseminated intravascular coagulation, multi-organ failure and neonatal death in up to 25% of cases.

Vacuum extraction (OR = 7.17; 95% CI: 5.43–10.25) and forceps delivery (OR = 2.66; 95% CI: 1.78–5.18) are risk factors for subgaleal haemorrhage [40]. The incidence after spontaneous vaginal deliveries is 4 per 10,000 [41] and ranges between 0 and 21% following vacuum extractions [12,22,41]. Maternal nulliparity, placement of vacuum cup over the sagittal suture close to infant's anterior fontanelle and failed vacuum extraction predispose to subgaleal haemorrhage [22].

Skull fractures can be caused by compression from forceps blades or from the skull pushing against the maternal bony pelvis and are usually linear, affecting the parietal bones, or depressed, forming the so-called 'ping-pong ball-type' fracture. A skull fracture must be suspected in any cephalhaematoma or subarachnoid haemorrhage. A registry of neonatal deaths attributable to intrapartum trauma revealed that cranial injury was almost always associated with physical difficulty at delivery, the use of instruments, poor judgement and persistence in continuing with the operative vaginal delivery in the presence of failure to progress or signs of fetal compromise [42].

Intracranial trauma

Intracranial haemorrhage occurs in approximately 5–6 per 10,000 live births and can be potentially fatal or cause lifelong disability. Forceps and vacuum delivery, precipitous delivery, prolonged second stage of labour, and macrosomia are recognized risk factors. Caesarean section after a failed attempt of operative vaginal delivery and the sequential use of vacuum and forceps are additional risk factors.

Epidural haemorrhage is a blood collection between a calvarial bone and its inner periosteum or between the periosteal membrane and the underlying outer dura fibrous stratum [43]. It is usually a result of injury to the middle meningeal artery, and is frequently associated with a cephalhaematoma or skull fracture. In neonates, the meningeal arteries are not embedded in the cranial bones and they are therefore less susceptible to injury. This probably explains the rarity of epidural haemorrhage in neonates, which accounts for approximately 2% of all cases of intracranial haemorrhage [44]. It is associated with difficult parturition and operative delivery in nulliparous women. It typically results from the mechanical forces exerted on the fetal head with or without the use of instruments. During labour an increased degree of moulding leading to excessive displacement of the skull bones may cause considerable injury to the dura matter.

Subdural haemorrhage is associated with mechanical compression and distortion of the fetal cranium,

tearing of veins and venous sinuses, and bleeding into the subdural space. The incidence is 2.9 per 10,000 after spontaneous delivery, 4.1 per 10,000 after caesarean section without labour, 8.0 per 10,000 after vacuum delivery, 9.8 per 10,000 after forceps delivery, 25.7 per 10,000 after caesarean section following failed instrumental vaginal delivery and 21.3 per 10,000 after combined vacuum and forceps delivery [9]. Subdural haematomas can also occur antenatally in utero and after uncomplicated vaginal deliveries.

Subarachnoid haemorrhage is most frequently caused by rupture of the small bridging vessels of the leptomeninges. The incidence of subarachnoid haemorrhage after spontaneous vaginal delivery is 0.1–1.3 per 10,000, after vacuum extraction 0.6–2.2 per 10,000, after forceps delivery 0.1–3.3 per 10,000 and after combined vacuum and forceps delivery 10.7 per 10,000 [9,28].

Nerve injury

The incidence of brachial plexus injury ranges from 0.13 to 3.6 per 1000 births. Risk factors include macrosomia, shoulder dystocia, operative deliveries, and malpresentation. Studies have shown that the risk of brachial plexus injury is higher in forceps deliveries than vacuum extractions [9,45], although other studies have shown that the risk between the two modes of delivery is similar [28]. There are three types of brachial plexus injury: injury to the upper plexus (C5–C7, Erb's palsy) accounts for approximately 90% of cases. Injury to C8–T1 (Klumpke's palsy) accounts for less than 1% of brachial plexus injury and injury to the entire plexus (approximately 10% of cases) results in a flaccid extremity with absent reflexes. The pathogenesis of injury often involves stretch injury when shoulder dystocia requires extreme lateral flexion and traction of the head. However, there are reports of injury that occurs when lateral flexion and traction of the head has not been applied, such as during precipitous deliveries or when there is injury to the posterior shoulder.

Facial nerve palsy is a rare complication of forceps deliveries with an incidence rate of 2.9–5 per 1000 forceps deliveries. However, one-third of facial nerve injuries occur in spontaneous delivery.

Laryngeal nerve injury causes vocal fold paralysis; 5–26% of congenital vocal fold paralysis is due to birth trauma. Forceps deliveries have been associated with an increased incidence.

Upper cervical spinal cord injury is estimated to complicate approximately 1 in 80,000 deliveries [46]. High cervical injuries are associated most often with forceps rotation of 90° or more from occipito-posterior or occipito-transverse position. Menticoglou *et al.* reported an incidence of spinal cord injury of approximately 0.7 per 1000 and suggested that these injuries are the result of 'unphysiological torsional forces' [25]. The injury is caused by longitudinal traction or rotation of the cord.

Retinal haemorrhage occurs more commonly in infants delivered by vacuum, compared to spontaneous deliveries or forceps-assisted deliveries [47,48]. However, the haemorrhage is transient with no apparent long-term developmental or any ophthalmological consequences.

Choice of instrument

The choice of forceps or vacuum should depend on the operator's experience, station, and the position of the fetal head. The instruments should be checked prior to application to ensure that the vacuum device is working and that the forceps blades match. There should be a willingness to abandon an operative delivery if there is difficulty in applying the instrument, if there is no appreciable descent with each pull, and if descent is not significant following three pulls of a correctly applied instrument and the baby has not been delivered after 15–20 min [14].

When one instrument has failed to effect delivery, sequential use of instruments offers the advantage of avoiding the complications of caesarean section at full dilatation with a low head, but increases the risks of fetal trauma [49,50]. Appropriate case selection, with careful decision-making, is of paramount importance. If the head has descended to the introitus, a sequential operative delivery is less likely to cause harm compared with the use of a second instrument when there is no or minimal descent.

Training

Adequate clinical experience and training are essential for the safe performance of operative deliveries and result in a significant decrease in maternal and neonatal morbidity. Experienced obstetricians demonstrate a higher level of competence with forceps manoeuvres than junior doctors. The decrease in number of forceps deliveries and increasing litigation has an impact on residents' training opportunities.

Vacuum delivery is perceived to be easier to learn than forceps; however, incorrect use of this device may result in increased failure rates and complications. Obstetric simulators have been designed to facilitate training and assessment of competencies of performing the manoeuvres. Traction force training using computer-assisted visual feedback can be useful in training practitioners to produce appropriate traction forces during obstetric forceps deliveries. The Royal College of Obstetricians and Gynaecologists recommends that the choice of the instrument should be appropriate to the clinical circumstances and the operator's skills, and only practitioners who are adequately trained, or who are under the supervision of trained practitioners, should undertake operative delivery [1].

References

1. Royal College of Obstetricians and Gynaecologists. *Operative Vaginal Delivery. Guideline No. 26.* Clinical green top guidelines. London: RCOG, 2005.

2. Kozak L J, Weeks J D. U.S. trends in obstetric procedures, 1990–2000. *Birth* 2002; **29**: 157–61.

3. Patel R R, Murphy D J. Forceps delivery in modern obstetric practice. *Br Med J* 2004; **328**: 1302–5.

4. Miksovsky P, Watson W J. Obstetric vacuum extraction: state of the art in the new millennium. *Obstet Gynecol Surv* 2001; **56**: 736–51.

5. Society of Obstetricians and Gynaecologists of Canada. Guidelines for operative vaginal birth. *J Obstet Gynaecol Can* 2004; **26**: 747–53.

6. Chalmers J A, Chalmers I. The obstetric vacuum extractor is the instrument of first choice for operative vaginal delivery. *Br J Obstet Gynaecol* 1989; **96**: 505–6.

7. Ben-Haroush A, Melamed N, Kaplan B, Yogev Y. Predictors of failed operative vaginal delivery: a single-center experience. *Am J Obstet Gynecol* 2007; **197**: 308e301–5.

8. Johanson R B, Menon B K. Vacuum extraction versus forceps for assisted vaginal delivery. *Cochrane Database Syst Rev* 2000; CD000224.

9. Towner D, Castro M A, Eby-Wilkens E, Gilbert W M. Effect of mode of delivery in nulliparous women on neonatal intracranial injury. *N Engl J Med* 1999; **341**: 1709–14.

10. American College of Obstetricians and Gynecologists. *Operative Vaginal Delivery.* Washington, DC: ACOG, 2000.

11. NICE. *Intrapartum Care. Care of Healthy Women and their Babies during Childbirth. Clinical Guideline.*

London: National Institute for Health and Clinical Excellence, 2007.

12. Simonson C, Barlow P, Dehennin N, *et al.* Neonatal complications of vacuum-assisted delivery. *Obstet Gynecol* 2007; **109**: 626–33.

13. McQuivey R W. Vacuum-assisted delivery: a review. *J Matern Fetal Neonatal Med* 2004; **16**: 171–80.

14. Edozien L C. Towards safe practice in instrumental vaginal delivery. *Best Pract Res Clin Obstet Gynaecol* 2007; **21**: 639–55.

15. Akmal S, Kametas N, Tsoi E, Hargreaves C, Nicolaides K H. Comparison of transvaginal digital examination with intrapartum sonography to determine fetal head position before instrumental delivery. *Ultrasound Obstet Gynecol* 2003; **21**: 437–40.

16. Sherer D M, Miodovnik M, Bradley K S, Langer O. Intrapartum fetal head position II: comparison between transvaginal digital examination and transabdominal ultrasound assessment during the second stage of labor. *Ultrasound Obstet Gynecol* 2002; **19**: 264–8.

17. Henrich W, Dudenhausen J, Fuchs I, Kamena A, Tutschek B. Intrapartum translabial ultrasound (ITU): sonographic landmarks and correlation with successful vacuum extraction. *Ultrasound Obstet Gynecol* 2006; **28**: 753–60.

18. Zahalka N, Sadan O, Malinger G, *et al.* Comparison of transvaginal sonography with digital examination and transabdominal sonography for the determination of fetal head position in the second stage of labor. *Am J Obstet Gynecol* 2005; **193**: 381–6.

19. Murphy D J, Liebling R E, Verity L, Swingler R, Patel R. Early maternal and neonatal morbidity associated with operative delivery in second stage of labour: a cohort study. *Lancet* 2001; **358**: 1203–7.

20. Johanson R, Menon V. Soft versus rigid vacuum extractor cups for assisted vaginal delivery. *Cochrane Database Syst Rev* 2000: CD000446.

21. Vacca A. Vacuum-assisted delivery. *Best Pract Res Clin Obstet Gynaecol* 2002; **16**: 17–30.

22. Boo N Y, Foong K W, Mahdy Z A, Yong S C, Jaafar R. Risk factors associated with subaponeurotic haemorrhage in full-term infants exposed to vacuum extraction. *Br J Obstet Gynaecol* 2005; **112**: 1516–21.

23. Whitlow B J, Tamizian O, Ashworth J, *et al.* Validation of traction force indicator in ventouse devices. *Int J Gynaecol Obstet* 2005; **90**: 35–8.

24. Vacca A. Vacuum-assisted delivery: an analysis of traction force and maternal and neonatal outcomes. *Aust NZ J Obstet Gynaecol* 2006; **46**: 124–7.

25. Menticoglou S M, Perlman M, Manning F A. High cervical spinal cord injury in neonates delivered with forceps: report of 15 cases. *Obstet Gynecol* 1995; **86**: 589–94.

26. Pallasmaa N, Ekblad U, Gissler M. Severe maternal morbidity and the mode of delivery. *Acta Obstet Gynecol Scand* 2008; **87**: 662–8.

27. Johanson R B, Rice C, Doyle M, *et al.* A randomised prospective study comparing the new vacuum extractor policy with forceps delivery. *Br J Obstet Gynaecol* 1993; **100**: 524–30.

28. Wen S W, Liu S, Kramer M S, *et al.* Comparison of maternal and infant outcomes between vacuum extraction and forceps deliveries. *Am J Epidemiol* 2001; **153**: 103–7.

29. Johnson J H, Figueroa R, Garry D, Elimian A, Maulik D. Immediate maternal and neonatal effects of forceps and vacuum-assisted deliveries. *Obstet Gynecol* 2004; **103**: 513–8.

30. Harkin R, Fitzpatrick M, O'Connell P R, O'Herlihy C. Anal sphincter disruption at vaginal delivery: is recurrence predictable? *Eur J Obstet Gynecol Reprod Biol* 2003; **109**: 149–52.

31. Damron D P, Capeless E L. Operative vaginal delivery: a comparison of forceps and vacuum for success rate and risk of rectal sphincter injury. *Am J Obstet Gynecol* 2004; **191**: 907–10.

32. Wu J M, Williams K S, Hundley A F, Connolly A, Visco A G. Occiput posterior fetal head position increases the risk of anal sphincter injury in vacuum-assisted deliveries. *Am J Obstet Gynecol* 2005; **193**: 525–8; discussion 528–9.

33. Rieger N, Schloithe A, Saccone G, Wattchow D. The effect of a normal vaginal delivery on anal function. *Acta Obstet Gynecol Scand* 1997; **76**: 769–72.

34. Nygaard I E, Rao S S, Dawson J D. Anal incontinence after anal sphincter disruption: a 30-year retrospective cohort study. *Obstet Gynecol* 1997; **89**: 896–901.

35. Dimpfl T, Hesse U, Schussler B. Incidence and cause of postpartum urinary stress incontinence. *Eur J Obstet Gynecol Reprod Biol* 1992; **43**: 29–33.

36. Arya L A, Jackson N D, Myers D L, Verma A. Risk of new-onset urinary incontinence after forceps and vacuum delivery in primiparous women. *Am J Obstet Gynecol* 2001; **185**: 1318–23; discussion 1323–4.

37. Liebling R E, Swingler R, Patel R R, *et al.* Pelvic floor morbidity up to one year after difficult instrumental delivery and cesarean section in the second stage of labor: a cohort study. *Am J Obstet Gynecol* 2004; **191**: 4–10.

38. Hayman R, Gilby J, Arulkumaran S. Clinical evaluation of a "hand pump" vacuum delivery device. *Obstet Gynecol* 2002; **100**: 1190–5.

39. Attilakos G, Sibanda T, Winter C, Johnson N, Draycott T. A randomised controlled trial of a new handheld vacuum extraction device. *Br J Obstet Gynaecol* 2005; **112**: 1510–15.

40. Gebremariam A. Subgaleal haemorrhage: risk factors and neurological and developmental outcome in survivors. *Ann Trop Paediatr* 1999; **19**: 45–50.

41. Uchil D, Arulkumaran S. Neonatal subgaleal hemorrhage and its relationship to delivery by vacuum extraction. *Obstet Gynecol Surv* 2003; **58**: 687–93.

42. O'Mahony F, Settatree R, Platt C, Johanson R. Review of singleton fetal and neonatal deaths associated with cranial trauma and cephalic delivery during a national intrapartum-related confidential enquiry. *Br J Obstet Gynaecol* 2005; **112**: 619–26.

43. Doumouchtsis S K, Arulkumaran S. Head injuries after instrumental vaginal deliveries. *Curr Opin Obstet Gynecol* 2006; **18**: 129–34.

44. Perlman J M. Brain injury in the term infant. *Semin Perinatol* 2004; **28**: 415–24.

45. Gilbert W M, Nesbitt T S, Danielsen B. Associated factors in 1611 cases of brachial plexus injury. *Obstet Gynecol* 1999; **93**: 536–40.

46. Mills J F, Dargaville P A, Coleman L T, Rosenfeld J V, Ekert P G. Upper cervical spinal cord injury in neonates: the use of magnetic resonance imaging. *J Pediatr* 2001; **138**: 105–8.

47. Berkus M D, Ramamurthy R S, O'Connor P S, Brown K, Hayashi R H. Cohort study of silastic obstetric vacuum cup deliveries: I. Safety of the instrument. *Obstet Gynecol* 1985; **66**: 503–9.

48. Williams M C, Knuppel R A, O'Brien W F, *et al.* Obstetric correlates of neonatal retinal hemorrhage. *Obstet Gynecol* 1993; **81**: 688–94.

49. Sadan O, Ginath S, Gomel A, *et al.* What to do after a failed attempt of vacuum delivery? *Eur J Obstet Gynecol Reprod Biol* 2003; **107**: 151–5.

50. Gardella C, Taylor M, Benedetti T, Hitti J, Critchlow C. The effect of sequential use of vacuum and forceps for assisted vaginal delivery on neonatal and maternal outcomes. *Am J Obstet Gynecol* 2001; **185**: 896–902.

Caesarean deliveries: indications, techniques and complications

Lisa Story and Sara Paterson-Brown

Introduction

Caesarean section (CS) is one of the most frequently performed surgical procedures in the United Kingdom, with almost a quarter of babies being delivered in this manner [1]. It is performed when it is perceived to be a safer method of delivery for the mother and/or the baby than delivery by the vaginal route. CS is being conducted increasingly frequently, drawing critical attention to where its rightful place should be, as unnecessary medicalization of childbirth is not without complication.

Junior doctors' hours have been dramatically reduced, as has their time in training, and this has led to major changes in day-to-day workings. Surgical technique for CS is learnt largely through an apprenticeship scheme of training, but this is becoming challenged by the breakdown in the 'team' structure of working. The newly introduced structured appraisals may help, but this chapter will try to address the standard surgical principles involved with CS, and also detail techniques to help avoid problems as well as how to overcome them.

Classification of CS and ITS indications

The traditional classification of CS as elective or emergency is too simplistic, making detailed comparisons impossible, and distinguishing between prelabour CS (which may be elective or emergency) and intrapartum CS (which are, by definition, emergency) is preferable. Furthermore, classifying the urgency of the procedure has been investigated [2], and the most consistent method recommended by the NCEPOD [3] and endorsed by the RCOG and RCA is detailed in Table 10.1. Thus prelabour CS could be any of the four categories of urgency, whilst intrapartum CS will only involve categories 1 and 2.

There are numerous indications for CS, but they can broadly be divided into those due to maternal and/or fetal factors. For ease of reference these are outlined in Table 10.2. The list is not exhaustive, but attempts to be structured and logical.

Procedure and surgical techniques
Pre-operative

All operations start with a decision to operate which involves discussion with the patient, appropriate consent, and then pre-operative preparation. The discussion should balance the pros and cons of the proposed CS with those of not doing it, and if CS is declined or refused (this distinction depends on the strength of the obstetrician's recommendations), such discussion should be clearly documented and, if possible, signed by the patient (similar documentation for Jehovah's Witnesses is more familiar to obstetricians, but the principles are the same). The promotion of 'patient choice' can be misinterpreted and risks the obstetrician standing back and not making their views clear: this passive role should be resisted, expert opinion and advice must be given, and the patient can then choose whether to follow it or not.

Consent

Informed consent should be obtained in a manner which clearly explains the reasons why CS is needed and the associated risks, distinguishing between those risks which are frequently occurring and those which may be unlikely but serious. The importance of good communication is essential and has been highlighted in the report *Safer Childbirth*. This not only encompasses communication with the patient, particularly those who are more vulnerable (for example, those

Best Practice in Labour and Delivery, ed. R. Warren and S. Arulkumaran. Published by Cambridge University Press.
© Cambridge University Press 2009.

Table 10.1 Classification of urgency of caesarean section.

Category	Indication
1	*Immediate threat to the life of the woman or fetus*
	e.g. for prelabour CS – abruption
	e.g. for intrapartum CS – uterine rupture
2	*Maternal or fetal compromise which was not immediately life-threatening*
	e.g. for prelabour CS – three previous CS with ruptured membranes and meconium-stained liquor
	e.g. for intrapartum CS – non-reassuring CTG when fetal blood sampling is not possible or contra-indicated
3	*No maternal or fetal compromise but needs early delivery*
	e.g. severe pre-eclampsia after waiting for steroids to work
4	*Delivery timed to suit the woman and staff*
	e.g. previous CS with fibroids and breech presentation at term

patients whose first language is not English, or those with social problems), but also communication within the team of health professionals [8]. Table 10.3 lists the serious risks highlighted in the RCOG guidelines for consent for CS [9].

Other significant risks include thromboembolic phenomena and sepsis, and may also include damage to the bowel, especially if there has been previous surgery. The increased risk of subsequent problems including repeat CS in future pregnancies should also be mentioned [9].

Timing of caesarean section

It is recommended that elective caesarean sections are conducted after 39 completed weeks: this optimizes fetal maturity (neonatal respiratory morbidity is half that at 38 weeks, i.e. less than 2%) while pre-empting spontaneous labour (risk approximately 10%) [10].

Blood tests/products

All women should have their haemoglobin checked prior to the procedure. Whilst routine group and saving/cross-matching of blood is not necessary, certain clinical situations may necessitate this; for example, if blood loss is anticipated to be excessive, if the woman is anaemic prior to the start of the procedure, if atypical antibodies are known to be present, or if local arrangements require this preparation.

In very high-risk cases, such as placenta praevia or suspected accreta, other pre-operative measures should also be considered: a senior obstetrician and anaesthetist should be present at the time of the operation; it may be wise to involve interventional radiologists; and a cell saver may be made available. Most importantly, the woman should have been fully counselled and consented for the different treatment options including the possibility of hysterectomy in selective cases. Adequate protocols should be present on every delivery suite for the event of massive obstetric haemorrhage.

Anaesthetic

All patients should be reviewed by the anaesthetist prior to surgery, and women who are at high risk of anaesthetic complications should have been highlighted and already seen in the antenatal period. The form of anaesthetic to be used will be discussed and decided on by the anaesthetist who is also responsible for discussing all anaesthetic risks and complications.

Intraoperative procedures

Patient preparation

The patient should be positioned supine with a left lateral tilt to minimize inferior vena cava compression by the gravid uterus, avoiding both maternal hypotension and subsequent reduced placental perfusion and fetal hypoxia. The bladder should be emptied with an indwelling catheter to minimize the risk of bladder injury intraoperatively, and to prevent over-distension of the bladder and urinary retention post-operatively. The abdomen should be cleaned and draped in a sterile manner, and if early skin–skin contact is planned the necessary adjustments should be made to the mother's clothing in advance of surgery to enable it.

Surgical principles

All surgery should be conducted using adequate but not excessive access with gentle handling of and respect to tissues and meticulous attention to haemostasis. Anatomical knowledge should be sound in order to avoid inadvertent damage, especially when pathology is encountered.

Table 10.2 Indications for caesarean section.

Pre-Labour			
Maternal	Surgical	Previous uterine surgery	Scar dehiscence is a significant risk associated with labouring with a scarred uterus following previous myomectomy, classical CS or more than two previous lower segment incisions. In the case of one previous lower segment incision there is an estimated 0.5% risk of scar rupture and maternal preference will influence the mode of delivery.
		Ovarian cyst	If a large ovarian cyst is present obstructing the pelvis, a CS will not only facilitate delivery of the baby but allow surgical treatment of the ovarian pathology.
		Previous anal sphincter damage	The risk of developing worsening faecal incontinence following previous sphincter damage may occur with a subsequent vaginal delivery. Women who are symptomatic or who have an abnormal endoanal ultrasound or manometry should be given the option of an elective caesarean section.
	Medical	Maternal disease	Certain maternal diseases may necessitate a CS such as Marfans disease with a dilated aortic root.
	Psychological	Maternal request	The reasons why the woman wishes to have a CS should be explored. The risks and benefits of the procedure and of planned labour and delivery should be explained in order to ensure the woman has made a fully informed decision. NICE guidelines suggest referring women for counselling should they describe a fear of childbirth and also state that a clinician has the right to refuse to perform a CS on grounds of maternal request alone [4].
Fetal	Mechanical	Breech	External cephalic version should be offered to women with a breech baby, but where this is unsuccessful or contra-indicated a CS may be indicated. The results of the Term Breech Trial indicate an improved short-term outcome for delivery of breech fetuses by caesarean section [5].
		Transverse lie	The cause of a transverse lie should always be assessed, as it may influence management and surgical access; for example, if it is due to placenta praevia or uterine or cervical fibroids.
	Risk of distress to fetus	Prematurity	A severely growth-restricted premature baby is vulnerable to the added stresses of labour, and may benefit from a prelabour CS. The timing of this in extremely premature babies is a more difficult decision. The GRIT trial evaluated the effect of delivering early to pre-empt terminal hypoxia versus delaying delivery to prolong gestation. Fetuses ranged from 24 to 36 weeks and the average length of delay was 4.9 days. There was no difference in overall mortality between the two groups [6].
		Multiple pregnancy	In uncomplicated diamniotic dichorionic twins, perinatal morbidity and mortality is increased for the second twin, but whether an elective CS improves outcomes remains uncertain, and NICE guidelines currently do not recommend routine CS. This is currently the subject of a multicentre trial. CS is recommended where the first twin presents as breech, in monoamniotic twins and in the case of higher-order births [4].

		Vasa praevia	This may be detected antenatally by ultrasound and Doppler. Elective CS is indicated to avoid rapid fetal exsanguination which is associated with tearing of the fetal vessels.
	Mother and baby	Placental abruption	Major placental abruption necessitates rapid delivery of the fetus by the quickest means possible to minimize morbidity and mortality to both mother and fetus.
		Placenta praevia	Major placenta praevia is an indication for CS. If minor praevia is present, the placental edge >2.5 cm from internal os, and the head is engaged vaginal delivery may be considered.
		Eclampsia	After cessation of fitting and stabilization of blood pressure it is necessary to expedite delivery. This is most likely to be by means of a caesarean section, especially in the preterm situation.
		Cardiac arrest	In the case of a maternal cardiac arrest where cardiopulmonary resuscitation (CPR) in the presence of left tilt has not been successful, evacuation of the uterus is required in order to reduce the oxygen demands on the mother, increase the efficiency of CPR and improve maternal chances of survival. The aim should be to empty the uterus within 5 min. Rapid delivery may also benefit the baby, but this is not the prime aim.
In labour	Fetal distress	Bradycardia/abnormal CTG	Fetal distress in labour may be an indication for delivery by CS. Fetal blood sampling reduces the rate of unnecessary caesarean sections for abnormal CTGs but a prolonged bradycardia requires immediate delivery.
		Cord prolapse	Prompt CS is generally required; however, instrumental delivery may be possible at full dilatation.
Maternal and fetal	Dystocia	Failure to progress	Delay in the first stage of labour occurs when the rate of cervical dilatation is less than 2 cm in 4 h or progress slows in multips. Other factors such as station and position of head and the strength of uterine contractions should also be evaluated. NICE guidelines state that in all cases where slow progress is suspected, amniotomy should be considered and the women should be re-examined after a further 2 h. If less than 1 cm further dilatation has been achieved, the woman should be re-evaluated to assess whether oxytocin may aid uterine contractions, particular care being taken in multips in order to exclude obstructed labour. The woman should be re-examined 4 h after oxytocin is started. If no progress is made or the woman shows signs of an obstructed labour, a CS should be offered [7].
		Cephalopelvic disproportion/ malposition	Absolute disproportion is rare, but relative disproportion due to a malposition (occipito-posterior) or a malpresentation (brow) is more common. If full dilatation has not been achieved a CS is required. If full dilatation has been achieved many malpositions are amenable to instrumental delivery, but if this is unsuitable or unsuccessful a CS is required.
	Other	Uterine rupture	Uterine rupture may result in massive haemorrhage for the mother and potentially hypoxia or death for the fetus, and an emergency CS is indicated.

Table 10.3 Serious risks associated with caesarean section [9].

	Risk	Frequency
Maternal risks	Hysterectomy	0.7–0.8%
	Need for surgery at later date	0.5%
	Bladder injury	0.1%
	Ureteric injury	0.03%
	Death	1/12,000
Fetal injury	Lacerations	2%
Future pregnancies	Increased risk of uterine rupture	0.4%
	Antepartum stillbirth	0.4%
	Placenta praevia/accreta in future pregnancies	0.4–0.8%

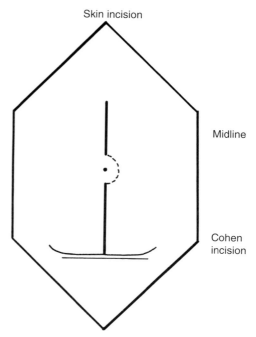

Figure 10.1 Diagram illustrating skin incisions for caesarean section

Skin incision and access to the peritoneal cavity

The skin incision should be made in one sweeping motion using the belly of the scalpel. It should be of an adequate size in order to give sufficient access and is usually about 12 cm long.

Three different types of skin incision can be used (Figure 10.1). Historically, a vertical midline skin incision was adopted; however, cosmetically, this scar is less acceptable and is associated with an increased incidence of postoperative wound discomfort, dehiscence, infection and hernia formation. It may still be necessary if access is required to the upper uterus or to other abdominal organs.

Two types of transverse lower abdominal incision can be used. These are the Pfannenstiel incision and the Cohen incision (Figure 10.1). These involve separating the rectus sheath from the underlying muscle and are therefore associated with an increased risk of haematoma formation. They do, however, heal well and have lower rates of wound dehiscence. When these incisions are extended laterally there is a risk of damage to the superficial circumflex iliac and superficial epigastric veins. Entry to the peritoneal cavity is achieved between the recti, and whichever entry is used, care should be taken not to hook the fingers laterally under these strap muscles as the inferior epigastric bundles lie between them and the peritoneum and are vulnerable to damage. The fingers should therefore be kept in the midline, exposing the peritoneum in a longitudinal plane.

With Pfannenstiel incisions, sharp dissection is used to open the anterior abdominal wall, whilst the Cohen incision uses blunt dissection (tearing of the tissues with fingers). The Cohen's incision is a quicker means of entry and is therefore the preferred technique when rapid access is needed [4]. There are clearly times when this rather crude method of entry is not appropriate; for example, after previous surgery where scarring is extensive and careful dissection is needed to identify structures and avoid inadvertent damage.

In cases where there is a previous CS scar, the decision regarding whether to go through the old scar or excise it completely will depend on its nature. It is usually best to excise the old scar, as this gives a better cosmetic result and is associated with improved wound healing; this is especially true with hypertrophic scars, but if it is keloid its margins should be left, as this generates less tissue reaction in the subsequent scar.

Exposure of and entry to the uterus

Once the peritoneal cavity has been opened the uterus should be assessed, including its rotation and the development of the lower segment. This is especially important when there is an abnormal lie, prematurity, fibroids or abnormal placentation, as a poorly formed lower segment will be vascular and thick, affording less access to the baby. The width of the lower segment (the distance between the broad ligaments) should be assessed relative to the size of the baby to decide if a transverse or longitudinal incision is most appropriate. In either case, the peritoneum needs to be reflected inferiorly before the uterine incision is made.

The visceral peritoneum of the uterovesical fold which overlies the lower segment of the uterus superior to the bladder should be lifted up, divided and opened with scissors. The lower peritoneal edge can then be separated carefully using a finger and reflected down, taking the bladder with it. Exposing the lower uterine segment is important, but over-zealous reflection of the bladder inferiorly can cause unnecessary trauma and bleeding and should be avoided. A Doyen's retractor should then be inserted, ensuring that the bladder is kept clear of the surgical field.

Before the uterine incision is made, it is essential that the assistant corrects any uterine rotation (usually dextro-rotation) by carefully placing one hand on one side of the woman's abdomen (usually the left).

Lower segment incision

The uterine incision should be made 2–3 cm below the upper edge of the uterovesical fold of peritoneum. This is especially important when the CS is performed at or near full dilatation, when the tendency is to go in too low, due to the stretched and ballooned out lower segment. A low entry in this situation risks extension of the uterine angles into the broad ligament, or even more dangerously it can risk entry into the vagina (inadvertent laparoelytrotomy) – both complications carry attendant risks to the ureters.

A superficial uterine incision should be made in the midline, curving up at each end. It should then be opened further in the midline over 1–2 cm with gentle cuts alternating with a sweep of the finger to clear the view until the membranes are reached. It is best to try to leave the membranes intact at this stage, as it avoids the risk of cutting the baby and maintains the liquor until the uterine incision is completed (particular attention is necessary where the membranes have already ruptured, in cases of oligohydramnios, breech presentations, advanced labour or after repeat CSs, where the lower segment can be very thin). Blunt

extension of the uterine incision superolaterally should then be performed using the fingers, as this is associated with less blood loss than sharp dissection. Occasionally, with a very thin scarred lower segment, tearing the incision can risk extension inferolaterally, and it may be more prudent to use scissors while protecting the baby with fingers from the other hand. The membranes should then be ruptured, taking great care to avoid cutting the baby.

In the case of an anterior placenta praevia the surgeon may choose to assess the placental site and cord insertion with ultrasound directly prior to the operation in order to plan the most appropriate access. On reaching the placenta, blunt dissection should follow: preferably the placenta should be gently pushed aside to access the membranes, but it may have to be entered digitally and the cord should be clamped quickly after delivery of the baby. The cord insertion should be avoided in all these manoeuvres. Placenta praevia can be associated with heavy blood loss, and it is essential that a senior doctor is present at delivery.

Delivering the baby

If the baby is cephalic the operator's right hand should be carefully inserted through the incision inferior to the baby's head and into the pelvis in order to cup the baby's head in the palm of the hand. The Doyen's retractor can then be removed and the head should be rotated to the occipito-transverse position and then subjected to gentle lateral flexion to deliver it into the wound. The assistant should then apply fundal pressure in order to facilitate delivery of firstly the head, then each shoulder gently in turn and then the trunk of the baby. Effecting delivery by the assistant using fundal pressure is important and minimal traction should be applied to the baby's head by the operator – neck and brachial plexus injuries are not confined to over-zealous traction at vaginal deliveries.

If the head is high and delivery is difficult, the Wrigley's forceps or Kiwi ventouse cup can be applied to gently guide out the baby's head. In cases where the head is deeply impacted in the pelvis (for example, in a CS at full dilatation) the operator should insert the hand as usual, and then wait until the uterus relaxes before trying to manipulate the head. Trying to dis-impact the head whilst there is a contraction is unlikely to work, will risk extension of the uterine angles, is likely to promote continued uterine tone, and may cause fetal trauma. If waiting does not help, then the anaesthetists can relax the uterus using a tocolytic such as terbutaline or GTN. In the unlikely event that there is still difficulty, an assistant may be able to dis-impact the head vaginally (again, this should not be attempted while the uterus is contracting). These CSs are at high risk of uterine tears, so careful inspection should be performed after delivery of the baby.

In cases where the baby is breech, if the legs are extended the operator's right hand can be cupped around the bottom and the breech delivered by lateral flexion coupled with fundal pressure from the assistant. Alternatively, a foot (recognized by the heel) can be held and the legs delivered first. In either situation the fetal back should be kept anterior, and completion of the delivery is again achieved by fundal pressure with minimal traction: the shoulders should be delivered with gentle rotation, in the same way as at a vaginal breech delivery, and the Mauriceau–Smellie–Veit technique can then be used to facilitate delivery of the head.

If the baby is transverse, a foot should be identified and the baby delivered as breech. In this circumstance, leaving the membranes intact for as long as possible will facilitate the internal rotation of the baby.

Midline and classical incisions

The classical CS incision involves entry to the uterus through an upper longitudinal uterine incision and is rarely used nowadays, except in some cases of placenta praevia accreta, where the placenta needs to be avoided by the incision altogether, or in some cases of fibroids. More commonly, a lower midline (De Lee) incision is indicated; for example, in extreme prematurity, where the lower segment is not yet formed, or with a transverse lie and prelabour rupture of membranes. In either case, checking uterine rotation before making the incision helps keep it in the midline.

Delivery of the placenta

The placenta should be delivered by controlled cord traction after the uterus has contracted and placental separation has occurred (expedited by the anaesthetist giving 5 iu of intravenous oxytocin). The uterus should be supported with the non-dominant hand during this procedure. Very rarely, the placenta does not separate despite the uterus being well contracted and a manual removal is required. Manual removal is associated with increased blood loss and risk of

infection, and therefore the operator should guard against impatience and certainly not perform manual removal if the uterus is not yet contracted, as this will increase blood loss considerably. If there are bleeding sinuses on the uterus these can be compressed using Green–Armitage clamps while awaiting placental separation.

If the placenta is morbidly adherent (placenta accreta) there are a variety of options: firstly, if the placenta has not been breached during uterine entry and delivery of the baby and no placental separation has occurred, the placenta may either be left in situ and the patient managed conservatively, or a hysterectomy may be preferred (depending on the pre-operative dialogue with the patient).

Secondly, if there is extensive haemorrhage from the placental bed after the placenta has been removed, a number of techniques may help gain control, including local infiltration with uterotonics, under-running bleeding areas with sutures, local pressure with a Rusch balloon, excising small areas of involved and bleeding myometrium, or embolization by intervention radiology. If these do not work, a hysterectomy may be necessary.

After delivery of the placenta, the uterine cavity should be checked to ensure it is empty; if the uterine angles are bleeding, they should be secured with Green–Armitage clamps before this is done.

Uterine closure

A blunt round-bodied needle minimizes the risk of needlestick injuries to both the operator and assistant. The suture material should be short-term absorbable due to the fact that the uterus involutes postnatally. A synthetic polyfilament such as vicryl is suitable.

The uterine angles should be identified carefully and tied securely. This can be facilitated using Green–Armitage clamps, which are also useful to clamp any bleeding sinuses, as mentioned above. It is rare to need to deliver the uterus to expose the angles, and this should not be done routinely as it increases discomfort, but it can be useful in selected cases. The anaesthetist should be warned before this is undertaken.

Although there is some debate regarding single-versus double-layer closure of the lower segment uterine incision, the evidence available to date favours the double-layer closure, as scar dehiscence is fivefold higher with a single-layer closure [11], and this is supported by NICE [4]. Closure of the uterus is

Two-layer closure of uterus

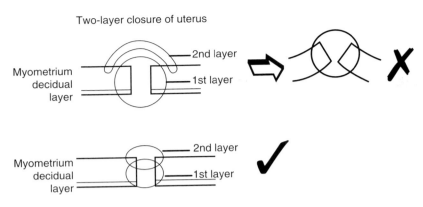

Figure 10.2 Diagram illustrating the correct technique for the two-layer closure of the uterine incision

currently being evaluated in a large multicentre UK trial – the CAESAR study.

The first layer of sutures picks up the uterine edges, but specific attention should be given to including the deep myometrium (with as little decidua as possible): a continuous locking technique is haemostatic and distributes the tension, making the suture less likely to cut through (especially useful with friable or thin lower segments). The second layer which consolidates the superficial borders of the myometrium affords further haemostasis, but also buries the first layer of sutures. It is not necessary to lock this second layer. Extra haemostatic sutures may be required if bleeding persists. The second layer is not just cosmetic, and bringing together adventitia from below and above the uterine incision purely to bury the first layer is illogical, can risk causing bleeding, and can hitch the bladder up towards the incision, making future surgery more treacherous (Figure 10.2).

Classical uterine incisions are normally repaired in three layers as they are much thicker. The principle to remember is that the dead space needs to be obliterated to achieve haemostasis and reduce the chance of haematoma formation. Sutures should be interrupted and absorbable. The final suture layer is best effected with a monofilament inert fine continuous locking suture to minimize adhesion formation.

The paracolic gutters should then be cleaned and the tubes and ovaries identified to ensure normal anatomy. Finally, a last check for haemostasis should be made, systematically checking both uterine angles, the suture line, under the Doyen's retractor where the peritoneum was reflected, then under the rectus sheath.

Drains and closure

Non-closure of the visceral and parietal peritoneum at caesarean section is recommended [12] and the routine use of a sub-rectus sheath wound drain in uncomplicated caesarean sections is not needed [13]. The use of drains is also being evaluated by the CAESAR trial. If a drain is needed in the peritoneal cavity, a soft large bore non-suctioned drain such as a Robinson drain is suitable. If a suction drain is to be used for the sub-rectus space, the parietal peritoneum should be closed to avoid direct communication of the suction drain with the abdomen contents.

The rectus sheath should be closed with a continuous stitch using an absorbable suture such as 1.0 Vicryl. Sutures should be placed 1 cm apart and 1 cm away from the wound edge in order to prevent hernia formation. This layer needs to be secure, but over-tightening causes postoperative pain: locking one or two sutures at even distances across the wound can help to distribute tension.

The subcutaneous tissue should be closed in women with more than 2 cm of subcutaneous fat to decrease the incidence of wound haematoma and infection. In slimmer patients it does not reduce the incidence of wound infection, but it may yet be anatomically sensible if, for example, an old scar has been excised and the wound edges are gaping. The point of this layer is to close the dead space and support the skin layer, so Scarpa's fascia should be deliberately included in it.

The low transverse skin incision used for CS is cosmetic and relatively comfortable, and therefore skin closure should be compatible with these principles. There is inadequate evidence as to the effects of different suture materials or methods of closure at CS [14], but a subcutaneous suture which can either be left in place (absorbable) or removed on day 4/5 (non-dissolvable) gives a good result. Staples are thought to cause more postoperative discomfort and a less-favourable cosmetic outcome and are not recommended.

Adjuncts to caesarean section

Antibiotics should be administered routinely at the time of operation. A single dose of a broad spectrum antibiotic such as Co-amoxiclav should be used.

All women should be given compression stockings, kept well hydrated and encouraged to mobilize after CS to minimize the risk of thromboembolism. Heparin thromboprophylaxis should be given if there are risk factors [15] and in accordance with local guidelines.

Careful documentation of the procedure and findings should be made in the notes as highlighted by *Safer Childbirth* [8].

Complications

Caesarean section is a major operation which can be associated with significant morbidity and mortality. Complications may be categorized into immediate, early and late.

Immediate
Anaesthetic

General anaesthesia can be associated with complications of intubation such as hypoxia, aspiration or failed intubation (the last occurring approx. 1 in 250–400 cases), awareness (resulting from an inadequate dose of anaesthesia or a drug error), or, as with any drug administration, anaphylaxis. Regional analgesia can also have immediate complications, including: hypotension, a total spinal anaesthetic, a dural puncture (which occurs in 0.5–1% of epidurals) and infection (the risk of meningitis is low, but spinal abscesses can form). Nerve damage secondary to epidural is rare and spinal cord damage should not occur as obstetric epidurals are sited below the cord. Other minor side effects include pruritis, nausea and vomiting, and shivering.

Haemorrhage

This can occur from the uterine edges, extended angles, or the placental bed, but as with vaginal delivery, the most common cause is uterine atony. Local protocols should be followed and uterotonic drugs should be administered, but if these fail, advanced techniques such as a Rusch balloon or a B lynch suture which provide tamponade may be helpful.

Damage to pelvic organs

The bladder is susceptible to damage when there has been previous pelvic surgery and adhesions. Bladder damage may be suspected anatomically if there is urine in the operating field, or when there is frank haematuria. If there is any doubt, the bladder can be distended (normal saline with or without methylene blue dye can be used) to see if there is a leak. An experienced operator should repair bladder damage: consultation should be sought with a urologist if damage is extensive. The principles of bladder repair are that it should be repaired in two layers (mucosa and then the submucosa and muscularis) using an absorbable suture such as vicryl. A large-bore non-suction drain should be placed in the uterovesical fold and a urinary catheter should be left in situ for 7–10 days. A cystogram may be performed before removing the catheter.

Ureteric injury is rare but possible if the uterine angle extends into the broad ligament, when it can be ligated during an attempt to control haemostasis. A urologist should be consulted immediately ureteric damage is suspected. A ureteric stent may be required and a peritoneal drain should be left in situ.

Bowel damage is rare but can occur on entry to the peritoneum if there has been previous surgery and adhesion formation. It should be covered with a wet pack and repaired after delivery of the baby and closure of the uterus. Injuries should be repaired by a general or colorectal surgeon using an absorbable suture material.

Fetal complications

Fetal injuries complicate a small proportion of CSs, with the most common being fetal laceration. Other trauma such as cephalohaematoma, clavicular fracture, brachial plexus injury, skull fracture and facial nerve palsy can occur and the baby should always be handled gently [16]. Neonatal respiratory morbidity may complicate CS due to iatrogenic prematurity, delay in the clearance of fluid from the fetal lungs, or a lack of the catecholamine surge experienced during vaginal delivery.

Early
Haemorrhage

Haemorrhage may occur in the early recovery period. This may be clearly evident if the patient is bleeding vaginally, into a drain or through the abdominal wound; however, it may also be concealed either intrauterine (a rising uterine fundus is the clue) or intraperitoneal. Tachycardia, oliguria or pallor should alert and a normal blood pressure should not reassure, as hypotension is a late sign. Urgent fluid resuscitation should be commenced, uterine atony should be treated and clots removed if present. If the uterus fails to respond or if the bleeding is intraperitoneal, early return to theatre is indicated.

Infective
Chest

Pain from abdominal surgery reduces mobility, deep breathing and coughing, which can predispose women to basal atelectasis and lower respiratory tract infection, especially if they had a general anaesthetic or are smokers. The patient may complain of cough, shortness of breath and pleuritic chest pain. If this is suspected, the chest should be auscultated, oxygen saturations monitored, a septic screen including a chest X-ray performed, and antibiotics commenced with physiotherapy. Care should be taken to exclude pulmonary embolism (see below).

Urine

Pyrexia postoperatively may also be attributable to a urinary tract infection. The patient may complain of dysuria or increased urinary frequency. Urine should consequently be checked with a urine dipstick and sent to the laboratory for sensitivity and culture.

Uterus

Endometritis occurs due to an infection of the endometrium. It may present with increased bleeding which may be offensive in nature, and there may be systemic symptoms associated with fever. The patient should be examined and resuscitated as needed. Retained products of conception are unlikely but not impossible after CS, and if symptoms do not settle with antibiotics an ultrasound examination may be helpful.

Wound

Wound haematomas, infection (superficial or deep), or dehiscence can occur. Factors which increase these risks include: obesity, diabetes, chorioamnionitis, corticosteroid use, or poor surgical technique with a casual attitude to haemostasis. Haematomas may resolve spontaneously with conservative management, but larger, more uncomfortable ones are best drained. If a wound infection is suspected the wound should be swabbed and a full septic screen performed.

This should be done before antibiotics are commenced if the woman is febrile. Imaging may be helpful in assessing whether there is a pelvic collection or haematoma which may require surgical drainage. Deep-seated infections that do not respond to antibiotic therapy may require surgical drainage or debridement.

Paralytic ileus

A paralytic ileus may occur postoperatively. The bowel may become adynamic, lacking in normal peristaltic contractions. Exacerbating factors include sepsis, hypokalaemia, hyponatraemia, uraemia, and certain drugs.

Pseudo-obstruction (Ogilvie's syndrome) is an acute functional obstruction of the distal colon, particularly found after CS, which is poorly recognized and has been associated with maternal deaths. Clinical features include abdominal distension and colicky pain, but absolute constipation may not occur depending on the level of the 'obstruction'. Bowel sounds tend to be tinkling but can be absent. The risk is of colonic rupture which tends to occur in the caecum or sigmoid, and tenderness in either iliac fossa is an ominous clinical sign. Management (in conjunction with a surgeon) is usually conservative, keeping the patient nil by mouth and giving intravenous fluids maintaining their electrolyte balance. An abdominal X-ray monitors the colonic distension and dilatation beyond 9–10 cm (or iliac fossa tenderness) suggests colonoscopic decompression may be required.

Thromboembolic disease

Women having a CS are at increased risk of venous thromboembolic disease (VTE) due to their pregnancy and surgery. Other risk factors include obesity, immobility, thrombophilia, smoking, family history, and previous history of VTE. It is the leading cause of maternal death in the United Kingdom [17], and substandard care is most commonly due to a failure to recognize the signs and symptoms or failure to implement appropriate thromboprophylaxis.

Late
Future fertility

Women who have had a CS are less likely than those who have had a vaginal delivery to have further children. Whether this is due to the surgery or the

Table 10.4 Placenta praevia and accreta associated with prelabour CS [20].

Prior CS	Number of women	Placenta accreta	TAH	% of cases of accreta in women with placenta praevia
0	6,201	15 (0.24%)	40 (0.65%)	3
1	15,808	49 (0.31%)	67 (0.42%)	11
2	6,324	36 (0.57%)	57 (0.9%)	40
3	1,452	31 (2.13%)	35 (2.4%)	61
4	258	6 (2.33%)	9 (3.49%)	67
≥5	89	6 (6.74%)	8 (8.99%)	

indication for the surgery is unclear. There appears to be a lesser desire for further children as well as a decreased ability to conceive [18]. If pregnancy is successful there is a greater association between having had a previous CS and stillbirth. The risk was found to be double in women who had had a previous CS than in women who had vaginal deliveries (2 per 1000 compared to 4 per 1000) [19]; however, this population of women form a higher-risk group which introduces bias.

Increased risk of scar rupture

The risk of uterine rupture is approximately 0.5% in subsequent labours. This may cause significant morbidity and mortality to both the mother and baby should it arise.

Placenta praevia

The more CS a woman has the greater the chance of placenta praevia in a future pregnancy, and the higher the risk that placenta accreta also occurs [20] (Table 10.4).

Adhesions

Any surgical procedure that involves entry to the peritoneal cavity can cause adhesions, making subsequent operative procedures more technically difficult and predisposing to other conditions such as bowel obstruction. These risks can be minimized by gentle, minimal handling of tissues, good haemostasis and non-closure of the peritoneum.

Hernia formation

Incisional hernias occur rarely with a Cohen's incision, but can follow button-holing of the sheath during its dissection off the recti to enter the abdomen.

Keloid scarring/endometriosis (rare)

A keloid scar may form over the incision site. Numerous therapies have been described to treat this proliferative fibrous reaction including steroid injections, surgical excision, radiotherapy, laser, imiquimod, silicone gel sheeting, and cryotherapy.

Endometriosis has been reported in CS scars: presenting with cyclical pain and swelling of the scar during menstruation, discharge may also be present. Ultrasound, CT and MRI may also help to facilitate the diagnosis. Treatment of choice remains surgical excision.

Fistula formation (very rare)

Vesicouterine fistula can occur as a complication of CS. It is more likely to occur if there has been previous extensive scarring and the bladder is tethered high with the uterine incision in close proximity to it. Presenting symptoms may include cyclical haematuria, amenorrhoea or continuous vaginal urinary leakage. Spontaneous healing has been reported in 5% of cases treated conservatively by means of catheterization for 4–8 weeks and hormonally induced amenorrhoea. Surgical management may be indicated.

Conclusion

The rate of caesarean section is increasing; however, the procedure is becoming safer due to the use of antibiotics, awareness of the need for thromboprophylaxis, and coherent delivery suite guidelines for the management of postpartum haemorrhage. There is, however, no place for complacency: the decision to perform each CS should be taken critically, balancing up the pros and cons for that particular individual. Meticulous planning and surgical attention to detail should help to minimize the risks of the procedure, and good analgesia and early mobilization should help limit postoperative morbidity. Local procedures should be in place to monitor CS practice in terms of indications for the procedure, standards of clinical care provided, and complications encountered. Active critical review should help to inform practice and capitalize on safety.

References

1. Royal College of Obstetricans and Gynaecologists Clinical Support Unit. *The National Caesarean Section Audit Report*. London: RCOG Press, 2001. Available online at: http://www.rcog.org.uk/resources/public/pdf/nscs_audit.pdf (accessed 30 January 2008).

2. Lucas D N, Yentis S M, Kinsella S M, *et al.* Urgency of caesarean section: a new classification. *J R Soc Med* 2000; **93**: 346–50.

3. NCEPOD. *Report of the National Confidential Enquiry into Perioperative Deaths 1992/1993*. London: NCEPOD, 1995.

4. National Institute of Clinical Excellence. *Clinical Guideline 13 Caesarean Section*. London: RCOG Press, 2004. Available online at: http://www.nice.org.uk/nicemedia/pdf/CG013fullguideline.pdf (accessed 30 January 2008).

5. Hannah M E, Hannah W J, Hewson S A, *et al.* Planned caesarean section versus planned vaginal birth for breech presentation at term: a randomised multicentre trial. Term Breech Trial Collaborative Group. *Lancet* 2000; **356**: 1375–83.

6. GRIT Study Group. A randomised trial of timed delivery for the compromised preterm fetus: short term outcomes and Bayesian interpretation. *Br J Obstet Gynaecol* 2003; **110**: 27–32.

7. National Institute of Clinical Excellence. *Clinical Guideline 55 Intrapartum Care*. London: RCOG Press, 2007. Available online at: http://www.nice.org.uk/nicemedia/pdf/IPCNICEGuidance.pdf (accessed 30 January 2008).

8. RCOG, RCM, RCA, RCPCH. *Safer Childbirth. Minimum Standards for the Organisation and Delivery of Care in Labour*. London: RCOG Press, 2007. Available online at: http://www.rcog.org.uk/resources/public/pdf/safer_childbirth_report_web.pdf (accessed 30 January 2008).

9. Welch C. *Caesarean Section*. RCOG Consent Advice 7. 2006. Available online at: http://www.rcog.org.uk/resources/Public/pdf/consent7_csection.pdf (accessed 30 January 2008).

10. Morrison J, Rennie J, Milton P. Neonatal respiratory morbidity and mode of delivery at term: influence of timing of elective caesarean section. *Br J Obstet Gynaecol* 1995; **102**: 101–6.

11. Bujold E, Bujold C, Hamilton E F, Harel F, Gauthier R J. The impact of a single-layer or double-layer closure on uterine rupture. *Am J Obstet Gynecol* 2002; **186**: 1326–30.

12. Bamigboye A A, Hofmeyr G J. Closure versus non-closure of the peritoneum at caesarean section. *Cochrane Database Syst Rev* 2003; **4**: CD000163.

13. Gates S, Anderson E R. Wound drainage for caesarean section. *Cochrane Database Syst Rev* 2005; **1**: CD004549.

14. Alderdice F, McKenna D, Dornan J. Techniques and materials for skin closure in caesarean section. *Cochrane Database Syst Rev* 2003; **2**: CD003577.

15. Nelson-Piercy C. *Thromboprophylaxis during Pregnancy, Labour and after Vaginal Delivery. RCOG Guideline No. 37*. 2006. Available online at: http://www.rcog.org.uk/resources/Public/pdf/green_top_28_thromboembolic_minorrevision.pdf (accessed 30 January 2008).

16. Alexander J M, Leveno K J, Hauth J, *et al.* Fetal injury associated with cesarean delivery. *Obstet Gynecol* 2006; **108**: 885–90.

17. CEMACH. *Saving Mothers' Lives*. London: CEMACH, 2007.

18. Jolly J, Walker J, Bhabra K. Subsequent obstetric performance related to primary mode of delivery. *Br J Obstet Gynaecol* 1999; **106**: 227–32.

19. Smith G C, Pell J P, Dobbie R. Caesarean section and risk of unexplained stillbirth in subsequent pregnancy. *Lancet* 2003; **362**: 1779–84.

20. Silver R M, Landon M B, Rouse D J, *et al.* Maternal morbidity associated with multiple repeat cesarean deliveries. *Obstet Gynecol* 2006; **107**: 1226–32.

Breech and twin delivery

Steve Walkinshaw

Approximately 3–4% of singleton births involve a breech presentation. Experience with vaginal breech birth is reducing in 'Westernized' healthcare settings. Twins account for an increasing proportion of births, usually around 1% but in some populations 2–3%, with contributions from both reproductive technology and increasing age. Like breech birth there has been a move towards caesarean section as mode of twin birth and a consequent reduction in exposure to the range of manoeuvres needed to manage the second twin.

Despite these trends, vaginal breech births and vaginal twin births occur regularly on the labour ward, and all practitioners will need both an understanding of the mechanisms of birth and skills in safe conduct of such births.

Breech birth
Breech birth at term

Whatever the criticisms of the Term Breech Trial [1], in most healthcare settings its publication accelerated the trend to elective caesarean birth for breech presentation at term. Overall the trial showed benefit in serious short-term outcomes, but no increased long-term morbidity in survivors. Although many have downplayed the importance of some of the transient short-term morbidity, common sense would dictate that most women would prefer their newborn infants not to suffer potentially avoidable trauma or admission to a neonatal unit. Data from Holland and Sweden [2,3], amongst others, have shown the predicted improvement in perinatal mortality following a move to elective caesarean birth, although French data did not support increased perinatal risk. Subsequent data from France [4] confirmed a lack of increased risk, particularly where very strict consensus guidelines

were in place, that was subtly different from the Term Breech vaginal birth guidance.

Others have debated the number needed to prevent harm. Hannah and Hofmeyr suggest 29 elective caesarean sections to avoid an adverse outcome, although for perinatal death it is nearer 200. The Dutch study [2] proposed a number needed to treat (NNT) of 175, and the Swedish study [3] proposed 400 for avoidance of perinatal mortality.

Maternal morbidity, either short- or medium-term, was not different in the Term Breech Trial, although elective caesarean clearly carries an increased risk for the mother. Villar et al. [5] showed risks of death of 4 in 10,000, risk of ICU admission of 2.7% and risk of hysterectomy of 3.5 per 1000 for women undergoing planned caesarean section compared with planned vaginal birth, results not dissimilar to a large US cohort. Risks in subsequent pregnancies include late stillbirth, placenta praevia accreta, and uterine rupture and its consequences. Dutch data [2] put this last risk as equivalent to that of the increase in perinatal mortality associated with vaginal breech birth. Risk to the baby from elective caesarean birth is not zero, as seen in the Term Breech data, and at all gestations up to 39–40 weeks there is an increased risk of neonatal respiratory distress.

This suggests that directive advising of elective caesarean birth for the term breech is not necessarily appropriate and that the more measured approach advised in the recent RCOG [6], ACOG [7] and RANZOG [8] guidelines is more useful.

External cephalic version (ECV)
Efficacy

Given the controversies the logical first step would seem to be to remove the problem by ECV. It has

Best Practice in Labour and Delivery, ed. R. Warren and S. Arulkumaran. Published by Cambridge University Press.
© Cambridge University Press 2009.

been an RCOG audit standard for some time to offer ECV to women with a diagnosed breech presentation at term.

There is significant reduction in the risk of caesarean section in women where there is an intention to undertake ECV (OR 0.55, 95% CI 0.33–0.91) with no increased risk to the baby [9]. Although high success rates were achieved in the trials, studies of practice show success rates nearer 50–60% (reviewed in reference [10]). Parity is the main factor that affects success, with nulliparous success rates around 1 in 3 and multiparous success rates around 2 in 3 or greater. Amniotic fluid volume may affect success, although there is no consensus on whether there should be an absolute cut-off for attempting the procedure. Maternal weight and height affect success and fetal weight (both macrosomia and small for gestation) may be a factor. Operator experience may play a role.

Reversion to breech occurs after successful ECV, with between 3 and 7% being reported for term ECV. Rates of over 20% have been reported for preterm ECV.

Techniques to improve success

Tocolysis and anaesthesia have been advocated to improve success rates. The most recent Cochrane review [11] shows a reduction in ECV failures with beta-agonist tocolysis (RR 0.74, 95% CI 0.64–0.87) and a reduction in caesarean section rate (RR 0.85, 95% CI 0.72–0.99). One further trial since this review confirms this efficacy. Others have used selective betamimetic treatment after failure of ECV without tocolysis [12], demonstrating reduction in caesarean section rates with this approach (RR 0.33, 95% CI 0.14–0.8). Sublingual nitroglycerine was not found to be effective in the systematic review, and in one subsequent large study. A trial comparing betamimetic with nitroglycerine tocolysis showed better success rates with betamimetic. One trial of fetal acoustic stimulation has shown fewer failures, but this requires further study. As yet, despite its popularity, there are no data on efficacy of calcium channel agents. Amnioinfusion has been advocated, but there is no evidence of efficacy. Some groups have used epidural and spinal analgesia. Overall there was no reduction in failure or caesarean section rates but there was heterogeneity of results, with the epidural studies suggesting benefit.

Various postural methods such as knee–elbow, knee–chest, Indian and Zilgrie positions have been advocated. Review of clinical trials shows no increase in the rate of cephalic births. Moxibustion, the use of burning herbs at acupoint BL 67 beside the outer corner of the fifth toenail, is not of benefit.

Safety

Systematic reviews of the randomized trials showed no increase in perinatal mortality or morbidity and other reviews of safety have been reassuring [13]. Transient fetal heart rate abnormalities occur in 5.7%, with persisting abnormal CTG in approximately 1 in 300. Placental abruption was very rare, occurring in 1 in 1000 cases. A detailed examination of perinatal deaths in series of ECV suggests a perinatal mortality of 1.6 per 1000. This is not different from the perinatal mortality of pregnancies between 37 and 40 weeks.

Overall the need for emergency birth occurs around 1 in every 200 attempts [10].

Contra-indication should be rare, being only 4% in one series. They would include recent antepartum haemorrhage, some uterine anomalies, abnormal cardiotocography, rupture of the membranes and multiple pregnancies in the antenatal period. Other factors such as suspected growth restriction or oligohydramnios might be relative contra-indications.

Uptake

Most women would choose ECV to allow vaginal delivery. However, more recent surveys have suggested a substantial minority of eligible women would decline ECV, opting for caesarean section. In part this may be a failure of education, and uptake can be increased by well-constructed information packages.

Conduct of ECV

There are no studies comparing different methods of performing ECV. Training is largely 'hands-on', although Burr and colleagues developed a model that has some promise.

A variety of healthcare professionals carry out ECV, including midwives. There are no studies comparing techniques, and practitioners should be able to vary their technique if necessary.

Table 11.1 Setting and preparation.

Regular service

Immediate access to operative birth

Ultrasound facilities

Fetal monitoring facilities

Comfortable bed with wedge

Establish fetal health (CTG)

Ultrasound examination – size, liquor, position, head flexion

Table 11.2 Conduct of ECV.

Ensure comfortable position (wedge or tilt, partial Trendelenburg)

Consider tocolysis

Disengage breech (palmar surface fingers pulling or modified Paulik's grip pushing) (Figure 11.1)

Manipulate breech laterally to encourage fetal flexion (forward somersault)

Consider use of other hand on fetal occiput to encourage flexion (Figure 11.2)

Continuous feedback on discomfort

If successful, place woman sitting upright

Auscultate or visualize fetal heart rate

If that fails, ask woman if she wishes a further attempt

Consider tocolysis if not used initially

Repeat procedure

When completed, repeat CTG

Check Rh (D) status and give appropriate dose Rh immunoglobin

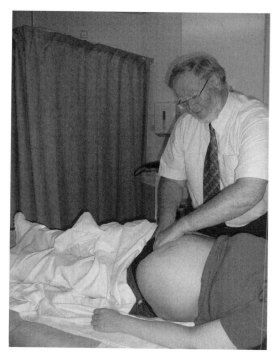

Figure 11.1 Displacement of the fetal breech at ECV using the 'one pole' method

Vaginal breech birth
Selection for vaginal breech birth

Practitioners need to be aware when considering vaginal breech birth that published studies usually work within guidance and exclusions. The Term Breech Trial had clear guidance for conduct of the vaginal birth arm of the trial [1] that were agreed by a consensus group. Other published studies have other exclusions [4] and have argued that selection and guidance for conduct can influence outcomes. See Table 11.3.

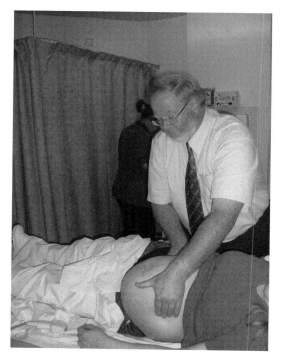

Figure 11.2 Flexing the fetal head after displacement of the breech

Table 11.3 Contra-indications (relative and absolute) to vaginal breech birth.

Other indication for caesarean birth

Footling breech or kneeling (feet below the buttocks) breech presentation

Known hyperextension of neck (ultrasound or clinical impression)

Large fetus (more than 4 kg)

Suspected fetal growth restriction

Previous caesarean section

Clinically inadequate pelvis

Lack of availability of experienced obstetrician

Insufficient throughput to maintain safety

Success is more likely if both the mother's pelvis and the baby are of average proportions, and Term Breech excluded fetuses known to be over 4 kg. The presentation should be either frank (hips flexed, knees extended) or complete (hips flexed, knees flexed but feet not below the fetal buttocks). Where presentation was not this, the risk of cord prolapse was 5.6% [6].

Hyperextension of the fetal head increases the risk of nuchal arms and head entrapment. Assessment of pelvic size is rarely carried out in modern practice, but should be considered if contemplating vaginal breech birth; there appears no advantage to formal pelvimetry, although a study of MR pelvimetry demonstrated a reduction in emergency but not overall caesarean births.

Neither presentation for the first time in labour nor previous caesarean birth are absolute contra-indications to vaginal breech birth, although the French groups have this as part of their consensus guideline.

There has been much debate about facilities and personnel. Subanalysis of the Term Breech Trial showed the absence of an experienced practitioner (variously defined) increased the risk of poor outcomes [6]. Analysis of the French multicentre study showed that a senior obstetrician was present in 95% of births [4].

The birth setting is more contentious. There are midwifery practitioners who conduct vaginal breech births and a number of case reports and individual stories, but no published series that allow a systematic assessment of either safety or success. At present any recommendation to women would need to be giving birth in a hospital setting. As contentious is whether size and throughput should matter. There is some evidence that adverse neonatal outcomes at caesarean birth for breech is higher (threefold) in units with less than 1000 births in a US setting; other studies in other pathologies such as vaginal birth after caesarean section have suggested similar trends. Logically teams working in smaller centres will have less exposure to vaginal breech birth, and need to consider whether they can safely support such requests.

Conduct of labour

The 7th Report of the Confidential Enquiry into Stillbirth and Deaths in Infancy [14] highlighted the need for senior involvement in supervising labour in intended or unexpected breech births. The Term Breech Trial and others have confirmed the importance of such involvement early.

The conduct of the first stage of labour does not need to be significantly different from other labours, with good support, adequate analgesia of a woman's choice and appropriate surveillance of the fetus.

There is no evidence that epidural analgesia is an advantage for breech birth. Similarly, the evidence supporting the use of continuous electronic fetal heart rate monitoring is no more robust for breech presentation as it is for general use, but most authorities advise its use. The CESDI report above was critical of the management of fetal monitoring. The data on fetal blood sampling from the buttock are too few to justify its use outside a research setting.

Induction of labour can be considered for a planned breech birth, as the evidence against is not substantial, but augmentation in current practice should be avoided unless there is careful review of uterine activity and labour progress at consultant/specialist level. One of the major differences between the Term Breech Trial protocol [1] and the French studies showing better outcome [4] is in the use of augmentation. Subgroup analysis of the trial suggested poorer outcomes if augmentation occurred [6], confirming the advice of the CESDI report [14]. See Table 11.4.

Table 11.4 First stage of labour.

Admission assessment (most senior staff available)
Fetal size, pelvic size, breech type, attitude fetal head
Inform consultant/specialist staff of admission
Advise continuous electronic fetal heart rate monitoring (EFM)
Discuss analgesia requirements; consider epidural analgesia
Oxytocin augmentation only after senior review and where clinically poor uterine activity (not simply for failure cervical dilatation)
Where EFM changes, senior review; fetal blood sampling not indicated
Careful review of descent as well as cervical progress

Table 11.5 Assisted breech birth.

Place in lithotomy when breech distending perineum
Consider episiotomy
Hands off the baby until the umbilicus appears (unless sacro-posterior)
Avoid handling the umbilical cord unless clearly under tension
If extended legs and do not deliver, flex the leg outwards using two or three fingers; no traction is needed
Allow spontaneous birth of the arms, then support the body if necessary
Encourage an assistant to carry out suprapubic pressure on the head to keep it flexed
If arms do not deliver and are flexed, then can use pelvic grip (Figure 11.3) to rotate baby to bring elbow into view and sweep arms out
Once arms are delivered, support the baby; do not let it 'hang'
Use forceps or Mauriceau–Smellie–Viet manoeuvre to deliver the head (Figures 11.4–11.6)

Conduct of breech birth

There are no recent data comparing safety or efficacy of the various techniques utilized in breech birth. Therefore debates on whether classical techniques are superior to Bracht manoeuvres, or whether forceps are superior to Mauriceau–Smellie–Viet techniques are simply personal debates. The last detailed comparison of Bracht techniques versus classical techniques was done in 1953 and actually recommended the Bracht technique. A study in 1991 showed some subtle neurodevelopmental differences in neonatal outcomes comparing classical and Bracht techniques. The techniques used by midwifery practitioners are essentially derived from Bracht.

The Mauriceau technique was compared with other techniques by one French group and showed no differences in neonatal outcomes. Older studies suggested improved neonatal outcomes where forceps were used for the after-coming head. Manoeuvres for difficulty with the arms, such as the classical method described by Kunzel and Kirschbaum [15], the method of Muller [15] or Lovset's manoeuvre [16], have never been compared.

Therefore there are only four general rules for birth of the breech:
- learn and become comfortable with one set of techniques;
- keep your hands to yourself until the umbilicus is delivered;
- use rotation not traction if in trouble;
- make sure an experienced practitioner is present, as well as anaesthetic and paediatric help

Assisted breech delivery

Breech birth in alternative birthing positions has never been formally assessed and the advice is to use the dorsal lithotomy position until such time as evidence appears for these alternatives. See Table 11.5.

Much of assisted breech birth is common sense and allowing normal birth to occur. Although episiotomy may not always be strictly necessary, particularly in a parous woman, it is advised in case more complex manoeuvres become necessary.

The manoeuvres to deliver the normal positions of the arms and legs require simple flexion and it should not be necessary to pull on the trunk to gain access.

There is debate on whether the baby should 'hang' near-vertically, as traditional teaching has it. Unsupported 'hanging' can result in uncontrolled birth of the head, and increases extension of the neck. It is best to support at an angle, resting the baby on the forearm.

Before attempting any of the manoeuvres to deliver the head, allow some time for the nape of the neck to become visible. Where using forceps, an assistant will be needed to support the body and

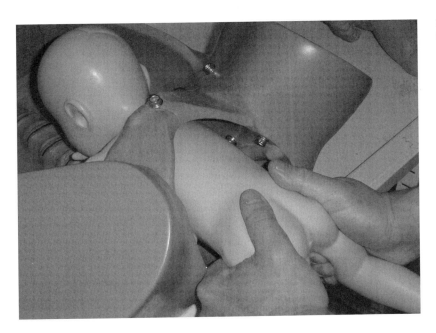

Figure 11.3 Pelvic grip for manipulation at vaginal breech birth

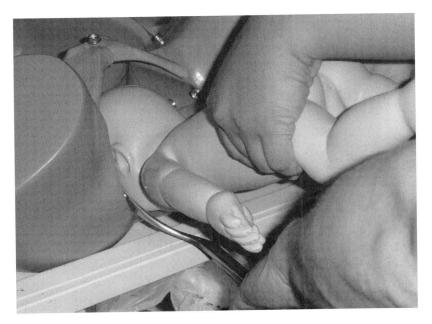

Figure 11.4 Forceps to the after-coming head

keep the arms out of the way. Wrigley's forceps are adequate for this task, unless Piper's forceps are available; these were designed for this task, having a longer shank (Figure 11.4).

The Mauriceau–Smellie–Viet manoeuvre requires draping of the baby over the forearm with the legs on either side. The classic description by Smellie, and before him, Gifford [16], involved placing a finger in the mouth, but current advice is that this is not necessary. The manoeuvre involves placing the index and middle fingers of one hand on either side of the fetal maxilla to allow some flexion, and the other hand placed on the back with the middle finger up the occiput. Birth is by flexion (Figures 11.5 and 11.6).

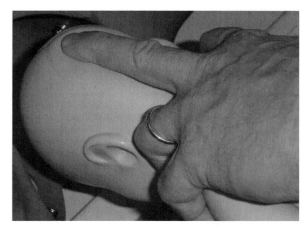

Figure 11.5 Upper hand position at Mauriceau–Smellie–Viet procedure

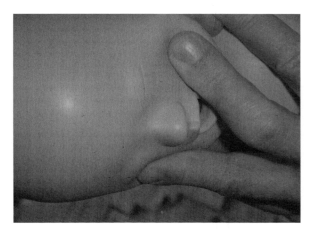

Figure 11.6 Lower hand position at Mauriceau–Smellie–Viet manoeuvre

Table 11.6 Bracht technique.

Place in lithotomy when breech distending perineum
Consider episiotomy
Hands off the baby until the umbilicus appears (unless sacro-posterior)
Avoid handling the umbilical cord unless clearly under tension
Abdominal then suprapubic pressure to maintain head flexion
Grasp the baby with the thumbs pressing the baby's thigh against its stomach and the rest of the hands over the sacral and loin area (pelvic grip)
Whilst the woman is pushing, gently rotate or lift the baby around the maternal symphysis, maintaining upwards movement but without traction (Figure 11.7).
Spontaneous birth of the legs and arms.
Mauriceau–Smellie–Viet or forceps for the head

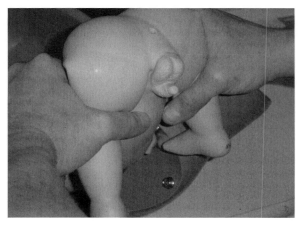

Figure 11.7 Initial rotation during Bracht technique

Bracht technique

This technique has been utilized for many years in mainland Europe [15]. It follows and exaggerates the planes of a spontaneous breech birth. The French studies showing better outcomes predominately use this technique. The key is the particular grasp of the baby, keeping the thighs flexed against the abdomen and then rotating the baby, using gentle pressure around the maternal symphyis. See Table 11.6 and Figure 11.7.

Manoeuvres for delay in delivery of the arms

This can present as either extended arms or where one or both arms are flexed behind the head. Careful observation of the shoulder blade should forewarn.

Lovset's manoeuvre

This manoeuvre was described in 1937.

It involves using the fact that the posterior shoulder will be lower in the pelvis.

Using the pelvic grip, the baby is rotated to an oblique position and gentle traction applied. The baby is then lifted in that plane to further encourage descent of the posterior shoulder and arm (Figure 11.8). The baby is then rotated through 180 degrees, presenting the arm under the symphysis, where it can be hooked out. The baby is then rotated through 180 degrees again to present the other shoulder and arm.

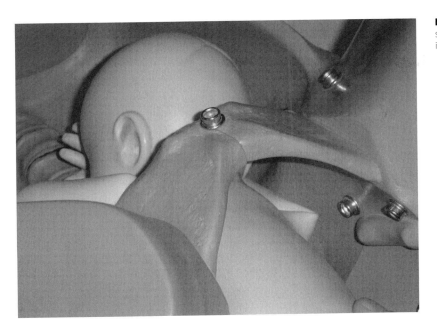

Figure 11.8 Lovset's manoeuvre showing entry of posterior shoulder into pelvis

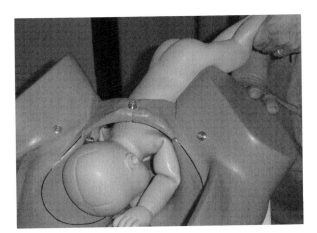

Figure 11.9 Classical arm manoeuvre showing entry of posterior shoulder into pelvis

Classical arm development

This uses similar principles to Lovset's approach by making the posterior shoulder available.

The baby is grasped by the feet and swung outwards and upwards in an oblique plane away from the shoulder of interest (Figure 11.9). The other hand is then inserted into the posterior vagina and along the arm. When sufficiently confident the arm is then swept across the chest and out. To deliver the other arm the baby is held along its sides and rotated through 180 degrees to bring the other shoulder into the posterior vagina. The 'swinging' manoeuvre is repeated to effect delivery of the other arm.

An alternative method has been suggested where the anterior arm is delivered first by swinging the baby in the opposite direction.

Nuchal arms

This should not happen and is usually a consequence of inappropriate traction. Where only one arm is involved, Lovset's manouoevre should be enough to free the arm.

An alternative method is simply to rotate, using the pelvic grip, in the direction the arm is pointing. This will usually bring the elbow under the symphysis.

When both arms are involved, management is difficult and one may have to try both rotations to see which is the most likely arm to be deliverable. Even in very skilled hands trauma is common.

Alternatively the classical technique described before can be successful for this.

Rotate (swing) the fetus towards the hand of the posterior nuchal arm and above the level of the maternal symphysis. This may result in delivery of the posterior arm, but if not it allows room for the occiput to slip below the elbow. A hand can be placed over the shoulder and behind the humerus to allow pressure on the humerus with delivery in front of the face.

If these manoeuvres fail, it is legitimate, in the author's opinion, to force the arm across the face to

Table 11.7 Head entrapment drill.

Call for anaesthetic support; prepare for caesarean birth

Check cervix is fully dilated; if not consider incision of cervix (4 and 7 o'clock)

Try combination of Mauriceau–Smellie–Viet and suprapubic pressure

Repeat with McRobert's position

Mid cavity forceps

Rotate and lift the body into a lateral position, apply suprapubic pressure to flex head into pelvis, then rotate back and continue with previous techniques

Symphysiotomy if adequate training

Caesarean section; use ventouse to aid extraction if necessary

deliver. Humeral or clavicular fractures are very likely, but will not cause long-term harm; perinatal hypoxia does.

Head entrapment

Other than advice on incising the cervix at 4 and 7 o'clock where entrapment is secondary to incomplete dilatation, there is little in the literature to guide clinicians on this rare but feared complication.

William Smellie's original description of the manoeuvre that bears his name was its use for a head trapped high in the pelvis.

Symphysiotomy is the classic technique that is suggested, although its morbidity in unskilled hands is formidable. More recently, case reports using McRobert's position have appeared, and there is logic in consideration of this position, where obstruction is above the symphysis. Smellie's manoeuvre or forceps should be able to deliver where the head is trapped in the mid pelvis. See Table 11.7.

Multiple birth
Multiple birth at term

There has been a steady increase in the proportion of multiple pregnancies delivered by elective caesarean birth. The most marked impetus came from Keily's review [17] of over 16,000 multiple births in New York, where he demonstrated increased overall neonatal mortality rates for infants weighing between

2501 and 3000 g and over 3001 g, and demonstrated intrapartum mortality rates that, although low (1.22 per 1000), were 3.5-times those of similar birthweight singleton infants. There remained debate over mode of birth, and particularly whether guidance could be tailored to presentation, birthweight or gestation.

The debate resurfaced in 2002 with publication of Scottish national data examining outcomes of 3874 twin pairs greater than 24 weeks' gestation. This found no difference in second twin outcomes for preterm twins by planned birth mode, but an increased risk, particularly of deaths attributed to anoxia or mechanical difficulties, in second twins from term pregnancies where birth was planned vaginal. They put the risk at around 1 in 350 for anoxia and 1 in 500 for mechanical problems. Smith *et al.* later refined these estimates in a larger study [18] over 8000 twin births at greater than 36 weeks' gestation. The absolute risk to the second twin of vaginal birth was 3.2 per 1000, with a relative risk (to elective caesarean birth) of 5. He suggested that 264 elective caesarean births were necessary to avoid a perinatal death due to anoxia or mechanical problems. In both studies birthweight discrepancy was the variable that seems associated with the highest risk.

Around this time, moves were underway to attempt a trial of planned caesarean versus planned vaginal birth for multiple pregnancy at term and a systematic review carried out by that team [19] did not demonstrate differences in mortality in the literature from 1980 to 2001. This group showed an increased rate of low 5-min Apgar scores, but increased overall neonatal morbidity associated with caesarean section. The Apgar score data were consistent with those found in a very large Scandinavian study.

US data were conflicting. The analyses by Wen and colleagues [20] in term pregnancies showed an increased risk of overall mortality and asphyxial mortality only in those infants born by caesarean section after vaginal birth of the first twin, with low rates overall (1 per 10,000 for caesarean birth and 2.4 per 1000 for vaginal then caesarean birth). There were no differences where both delivered vaginally. The rate of second twin caesarean section was 9.45%. Data in a subsequent paper showed the same findings for low 5-min Apgar scores and an increased risk (3.4-fold, absolute risk 2.9 per 1000) for neonatal seizures for the group where the second twin was born by caesarean section after vaginal birth of the first twin. The differences were less stark than the Scottish cohort, although there were key methodological problems in the US data set.

In contrast the massive study by Sheay *et al.* [21] of over 290,000 twin pregnancies from national data sets showed no difference in neonatal mortality between twins 1 and 2, even when broken down into birth-weight groups. Looking at their data by mode of birth, there was a significant increase in neonatal deaths at vaginal birth, but odds ratios were only 1.08. These data were not controlled for gestation or birthweight. Examination of cause of death (through ICD coding) showed no differences in deaths coded as intrauterine hypoxia or birth asphyxia. The conclusions here were that alleged increases in mortality for second twins were not demonstrable.

Nova Scotian data, from a well-validated data set, followed [22], although looking at composite outcomes. This data set showed a threefold increase in composite perinatal morbidity for the second twin in planned vaginal births, with no differences in outcomes by birth order when planned caesarean birth. The relative presentation of twins did not seem to influence outcomes, but once again inter twin size difference did. The odds of poor outcome were 3.75-times greater where twin 2 was more than 20% larger than twin 1. In detailed subanalyses asphyxia (5-min Apgar score less than 3, cord artery pH less than 7 or base deficit more than 12 mmol/l) was 2.5-times commoner in second twins.

Smith *et al.* [23] re-entered the debate with a study of twin deaths from England, Wales and Northern Ireland. Using the perinatal death reporting system he showed no differences linked to mode of birth for births less than 36 weeks' gestation, but a relative risk of perinatal death secondary to anoxia of 3.4 for second twins where birth was planned vaginally.

The conclusions that can be drawn from the data on twins and elective caesarean birth are much less clear than for term breech, and ultimately the answer will need to be sought from randomized trials. One medium-sized trial has been completed but not yet published, and the large trial co-ordinated by the Toronto group is still recruiting. The issues of maternal morbidity, both immediate and long-term, are not dissimilar from the arguments in term breech, and will ultimately need to be factored into any decision process. National guidelines reflect this uncertainty [24,25].

Vaginal twin birth
Selection
Approximately 40% of twins will present at birth as vertex–vertex, 40% as vertex–non-vertex and 20% with the first twin non-vertex. Given the data on singleton breech births, it would seem logical to recommend elective caesarean section where the presenting twin is breech or transverse, although published data do not show large differences in outcomes where labour occurs. Interlocking of twins is extraordinarily rare (1/600–800) and should not be used to influence choice of mode of birth.

There is general agreement that mono-amniotic twins should be delivered by elective caesarean section, and a growing consensus that this should take place around 32 weeks' gestation.

The only other group where caesarean section might be considered with a vertex first twin is where the second twin is significantly larger than the first. In a number of studies, morbidity appears greater if the second twin is 20–25% larger or where the absolute difference is more than 250 g [26].

Available evidence suggests that vaginal birth of twins after caesarean section does not carry additional risk compared with vaginal birth after caesarean section in singleton pregnancies [27], and although most practitioners would suggest caesarean birth, women should have a choice.

Conduct of labour

Birth in a hospital setting is recommended for twin birth, and the key areas are preparation and the presence of skilled practitioners.

The conduct of labour and the support provided during labour should conform to usual standards.

Fetal monitoring

Most texts recommend continuous electronic fetal heart rate monitoring, although there is no specific evidence to support this [24,25,28]. There needs to be certainty that two separate heart rates are being monitored, and this may involve the use of ultrasound to pick out both fetal heart positions. Where external monitoring has been used for both twins, very high signal loss rates have been reported (up to 33% in the first stage and 60% in the second stage), and there is a strong case for early amniotomy and direct fetal scalp electrode monitoring of the first twin. More regular monitoring of the maternal heart rate is wise to ensure no confusion.

Analgesia

All options should be available although most authorities recommend earlier or elective use of epidural analgesia [24,25,27]. The logic of this argument is that vaginal operative birth rates are high (8% in one study where the first twin delivered spontaneously), internal manipulation may be needed, and that caesarean section for the second twin may occur (6% in one study where the first twin delivered spontaneously).

There is evidence that the length of the first stage of labour is prolonged by about 1 h, but no evidence that the interval between births of the twins is increased.

As in singleton labour, maternal informed choice should be paramount.

Oxytocin augmentation

There is no evidence that the use of oxytocin to augment poor progress in the first stage of labour is contra-indicated for twin labour and it should be considered for similar indications to singleton labour. See Table 11.8.

Table 11.8 First stage of labour.

Assess presentation and relative size of twins
Non-cephalic presentation: recommend caesarean birth
Twin 2 larger by 20–25%: consider caesarean birth
Care co-ordinated by senior staff
Intravenous access
Continuous one-to-one midwifery care
Continuous electronic fetal heart rate monitoring
More frequent maternal pulse estimate
Twin 1 by direct ECG as soon as feasible
Consider early offer of epidural analgesia
Use oxytocin under senior supervision for usual indications
Prepare for the second stage and birth
Ultrasound equipment
Access to obstetric theatre
Prepare oxytocin infusion
Have tocolytic agent available

Conduct of birth

Where the first twin is cephalic then birth should follow the usual guidance for the length of the second stage and the indications for operative birth.

Once the first twin is born, the presentation of the second twin should be sought by abdominal palpation followed by digital vaginal examination and by ultrasound if there is uncertainty. Where the lie is longitudinal it should be stabilized by an assistant.

Use of oxytocin

Many recommend the immediate use of oxytocin following the birth of the first twin, to ensure that the second enters the pelvis and to shorten the birth interval [24,27]. There is little concrete evidence for this outside its logical use where uterine contractions cease. There are some data suggesting a reduction in birth interval and this may be an advantage. It is important that an infusion has been prepared in advance. Where the lie of the second twin is longitudinal, there is a better argument for oxytocin use as soon as possible.

Use of tocolysis

Where the lie of the second twin is not longitudinal or where the presentation is high, then internal manipulation or ECV may be needed. For this to be successful and safe, the uterus needs to be relaxed. This may be achieved by switching off any oxytocin infusion in progress, or by giving tocolysis [29].

The most frequently used acute tocolytic is terbutaline, either as 250 μg subcutaneously, or given intravenously over 5 min. Other options include atosiban, 6.75 mg given over 1 min. These are both effective but give a relatively sustained uterine relaxation, which may be a disadvantage. There is growing experience with intravenous nitroglycerine, which has a very short half-life (2 min). A dose of 200 μg is normally enough, but more can be given safely. The major drawback is hypotension, and the anaesthetist needs to be prepared for this prior to administration.

Inter twin delivery interval

There is continuing debate on whether arbitrary time constraints need to be applied to the interval between the birth of the twins where fetal heart rate monitoring is reassuring. Traditional teaching was that the birth of the second twin should be achieved within

30 min of the first. Data following the introduction of electronic fetal heart rate monitoring showed no differences in measures of short-term morbidity [27]. There is a linear decrease in cord artery pH with an increasing interval that reaches statistical but not clinical significance by 30 min. Others have shown increasingly frequent neonatal acidosis (cord artery pH less than 7.0 or base deficit greater than 12 mmol/l) with longer time intervals [30,31]. In one study the rate was 27% after 30 min, and in another the difference in severe acidosis reached statistical significance at 60 min.

Adding to the debate are data that suggest that longer inter twin intervals are associated with increasing second twin caesarean section rates – the studies showing a six- to eightfold increase after 30–60 min.

Overall the data suggest that sooner is better and that a relaxed approach to the interval may be unwise.

Birth of the non-vertex second twin

There is no substantive randomized evidence to guide the clinical decision between ECV, internal podalic version (IPV) and breech extraction, and caesarean section where the second twin requires manipulation (Table 11.9). Reviews of non-randomized studies, however, seem reasonably consistent [27,28], showing higher vaginal birth rates (97% compared with 45% in singleton breeches) without any excess of injury or perinatal hypoxia when IPV is used. Similarly, outcomes appear as good where IPV is used as compared to caesarean section, although there are less data. The emerging data on maternal morbidity when caesarean section is carried out at full dilatation would also suggest that liberal use of caesarean section for the second non-vertex twin, before or after ECV, would not be an advantage.

Skills and preparation are the key elements for these procedures. ECV is a more common procedure and it is likely that this approach will find most favour. Provided there is good uterine relaxation, success in 30–50% of cases might be expected.

Skills in IPV are less, and may be falling worldwide. One study in India showed a halving of the use of IPV for second transverse twins over a 12-year period.

The key elements for successful IPV are good tocolysis and patience. The approach where the membranes are left intact is now favoured since the studies of Rabinovici in the 1980s [32]. Skills and drills can be useful, but best preparation is to practise the initial

Table 11.9 Internal podalic version and breech extraction.

Requirements

Continuous fetal heart rate monitoring

Uterine relaxation (including tocolysis)

Adequate analgesia

Immediate access to obstetric theatre

Ultrasound equipment

Technique

Grasp the anterior or both feet through the membranes

Use other hand to guide fetal head to longitudinal lie

Gentle continuous traction towards introitus

Continuous pressure on abdomen to flex the fetal head (as in vaginal breech birth by Bracht technique; some may find it easier to use an assistant)

Leave membranes intact until feet either below the level of the ischial spines or at introitus

Once the umbilicus is delivered, proceed using either Bracht manoeuvres or Lovset's manoeuvre to deliver the arms

Birth of the head using conventional techniques

techniques (see below) during caesarean section for transverse lie or for twins.

Where the membranes are already ruptured and the lie is transverse or oblique, ECV may not be possible. An experienced practitioner using good uterine relaxation techniques may be able to achieve birth with IPV, but if uterine relaxation cannot be readily achieved or if the practitioner does not feel sufficiently competent under these circumstances, then caesarean section should be undertaken. Where the membranes rupture early in the process of attempted IPV, usually because of inadequate uterine relaxation, it may be possible to continue provided the operator still has hold of the foot and there is good uterine relaxation, but attempts should not be prolonged or vigorous. The procedure can continue even if after membrane rupture the arm prolapses, as it will gradually move upwards with steady traction.

Preterm breech and twin birth

There is a separate debate on whether or not caesarean section should be recommended for preterm

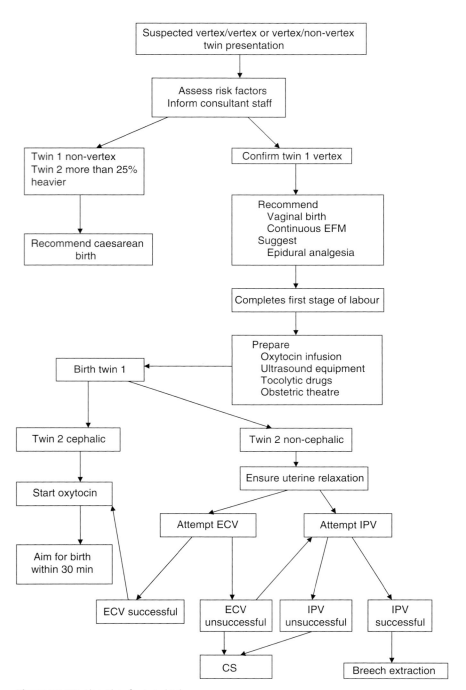

Figure 11.10 Algorithm for twin birth

breech presentation and for preterm twins. The conduct of labour or birth is not different to that described above (Figure 11.10).

The majority of earlier studies do not support a policy of caesarean section for the preterm breech presentation [28]. However, one detailed audit in the UK of births between 27 and 28 weeks' gestation suggested increased mortality for breech presentations at these gestations born vaginally (22.6% compared with 13.5% for births by caesarean section) [33].

More recent population studies from the US [34] have shown marked increased risk for mortality, trauma and birth asphyxia for all birthweight categories between 500 and 2500 g. Recent Swedish data have also shown increased mortality for vaginal preterm breech birth, although of lesser magnitude than the US data [35]. All of these types of studies are prone to selection bias, but argue caution in the selection of mode of birth for the preterm breech.

A number of studies, including one with long-term follow-up [36], have shown no advantage to caesarean preterm birth based on gestation or birth-weight cut-offs [28] for multiple births. Others [37] suggested advantages to caesarean birth in terms of mortality and morbidity where the birthweights were less than 1000 g, but not above this limit. Taken overall there do not seem to be strong grounds for elective caesarean birth or caesarean section during labour simply on gestation or estimated fetal weight grounds.

References

1. Hannah M E, Hannah W J, Hewson S A, Hodnett E D, Saigal S, Willan A R for the TBT Group. Planned caesarean section versus planned vaginal birth for breech presentation at term: a randomised multicentre trial. *Lancet* 2000; **356**: 1375–83.

2. Rietberg C C, Elferink-Stinkens P M, Visser G H A. The effect of the Term Breech Trial on medical intervention behaviour and neonatal outcome in The Netherlands: an analysis of 35,453 term breech infants. *Br J Obstet Gynaecol* 2005; **112**: 205–9.

3. Swedish Collaborative Breech Study Group. Term breech delivery in Sweden: mortality relative to fetal presentation and planned mode of delivery. *Acta Obstet Gynecol Scand* 2005; **84**: 593–601.

4. Vendittelli F, Pons J C, Lennery D, Mamelle N. Obstetricians of the AUDIPOG Sentinel Network. The term breech presentation: neonatal results and obstetric practices in France. *Eur J Obstet Gynecol Reprod Biol* 2006; **125**: 176–84.

5. Villar J, Carroli G, Zavaleta N, *et al.* Maternal and neonatal individual risks and benefits associated with caesarean delivery: multicentre prospective study. *Br Med J* 2007; **335**: 1025–7.

6. Hofmeyr G J, Impey L. *The Management of Breech Presentation.* RCOG Guideline no. 20b London: RCOG, 2006.

7. ACOG Committee Opinion No. 340. Mode of term singleton breech delivery. *Obstet Gynecol* 2006; **108**: 235–7.

8. Royal Australian and New Zealand College of Obstetricians and Gynaecologists. Breech deliveries at term: College Statement No. C-Obs 11 2005.

9. Hofmeyr G J, Kulier R. External cephalic version for breech presentation at term. *Cochrane Database Syst Rev.* 1996; **2**: Art. No.: CD000083. DOI: 10.1002/14651858.CD000083.

10. Impey L, Hofmeyr G J. *External Cephalic Version and Reducing the Incidence of Breech Presentation.* RCOG guideline No. 20a. London: RCOG, 2006.

11. Hofmeyr G J, Gyte G. Interventions to help external cephalic version for breech presentation at term. *Cochrane Database Syst Rev.* 1996; **3**: Art. No.: CD000184. DOI: 10.1002/14651858.CD000184.pub2.

12. Impey L, Pandit M. Tocolysis for repeat external cephalic version in breech presentation at term: a randomised, double-blinded, placebo-controlled trial. *Br J Obstet Gynaecol* 2005; **112**: 627–31.

13. Collaris R J, Guid Oei S. External cephalic version: a safe procedure? A systematic review of version-related risks. *Acta Obstet Gynecol Scand* 2004; **83**: 511–8.

14. Confidential Enquiry into Stillbirths and Deaths in Infancy. *Breech Presentation at the Onset of Labour. 7th Annual Report*, London: Maternal and Child Health Consortium, 2000; 25–40.

15. Kunzel W, Kirschbaum M. Management of vaginal delivery in breech presentation at term. In: *European Practice in Gynaecology and Obstetrics. Breech Delivery.* Paris: Elsevier, 2002; 99–126.

16. Breech delivery. In: Baskett T F, Calder A A, Arulkumaran S, eds. *Munro Kerr's Operative Obstetrics.* London: Saunders Elsevier, 2007; 181–94.

17. Keily J L. The epidemiology of perinatal mortality in multiple births. *Bull NY Acad Med* 1990; **66**: 618–37.

18. Smith G C, Shah I, White I R, Pell J P, Dobbie R. Mode of delivery and the risk of delivery-related perinatal death among twins at term: a retrospective cohort study of 8073 births. *Br J Obstet Gynaecol.* 2005; **112**: 1139–44.

19. Hogle K L, Hutton E K, McBrien K A, Barrett J F R, Hannah M E. Cesarean delivery for twins: a systematic review and meta-analysis. *Am J Obstet Gynecol* 2003; **188**: 220–7.

20. Wen S W, Fung K F F, Oppenheimer L, *et al.* Neonatal mortality in second twin according to cause of death, gestational age, and mode of delivery. *Am J Obstet Gynecol* 2004; **191**: 778–83.

21. Sheay W, Ananth C V, Kinzler W L. Perinatal mortality in first- and second-born twins in the United States. *Obstet Gynecol* 2004; **103**: 63–70.

22. Armson B A, O'Connell C, Persad V, *et al.* Determinants of perinatal mortality and serious neonatal morbidity in the second twin. *Obstet Gynecol* 2006; **108**: 556–64.

23. Smith G C, Fleming K M, White I R. Birth order of twins and risk of perinatal death related to delivery in England, Northern Ireland, and Wales, 1994–2003: retrospective cohort study. *Br Med J* 2007; **334**: 576–8.

24. SOGC Consensus Statement No. 91. Management of Twin Pregnancies. July 2000.

25. Barrett J F R. Management of labour in multiple pregnancies. In: Kilby M, Baker P, Critchley H, Field D, eds. *Multiple Pregnancy*. London: RCOG Press, 2006; 223–234.

26. Williams K P, Galerneau F. Intrapartum influence on caesarean delivery in multiple gestation. *Acta Obstet Gynecol Scand* 2003; **82**: 241–5.

27. Cruikshank D P. Intrapartum management of twin gestations. *Obstet Gynecol* 2007; **109**: 1167–76.

28. Barrett J F R, Knox Ritchie W. Twin delivery best practice and research. *Clin Obstet Gynaecol* 2002; **16**: 43–56.

29. Procedures and techniques. Acute tocolysis. In: Baskett T F, Calder A A, Arulkumaran S, eds. *Munro Kerr's Operative Obstetrics*. London: Saunders Elsevier, 2007; 285–88.

30. Oppenheimer E P, Yang Q, Wen S W, Fung K, Walker M. Relationship between inter twin delivery interval and metabolic acidosis in the second twin. *Am J Perinatol* 2006; **23**: 481–5.

31. Leung T Y, Tam W H, Leung T N, Lok I H, Lau T K. Effect of twin-to-twin delivery interval on umbilical cord blood gas in the second twins. *Br J Obstet Gynaecol* 2002; **109**: 63–7.

32. Rabinovici J, Barkai G, Reichman B, Serr D M, Mashiach S. Internal podalic version with unruptured membranes for the second twin in transverse lie. *Obstet Gynecol* 1988; **71**: 428–30.

33. Confidential Enquiry into Stillbirths and Deaths in Infancy. *Survival Rates of Babies Born between 27 and 28 weeks' Gestation in England, Wales and Northern Ireland 1998–2000. 8th Annual Report.* London: Maternal and Child Health Consortium, 2002; 83–100.

34. Robilio P A, Boe N H, Danielsen B, Gilbert W M. Vaginal vs. cesarean delivery for preterm breech presentation of singleton infants in California: a population-based study. *J Reprod Med* 2007; **52** (6): 473–9.

35. Hebst A, Kallen K. Influence of mode of delivery on neonatal mortality and morbidity in spontaneous preterm breech delivery. *Eur J Obstet Gynecol Reprod Biol* 2007; **133**: 25–9.

36. Rydhstrom H. Prognosis for twins with birth weight less than 1500 g: the impact of caesarean section in relation to fetal presentation. *Am J Obstet Gynecol* 1999; **163**: 528–33.

37. Zhang J, Bowes W A, Grey T W, McMahon M J. Twin delivery and neonatal and infant mortality: a population-based study. *Obstet Gynecol* 1996; **88**: 593–8.

Cord prolapse and shoulder dystocia

Joanna Crofts, Timothy Draycott and Mark Denbow

Umbilical cord prolapse
Definition and incidence

Cord prolapse is the descent of the umbilical cord through the cervix alongside, or past, the fetal presenting part in the presence of ruptured membranes. The incidence is between 0.1 and 0.6% and 1% in breech presentation [1].

Pathophysiology of cord prolapse

Cord prolapse most commonly occurs after the amniotic membranes rupture (spontaneously or artificially) where the fetal presenting part is poorly applied to the maternal cervix. The umbilical cord may subsequently be compressed, compromising the fetal blood supply.

Risk factors

Most risks factors for cord prolapse are associated with a poorly applied fetal presenting part (Table 12.1).

A stepwise multivariate logistic regression model study of 456 cases of cord prolapse in a delivery population of 121,227 women [2] identified independent risk factors for cord prolapse (odds ratio [95% confidence interval]):

- malpresentation (5.1 [4.1–6.3]),
- polyhydramnios (3.0 [2.3–3.9]),
- true knot of the umbilical cord (3.0 [1.8–5.1]),
- preterm delivery (2.1 [1.6–2.8]),
- induction of labour (2.2 [1.7–2.8]),
- grandmultiparity (1.9 [1.5–2.3]),
- lack of prenatal care (1.4 [1.02–1.8]), and
- male gender (1.3 [1.1–1.6]).

A case control study of 709 cases of cord prolapse and 2407 randomly selected controls found that infants affected by cord prolapse were more likely to weigh less than 2500 g (4.8 [3.7–6.2]) and to be born prematurely (2.9 [2.2–3.7]). Other risk factors included second twin (5.0 [3.3–11.7]) and breech presentation (birth weight-adjusted 2.5 [1.7–3.9]) [3]. Expectant management of preterm ruptured membranes is also associated with cord prolapse [1].

Obstetric interventions (amniotomy, fetal scalp electrode application, external cephalic version and amnioreduction) are associated with an increased risk of umbilical cord prolapse, especially in the presence of a high presenting part.

Prediction

Ultrasound has been proposed as a method of detecting cord presentation and therefore predicting pregnancies at greatest risk of cord prolapse. However, there is currently insufficient evidence to support such practice [1].

Prevention

The RCOG recommends that women with transverse, oblique or unstable lie should be offered elective admission to hospital at 37 weeks (or sooner if there are signs of labour or suspicion of ruptured membranes) [1]. Elective admission does not prevent cord prolapse; however, if cord prolapse does occur in hospital, immediate diagnosis and emergency treatment is possible, thereby improving neonatal outcome. Women with a transverse, oblique or unstable lie should be offered an elective caesarean section at term. Alternative management would be to conservatively manage until spontaneous onset of labour and

Table 12.1 Risk factors for cord prolapse.

Antenatal	Intrapartum
Breech presentation	Amniotomy (especially with a high presenting part)
Unstable lie	Prematurity
Oblique or transverse lie	Breech presentation
External cephalic version	Second twin
Amnioreduction	Amnioinfusion
Expectant management of prelabour rupture of membranes	Fetal scalp electrode application
Male fetus	Disimpaction of the fetal head during rotational assisted delivery
Previous cord prolapse	

to re-evaluate the lie and presentation at this point. An emergency caesarean section is indicated if labour or ruptured membranes are associated with an abnormal lie, or if the cord is palpated below the presenting part on vaginal examination during labour; in this situation, artificial rupture of membranes should be avoided [1].

Any obstetric intervention after the membranes have ruptured (application of fetal scalp electrode, manual rotation of vertex, internal podalic version) carries a risk of cord prolapse, and upwards displacement of the presenting part after membrane rupture should therefore be minimized. Fundal pressure or stabilization of a longitudinal lie may reduce the risk of cord prolapse during artificial rupture of the membranes if the vertex is high. Artificial rupture of membranes should be avoided whenever possible if the presenting part is unengaged and mobile; if it becomes necessary, it should be performed in, or near, the operating theatre with facilities to perform an immediate emergency caesarean section if required.

Management
Recognition of cord prolapse
Cord prolapse should be suspected when there is an abnormal fetal heart rate pattern (e.g. bradycardia, decelerations) in the presence of ruptured membranes, particularly if such changes commence soon after membrane rupture. A speculum and/or a digital vaginal examination should be performed when cord prolapse is suspected, regardless of gestation. Mismanagement of abnormal fetal heart rate patterns is one of the commonest aspects of substandard care identified in cord prolapse associated with perinatal death [1].

Call for help
As soon as cord prolapse is diagnosed, urgent help should be called immediately, including (if possible) a senior midwife, additional midwifery staff, the most experienced obstetrician available, an anaesthetist, the theatre team, and a neonatologist.

If cord prolapse occurs outside hospital, an emergency ambulance should be called immediately to transfer the patient to an appropriate obstetric unit. Even if delivery appears imminent, a paramedic ambulance should still be called in case of neonatal compromise at birth.

When help arrives 'cord prolapse' should be clearly stated so that all in attendance immediately understand the problem. Staff outside the obstetric unit (midwives, ambulance staff, General Practitioners) should liaise directly with the obstetric unit, clearly stating they are transferring in a patient with a cord prolapse, giving an estimated time of arrival at hospital, so that the appropriate hospital staff are aware, and preparations can be made to ensure timely delivery on arrival at hospital.

Prepare for immediate delivery and minimize cord compression
As soon as cord prolapse has been recognized, cord compression should be minimized and preparations should be made for immediate, emergency delivery. Unless the cervix is fully dilated, delivery should be by emergency caesarean section [1].

Reducing cord compression
There are several methods described to minimize compression of the cord between the cervix and presenting part.

Digital elevation
When cord prolapse is diagnosed, the presenting part should be digitally elevated away from the cord by maintaining the examination hand within the vagina and applying upwards pressure on the presenting part. Handling of the cord should be kept to a minimum to reduce the risk of cord vasospasm.

Maternal positioning

The presenting part may be displaced away from the prolapsed cord using different maternal positions: knee–chest position (woman kneeling on bed with her head down and pelvis in the air), or tilting the bed so that the foot of the bed is steeply raised with the mother lying in the left lateral position.

Bladder filling

If the decision-to-delivery interval is likely to be prolonged, particularly if it involves ambulance transfer, elevation of the presenting part through bladder filling may be helpful [4]. The bladder should be catheterized with an indwelling urinary catheter and filled with 500–700 ml of fluid by connecting a bag of intravenous fluid to the catheter and clamping the catheter once 500–750 ml have been instilled. It is essential to empty the bladder just before attempted delivery, be it vaginal or caesarean section.

When bladder filling was first described there was one neonatal death in 28 cases, with a decision-to-delivery interval of 25–115 min [4]. Two subsequent studies of a total of 112 cases of cord prolapse managed with bladder filling reported no fetal deaths despite an average diagnosis-to-delivery interval of over 30 min [1].

Assess fetal well-being

The fetus should be continuously monitored once cord prolapse has been diagnosed, if possible. If there is no audible fetal heart an ultrasound scan should be performed as soon as possible to confirm fetal viability.

Prepare for immediate delivery

Wide-bore intravenous access should be established and blood taken for full blood count and group and save. Whilst preparing for immediate delivery, the fetal condition should be optimized. If a syntocinon infusion is running, this should be stopped and a 500 ml bolus of intravenous fluid given. Tocolysis to inhibit uterine contractions can be considered, e.g. terbutaline sulphate 0.25 mg subcutaneously. However, although terbutaline has been demonstrated to reduce contractions and abolish bradycardia in the absence of cord prolapse, there is no direct evidence that it is of benefit during cord prolapse. Manipulation of the cord or exposure to air may cause reactive vasoconstriction and fetal hypoxia–acidosis, therefore some authorities advise that swabs soaked in warm saline wrapped around the cord may be beneficial, but there are no data to support or refute this [1].

Although the measures described above may be useful during preparation for delivery, delivery should not be delayed by them.

Delivery

Emergency caesarean section is the recommended mode of delivery when vaginal delivery is not imminent. Caesarean section is associated with lower perinatal mortality and low Apgar score at 5 min compared to spontaneous vaginal delivery. However, when vaginal delivery is imminent, outcomes appear to be similar or better with vaginal delivery [1].

There is poor correlation between the decision-to-delivery interval and umbilical cord pH. Neonatal outcomes after emergency caesarean section occurring up to 60 min from decision appear to be no worse than those following immediate delivery, in cases without a non-resolving bradycardia. However, a caesarean section should be performed within 30 min (category 1) if there are fetal heart rate abnormalities associated with cord prolapse. A caesarean section of urgency category 2 is appropriate in cases where the fetal heart rate is reassuring [1].

In the majority of cases, regional, rather than general, anaesthesia may be used; however, prolonged and repeated attempts at regional anaesthesia must be avoided. The presenting part should be kept elevated while the anaesthesia is undertaken. Clear communication about the urgency and timing of delivery is required between the obstetric and anaesthetic team to ensure the safest method of anaesthesia for both mother and fetus.

Vaginal birth can be attempted at full dilatation when it can be accomplished within 20 min or less from diagnosis, and ideally within 10 min. Ventouse or forceps delivery should only be considered if the prerequisites for operative delivery are met. In general, poor fetal outcomes are associated with more difficult attempts at achieving vaginal birth. In multiparas, or for second twins, a ventouse extraction may be attempted by experienced operators at 9 cm dilatation when there is cord prolapse with severe CTG abnormalities and delivery is considered easily achievable. Breech extraction may be performed under some circumstances, e.g. after internal podalic version for the second twin or when delivery is imminent in singleton breech presentation.

Neonatal resuscitation

An experienced neonatal team must be present at delivery to ensure full cardiorespiratory support is given, if required, to the neonate.

Documentation

Documentation should include the time cord prolapse occurred, the time help was called and arrived, methods used to alleviate cord compression, the decision to deliver and delivery times, and method of delivery.

Neonatal morbidity and mortality associated with cord prolapse

The perinatal mortality rate associated with cord prolapse has declined over the last century. However, the mortality rate over the past few decades has remained static: 36–162 per 1000 [1], with cases of cord prolapse appearing consistently in perinatal mortality enquiries. Birth asphyxia (due to cord compression preventing venous return to the fetus and arterial vasospasm secondary to exposure to vaginal fluids and/or air) may result in hypoxic–ischaemic encephalopathy, cerebral palsy or neonatal death. Prematurity and congenital malformation account for the majority of adverse outcomes associated with cord prolapse in hospital, but birth asphyxia and perinatal death does occur in normally formed term babies following cord prolapse.

Shoulder dystocia
Definition and incidence

Shoulder dystocia is a vaginal cephalic delivery that requires additional obstetric manoeuvres to deliver the fetus after gentle downward traction has failed. Shoulder dystocia occurs when either the anterior, or less commonly the posterior, fetal shoulder impact on the maternal symphysis or the sacral promontory, respectively, preventing delivery of the body after delivery of the fetal head. The incidence of shoulder dystocia in the largest series (34,800–267,228 births) is between 0.58 and 0.70% [5].

Pathophysiology of shoulder dystocia

In the majority of women the antero-posterior diameter of the pelvic inlet is narrower than the oblique or transverse diameter. Shoulder dystocia occurs when the diameter of the maternal pelvis through which the fetal shoulders attempt to pass is less than the bisacromial length of the fetus, usually when the fetal shoulders do not rotate to the wider oblique diameter.

Antenatal risk factors for shoulder dystocia
Macrosomia

The greater the fetal birthweight, the higher risk of shoulder dystocia [5]. A review of 175,886 vaginal births of infants born to non-diabetic mothers reported rates of shoulder dystocia of 5.2%, 9.1%, 14.3% and 29.0% in infants weighing 4000–4250 g, 4250–4500 g, 4500–4750 g, and 4750–5000 g, respectively [6]. Infants weighing over 4000 g are significantly more likely to suffer shoulder dystocia compared to those weighing less than 4000 g (11.1% and 0.6%, respectively) [7].

Previous shoulder dystocia

Previous shoulder dystocia is a risk factor for recurrent shoulder dystocia. The recurrence rate is reported to be approximately 15% [5]. However, rates may be underestimated due to selection bias; elective caesarean section may be performed in some pregnancies following shoulder dystocia.

Maternal diabetes mellitus

Maternal diabetes mellitus increases the risk of shoulder dystocia [5]. Infants of diabetic mothers have a three- to fourfold increased risk of shoulder dystocia compared to infants of non-diabetic mothers for the same birthweight. Diabetes increases the risk of shoulder dystocia by more than 70% [6].

Instrumental delivery

Compared to a spontaneous delivery, shoulder dystocia is approximately twice as likely to occur with instrumental delivery [6].

Maternal obesity

Shoulder dystocia is associated with obesity; however, obese women tend to have larger babies and the association may be due to fetal macrosomia, rather than maternal obesity per se. In a study which controlled for potential confounding effects of other variables associated with obesity, there was no significant increase in the risk of shoulder dystocia associated with maternal obesity (odds ratio 0.9 [95% CI 0.5, 1.6]) [8].

Parity

There appears to be no relationship between parity and shoulder dystocia.

Gestational age

Studies investigating births between 37 and 43 weeks' gestation suggest there is no significant difference in the gestational age at delivery of births complicated by a shoulder dystocia and births without shoulder dystocia.

Intrapartum risks

The risk of shoulder dystocia is increased in any labour in which progress is slow (prolonged first stage, prolonged second stage, use of syntocinon for augmentation of labour).

Prediction

Macrosomia alone is a weak predictor of shoulder dystocia. The majority of infants with a birth weight of $\geq$4500 g do not develop shoulder dystocia [9] and, equally importantly, 30–48% of shoulder dystocia occurs in infants with a birth weight <4000 g [9]. Furthermore, antenatal detection of macrosomia is poor. Clinical fetal weight estimation is unreliable; third trimester ultrasound scans have at least a 10% margin for error for actual birth weight and sensitivity of just 60% for macrosomia (>4500 g) [9].

A retrospective review of 267,228 vaginal births reported that even the most powerful predictors for shoulder dystocia have a sensitivity of just 12% and positive predictive value of under 5% [10]. The majority of cases of shoulder dystocia occur with women with no risk factors. Shoulder dystocia is, therefore, an unpredictable and largely unpreventable event. Clinicians should be aware of existing risk factors, but must always be alert to the possibility of shoulder dystocia with any delivery [9].

Prevention

Shoulder dystocia can only be prevented by caesarean section. However, a decision analysis model estimated that an additional 2345 caesarean deliveries would be required to prevent one permanent injury from shoulder dystocia [11]. Estimation of fetal weight is unreliable, and the large majority of macrosomic infants do not experience shoulder dystocia, therefore elective caesarean section is not recommended in cases of suspected fetal macrosomia [9]. However, elective caesarean section should be considered for a woman with diabetes and suspected fetal macrosomia (estimated fetal weight >4500 g), reflecting the higher incidence of brachial plexus injury in this subgroup, and may be considered if the estimated fetal weight is over 5000 g in non-diabetic pregnancies.

Management

There are numerous techniques described that can be used to relieve shoulder dystocia. The Royal College of Obstetricians and Gynaecology have published an evidence-based algorithm for the management of shoulder dystocia [9].

There is no evidence that one manoeuvre is superior to another. The algorithm begins with simple measures, which are often effective, and leads progressively to more-invasive manoeuvres.

Recognition of shoulder dystocia

There may be difficulty with delivery of the face and chin. When the head delivers it remains tightly applied to the vulva, retracts and depresses the perineum – the 'turtle-neck' sign. There may be a failure of restitution and the anterior shoulder then fails to deliver with routine traction.

Call for help

As soon as shoulder dystocia is suspected help must be summoned immediately. Help should include (if possible) a senior midwife and additional midwifery staff, the most experienced obstetrician available, and the neonatologist. If shoulder dystocia is not resolved quickly then the obstetric consultant and anaesthetist should be urgently called.

Clearly state the problem

'Shoulder dystocia' should be clearly stated as help arrives so that attendants immediately understand the problem.

Maternal pushing should be discouraged as it may increase the impaction of the shoulders, and will not resolve the dystocia.

McRoberts' position

McRoberts' position (hyperflexion of the maternal legs) is the most widely advocated first-line manoeuvre

135

and was first described in 1983 [12]. McRoberts' position increases the relative antero-posterior diameter of the pelvic inlet by rotating the maternal pelvis cephaloid and straightening the sacrum relative to the lumbar spine. The reported success rate is between 40 and 90% [5]. McRoberts' position is associated with less neonatal trauma than other resolution manoeuvres; however, this may be because more severe cases of shoulder dystocia, which are more likely to result in injury, often require more than one resolution manoeuvre.

There is no evidence that using McRoberts' position in anticipation of shoulder dystocia is helpful, therefore prophylactic McRoberts' positioning is not recommended [9].

To perform McRoberts' position, the mother should be laid flat and her legs hyperflexed against her abdomen by an assistant on each side. Routine traction (the same degree of traction applied during a normal delivery) should be applied to the fetal head. If the shoulders are not released an additional resolution manoeuvre should be attempted.

Suprapubic pressure

Suprapubic pressure (or Rubin's I manoeuvre) was first described by Rubin [13] in 1964, and improves the rate of shoulder dystocia resolution when used in combination with McRoberts' manoeuvre. The aim is to reduce the diameter of the fetal shoulders (the bisacromial diameter) by adduction and rotate the shoulders into the wider oblique angle of the maternal pelvis.

Suprapubic pressure should be applied superior to the maternal symphysis pubis in a downward and lateral direction by an assistant from the side of the fetal back (if this is known) to adduct the shoulders. Again, if the anterior shoulder is not released with suprapubic pressure and routine traction, a further manoeuvre should be attempted.

Evaluate the need for an episiotomy

An episiotomy will not relieve the bony obstruction that causes shoulder dystocia and therefore by itself will not resolve the dystocia. However, an episiotomy may be required to improve access to the pelvis, facilitating internal vaginal manoeuvres.

Internal manoeuvres

There are two categories of internal manoeuvres that can be performed – internal rotation, and delivery of the posterior arm. There is no evidence that one should be performed before the other. All internal manoeuvres start with the same action – gaining access to the pelvis; this should be gained posteriorly as the potential space in the pelvis is the sacral hollow. The whole hand (including the thumb) should be inserted into the vagina posteriorly.

Internal rotational manoeuvres

The aims of internal rotation are to:

(i) move the fetal shoulders out of the narrowest diameter of the pelvis (the anterior-posterior) and into a wider diameter (the oblique or transverse) – Woods' screw and Rubin II;

(ii) reduce the fetal bisacromial diameter – Rubin II; and

(iii) utilize the pelvic anatomy: as the shoulders rotate they descend through the pelvis due to the pelvic bony architecture – Woods' screw.

Woods' screw

Woods and Westbury described internal rotation of the fetal shoulder as a mechanism to resolve shoulder dystocia in 1942 [14]. The fetus in shoulder dystocia is described to be acting as a screw which has the greatest resistance to its release by a direct pull.

Woods' screw involves pressure on the anterior aspect of the posterior fetal shoulder to rotate the fetal shoulders out of the anterior-posterior diameter into the wider oblique or transverse diameter of the maternal pelvis. If required, the rotation can be continued through 180° (until the original posterior shoulder becomes the new anterior shoulder) taking advantage of the pelvic anatomy; due to the 'threads' in the maternal pelvis the fetal shoulders move down through the pelvis during the rotation, and the new fetal anterior shoulder should be below the maternal symphysis pubis and free from obstruction.

Rubin II

Rubin [13] described a 'Two-maneuver program' for shoulder dystocia management in 1964. The first manoeuvre, Rubin I, is suprapubic pressure. The second stage of manoeuvres involves internal rotation of the fetal shoulders by pressure on the posterior aspect of the posterior (or anterior) fetal shoulder. Rubin describe this manoeuvre as: 'inserting the fingers of one hand vaginally behind whichever shoulder is more readily accessible (usually the posterior) and pushing the shoulders toward the fetus' chest'.

Pressure on the posterior aspect of the fetal shoulder produces adduction which reduces the bisacromial diameter (compared with Woods' screw, which abducts the fetal shoulders).

Rotation can be most easily achieved by pressing on the anterior or posterior aspect of the posterior shoulder. Pressure on the posterior aspect of the posterior shoulder has the added benefit of adducting the shoulders and reducing the shoulder diameter. Rotation should move the shoulders into the wider oblique diameter, resolving the shoulder dystocia, so delivery becomes possible with routine traction. If delivery does not occur, the pressure can be continued and the shoulders rotated through 180°.

If pressure in one direction is not effective, efforts should be made to rotate the shoulders in the opposite direction by pressure on the opposite aspect of the fetal posterior shoulder. If pressure on the posterior shoulder is unsuccessful, pressure can be applied to the anterior fetal shoulder.

An assistant providing suprapubic pressure may help during attempted internal rotation. The person performing internal rotation needs to ensure suprapubic pressure is applied in the correct direction and rotation is with, not against, each other.

Delivery of the posterior arm

Delivery may also be facilitated by delivery of the posterior arm, described by Barnum in 1945 [15]. The rationale is that by delivering the posterior arm the diameter of the fetal shoulders is narrowed by the width of the arm, providing enough room to resolve the shoulder dystocia.

If the fetal arms are flexed the posterior fetal hand and forearm will be encountered on entry into the sacral hollow and the fetal wrist can be grasped by the accoucheur's fingers and thumb. The posterior arm can then be removed from the maternal pelvis by gentle traction in a straight line, in so doing, the fetal arm will be swept across the fetal face. Once the posterior arm has delivered, gentle traction can be applied to the fetal head; if the shoulder dystocia has resolved the fetus should be delivered easily. However, if despite delivering the posterior arm, the shoulder dystocia has not resolved, the fetus can be rotated through 180° with traction across the fetal chest. The posterior shoulder will become the new anterior shoulder and will be below the symphysis pubis, resolving the dystocia.

The posterior arm is more difficult to deliver if it is straight, as the arm needs to be flexed before the wrist can be grasped. To flex the posterior arm it should be followed down to the elbow, and pressure and counter-pressure applied to the antecubital fossa and back of the forearm. Traction on the upper arm should be avoided as it is likely to result in humeral fracture.

All-fours position

The all-fours manoeuvre may dislodge the anterior shoulder and facilitate access to the posterior shoulder to enable internal manoeuvres to be performed. In 82 reported cases the success rate was 83% without the need for additional manoeuvres and with few injuries to mothers and babies. The mother should be asked to transfer onto her hands and knees, and gentle traction should be applied to the fetal head to determine if the shoulders have been released. It may be difficult for some mothers to assume this position, particularly with an epidural block.

Additional manoeuvres

Surgical manoeuvres such as cephalic replacement followed by caesarean section and symphysiotomy are uncommon and have serious potential maternal morbidity. They are considered to be last-resort measures and should only be performed if the fetal heart beat is still present [9].

Zavanelli manoeuvre

Cephalic replacement of the head and subsequent delivery by caesarean section was first performed by Zavanelli. In a case series of 59, cephalic replacement was unsuccessful in 6 cases (10%), and 2 mothers (3%) suffered a ruptured uterus. Furthermore, two (3%) babies died, and of the survivors, two (4%) babies had permanent neurological injury and five (9%) experienced a permanent brachial plexus injury. It is important to note that the uterus retracts after delivery of the fetal head, so tocolysis is required prior to unrestituting, flexing and replacing the fetal head into the uterine cavity.

Symphysiotomy

Symphysiotomy is the surgical division of the symphyseal ligament to increase pelvic dimensions. It is associated with high incidence of serious maternal morbidity, including urethral and bladder injury,

137

infection, pain and long-term walking difficulty, and poor neonatal outcome.

What not to do

It is instinctive to apply traction to the fetal head in an attempt to deliver the baby. However, strong downward traction on the fetal head is associated with neonatal trauma, including permanent brachial plexus injury. Traction will not resolve the dystocia and traction above that used during a normal delivery should be avoided. Evidence suggests that traction applied quickly with a 'jerk', rather than applied slowly, may be more damaging to the nerves of brachial plexus; therefore traction should be applied slowly, carefully and in an axial direction.

Fundal pressure has been described as a manoeuvre in the management of shoulder dystocia; indeed, fundal pressure is described by both Woods [14] and Rubin [13] in their original description of internal rotational manoeuvres. However, a study in 1987 reported fundal pressure, in the absence of other manoeuvres, was associated with a 77% complication rate, including uterine rupture [16] and brachial plexus injury in the neonate. Therefore, fundal pressure is no longer a recommended manoeuvre in the management of shoulder dystocia and should not be used.

Documentation

A review of fatal cases of shoulder dystocia in the United Kingdom reported the sequence of events during delivery was often inadequately recorded and stressed the need for a clear, complete, contemporaneous record of the sequence of events. The RCOG shoulder dystocia guideline suggests that a proforma may be helpful in documenting key events after delivery [9]. Documentation should include time of delivery of the head and body, manoeuvres performed (with timings and sequence), anterior fetal shoulder at the time of the dystocia, degree of traction applied, staff in attendance and the time they arrived, fetal condition at birth (including cord pH measurements) and an explanation to the parents.

After the birth

Shoulder dystocia is a frightening and potentially traumatic experience for the mother and her attending family. It is important to inform the parents what is happening and give the mother clear instructions during the emergency. The birth and the reason for the use of manoeuvres should be discussed after delivery.

Any baby with a suspected injury following shoulder dystocia should be immediately reviewed by a neonatologist. In the UK the Erb's Palsy Group is an excellent source of information and supports families and healthcare practitioners caring for children with brachial plexus injuries (www.erbspalsygroup.co.uk).

A woman who has had a previous shoulder dystocia should be referred to a consultant-led antenatal clinic in subsequent pregnancies to discuss antenatal care and mode of delivery.

Maternal morbidity associated with shoulder dystocia

There is significant maternal morbidity associated with shoulder dystocia; particularly postpartum haemorrhage (11%) and third- and fourth-degree perineal tears (3.8%). Many women also experience psychological trauma and guilt following shoulder dystocia, especially if their child has suffered a birth injury.

Neonatal morbidity and mortality associated with shoulder dystocia
Brachial plexus injury

The brachial plexus is the most complex structure in the peripheral nervous system conveying motor, sensory and sympathetic nerve fibres to the arm and shoulder. The brachial plexus contains five roots (C5–C8, T1) which terminate in five main peripheral nerves. Sympathetic nerve fibres from the first thoracic root provide the autonomic nerve supply to the head, neck and upper limbs, and control sweat glands, pupil dilatation and eyelid movement.

The brachial plexus is vulnerable to trauma due to its large size, superficial location and position between two highly mobile structures, the neck and arm. The incidence of brachial plexus injury (BPI) in the United Kingdom and Republic of Ireland in 1998–1999 was 1 in 2300 live births [17]. The proportion of BPIs reported to be permanent, an injury lasting more than 12 months, ranges between 8 and 12%; a rate of approximately 1 permanent injury per 10,000 births.

Risk of brachial plexus injury

BPIs are associated with shoulder dystocia with a wide incidence range: 8.5–32% of shoulder dystocias [18]. BPI in association with shoulder dystocia has been found repeatedly to occur regardless of the procedure used to disimpact the shoulder [5], and appears to be independent of the experience of the accoucheur conducting the delivery.

BPIs, however, have been reported to arise without concomitant shoulder dystocia in up to 47% of cases [9], indicating that injury can occur without recognized shoulder dystocia.

BPI is nearly 20 times more common in infants of diabetic mothers compared to those of non-diabetics. Assisted vaginal delivery and increased birth weight are also associated with a significantly increased risk compared to spontaneous vaginal delivery [17,19]. Conversely, delivery by caesarean section appears protective. As with shoulder dystocia, the risk factors for BPI are not independent and accurate prediction of pregnancies at risk is currently not possible.

Classification of brachial plexus injury

Erb's palsy

Erb's palsy, or upper BPI, is the most common form of BPI with a frequency of 73–86% [20]. The affected cervical nerve roots are the fifth (C5) and sixth (C6), with the seventh cervical root (C7) sometimes also involved. The classic Erb's palsy posture is a result of paralysis or weakness in the shoulder muscles, the elbow flexors, and the forearm supinators. The affected arm hangs down and is internally rotated, extended, and pronated. If C7 is involved, the wrist and finger extensors are also paralysed. The loss of extension causes the wrist to flex and the fingers to curl up in the 'waiter's tip position'. Full functional recovery is reported to occur in 65–90% of cases; the prognosis is worse with C7 involvement [20].

Klumpke's palsy

Klumpke's palsy, an isolated lower BPI, is rare, accounting for 0.6–2% of obstetric BPIs [20]. The affected cervical nerve roots are the eighth cervical (C8) and first thoracic (T1), with occasional C7 involvement. Klumpke's palsy is characterized by weakness of the triceps, forearm pronators, and wrist flexors. The classic physical findings are a 'claw-like' paralysed hand with good elbow and shoulder function.

Full functional recovery is reported to occur in less than 50% of cases [20].

Total brachial plexus injury

Complete involvement of the brachial plexus occurs in approximately 20% of BPIs [20]. The entire plexus from C5 to T1 is involved, with total sensory and motor deficits of the entire arm, resulting in a paralysed arm with no sensation. Horner's syndrome, caused by sympathetic nerve injury, resulting in contraction of the pupil and ptosis on the affected side, may also be present with a total brachial plexus injury and is associated with a worse prognosis. Full functional recovery is very rare without surgical intervention.

Other fetal injuries

Other reported fetal injuries include fractures of the humerus and clavicle, pneumothoraxes and hypoxic brain damage.

Recommendations and requirements for shoulder dystocia training

There is a need for shoulder dystocia training. Poor outcomes following shoulder dystocia are commonly a result of inappropriate clinical management. The 5th Confidential Enquiries into Stillbirths and Deaths in Infancy in England and Wales found grade three suboptimal care in 66% of neonatal deaths following shoulder dystocia. In 2003 the NHS Litigation Authority produced a report on the 264 claims for obstetric brachial plexus injury (OBPI) in England. Medico-legal experts judged 46% (72/158) of the reviewed cases to involve substandard care. The most common criticism related to failure to carry out standard shoulder dystocia resolution manoeuvres. A recently published study found only 43% of midwives and doctors were able to successfully manage a severe shoulder dystocia simulation prior to training.

Poor neonatal outcome following shoulder dystocia is associated with a lack of staff confidence and competence managing this unpredictable and largely unpreventable condition. Therefore, training for the management of shoulder dystocia might be the most effective means of reducing the associated morbidity and mortality. The 5th CESDI Report recommended a 'high level of awareness and training for all birth attendants' as 'professionals will be exposed to it [shoulder dystocia] relatively infrequently, but urgent action is needed when it does occur'. Annual shoulder dystocia training is a mandatory requirement in the maternity Clinical Negligence Scheme for Trusts in the UK.

Practical training for shoulder dystocia management using specifically designed mannequins has been associated with increased knowledge and performance in the management of simulated shoulder dystocia. Furthermore, a recently published retrospective study of real life shoulder dystocias in one hospital over a nine year period demonstrated improved clinical management and a significant reduction in neonatal injury at birth from 9.3% pre-training to 2.3% after the introduction of training [21].

References

1. Royal College of Obstetricians and Gynaecologists. *Green Top Guideline: Management of Cord Prolapse.* London: RCOG, 2008.

2. Kahana B, *et al.* Umbilical cord prolapse and perinatal outcomes. *Int J Gynecol Obstet* 2004; **84**: 127–32.

3. Critchlow C W, *et al.* Risk factors and infant outcomes associated with umbilical cord prolapse: a population-based case-control study among births in Washington State. *Am J Obstet Gynecol* 1994; **170**: 613–8.

4. Katz Z, *et al.* Management of labor with umbilical cord prolapse: a 5-year study. *Obstet Gynecol* 1988; **72**: 278–81.

5. Gherman R B. Shoulder dystocia: an evidence-based evaluation of the obstetric nightmare. *Clin Obstet Gynecol* 2002; **45**: 345–62.

6. Nesbitt T S, Gilbert W M, Herrchen B. Shoulder dystocia and associated risk factors with macrosomic infants born in California. *Am J Obstet Gynecol* 1998; **179**: 476–80.

7. Nocon J J, *et al.* Shoulder dystocia: an analysis of risks and obstetric maneuvers. *Am J Obstet Gynecol* 1993; **168**: 1732–7; discussion 1737–9.

8. Robinson H, *et al.* Is maternal obesity a predictor of shoulder dystocia? *Obstet Gynecol* 2003; **101**: 24–7.

9. Royal College of Obstetricians and Gynaecologists. *Shoulder Dystocia: Green-top Guideline.* London: RCOG, 2005.

10. Ouzounian J G, Gherman R B. Shoulder dystocia: are historic risk factors reliable predictors? *Am J Obstet Gynecol* 2005; **192**: 1933–5.

11. Rouse D J, Owen J. Prophylactic cesarean delivery for fetal macrosomia diagnosed by means of ultrasonography – A Faustian bargain? *Am J Obstet Gynecol* 1999; **181**: 332–8.

12. Gonik B, Stringer C A, Held B. An alternate maneuver for management of shoulder dystocia. *Am J Obstet Gynecol* 1983; **145**: 882–4.

13. Rubin A. Management of shoulder dystocia. *J Am Med Assoc* 1964; **189**: 835–7.

14. Woods C E, Westbury N Y. A principle of physics as applicable to shoulder delivery. *Am J Obstet Gynecol* 1942; 796–804.

15. Barnum C G. Dystocia due to the shoulders. *Am J Obstet Gynecol* 1945; **50**: 439–42.

16. Gross T L, *et al.* Shoulder dystocia: a fetal–physician risk. *Am J Obstet Gynecol* 1987; **156**: 1408–18.

17. Evans-Jones G, *et al.* Congenital brachial palsy: incidence, causes, and outcome in the United Kingdom and Republic of Ireland. *Arch Dis Child Fetal Neonatal Ed* 2003; **88**: F185–9.

18. Christoffersson M, *et al.* Shoulder dystocia and brachial plexus injury: a case-control study. *Acta Obstet Gynecol Scand* 2003; **82**: 147–51.

19. Chauhan S P, *et al.* Brachial plexus injury: a 23-year experience from a tertiary center. *Am J Obstet Gynecol* 2005; **192**: 1795–800.

20. Benjamin K. Distinguishing physical characteristics and management of brachial plexus injuries. *Adv Neonat Care* 2005; **5**: 240–51.

21. Draycott, T. J. *et al.*, Improving neonatal outcome through practical shoulder dystocia training. *Obstet Gynecol*, 2008. **112**(1): 14–20.

Chapter

13

Antepartum haemorrhage

Neelam Potdar, Osric Navti and Justin C. Konje

Introduction

Antepartum haemorrhage (APH) is defined as any bleeding from the genital tract between the 24th week of pregnancy and the onset of labour. This definition of gestational age is based on the UK professional guidance for viability cut-off point of 24 weeks [1]. APH complicates 2–5% of all pregnancies [2] and is associated with significant maternal and perinatal morbidity and mortality. Globally, obstetric haemorrhage remains one of the most important causes of maternal mortality, accounting for 11% of maternal deaths. In the 2003–2005 Confidential Enquiry into Maternal and Child Health Report (CEMACH), mortality rate due to obstetric haemorrhage was 0.66 per 100,000 maternities [3]. The WHO estimates a 1% case fatality rate for the 14 million annual cases of obstetric haemorrhage [4].

Aetiology

There are numerous causes for APH (Table 13.1), although a cause is identified in approximately half the cases only. Bleeding from the placental bed is the commonest cause, and in some cases a local cause in the genital tract can be ascertained.

Diagnosis and management

APH by nature is unpredictable, and the bleeding at presentation can be significant or non-substantial. Ideally, management of any patient with APH should be in a hospital with adequate facilities for transfusion, delivery by caesarean section, and neonatal intensive care. Initial management includes history-taking, evaluation of the general condition, initiation of appropriate investigations and treatment.

History

This must include the amount, character and duration of bleeding. It is also important to ascertain if there is any associated abdominal pain or regular uterine contractions. Initiating or contributory factors such as trauma or coitus should be excluded. The gestational age as confirmed by either a booking ultrasound scan or last menstrual period and information regarding placental site should be obtained. Additional useful information includes history of number of past bleeding episodes, ruptured membranes, past obstetric history, and cervical smear history.

Physical examination

This is aimed at assessing both maternal and fetal conditions and includes a general examination for evidence of shock (pallor, restlessness, cold–clammy extremities and poor skin perfusion); assessing maternal pulse, respiratory rate and blood pressure. Abdominal examination includes fundal height measurement, consistency of uterus (soft or firm), presence of tenderness, palpable uterine contractions, fetal lie, presentation and viability. Vulval inspection should include an assessment of the amount of bleeding and determination of whether or not the bleeding is continuing. A speculum examination is essential, but should only be done after placenta praevia has been excluded. In the past, the Apt test was performed if the bleeding was thought to be of fetal origin. The test is based on the principle that fetal haemoglobin is alkali-stable versus adult haemoglobin which denaturates on alkali exposure. It is now performed rarely.

Initial management and investigations

The initial assessment/resuscitation and investigations is generic for all types of APH, with further

---

Best Practice in Labour and Delivery, ed. R. Warren and S. Arulkumaran. Published by Cambridge University Press.
© Cambridge University Press 2009.

Table 13.1 Causes of antepartum haemorrhage.

	Causes	Incidence (%)
Placental	Placenta praevia	31
	Placental abruption	22
	Vasa praevia	0.5
Unclassified	Marginal	28
Genital tract	Cervicitis	4.0
	Trauma	3.0
	Vulvovaginal varicosities	0.5
	Genital infections	0.5
	Genital tumours	0.5
	Others	10.0

Table 13.2 Grading of placenta praevia.

Grade	Description
I	Placenta is in the lower segment, but the lower edge does not reach the internal os
II	Lower edge of the placenta reaches but does not cover the internal os
III	Placenta covers the internal os partially
IV	Placenta covers the internal os completely

treatment tailored according to the severity of bleeding, gestational age of the pregnancy and the cause of bleeding. These should include the following.

1. Access to intravenous line with one or two wide-bore cannulae (preferably size 14–16 French gauge).
2. Obtaining blood for a full blood count, urea and electrolytes, group and save and holding of serum for potential cross-match depending upon the severity of bleeding. In the presence of heavy bleeding, at least 4 units of blood should be cross-matched. If placental abruption is suspected a coagulation profile should also be checked. Other tests include a Kleihauer–Betke test on maternal blood and urine dipstick for protein.
3. Administration of intravenous fluids if bleeding is continuing or the woman is haemodynamically compromised. Crystalloids are preferred over colloids, but if given in such circumstances, it is restricted to a maximum of 1500 ml (RCOG Green Top Guideline on Blood Transfusion) [5]. Consideration should be given to transfusing O Rhesus (D) negative blood where cross-matching is delayed.
4. An ultrasound scan assessment to confirm placental site once the feto-maternal status is satisfactory. This may not always be necessary.

Subsequent management (conservative or immediate) will depend on the feto-maternal condition and the gestational age. These will be discussed under the various types of APH.

Placenta praevia

Placenta praevia is defined as a placenta inserted partially or wholly in the lower uterine segment. If the placenta lies over the cervical os, it is considered as major praevia. Traditionally, different grades have been defined based on the relationship of the placenta to the internal cervical os (Table 13.2). In clinical practice, ultrasound definitions with relation to the cervical os are more commonly used (Figure 13.1).

The prevalence of clinically identified placenta praevia is approximately 4–5/1000 pregnancies [6]. The exact aetiology of placenta praevia is unknown, but it has been shown to be associated with increasing maternal age, parity, smoking, in-vitro fertilization, multiple pregnancy and previous caesarean section. A single caesarean section increases the risk of placenta praevia by 0.63%, whereas two previous caesarean sections confer a twofold increased risk in a subsequent pregnancy [7].

Clinical implication

Placenta praevia can lead to varying degrees of maternal haemorrhage at different gestations, with a significant impact on materno-fetal well-being.

Maternal risks include the following.

i. Maternal mortality: primarily due to haemorrhage, has reduced from 5% to less than 0.1% since the use of conservative management [8].
   In the last CEMACH report, three maternal deaths were reported secondary to placenta praevia [3].
ii. Postpartum haemorrhage: this occurs due to inadequate occlusion of the sinuses in the lower uterine segment at the site of the placental bed.
iii. Placenta accreta: occurs in approximately 15% of cases with placenta praevia.

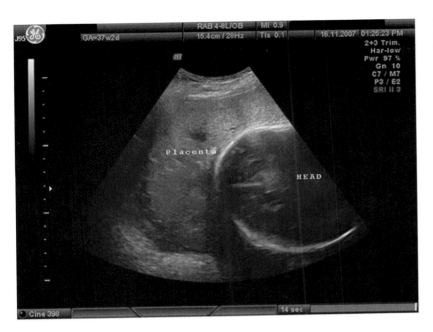

Figure 13.1 Ultrasound image of placenta praevia covering internal cervical os

iv. Air embolism: this is possible if the sinuses in the placental bed are torn.

v. Postpartum sepsis: often secondary to ascending infection.

vi. Recurrence: after one previous placenta praevia the recurrence rate is approximately 4–8%.

Fetal risks include the following.

i. Perinatal mortality: is primarily due to prematurity. Previously, the perinatal mortality for cases presenting between 27 and 32 weeks was approximately 20%; however, with conservative management and improved neonatal care this has dropped to 42–81/1000 [9]. In women with placenta praevia, the odds ratios for having a preterm delivery, need for neonatal intensive care and low birth weight are 27.7, 3.4 and 7.4, respectively [10].

ii. Fetal growth restriction: can occur in approximately 16% of cases and is more likely in women with recurrent bleeding episodes.

iii. Major congenital malformations: reports indicate a doubling in women with placenta praevia. The most common are those of the central nervous, cardiovascular, respiratory and gastrointestinal systems.

iv. Unexpected fetal death secondary to vasa praevia or severe maternal haemorrhage can occur.

v. Other associated risks are fetal malpresentation, fetal anaemia, umbilical cord prolapse and cord compression.

Diagnosis
Clinical

Placenta praevia characteristically presents with painless vaginal bleeding. The initial bleed in more than 50% of cases occurs prior to 36 weeks' gestation. In some cases, threatened miscarriage in early pregnancy precedes the bleeding due to placenta praevia. It is not uncommon for the bleeding episodes to be recurrent in most cases, with the severity of subsequent episodes usually being greater than the previous one.

The absence of abdominal pain is regarded as a significant differentiating feature between placenta praevia and abruption, although 10% of women with placenta praevia will have a co-existing abruption. Since most women undergo a second trimester ultrasound scan and placental localization, low-lying placentae should have been diagnosed. Other findings on abdominal examination include malpresentation of the fetus, which occurs in about 35% of cases [9]. Vaginal examination is avoided in known cases of placenta praevia as speculum or digital examination may further aggravate bleeding. Historically, in suspected placenta praevia cases with mild to moderate bleeding and delivery being considered, a digital vaginal examination was performed in theatre with or without anaesthesia. This 'double set-up examination' allowed immediate access to caesarean section, if the placental edge was felt on examination or there was vaginal bleeding [11]. With the advent of better imaging modalities this approach is rarely undertaken; however, in the parts of the world where ultrasound is not routinely available, it can be useful.

Screening for low-lying placenta

Various radiological methods have been used in the past to localize the placenta, including soft tissue placentography, radioisotope radiography, pelvic angiography, and thermography. Currently the gold standard for localizing low-lying placenta is ultrasound scan, with an emerging role for magnetic resonance imaging (MRI). Transabdominal ultrasound scan has a high false-positive rate for detection of low-lying placentae, whereas transvaginal scanning is safe in the presence of placenta praevia and is more accurate. In most obstetric units in the UK, fetal anomaly screening is undertaken between 20 and 24 weeks of pregnancy and this includes documentation on placental localization. This examination is used to predict the likelihood of placenta praevia at term. Women with low-lying placenta at 20–24 weeks are offered a repeat scan between 34 and 36 weeks of gestation to confirm the diagnosis. In cases with asymptomatic suspected major placenta praevia, a transvaginal scan is performed at 32 weeks, to confirm the diagnosis and allow planning for third trimester management. A few studies have shown that before 24 weeks' gestation, the placenta can be low-lying in 28% of the cases, but by term only 3% of these are low-lying [8,9]. This is because the placenta 'migrates' to the upper uterine segment as the pregnancy advances. The mean rate of placental migration is about 5.4 mm per week. In recent years, ultrasound has been used to predict the likelihood and extent of placental migration, and the occurrence of placenta praevia at term. Studies using transvaginal ultrasound have shown that unless the placental edge is reaching the internal cervical os at mid-pregnancy, placenta praevia is unlikely to be present at term [12,13]. Oppenheimer et al. showed that at mid trimester, if the placental edge overlapped the internal cervical os by >2 cm, placental migration did not occur. When the placental edge was >2 cm away from the internal

os, migration always occurred; whereas if the edge was <2 cm from the os, placental migration occurred in 88.5% of cases [14]. The significance of the shape of the placental edge to predict placental migration has also been studied. A thick placental edge, defined as thickness of 1 cm or more, within 1 cm from the edge and/or an angle between the basal and chorionic plate of >45° is associated with a lesser chance of placental migration [15].

A false negative scan for a low-lying placenta has been reported in 7% of cases. This is primarily seen when the placenta is posterior, the bladder is full, the fetal head obscures the placental margin or the operator fails to scan the lateral uterine wall [16].

Management options

These are either (a) immediate delivery, or (b) expectant management, both of which are influenced by the severity of haemorrhage, fetal well-being and gestational age.

Immediate delivery

Where there is severe life-threatening haemorrhage, irrespective of the gestational age, caesarean section is the only delivery option. With mild to moderate bleeding occurring after 34 weeks' gestation, delivery should be planned after stabilizing the maternal condition.

Expectant management

In cases where the bleeding is small and self-limiting, expectant management has a role. This provides time to achieve fetal maturity, thereby reducing perinatal morbidity and mortality. Another advantage is that in some cases with advancing gestation, the placenta migrates and vaginal delivery might be considered reasonable. There has been controversy regarding the expectant management as inpatient or outpatient. Cotton et al. reported no difference in the perinatal or maternal mortality rates in cases managed either at home or in the hospital [9], whereas others have reported an increase in the neonatal morbidity with those managed at home. For women with asymptomatic placenta praevia, conservative management at home is becoming increasingly acceptable [17]. The RCOG in the UK has recommended that women with major placenta praevia who have previously bled should be admitted and managed as inpatients from

34 weeks of gestation [18]. Those with major praevia who have never bled and are asymptomatic require careful counselling before being offered outpatient care. These cases require close proximity with the hospital and the constant presence of a companion. During expectant management, preterm delivery is a major problem, with approximately 40% occurring before 37 weeks [19]. About 88.2% of women with placenta praevia undergo caesarean section before term [10]. Furthermore, the use of tocolysis for uterine contractions with vaginal bleeding is controversial. In the presence of co-existing abruption, the use of tocolysis can mask features of hypovolaemia. Others have shown reduced perinatal morbidity and mortality with the use of tocolysis in preterm labour and placenta praevia [20]. Similarly, the use of cervical cerclage to reduce bleeding and prolong pregnancy is not recommended as sufficient evidence is lacking.

Liberal use of blood transfusion has been advocated in cases with excess bleeding. The aim is to optimize oxygen supply to the fetus and restore maternal blood volume with haemoglobin of at least 10 g/dl and a haematocrit of 30%. If the bleeding settles, conservative management can be continued on an inpatient basis. Once a significant bleeding episode has occurred, four units of cross-matched blood should be made readily available. Where indicated, maternal steroids should be administered for fetal lung maturity. With prolonged inpatient care, immobility thromboprophylaxis should be encouraged and delivery planned around 38 weeks' gestation.

Mode of delivery

This is determined by the clinical state of the patient, fetus and the ultrasound findings. Caesarean section is the recommended method for major placenta praevia, whereas vaginal delivery may be possible with minor degrees. Currently, as the diagnosis of praevia is based on ultrasound findings, the distance of the placental edge from the internal os can guide decision-making. The Royal College of Obstetricians and Gynaecologists (RCOG) have recommended that the placenta needs to be at least 2 cm from the cervical os for an attempted vaginal delivery [18]. Bhide et al. [21] have suggested that if the placental edge is further than 2 cm from cervical internal os but within 3.5 cm, vaginal delivery can be attempted. In the UK, the RCOG recommends that for a planned caesarean section for placenta praevia, a consultant obstetrician

and anaesthetist should be present within the delivery suite. In case of emergency, consultant staff should be alerted and attend as soon as possible. Specialized multidisciplinary personnel such as the haematologist and interventional radiologist should be informed and their help sought promptly if required. The American College of Obstetricians and Gynaecologists and the Royal Australian and New Zealand College of Obstetricians and Gynaecologists are of the consensus that, when hysterectomy is anticipated, consent should include the same [22,23]. If the patient is not actively bleeding and is in a stable condition, an experienced anaesthetist may consider regional anaesthesia, otherwise general anaesthesia is used. For all cases, whether elective or emergency, cross-matched blood is kept available and the amount depends upon the clinical features of the individual case and availability of the local blood bank services. If the woman has atypical antibodies, specific arrangements for appropriately typed blood should be made with the blood bank. There is no evidence to support the use of autologous blood transfusion in the management of placenta praevia, although cell salvage can be considered for certain high-risk cases. The uterine incision in placenta praevia is usually made in the lower segment; however, in difficult cases it may be converted to a T-, J-, or U-shaped incision. In the presence of an anterior placenta, the approach can be of either going through the placenta to deliver the baby or identifying the placental edge and going through the membranes above or below it. Tearing or cutting through the placenta should be avoided, as there is a risk of fetal vessels being torn. Inevitably, the placental bed sinuses bleed as the lower segment is less muscular with reduced ability for retraction. Where uterotonics are not effective, figure of eight haemostatic sutures can be applied to the placental bed. Other modalities shown to be effective include intramyometrial prostaglandins, intrauterine hydrostatic balloon, and uterine brace sutures. In uncontrolled bleeding, an early decision may be required for uterine or internal iliac artery ligation or even hysterectomy. Embolization of the uterine arteries has been shown to be extremely useful in selected cases. Where the placenta is morbidly adherent, it can be left in situ with prophylactic or therapeutic uterine artery embolization or internal iliac artery ligation. The use of methotrexate tends to vary from centre to centre. Successful pregnancies have been reported thereafter, although in some cases there is a risk of subsequent haemorrhage and need for hysterectomy [24].

Vasa praevia

Vasa praevia is a rare condition where the fetal blood vessels traverse the fetal membranes in the lower part of the uterus, unsupported by placental tissue or the umbilical cord. It occurs in 1 per 6000 deliveries [25] and is associated with high perinatal mortality. As the fetal vessels precede the presenting part, they may rupture before or during labour, leading to fetal blood loss. Before the widespread use of ultrasound, vasa praevia was diagnosed retrospectively and perinatal mortality was high. Characteristic ultrasound features for the diagnosis of vasa praevia include echogenic parallel or circular lines near the cervix representing the umbilical cord, which can be further confirmed by Doppler and transvaginal scan [26]. It is important to diagnose these cases antenatally and offer elective caesarean section at term.

Placenta percreta/accreta

Placenta accreta or the morbidly adherent placenta occurs due to abnormalities in implantation. It is associated with a high maternal morbidity and mortality. In the United Kingdom Obstetric Surveillance Study (UKOSS) of women requiring peripartum hysterectomy, 38% had a morbidly adherent placenta (placenta accreta or increta) [27]. The prevalence is higher if the placenta is low-lying or if there is a prior scar on the uterus. An anterior low-lying placenta with a history of prelabour caesarean section is more likely to be morbidly adherent, and for such cases the index of suspicion should be high. Recent reports suggest antenatal diagnosis on ultrasound scan with a high positive predictive value for placenta accreta [28]. Three-dimensional colour power Doppler has been used for diagnosis with a positive predictive value of 87.5% [29]. One of the specific recommendations of the 2007 CEMACH report is that women with previous caesarean section should have the placental site determined by ultrasound scan. MRI has a poor sensitivity of about 38% and is still considered as a research tool [30]. The management of morbidly adherent placenta requires multidisciplinary care and planning in the antenatal and intrapartum period. Interventional radiology may be useful in these cases and the RCOG has produced guidelines on the subject (Good Practice Guidelines No. 6, June 2007) [31].

Table 13.3 Grading of abruption.

Grade	Description
0	Asymptomatic – small retroplacental clot
1	External vaginal bleeding present. Uterine tenderness and tetany may be present. No sign of maternal shock or fetal distress
2	External vaginal bleeding may or may not be present. No signs of maternal shock, but fetal distress is present
3	External bleeding may or may not be present. Marked uterine tetany, a board-like rigidity on palpation. Persistent abdominal pain, maternal shock and fetal distress are present. Coagulopathy may become evident in 30% of cases.

Placental abruption

Placental abruption is the most common cause of bleeding in the second and third trimesters of pregnancy. It is defined as the partial or complete premature separation of a normally situated placenta. It complicates approximately 0.3–1% of births [32,33], although temporal trends in some countries have shown an increase in the rates of abruption [34,35]. The wide variation in the reported incidence reflects discrepancy in the clinical and histological diagnosis. Histologic evidence of abruption was seen in 3.8% [36] to 4.5% [37] of routinely examined placentae, suggesting small episodes are more common than the clinical diagnosis. In addition, the incidence of abruption is highest at 24–26 weeks' gestation, and decreases with advancing gestational age [34].

Placental abruption in 65–80% of cases is 'revealed', where the blood tracks between the membranes and the decidua, and escapes into the vagina. In the other 20–35% of cases, abruption is 'concealed', and the blood accumulates behind the placenta with no obvious external bleeding. Traditionally, four grades of placental abruption have been described (Table 13.3); the most severe grade is reported in 0.2% of pregnancies.

Risk factors and aetiopathogenesis

The exact aetiology of placental abruption is unknown, although haemorrhage at the deciduo-placental interface and acute vasospasm of the small blood vessels seems to precede the placental separation. Vascular thrombosis can also lead to decidual necrosis and venous haemorrhage. Recently, reduced expression of specific placental cell membrane protein has been seen in labours complicated by placental abruption [38].

Direct trauma to the abdomen can cause a shearing force, leading to acute placental separation. This mechanism also explains placental separation with sudden intrauterine decompression, following membrane rupture in cases of polyhydramnios or after the delivery of the first twin. Cocaine and drug abuse cause placental vasoconstriction, leading to abruption. Maternal smoking doubles the risk of abruption, whereas if both parents smoke the risk is increased fivefold [35]. A dose–response relationship has been demonstrated between the number of cigarettes smoked and the risk of placental abruption. In addition, women who stop smoking early in pregnancy have the same risk of placental abruption as women who have never smoked. Other risk factors include previous caesarean section, bleeding in early pregnancy, an elevated second trimester maternal serum alpha-fetoprotein (10-fold increased risk of abruption) [39] and second trimester notching of the uterine artery Doppler [40]. Pre-eclampsia is associated with a 2.7-fold increased risk of placental abruption [35]; chronic hypertension, pregnancy-induced hypertension, premature rupture of membranes and previous caesarean section are other risk factors. The association between thrombophilia and abruption is controversial; therefore, in women with placental abruption without a known cause, thrombophilia screening should be considered.

Clinical implication

Since the degrees of placental abruption vary from non-substantial vaginal bleeding with minimal or nil consequence to substantive or massive abruption leading to marked perinatal morbidity and mortality, the clinical implication will depend on the severity of the bleeding.

Maternal risks include the following.

i. Maternal mortality: is about 1%. In the last CEMACH Report (2003–2005), two maternal deaths were due to placental abruption. Although severe haemorrhage is usually the cause of mortality, disseminated intravascular coagulation (DIC) itself can cause severe bleeding, renal failure and death.

ii. Hypovolaemic shock: is due to an underestimation of the blood loss with concealed bleeding within the myometrium.

iii. DIC.

iv. Renal tubular necrosis: occurs secondary to acute hypovolaemia and cortical necrosis can result from DIC. This can lead to chronic renal failure.

v. Postpartum haemorrhage: occurs due to DIC or 'couvelaire uterus' where concealed bleeding has tracked within the myometrium, impairing its ability to contract.

vi. Feto-maternal haemorrhage: can occur, therefore all Rhesus (D) negative cases should undergo the Kleihauer–Betke test and anti-D immunoglobulin administered within 72 h to prevent sensitization. Repeated doses will be dependent on the size of the feto-maternal bleed as determined by the Kleihauer–Betke test.

Fetal risks include the following.

i. Increased perinatal mortality (OR=30.0, 95% CI 19.7–45.6) [33]. In a US population-based cohort, the perinatal mortality in pregnancies complicated by placental abruption was 14-fold higher than all other births [41]. This is attributed primarily to preterm birth, as abruption is an important indication for iatrogenic preterm delivery. In a fetus delivered after an abruption, there is a 10-fold increased risk of developing periventricular leukomalacia [42].

ii. Fetal growth restriction: is reported in about 80% of the fetuses born before 36 weeks' gestation.

iii. Major congenital malformations: are increased threefold, and most involve the central nervous system [2].

iv. Fetal anaemia: can occur due to severe fetal bleeding, and transient coagulopathies have been noted in neonates born to women with placental abruption.

Diagnosis

Clinical

Diagnosis is usually made based on the clinical symptoms and signs. In milder forms, this is made after delivery, when a retroplacental clot is identified or reported after placental histology. The classical presentation is with vaginal bleeding, abdominal pain and uterine contractions. Vaginal bleeding is seen in

70–80% of cases, although the amount of revealed bleeding correlates poorly with the degree of abruption. In about 50% of cases vaginal bleeding occurs after the 36th week of gestation, and as labour is a precipitating factor nearly 50% of patients with placental abruption are in established labour. Abdominal pain probably indicates extravasation of blood into the myometrium, and in some cases pain can be sudden, sharp and severe. Patients may present with symptoms of shock, including nausea, thirst, anxiety and restlessness. At times pain due to placental abruption can be difficult to differentiate from uterine contractions, which in placental abruption are frequent, with a rate of over 5 in 10 min. In addition to the above symptoms, the patient may complain of absent or reduced fetal movements.

Examination, in severe cases, may demonstrate features of hypovolaemic shock with marked tachycardia. Pre-existing hypertension may mask true hypovolaemia, therefore blood pressure reading in itself is not a reliable sign. Abdominal palpation may reveal a woody-hard, tender uterus, with high-frequency, low-amplitude uterine contractions. There may be difficulty in palpating the fetus and locating the fetal heart in such cases. Depending upon the degree of placental separation, the fetal heart rate may be normal, show signs of distress, or be absent where the fetus is dead. The cardiotocogram can show recurrent variable or late decelerations, reduced variability, a sinusoidal pattern, or even bradycardia. Stillbirths have been reported where there is greater than 50% placental separation [32]. Vaginal examination is likely to reveal blood and the presence of blood clots; in cases complicated with coagulopathy (35–38%), there may be dark-coloured blood with an absence of clotting. With ruptured membranes, blood-stained liquor can be seen and, more often, labour tends to proceed rapidly.

Ultrasonography

The role of ultrasound in the diagnosis of placental abruption is controversial. In cases of acute revealed abruption there may be no specific ultrasound findings. It has a role in identifying coincident placenta praevia and can be used for monitoring cases expectantly, and help with the timing of delivery. The parameters that can be assessed are location of haematoma, variation in size and fetal growth. Nyberg *et al.* [43] have described ultrasound appearances of acute abruption varying from hyperechoic to isoechoic when compared to the placenta. As the clot resolves, appearances become hypoechoic within a week and sonolucent within 2 weeks. Another study has shown ultrasound sensitivity of 80% and specificity of 92% for the diagnosis of abruption [44]. The appearances include pre-placental collection under the chorionic plate, jelly-like movement of the chorionic plate with fetal activity, retroplacental collection, marginal haematoma, subchorionic haematoma, increased heterogenous placental thickness of more than 5 cm in perpendicular plane, and intra-amniotic haematoma.

Management options

As the clinical presentation is variable, management options need to be individualized and are guided by the severity of abruption, gestational age, and the maternal and fetal condition. Whilst aggressive management is needed for more severe cases, a conservative approach should be adopted for milder forms. After the general management described earlier in this chapter, specific measures to be considered are as described below.

Expectant management

In mild abruption presenting between 24 and 34 weeks' gestation, and where the maternal–fetal condition is stable, conservative management should be the option of choice. Preterm delivery is a major cause for perinatal death, and if possible all attempts should be made to prolong the gestation at delivery. These patients need close monitoring for signs of worsening abruption and deterioration in fetal well-being. Steroids should be administered for fetal lung maturity and serial ultrasound scans performed to assess fetal growth, and in cases with retroplacental clot, the size of the haematoma. For expectant management, initial hospitalization and assessment of the maternal and fetal condition is reasonable; further outpatient management has a role provided the maternal–fetal condition remains stable. Timing of delivery depends upon vaginal bleeding, fetal condition and the gestational age. With recurrent bleeding episodes and a satisfactory fetal assessment, induction at 37–38 weeks' gestation is recommended. Delivery should be organized at centres with appropriate neonatal facilities and the parents should be counselled regarding the potential treatments and outcomes for the neonate.

In cases of prematurity, mild abruption and uterine contractions, the use of tocolytics is controversial. Their use has traditionally been contraindicated, for they can worsen the process of abruption. β-Sympathomimetics such as terbutaline can cause tachycardia and therefore mask the clinical signs of further blood loss. Some studies have used tocolytics with abruption, achieving a mean latency period to delivery of 12.4 and 18.9 days, respectively [45,46]. In mild and stable cases of placental abruption, which are remote from term, it seems reasonable to use tocolytics with caution. Tocolytics may allow time for steroid administration to promote fetal lung maturity and newer tocolytics with milder side effect profiles can be used.

Immediate delivery

This depends upon the severity of the placental abruption and fetal survival. In cases of fetal death, regardless of the gestation, and in the absence of other contra-indications, e.g. haemodynamic instability, it is prudent to aim for a vaginal delivery. Once the initial resuscitation has been initiated, amniotomy is frequently sufficient to induce labour and delivery is achieved fairly rapidly. In some cases syntocinon augmentation may be needed, which must be administered cautiously because of the risk of hyperstimulation and consequent uterine rupture.

When the fetus is alive, at or near-term, prompt delivery is indicated. The decision regarding the mode of delivery is guided by the fetal and maternal well-being. In addition, in severe cases the fetal outlook is poor not only for the immediate survival, but about 15% of liveborn infants do not survive [47].

Where there is evidence of fetal compromise and delivery is not imminent, caesarean section should be performed immediately once maternal resuscitation has been commenced. Longer decision-delivery intervals are associated with poor perinatal outcomes [48]. Studies have suggested better perinatal outcomes with caesarean section rather than vaginal delivery [48,49]. However, emphasis must be placed on stabilizing the maternal condition as the presence of coagulopathy contributes to considerable maternal morbidity and mortality, especially with surgery.

In mild to moderate cases of placental abruption at term, with no fetal compromise, vaginal delivery is a reasonable option. Prostaglandins can be used for cervical ripening with extreme caution in order to avoid tetanic uterine contractions. Where possible, amniotomy is performed to hasten delivery, with syntocinon augmentation if needed. Continuous electronic fetal monitoring should be performed to identify early abnormal fetal heart rate patterns, as the perinatal mortality is likely to be higher with vaginal delivery in the absence of continuous fetal monitoring.

Management of complications

Major complications include haemorrhagic shock, DIC, renal tubular or cortical damage, and postpartum haemorrhage.

Haemorrhagic shock

This usually occurs when the blood loss is in excess of 1000–1500 ml. Blood loss is often underestimated as a result of concealed haemorrhage and variation in clinical judgement. For guidance, trebling the volume of visible blood clot provides a rough estimate of the blood loss. Resuscitation is aimed at restoring the circulating blood volume for adequate tissue perfusion. Four to six units of blood should be cross-matched and urgent blood sent for full blood count, coagulation profile, renal and liver function tests. The initial haemoglobin and haematocrit can be deceptively high because of haemoconcentration. While waiting for cross-matched blood, colloids can be used as plasma expanders; dextrose is avoided as it interferes with clotting and blood cross-matching. In emergent situations, uncrossed Rhesus O negative blood can be transfused. Fluid replacement should be monitored closely to avoid overloading. This can be done by monitoring maternal pulse, blood pressure, jugular venous pulse and hourly urine output. An indwelling urethral catheter should be passed and urinary output should be at least 30 ml/h. With severe haemodynamic compromise, especially in the presence of pre-eclampsia, the central venous pressure (CVP) line should be used. Measurement of the pulmonary capillary wedge pressure via a Swan–Ganz catheter reflects circulatory adequacy better than CVP, but its use depends upon the expertise and facilities. Complications from massive blood transfusion (transfusion in excess of one and a half times the patient's blood volume, or 10 or more units) should be looked out for. These can be hyperkalaemia, hypocalcaemia, thrombocytopaenia and other clotting disorders. Hyperkalaemia presents clinically with confusion, lethargy and cardiac monitoring showing bradycardia, characteristic T-wave changes with conduction defects and ultimately ventricular arrest. Hypocalcaemia presents with tingling in hands and feet, painful cramps and positive Trousseau's and Chvostek's sign. Platelet transfusion is considered if the platelet count is less than $50,000/mm^3$ and fibrinogen replacement if levels fall below 100 mg/ml.

Disseminated intravascular coagulation

This occurs more commonly with severe abruption and is seen in 10% of cases. The mechanism involves release of tissue thromboplastin from the site of placental injury, which activates widespread coagulation with consumptive coagulopathy. Fibrinolysis of the clots increases the fibrin degradation products, which also act as anticoagulants.

Based on the coagulation profile, Letsky has classified DIC into three stages [50]. In stage 1 (compensated phase), there are raised fibrinogen degradation products (FDPs) and increased soluble fibrin complexes; in stage 2 (uncomplicated progression) there is a fall in fibrinogen levels, platelet count and factors V and VII. In stage 3 (complicated phase, with haemostatic failure) the fibrinogen levels and platelet count are very low, with high fibrinogen degradation products. The findings are of a normal bleeding time, abnormal clot retraction, thrombocytopenia, elevated FDP levels, normal to prolonged PT and PTT, low fibrinogen levels and short thrombin time.

The ultimate treatment in the presence of DIC is delivery of the fetus and the placenta, as spontaneous resolution can occur only after delivery. After the initial diagnosis, management involves liasing with the haematologists and anaesthetists, and replacing the lost blood volume and the consumed clotting factors. Fresh frozen plasma, cryoprecipitate and platelets are the products of choice. Fresh plasma is preferred as it is rich in factors V and VII, the fibrinogen content of fresh frozen plasma (1 g/unit) is four times that of cryoprecipitate (0.25 g/unit). Cryoprecipitate is rich in factors VII and XII. If the patient needs to undergo surgery, platelets can be given if the count is less than $50,000/mm^3$. In addition, use of heparin in DIC is controversial. In early stages and in cases where there is distal organ microvascular plugging, heparin can be used, whereas in severe cases heparin is contra-indicated. Similarly,

antifibrinolytic agents can precipitate unchecked intravascular coagulation. Where surgery is required, general anaesthesia is preferred as opposed to regional anaesthesia due to the risk of haemorrhage in the dural and epidural space, and the worsening of shock secondary to sympathetic outflow blockade leading to hypotension.

Renal failure

Tubular renal necrosis occurs secondary to hypovolaemia, and cortical necrosis can be caused by microvascular clotting in the renal vasculature. Oliguria in the first 12 h after placental abruption is common and is not necessarily associated with renal damage. Fluid replacement should be monitored closely and renal function assessed by serum biochemistry. Diuretics should be used with caution in consultation with renal physicians.

Postpartum haemorrhage

This complicates 25% of cases and a contributing factor is poor myometrial contractility secondary to couvelaire uterus and the presence of DIC. Initial management involves the use of oxytocics, ergometrine, prostaglandins, blood transfusion, and rapid correction of coagulopathy. If these measures fail, intrauterine balloon compression, uterine brace suture, internal iliac artery ligation, and hysterectomy are other available treatment options.

Subsequent pregnancy after placental abruption

Optimal counselling and support through subsequent pregnancy should be provided. There is a 15% recurrence rate after one previous abruption and increases to 20% after two previous episodes [51]. In addition, there is an increased risk of recurrence for other pregnancy complications. Pre-conception counselling is essential to encourage smoking and cocaine cessation, and to obtain good blood pressure control where needed. With previous severe abruption, use of low-dose aspirin from as early as 5 weeks of pregnancy has shown some benefit in reducing the complications. In cases with confirmed inherited thrombophilias, relevant thromboprohylaxis is indicated in subsequent pregnancies.

References

1. Bottomley V. House of Commons Hansard. 1990: Col 173.

2. Green J. Placenta abnormalities: placenta praevia and abruptio placentae. In: Creasy R K, Resnik R, eds. *Maternal Fetal Medicine: Principles and Practice.* Philadelphia: W. B. Saunders, 1989.

3. Confidential Enquiry into Maternal and Child Health (CEMACH). *Saving Mothers' Lives: Reviewing Maternal Deaths to make Motherhood Safer 2003–2005. The Seventh Report of the Confidential Enquiries into Maternal Deaths in the United Kingdom,* 2007.

4. AbouZahr C. Global burden of maternal death and disability. *Br Med Bull* 2003; **67**: 1–11.

5. Royal College of Obstetricians and Gynaecologists. *Blood Transfusion in Obstetrics.* RCOG Green Top Guideline No. 47. London: RCOG, 2007.

6. Faiz A S, Ananth C V. Etiology and risk factors for placenta previa: an overview and meta-analysis of observational studies. *J Matern Fetal Neonatal Med* 2003; **13**: 175–90.

7. Getahun D, Oyelese Y, Salihu H M, Ananth C V. Previous cesarean delivery and risks of placenta previa and placental abruption. *Obstet Gynecol* 2006; **107**: 771–8.

8. Hibbard B. M. Bleeding in late pregnancy. *Principles of Obstetrics.* Butterworth Heinemann, 1988.

9. Cotton D B, Read J A, Paul R H, Quilligan E J. The conservative aggressive management of placenta praevia. *Am J Obstet Gynecol* 1980; **137**: 687–95.

10. Papinniemi M, Keski-Nisula L, Heinonen S. Placental ratio and risk of velamentous umbilical cord insertion are increased in women with placenta previa. *Am J Perinatol* 2007; **24**: 353–7.

11. Konje J C Taylor D J. Bleeding in late pregnancy. In: James D K, Steer P J, Weiner C P, Gonik B, eds. *High Risk Pregnancy: Management Options,* 2nd edn. Philadelphia: Saunders, 1999.

12. Taipale P, Hiilesmaa V, Ylostalo P. Transvaginal ultrasonography at 18–23 weeks in predicting placenta previa at delivery. *Ultrasound Obstet Gynecol* 1998; **12**: 422–5.

13. Becker R H, Vonk R, Mende B C, Ragosch V, Entezami M. The relevance of placental location at 20–23 gestational weeks for prediction of placenta previa at delivery: evaluation of 8650 cases. *Ultrasound Obstet Gynecol* 2001; **17**: 496–501.

14. Oppenheimer L, Holmes P, Simpson N, Dabrowski A. Diagnosis of low-lying placenta: can migration in the third trimester predict outcome? *Ultrasound Obstet Gynecol* 2001; **18**: 100–2.

15. Ghourab S. Third-trimester transvaginal ultrasonography in placenta previa: does the shape of the lower placental edge predict clinical outcome? *Ultrasound Obstet Gynecol* 2001; **18**: 103–8.

16. Laing F C. Placenta previa: avoiding false-negative diagnoses. *J Clin Ultrasound* 1981; **9**: 109–13.

17. Rosen D M B, Peek M J. Do women with placenta praevia without antepartum haemorrhage require hospitalisation. *Austral N Z J Obstet Gynaecol* 1994; **34**: 130–4.

18. Royal College of Obstetricians and Gynaecologists. *Placenta Praevia and Placenta Praevia Accreta: Diagnosis and Management.* RCOG Greentop Guideline No. 27 London: RCOG, 2005.

19. Brenner W E, Edelman D A, Hendricks C H. Characteristics of patients with placenta previa and results of 'expectant management'. *Am J Obstet Gynecol* 1978; **132**: 180–91.

20. Silver R, Depp R, Sabbagha R E, Dooley S L, Socol M L, Tamura R K. Placenta praevia: aggressive expectant management. *Am J Obstet Gynaecol* 1984; **150**: 15–22.

21. Bhide A, Prefumo F, Moore J, Hollis B, Thilaganathan B. Placental edge to internal os distance in the late third trimester and mode of delivery in placenta praevia. *Br J Obstet Gynaecol* 2003; **110**: 860–4.

22. American College of Obstetricians and Gynecologists. ACOG committee opinion. Placenta accreta. No. 266. *Int J Gynaecol Obstet* 2002; **77**: 77–8.

23. Royal Australian and New Zealand College of Obstetricians and Gynaecologists. Statement: Placenta accreta. Statement no. C-Obs 20. 2003.

24. Kayem G, Davy C, Goffinet F, Thomas C, Clement D, Cabrol D. Conservative versus extirpative management in cases of placenta accreta. *Obstet Gynecol* 2004; **104**: 531–6.

25. Lee W, Kirk J S, Comstock C H, Romero R. Vasa previa: prenatal detection by three-dimensional ultrasonography. *Ultrasound Obstet Gynecol* 2000; **16**: 384–7.

26. Oyelese Y, Catanzarite V, Prefumo F, *et al.* Vasa previa: the impact of prenatal diagnosis on outcomes. *Obstet Gynecol* 2004; **103**: 937–42.

27. Knight M. Peripartum hysterectomy in the UK: management and outcomes of the associated haemorrhage. *Br J Obstet Gynaecol* 2007; **114**: 1380–7.

28. Comstock C H, Love J J, Jr, Bronsteen R A, *et al.* Sonographic detection of placenta accreta in the second and third trimesters of pregnancy. *Am J Obstet Gynecol* 2004; **190**: 1135–40.

29. Chou M M, Tseng J J, Ho E S, Hwang J I. Three dimensional color power Doppler imaging in the assessment of uteroplacental neovascularisation in

placenta praevia increta/percreta. *Am J Obstet Gynecol* 2002; **187**: 515–6.

30. G Lam J K, McMahon M. Use of magnetic resonance imaging and ultrasound in the antenatal diagnosis of placenta accreta. *J Soc Gynecol Investigation* 2002; **9**: 37–40.

31. Royal College of Obstetricians and Gynaecologists. *The Role of Emergency and Elective Interventional Radiology in Postpartum Haemorrhage*. RCOG Good Practice Guideline No. 6. London: RCOG, 2007.

32. Ananth C V, Berkowitz G S, Savitz D A, Lapinski R H. Placental abruption and adverse perinatal outcomes. *J Am Med Assoc* 1999; **282**: 1646–51.

33. Sheiner E S-V I, Hallak M, Hadar A, *et al.* Placental abruption in term pregnancies: clinical significance and obstetric risk factors. *J Matern Fetal Neonatal Med* 2003; **13**: 45–9.

34. Oyelese Y, Ananth C V. Placental abruption. *Obstet Gynecol* 2006; **108**: 1005–16.

35. Tikkanen M, Nuutila M, Hiilesmaa V, Paavonen J, Ylikorkala A. Clinical presentation and risk factors of placental abruption. *Acta Obstet Gynecol Scand* 2006; **85**: 700–5.

36. Bernischke K, Gille J. Placental pathology and asphyxia. In: Gluck L, ed. *Intrauterine Asphyxia and the Developing Fetal Brain*. Chicago, IL: Yearbook Medical Publishers, 1977.

37. Fox H. *Pathology of the Placenta*. London: W.B. Saunders, 1978.

38. Wicherek L, Klimek M, Dutsch-Wicherek M, Kolodziejski L, Skotniczny K. The molecular changes during placental detachment. *Eur J Obstet Gynecol ReprodBiol* 2006; **125**: 171–5.

39. Katz V L C N, Cefalo R C. Unexplained elevations of maternal serum alpha-fetoprotein. *Obstet Gynecol Surv* 1990; **45**: 719–26.

40. Harrington K, Cooper D, Lees C, Hecher K, Campbell S. Doppler ultrasound of the uterine arteries: the importance of bilateral notching in the prediction of pre-eclampsia, placental abruption or delivery of a small-for-gestational-age baby. *Ultrasound Obstet Gynecol* 1996; **7**: 182–8.

41. Ananth C V, Wilcox A J. Placental abruption and perinatal mortality in the United States. *Am J Epidemiol* 2001; **153**: 332–7.

42. Gibbs J M, Weindling A M. Neonatal intracranial lesions following placental abruption. *Eur J Pediatr* 1994; **153**: 195–7.

43. Nyberg D A, Cyr D R, Mack L A, Wilson D A, Shuman W P. Sonographic spectrum of placental abruption. *Am J Roentgen* 1987; **148**: 161–4.

44. Yeo L, Ananth C V, Vintzileos A. Placenta abruption. In: Sciarra J, ed. *Gynaecology and Obstetrics*. Hagerstown, MD: Lippincott, Williams & Wilkins, 2004.

45. Bond A L, Edersheim T G, Curry L, Druzin M L, Hutson J M. Expectant management of abruptio placentae before 35 weeks gestation. *Am J Perinatol* 1989; **6**: 121–3.

46. Towers C V, Pircon R A, Heppard M. Is tocolysis safe in the management of third-trimester bleeding? *Am J Obstet Gynecol* 1999; **180**: 1572–8.

47. Abdella T N, Sibai B M, Hays J M, Anderson G D. Relationship of hypertensive disease to abruptio placentae. *Obstet Gynecol* 1984; **63**: 365–70.

48. Kayani S I, Walkinshaw S A, Preston C. Pregnancy outcome in severe placental abruption. *Br J Obstet Gynaecol* 2003; **110**: 679–83.

49. Witlin A G, Sibai B M. Perinatal and maternal outcome following abruptio placentae. *Hypertens Pregnancy* 2001; **20**: 195–203.

50. Letsky E A. Disseminated intravascular coagulation. *Best Pract Res Clin Obstet Gynaecol* 2001; **15**: 623–44.

51. Rasmussen S, Irgens L M, Dalaker K. Outcomes of pregnancies subsequent to placental abruption: a risk assessment. *Acta Obstet Gynecol Scand* 2000; **79**: 496–501.

Management of the third stage of labour

Pina Amin and Audrey Long

The third stage of labour is the time from the birth of the baby to the delivery of the placenta and membranes. Once a woman is delivered of a healthy infant, all else including the delivery of the placenta pales into relative insignificance. More women die from accidents of the third stage than of any other stage of labour. In the majority of cases, the third stage is uneventful. However, in a small number of cases, severe complications can occur without any notice. This risk continues for some period after delivery of the placenta. Although in the United Kingdom death rate due to postpartum haemorrhage has not risen in the last triennium [1], it accounts for 25% of maternal deaths in the developing world.

Physiology of the third stage of labour
Placental separation

The uterus diminishes rapidly in size during birth of the baby. The retraction is effected by all three layers of uterine muscle fibres. The average diminution in length of the uterus from the onset of birth to its completion is 6.5 inches in 5 min. This is achieved by myometrial retraction, which is a unique characteristic of the uterine muscle to maintain its shortened length following each successive contraction. This continued retraction results in thickening of myometrium, reduction of uterine volume and shrinkage of placental bed. The non-contractile placenta is undermined, detached and propelled into the lower uterine segment. This process is usually completed within 4.5 min of delivery of the baby [2]. The second mechanism of separation is through haematoma formation. This occurs due to venous occlusion and vascular rupture in the placental bed caused by uterine contractions.

Haemostasis

The placental bed at term is perfused with a blood flow of 500–700 ml/min. The blood vessels penetrating the uterus to supply the placental bed are surrounded by the interlacing muscle fibre of the myometrium. Contraction of these muscle fibres compresses the blood vessels like 'living ligatures'. Retraction of the muscle fibre keeps the vessels closed. A vivid demonstration of this physiologic control of bleeding is seen at caesarean section when the emptied uterus becomes thick, firm and pale. In addition to uterine muscle contraction, fibrinous thrombi formation occurs in maternal sinuses, which also helps achieve haemostasis by sealing the small sinuses in the uterine wall.

Signs of placental separation

1. The most reliable sign is the lengthening of the umbilical cord as the placenta separates and is pushed into the lower uterine segment by progressive uterine contractions. Placing a clamp on the cord near the perineum makes it easier to appreciate this lengthening. Traction on the cord should not be applied without countertraction on the uterus above the symphysis, otherwise, one may mistake cord lengthening due to impending prolapse or inversion of uterus.
2. The uterus takes on a more globular shape and becomes firmer. This occurs as the placenta descends into the lower segment and the body of the uterus continues to retract. This change may be difficult to appreciate clinically.
3. A gush of blood occurs. The retro placental clot is able to escape as the placenta descends to the lower uterine segment. The retro placental clot usually forms centrally and escapes following

Best Practice in Labour and Delivery, ed. R. Warren and S. Arulkumaran. Published by Cambridge University Press.
© Cambridge University Press 2009.

complete separation; however, if the blood can find a path to escape, it may do so before complete separation and thus is not a reliable indicator of complete separation. This occurrence is sometimes associated with increased bleeding and a prolonged third stage, with the delivery of the leading edge of the placenta and maternal surface first (the Matthews Duncan method), rather than the cord insertion and fetal surface, which is more common (the Schultze method).

Vaginal examination and assessment of the perineum after the birth of the baby

Although an assessment of the vagina and perineum can be carried out prior to delivery of the placenta, a more thorough, detailed look should be carried out after placental delivery. The labia and perineum should be evaluated for any lacerations or haematomas. This examination is especially important following an operative delivery. If there are lacerations around the urethra, consideration should be given to insertion of an indwelling urinary catheter. Consideration for an indwelling catheter should also be given in the case of instrumental delivery involving regional analgesia. The vagina and cervix should be inspected routinely for laceration following instrumental delivery.

Third stage

Expectant management

This is often described as physiological. Following delivery of the baby, the cord is not clamped and cut until pulsations have ceased. The placenta is delivered with maternal effort aided only by gravity, nipple stimulation or breast feeding. This method is commonly practised in Northern European countries, the USA and Canada [3,4]. This method results in a longer third stage of labour and increased risk of postpartum haemorrhage [5,6]. In the 'Bristol third stage trial', women and midwives commented adversely about the length of the third stage with expectant management [7]. Women may choose this method as it is non-interventional, but current evidence would suggest we should advise women about the advantages of active management.

Active management

This involves the administration of oxytocic drugs, usually with the delivery of the anterior shoulder,

although variations in practice involve administration after delivery of the baby or placenta. This is followed by early clamping of the umbilical cord and controlled cord traction (CCT). There are two methods of CCT. The Brandt Andrews manoeuvre is most commonly employed in UK practice. This involves one hand on the lower abdomen which secures the uterine fundus to prevent inversion and steady traction on the cord with the other hand. The second is the Crede manoeuvre in which the hand holding the cord is fixed, and the hand on the lower abdomen applies upward traction. Use of fundal pressure to deliver the placenta is also described, although this may cause pain, haemorrhage and increase the risk of uterine inversion [8].

Current evidence is unclear as to the best timing of cord clamping; delayed clamping reduces neonatal anaemia and increases neonatal jaundice. It is not clear whether this has benefits. It is also unclear as to whether draining cord blood after clamping has benefits in reducing the length of third stage [9].

Management at caesarean section

Delivery of the placenta at caesarean section should be by CCT following administration of oxytocic drugs. Manual removal is associated with increased risk of postpartum haemorrhage and infection.

Uterotonic drugs used in the third stage of labour (Table 14.1)

Ergot alkaloids (ergometrine, methylergometrine) are usually given intravenously (IV) or intramuscularly (IM). The usual dose is 250–500 mcg. The oral forms are unstable and have unpredictable effects. They are effective in reducing postpartum haemorrhage (PPH), but are associated with increased vomiting, pain and elevation of blood pressure. They are contra-indicated in the presence of hypertension, cardiac disease, and other vascular conditions such as migraine [10].

Oxytocin is usually given IV or IM as a bolus. There are no adverse maternal haemodynamic responses to IV bolus of 5 IU. Infusion is less effective at preventing PPH, but may be used following initial bolus for prophylaxis or treatment of PPH. It is well tolerated and can be safely used for all women.

Syntometrine® combines 5 IU oxytocin with 0.5 mg ergometrine. It is associated with a small reduction in the risk of PPH 500–1000 ml compared to oxytocin alone. However, there is also an increase in maternal side effects (increased blood pressure, nausea and vomiting) [11].

Carbetocin is a long-acting oxytocin. Its effect is related to dose, but the usual dose is 100 mcg IV. In comparison to oxytocin it is associated with less need for additional uterotonic agents and uterine massage. However, current evidence does not suggest that it is better than oxytocin alone at preventing PPH [12]. It may have a role in women at high risk of PPH.

Misoprostol is an analogue of prostaglandin E1. There has been much interest in this as a uterotonic agent, as it is cheap, stable and can be given orally. It has been shown to be effective at preventing PPH, but is less effective compared with oxytocin, and is associated with side effects including shivering and pyrexia [13]. These side effects are less when it is given rectally [14]. It can be used in women where ergometrine is contra-indicated. The usual dose would be 600 mcg orally or 800 mcg rectally. In the developing world it is likely to have a very useful role in the management of the third stage. However, in the developed world, it is unlikely to replace oxytocin as the first-line uterotonic.

Carboprost is an analogue of prostaglandin F2α. It is usually given IM or direct into the myometrium, which is invasive. The usual dose is 250 mcg repeated at intervals of not less than 15 min, to a maximum dose of 2 mg. There is insufficient evidence to support its use in routine active management; however, it will continue to have a role in the treatment of PPH.

Intraumbilical oxytocin is usually given as a bolus of 10 IU oxytocin diluted to 20 ml with normal saline and given into the proximal umbilical cord. There have been a number of trials looking at prevention of PPH which have shown no significant benefit, although there is some evidence that it reduces the need for manual removal of the placenta when delivery of the placenta is delayed [15,16].

In conclusion, management of the third stage should be active, with 10 IU oxytocin IM or 5 IU IV at delivery of anterior shoulder, early cord clamping and CCT by the Brandt Andrews method.

Table 14.1 Drugs used for the third stage of labour.

Agent	Dose	Route	Side effects	Contra-indications	Comments
Oxytocin	10 IU 5 IU	IM IV	Few	None	Effective, relatively cheap, can be repeated. Protection from light and needs cold storage conditions
Ergometrine	250 mcg	IM or IV	Nausea, vomiting hypertension	Pre-eclampsia, hypertension, cardiac, migraine	Needs cold storage conditions and protection from light
Syntometrine®	5 IU Syntocinon/ 0.5 mg Ergometrine	IM	Nausea, vomiting hypertension	Pre-eclampsia, hypertension, cardiac, migraine	Needs storage conditions and protection from light
Carbetocin	100 mcg	IV			Long-acting
Carboprost	250 mcg	IM	Bronchospasm	Asthma	Can be given into the myometrium
Misoprostol	600 mcg	PO	GI disturbance, shivering, pyrexia		Cheap, stable, no special storage conditions
	800 mcg	PR			
Intraumbilical oxytocin	10 IU in 20 ml saline	Umbilical	None	None	May reduce manual removal, uncertain effect on PPH

Retained placenta

The third stage of labour is diagnosed as prolonged if not completed within 30 min of the birth of the baby with active management and 60 min with physiological management [17]. Severe postpartum haemorrhage is related to a prolonged third stage of labour of more than 30 min. A prospective study (2) of 6588 women delivered vaginally showed that a third stage longer than 18 min is associated with significant risk of postpartum haemorrhage. After 30 min the odds of having postpartum haemorrhage are six times higher than before 30 min.

Ensuring the bladder is empty may speed the delivery of the placenta and aid in the assessment and control of the uterus.

Intravenous access should always be secured in women with retained placenta, and blood taken for full blood count and group and save serum. Intravenous infusion of oxytocin to assist the delivery of the placenta is practised, but its efficacy is not known. Comparison between intraumbilical injection of oxytocin, 10 IU in 20 ml of saline and expectant management or saline injection alone, suggest this practice reduces the need for manual removal of placenta [17]. This intervention seems reasonable in stable women with minimal bleeding while preparation for a manual removal is being made.

Causes of retained placenta

The placenta separates at the physiologic plane of cleavage formed by the vascular network between the basal plate and the uterine wall. In some pregnancies, this physiologic plane of cleavage is lacking, which results in the failure of placental separation after the birth of the baby. Partial or total absence of the decidua basalis and imperfect development of Nitabuch's layer allows the chorionic villi to invade into the myometrium.

The degree of placental invasion varies, and the placental villi may adhere to (accreta), invade into (increta) or penetrate through (percreta) the myometrium. The cause of this defect is not well understood, but is usually associated with areas of previously scarred endometrium. Placenta accreta has affinity for multiparous women with advanced age. The two most important risk factors for placenta accreta are a known placenta praevia and a prior caesarean delivery.

Risk factors for retained placenta

- Previous caesarean delivery.
- Previous uterine curettage.
- History of uterine infection.
- Uterine fibroids.
- Previous manual removal of placenta.
- Premature delivery.

Sometimes, the placenta may have separated but is retained due to uterine atony or uterine constriction ring.

Management of retained placenta

The retained or partially detached placenta interferes with uterine contraction and retraction and leads to bleeding. Manual removal of the placenta is performed with a level of analgesia that matches the clinical urgency of the situation. Either regional block or general anaesthesia can be used after discussion and consent from the woman. Cessation of any oxytocin infusion or the administration of uterine relaxants to promote uterine exploration and manual removal is rarely required and may lead to increased bleeding. Ultrasound and Doppler flow study may be useful in the hands of an experienced operator in selected cases.

The woman with a retained placenta can be clinically shocked, having had postpartum haemorrhage. Adequate resuscitation is mandatory before attempting manual removal. This should include appropriate intravenous fluids. Assessment for requirement of blood products is made by an experienced anaesthetist and obstetrician after careful consideration of the clinical condition and estimated blood loss.

Technique of manual removal of the placenta

An elbow-length glove is worn and attention is paid to asepsis. The woman is put in the lithotomy position. The perineum is prepared aseptically. The vaginal hand is lubricated to facilitate easier entry. The hand is passed in the vagina and through the cervix into the lower segment of uterus, following the umbilical cord shown in Figure 14.1. Care is taken to minimize the profile of the hand as it enters, keeping the thumb and finger together in the shape of a cone to avoid trauma.

Control of the uterine fundus with the other hand is essential. If the placenta is encountered in the lower segment, it is removed, if not, the placental edge is

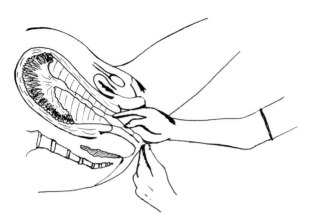

Figure 14.1 Insertion of hand in the uterus following the umbilical cord

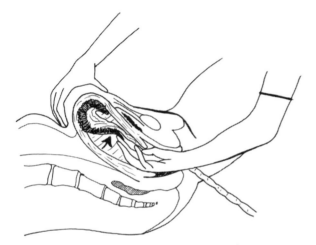

Figure 14.2 Creating plane between placenta and uterus

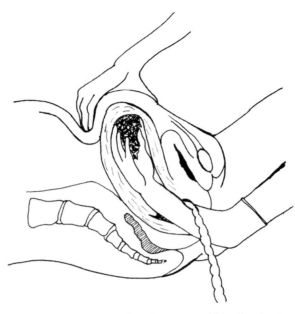

Figure 14.3 Placenta in palm prior to removal from the uterus

sought. Once found, the fingers gently develop the space between the placenta and uterus and shear off the placenta (Figure 14.2).

The placenta is pushed to the palmar aspect of the hand and when it is entirely separated, the hand is withdrawn with the placenta in the palm, as in Figure 14.3. If the placenta does not separate from the uterine surface by gentle lateral movement of the fingertips at the line of cleavage, suspect placenta accreta. Call for expert help to confirm the findings. If necessary, consider laparotomy with a view to hysterectomy.

Ensure that an oxytocin infusion is commenced and running, rapid enough to maintain the contraction of the uterus once the placenta is removed, and perform uterine massage. Care must be taken to tease out the membranes. Once the uterine contractions are established, examine the placenta and membrane to determine whether further exploration of the uterine cavity is necessary. A vessel leading to the edge of the membrane suggests a retained succenturiate lobe. As a rule of thumb, the membranes should be large enough to cover the placenta one and a half times.

Postpartum care

Maternal postpartum observation should be tailored to the need for timely identification of signs of excessive blood loss, including hypotension and tachycardia. Maternal vital signs and the amount of vaginal bleeding should be evaluated continuously. The uterine fundus should be identified and massaged, and its size and degree of contraction noted [18].

Women with anaemia are particularly vulnerable, since they may not tolerate even a moderate amount of blood loss. Women with inherited coagulopathies require individualized treatment, as their risks for bleeding extend beyond the first 24 h after delivery. In women with infective risks or where infection may worsen the maternal condition, a single dose of prophylactic antibiotics is given [19]; ampicillin 2 g IV plus metronidazole 500 mg IV or cefazolin 1 g IV plus metronidazole 500 mg IV.

Women at risk of postpartum haemorrhage

Women with risk factors for postpartum haemorrhage should be advised to give birth in an obstetric

157

unit where more emergency treatment options are available.

Close observation for signs of bleeding following delivery is necessary in such women.

Antenatal risk factors include the following.

- Previous retained placenta or PPH.
- Maternal haemoglobin below 8.5 g/dl at onset of labour.
- Body mass index greater than 35 kg/m^2.
- Grand multiparity (parity 4 or more)
- Antepartum haemorrhage.
- Overdistension of the uterus (for example, multiple pregnancy, polyhydramnios or macrosomia).
- Existing uterine abnormalities, e.g. fibroids.
- Maternal age (35 years or over).

Risk factors in labour include:

- induction of labour;
- prolonged first, second or third stage of labour;
- oxytocin use;
- precipitate labour; and
- operative birth.

In two-thirds of cases, postpartum haemorrhage occurs without any risk factors. Hence vigilance is required by staff caring for women in labour.

Prevention of postpartum haemorrhage is much easier than its treatment

Every birth attendant needs to have the knowledge, skills and critical judgement to carry out active management of the third stage of labour as well as access to required supplies and equipment. Incorporation of guidelines for the active management of the third stage of labour and prevention of postpartum haemorrhage into local guidelines is essential. The skills in the management of a complicated third stage of labour should be updated regularly by conduction of 'obstetric drills' similar to other obstetric emergencies. National professional associations and government bodies play an important role in addressing legislative and other barriers that impede the prevention and treatment of postpartum haemorrhage. It is also important to provide adequate education to the public – mothers and their families – for prevention of postpartum haemorrhage.

Errors in the management of the third stage and their sequelae

Attempts to deliver a placenta that is not completely separated may cause partial separation and retained products. It may also cause uterine inversion. Mismanagement of the third stage of the labour with excessive cord traction and fundal pressure is responsible for uterine inversion in the majority of cases.

There is an ever-present danger of uterine rupture during the manual removal of placenta. This usually occurs if the operator fails to push the fundus down on to the vaginal hand. The inexperienced operator may mistake the lower segment for the uterine cavity and grasp the upper segment, mistaking it for the placenta. Further trauma to the lower segment may be the result of trying to force the hand through the retraction ring.

Retained placenta under special circumstances

Morbidly adherent placenta such as placenta accreta, placenta increta and placenta percreta as mentioned earlier occur due to abnormal placentation and defective basalis layer due to previous scarring. The incidence of morbidly attached placenta is rising due to the rising rate of caesarean delivery.

The risk of placenta accreta rises sharply in mothers who have had two or more previous caesarean section who are aged 35 years or over and having an anterior or central placenta praevia. Women with previous uterine trauma in the form of uterine curettage and uterine perforation are also at risk of morbidly adherent placenta.

Placenta accreta is usually diagnosed when difficulty is encountered during delivery of the placenta and manual removal has to be performed. With a high index of suspicion, placenta accreta and its variants can be diagnosed antenatally in the above-mentioned high-risk women. When a diagnosis of placenta praevia is made, colour flow Doppler ultrasonography should be performed, as it has higher sensitivity and specificity compared to Magnetic Resonance Imaging [20]. Where antenatal imaging is not possible locally, such women should be managed as if they have placenta accreta until proven otherwise. Bilateral internal iliac artery occlusion balloon can be placed prior to commencement of caesarean section. At caesarean section, after the delivery of the baby, uterine arterial embolization could be carried out via pre-inserted catheters and hysterectomy performed if there is continued blood loss. All these require careful organization and multidisciplinary team approach by obstetrician, radiologist, anaesthetist and vascular surgeon.

Placenta increta/percreta can be managed conservatively in highly selected cases, where there is minimal bleeding and the woman desires to preserve her fertility. This involves delivering the baby via an upper segment vertical incision and leaving the placenta behind. The conservative management requires rigorous follow-up until complete resorption of the placenta occurs. Undetectable bHCG values do not seem to guarantee complete resorption of retained placental tissue. Close monitoring for signs and symptoms of infection and coagulopathy is necessary. In the case of major haemorrhage which usually [20] occurs 10–14 days after delivery, hysterectomy should not be delayed. Careful counselling of the woman is extremely important.

Placenta percreta can invade the urinary bladder and usually requires surgery, which may include partial resection of the bladder.

Conclusion

The majority of women will have an uneventful third stage of labour. However, it can be very unforgiving in a minority, hence careful management by an experienced clinician is crucial.

References

1. CEMACH. Saving Mothers' Lives 2003–2005. *Confidential Enquiry into Maternal and Child Health.* 2007.

2. Magann E F, Evans S, Chauhan S P, Lanneau G, Fisk A D, Morrison J C. The length of the third stage of labor and the risk of postpartum hemorrhage. *Obstet Gynecol* 2005; **105**: 290–3.

3. McDonald S. Management of the third stage of labor. *J Midwifery Womens Hlth* 2007; **52**: 254–61.

4. Winter C, Macfarlane A, Deneux-Tharaux C, *et al.* Variations in policies for management of the third stage of labour and the immediate management of postpartum haemorrhage in Europe. *Br J Obstet Gynaecol* 2007; **114**: 845–54.

5. Chong Y S, Su L L, Arulkumaran S. Current strategies for the prevention of postpartum haemorrhage in the third stage of labour. *Curr Opin Obstet Gynecol* 2004; **16**: 143–50.

6. Prendiville W J, Harding J E, Elbourne D R, Stirrat G M. The Bristol third stage trial: active versus physiological management of third stage of labour. *Br Med J* 1988; **297**: 1295–300.

7. Harding J E, Elbourne D R, Prendiville W J. Views of mothers and midwives participating in the Bristol randomized, controlled trial of active management of the third stage of labor. *Birth* 1989; **16**: 1–6.

8. Pena-Marti G, Comunian-Carrasco G. Fundal pressure versus controlled cord traction as part of the active management of the third stage of labour. *Cochrane Database Syst Rev* 2007; **4**: CD005462.

9. Soltani H, Dickinson F, Symonds I. Placental cord drainage after spontaneous vaginal delivery as part of the management of the third stage of labour. *Cochrane Database Syst Rev* 2005; **4**: CD004665.

10. Liabsuetrakul T, Choobun T, Peeyananjarassri K, Islam Q M. Prophylactic use of ergot alkaloids in the third stage of labour. *Cochrane Database Syst Rev* 2007; **2**: CD005456.

11. McDonald S, Abbott J M, Higgins S P. Prophylactic ergometrine–oxytocin versus oxytocin for the third stage of labour. *Cochrane Database Syst Rev* 2004; **1**: CD000201.

12. Su L L, Chong Y S, Samuel M. Oxytocin agonists for preventing postpartum haemorrhage. *Cochrane Database Syst Rev* 2007; **3**: CD005457.

13. Gulmezoglu A M, Forna F, Villar J, Hofmeyr G J. Prostaglandins for preventing postpartum haemorrhage. *Cochrane Database Syst Rev* 2007; **3**: CD000494.

14. Khan R U, El-Refaey H. Pharmacokinetics and adverse-effect profile of rectally administered misoprostol in the third stage of labor. *Obstet Gynecol* 2003; **101**: 968–74.

15. Habek D, Franicevic D. Intraumbilical injection of uterotonics for retained placenta. *Int J Gynaecol Obstet* 2007; **99**: 105–9.

16. Ghulmiyyah L M, Wehbe S A, Saltzman S L, Ehleben C, Sibai B M. Intraumbilical vein injection of oxytocin and the third stage of labor: randomized double-blind placebo trial. *Am J Perinatol* 2007; **24**: 347–52.

17. Intrapartum care – care of healthy women and their babies during childbirth National Collaborating Centre for Women's and Children's Health – Commissioned by NICE. 2007.

18. ACOG. Guideline for Perinatal Care. 2007; 6th edition.

19. WHO. Managing complications in pregnancy and childbirth. *A Guide for Midwives and Doctors.* WHO, 2003.

20. RCOG. *Placenta Praevia and Placenta Praevia Accreta: Diagnosis and Management.* Green Top Guideline. Number 27. London: RCOG, 2005.

Postpartum haemorrhage (PPH)

Nutan Mishra and Edwin Chandraharan

Introduction

It is estimated that about 600,000 women die each year due to pregnancy and childbirth (direct causes), or those aggravated or complicated by pregnancy (indirect causes). Primary postpartum haemorrhage (PPH) is the most common cause of direct maternal death in the developing world. Even in the developed world, where PPH is the fifth leading cause of direct maternal death, it is the commonest cause of severe maternal morbidity. In global terms, haemorrhage remains one of the most important causes of maternal mortality and accounts for 11% of all maternal deaths. The World Health Organization (WHO) estimates a 1% case fatality rate for the 14 million annual cases of obstetric haemorrhage. As a conservative estimate, some 140,000 deaths each year could be prevented, if the women themselves had been given an understanding of the possible warning signs of bleeding, the knowledge and ability to seek skilled maternity care, at least at delivery, and had access to functioning emergency obstetric services [1].

By definition, PPH refers to a blood loss of more than 500 ml (or 1000 ml during a caesarean section) after the delivery of the fetus. However, this is an 'arbitrary' value, as patients with a low Body Mass Index (BMI) may have a low blood volume (70 ml/kg), and women who are anaemic may have fewer physiological reserves. Hence, they may not tolerate even 500 ml of blood loss and may decompensate much earlier. Massive postpartum haemorrhage refers to the loss of 30–40% (generally over 2 l) of the patient's blood volume resulting in changes in the haemodynamic parameters.

Complications include haemorrhagic shock, disseminated intravascular coagulopathy (DIC), adult respiratory distress syndrome, renal failure, hepatic failure, loss of fertility, pituitary necrosis (Sheehan syndrome), and maternal death [2].

Postpartum haemorrhage is often unpredictable, although many risk factors have been identified [2]. Abnormalities of one or a combination of four basic processes (Four T's): uterine atony (Tone); retained placenta, membranes, or blood clots (Tissue); genital tract trauma (Trauma); or coagulation abnormalities (Thrombin) usually account for PPH.

Causes of PPH (primary or secondary)

Hypotonia/atonia

- Uterine atony.
- Placenta praevia.
- Uterine inversion.
- Uterine overdistension – polyhydramnios, multiple pregnancy, fibroids.

Trauma

- Genital tract injury including broad ligament haematoma.
- Uterine rupture.
- Surgical – caesarean sections, angular extensions, episiotomy.

Tissue

- Retained placenta or products of conception.

Coagulation failure

- Placental abruption.
- Pre-eclampsia.
- Septicaemia/intrauterine sepsis.
- Existing coagulation abnormalities.

Best Practice in Labour and Delivery, ed. R. Warren and S. Arulkumaran. Published by Cambridge University Press.
© Cambridge University Press 2009.

Risk factors for PPH [2]

- Prolonged labour.
- Augmented labour.
- Rapid labour.
- History of PPH.
- Episiotomy.
- Pre-eclampsia.
- Overdistension of the uterus (multiple pregnancy, polyhydramnios).
- Operative delivery.
- Chorioamnionitis.
- Maternal obesity.

Primary postpartum haemorrhage (primary PPH)

This refers to excessive bleeding (>500 ml) from the genital tract that occurs within the first 24 h of delivery. It could be due to any of the causes mentioned above. In general, it is due to the 4T's – Tone (80%), Tissue (retained products), Thrombin (coagulopathy) and Trauma (genital tract injury, including uterine rupture).

Secondary PPH

Excessive bleeding that occurs after 24 h (usually 1–2 weeks) after delivery is termed secondary PPH. The commonest cause is infection (endometritis) that is often secondary to retained products of conception. Hence, management includes antibiotics to treat infection and evacuation of retained products (if present) to eliminate the focus of infection.

Haemodynamic changes in massive postpartum haemorrhage

Pregnancy is associated with physiological changes in various systems, including haematology. The plasma volume and the red cell mass increase by approximately 40 and 25%, respectively [3], and this increases the ability of a pregnant woman to withstand the effects of obstetric haemorrhage.

Young, fit and healthy women can withstand and compensate for the blood loss without any demonstrable cardiovascular changes. Hypotension, dizziness, pallor, and oliguria may not occur until blood loss is substantial. At this stage she would have lost at least 30% of her blood volume. A 'rule of 30' has

Table 15.1 'Rule of 30' for massive obstetric haemorrhage.

Systolic blood pressure	Falls by 30 mmHg
Pulse	Increased by 30 beats/min
Haemoglobin	Falls by 30% (approx 3 g/dl)
Haematocrit	Falls by 30%
Estimated blood loss	30% of the estimated blood volume
	(70 ml/kg in adults)
	(100 ml/kg during pregnancy)

been proposed to help assess the degree of obstetric haemorrhage [4]. According to this rule, if the systolic blood pressure of the patient falls by 30 mmHg, pulse rises by 30 beats/min, haemoglobin (Hb) and haematocrit drop by 30%, then it is most likely that the patient may have lost approximately 30% of her blood volume (Table 15.1).

An acute and severe blood loss can lead to rapid decompensation and cardiovascular failure. Severity depends on body weight (i.e. BMI), pre-haemorrhage haemoglobin level and the presence of other co-morbidities.

For instance, a blood loss of 1.5 l may cause a severe shock in a woman weighing 48 kg, but only a mild shock in a women weighing 84 kg. As more time elapses between the onset of severe shock and resuscitation, the percentage of surviving patients decreases because metabolic acidosis may ensue. A window of opportunity often exists in which, if treatment is commenced, the outcome may be optimal. This is often termed 'The Golden Hour' and refers to the time in which resuscitation must begin to ensure the best chance of survival. The probability of survival decreases sharply after the first hour, if the patient is not effectively resuscitated.

Management (Table 15.2)

Management of PPH involves recognition (i.e. prompt diagnosis), resuscitation to ensure maternal haemodynamic stability, and identification and treatment of the underlying cause. In massive postpartum haemorrhage, a multidisciplinary approach is essential and the presence and advice of senior obstetrician, midwife, anaesthetist and haematologist are vital.

Table 15.2 'HAEMOSTASIS': a management algorithm for postpartum haemorrhage.

H – Ask for HELP and hands on the uterus (uterine massage)

A – Assess and resuscitate

E – Establish aetiology, ensure availability of blood and ecbolics

M – Massage uterus

O – Oxytocin infusion/prostaglandins – IV/per rectal/IM/ intramyometrial

S – Shift to theatre – aortic pressure or anti-shock garment/bimanual compression as appropriate

T – Tamponade ballon/uterine packing – after exclusion of tissue and trauma

A – Apply compression sutures – B-Lynch/modified

S – Systematic pelvic devascularization – uterine/ ovarian/quadruple/internal iliac

I – Interventional radiology and, if appropriate, uterine artery embolization

S – Subtotal/total abdominal hysterectomy

Services of ancillary staff (porters, receptionist, theatre staff) should be sought to ensure optimum care. When severe haemorrhage occurs, it is good practice to seek help from colleagues with gynaecological surgical experience, as complex surgical procedures may be required to arrest bleeding [1]. An initial assessment regarding the degree of blood loss and the severity of the haemodynamic instability is vital and it is always better to overestimate the blood loss and to anticipate the possibility of further bleeding.

The degree of pallor, level of consciousness, vital signs (pulse, blood pressure, respiration and temperature) and, if facilities are available, oxygen saturation should be monitored. A management algorithm for this serious and potentially fatal condition has been proposed [5]. The mnemonic 'HAEMOSTASIS' spells out the suggested actions that may facilitate the management of atonic PPH in a logical and stepwise manner [5].

Resuscitation of the patient and identification of the specific causes of PPH to institute immediate appropriate management should be carried out simultaneously, so as to avoid any delay in correcting hypovolumia.

Resuscitation

Resuscitation involves attention to Airway, Breathing and Circulation (ABC). Securing the airway and ensuring adequate oxygenation are paramount. This should be followed by replacement of blood volume to restore the oxygen carrying capacity of blood. Investigations to determine the degree of blood loss and the integrity of the coagulation system as well as monitoring of the vital signs should be carried out.

Two large-bore (14G) intravenous cannulae should be inserted and blood should be taken for investigations. These include full blood count (FBC), clotting profile, urea and electrolytes, and grouping and cross-matching. Rapid fluid infusion with crystalloids and colloids should be carried out until cross-matched blood is available. Crystalloids (0.9% normal saline, or Hartman's solution) are preferred over colloids, as the latter are associated with a 4% increase in the absolute risk of maternal mortality compared with crystalloids [6]. Colloids may also interfere with cross-matching and platelet function. If they are used, the maximum recommended dosage of colloids is 1500 ml in 24 h.

It is vital to try to identify a cause while resuscitation is being carried out to save valuable time. The single most common cause of haemorrhage is uterine atony, which accounts for about 80% of PPH. Hence, the bladder should be emptied to aid uterine contractions and a bimanual pelvic examination should be performed. The finding of the characteristic soft, poorly contracted (boggy) uterus suggests atony as a causative factor. The uterine contractions can be enhanced by uterine massage or bimanual compression. Both of these may help reduce blood loss, expel blood and clots, and allow time for other measures to be implemented. Once atonic uterus has been identified as the cause of PPH, measures should be taken to ensure optimum uterine contraction and retraction. These include the use of pharmacologic agents, use of uterine balloon tamponade, interventional radiology (uterine artery embolization) and surgical measures (exploratory laparotomy, uterine compression sutures, ligation of blood vessels, and total or subtotal hysterectomy), if needed.

If bleeding persists despite measures to correct uterine atony, other causes must be considered. Even if atony persists, there may be other contributing or co-existing factors such as a retained placenta, a tear

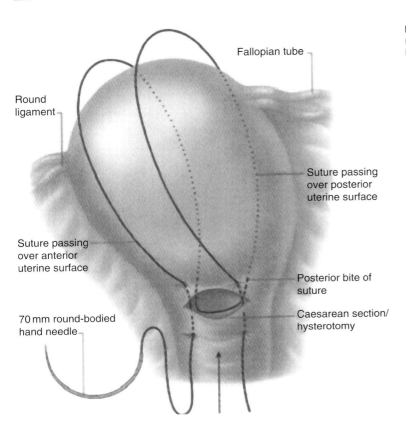

Figure 15.1 B-Lynch compression suture. (Reproduced with permission: Sapiens Publishing, 2006). (See colour plate section.)

of the vaginal wall or cervix, a vulval or paravaginal haematoma, a uterine scar rupture, disseminated intravascular coagulation (DIC), and, rarely, amniotic fluid embolism.

One should be aware of possible concealed bleeding, which may be intrauterine, intraperitoneal, within the broad ligament and/or paravaginal tissues. Lacerations should be ruled out by careful visual assessment of the lower genital tract. Adequate exposure, assistance, good lighting, availability of appropriate instruments and effective anaesthesia are necessary for identification and proper repair of lacerations. Therefore, transfer to a well-equipped operating theatre may be required to satisfy the above criteria.

Restoration of the oxygen carrying capacity of the blood and correction of any derangements in coagulation by blood transfusion and the use of blood products should be considered. This is especially so in cases of massive PPH, where more than 30% of blood volume is lost, as further bleeding may result in hypoxia and metabolic acidosis that may affect the vital organs. Furthermore, the clotting factors may be lost along with excessive blood loss ('washout phenomenon'). Until cross-matched blood is available, O negative or uncross-matched group-specific blood may be transfused, if there were no abnormal antibodies in the recipient's blood. Massive obstetric haemorrhage protocols should be used early and adhered to [1]. In special circumstances, auto-transfusion (or cell salvaging) may be considered, although during a caesarean section this carries a theoretical risk of amniotic fluid embolism and infection. Auto-transfusion involves collection of maternal blood and the use of a cell-saver device (Figure 15.1) to wash and filter the blood to remove the leukocytes and re-infuse the red cells [7]. However, it is important to appreciate that auto-transfusion and other blood products may not be acceptable to some patients. Hence, anaesthetists and haematologists should be involved very early to ensure optimum fluid management.

Apart from intravenous (IV) crystalloids, colloids, blood and oxytocin, the infusion of blood products needs to be considered. In massive obstetric blood loss, rapid infusion of fresh frozen plasma (FFP) may be required to replace clotting factors other than platelets. The development of a dilutional coagulopathy should be avoided, if at all possible by early use of FFP and other blood products as required [1]. It is recommended that with every 6 units of blood transfusion, 1 l of FFP should be administered (15 ml/kg). Hence, four to five bags of FFP are required, as each bag contains about 200–250 ml of FFP. Platelet count should be maintained above 50,000 by infusing platelet concentrates, if indicated. Cryoprecipitate may also be needed if the patient develops DIC and her fibrinogen drops to less than 1 g/dl (10 g/l).

Pharmacological treatment of postpartum haemorrhage

Current evidence suggests that uterotonics including oxytocin, ergometrine, and 15-methyl prostaglandin F2 alpha (intramyometrial or intramuscular) are effective measures to achieve haemostasis and to avoid surgical intervention in the majority of cases of atonic PPH [8]. Syntocinon (10 units) can be administered as a slow IV bolus. Syntometrine is considered to be more effective than oxytocin in causing tonic uterine contraction to arrest bleeding, but is associated with more side effects. Carbetocin, a long-standing oxytocin agonist, appears to be a promising agent for the prevention of PPH. The potential advantage of intramuscular carbetocin over intramuscular oxytocin is its longer duration of action. Its relative lack of gastrointestinal and cardiovascular side effects may also prove advantageous, as compared with syntometrine. Despite these advantages, it is not widely used in clinical practice, as it is more expensive compared to syntometrine [9].

Syntocinon 40 units can be added to 500 ml of normal saline and infused at a rate of 125 ml/h (i.e. 10 units of syntocinon/h). Oxytocin is produced in the hypothalamus and stored in the posterior pituitary gland, along with anti-diuretic hormone (ADH). It does have some ADH-like action and may cause retention of fluid. Therefore, it is important to avoid fluid overload, as fatal pulmonary and cerebral oedema with convulsions due to dilutional hyponatraemia has been reported with injudicious use of oxytocin. Hence, careful monitoring of fluid input and output is essential, if oxytocin is infused in large amounts.

Prostaglandins cause smooth muscle contraction and are invaluable in the management of atonic PPH. They are not recommended as prophylaxis of PPH due to their adverse gastrointestinal side effects. Hemabate (15-methyl prostaglandin 2 alpha) 250 μg can be administered intramuscularly. The dose can be repeated every 15 min for a maximum of eight doses (2 mg) [2]. However, it is advisable to move the patient to the theatre if profuse bleeding persists after three doses of hemabate. Intramyometrial injection of hemabate has been tried [10], but recent studies have questioned its effectiveness. Serious complications, including severe hypotension and cardiac arrest, have been reported with intramyometrial prostaglandin administration, likely due to inadvertent injection into uterine veins. Hence, the plunger of the syringe should be withdrawn to ensure that the needle is not inside a vein, prior to injection. If the PPH is unresponsive to ergometrine or oxytocin, rectal misoprostol (800–1000 μg) may be tried [2]. This is a valuable option in developing countries due to its low cost and relatively easier storage. Four to five tablets (200 mcg each) of misoprostol are administered rectally. Diarrhoea and other gastrointestinal side effects are common complications.

Surgical management of intractable postpartum haemorrhage

A recent systematic review concluded that there is no evidence to suggest that any one method is superior in the management of severe PPH [11].

A combination of measures (i.e. a 'multipronged attack') to combat postpartum haemorrhage is likely to be the most effective. The entire clinical situation should be considered; the degree of haemodynamic instability of the patient, the rapidity of blood loss and the likelihood of further loss, the availability of resources, and the experience and skill of the clinician would determine the surgical management.

Tamponade or uterine packing

Tamponade of the uterus can be effective in decreasing haemorrhage secondary to uterine atony, especially when uterotonics fail to cause sustained uterine contractions and satisfactory control of haemorrhage after vaginal delivery [2]. Balloon tamponade is the least invasive and most rapid approach and it would be logical to use this as first step in the management, when initial medical management fails to arrest bleeding [11]. It also allows adequate time to correct the coagulopathy if present. Senior obstetric input should be sought, as further surgical measures may be necessary if uterine tamponade fails to arrest haemorrhage. A multidisciplinary approach is essential with inputs from anaesthetists and a haematologist, and the high-dependency or intensive care unit should be alerted.

Uterine packing with gauze requires careful layering of the material back and forth from one cornu to the other using a sponge stick, packing back and forth, and ending with the extension of the gauze through the cervical os [2]. The same effect can be derived more easily using a Foley catheter, Sengstaken–Blakemore oesophageal catheter (SBOC), or the Rusch urological hydrostatic balloon [11]. The 'Bakri SOS' balloon has been designed especially for tamponade within the uterine cavity in cases of PPH secondary to uterine atony. The balloon is inserted through the cervix into the endometrial cavity, with the aid of a sponge holding forceps to steady the tip of the balloon. The procedure is often straightforward and takes only a few minutes. It arrests the bleeding and may prevent coagulopathy due to massive blood loss, and hence may alleviate the need for further surgical procedures.

About 300–400 ml of saline or sterile water may need to be injected to distend the balloon of the catheter, in order to exert the desired counter-pressure to stop bleeding from the uterine sinuses. In developing countries, if these catheters are not freely available, uterine packing could be tried with sterile gauze. Success with a condom used as a balloon tied to a plastic or Foley's catheter has been reported from Bangladesh. Apart from helping to arrest haemorrhage and providing additional time to correct coagulopathy, tamponade is likely to help avoid a laparotomy and hysterectomy and thus may help preserve future fertility.

Exploratory laparotomy is indicated when uterotonic agents, with or without tamponade, fail to control bleeding in a patient, who has given birth vaginally. The decision to perform a laparotomy may need to be considered earlier if the haemodynamic instability ensues, or if uterine scar rupture is suspected clinically. There is an argument for a midline vertical abdominal incision to optimize exposure, especially if internal iliac artery ligation is contemplated or in an obese patient. However, the type of incision depends on the preference, skill and experience of the operator as well as the clinical situation.

Consent for examination under anaesthesia, tamponade, laparotomy and hysterectomy should have been obtained as the patient is being moved to the theatre. This may not always be feasible due to the patient's condition or her level of consciousness. In such cases, treatment should be carried out in the patient's best interest to save life. Although informed consent for any procedure cannot be provided by others on behalf of a competent adult, it is good practice to inform her next of kin of the possibility of laparotomy and its sequelae if the patient is unable to give an informed consent due to collapse. Their agreement or consent helps to prevent misunderstanding regarding the need for such treatment. Laparotomy allows for direct visualization and access to the uterus as well as to the pelvic vasculature.

Factors that are likely to determine the need for further measures include the amount of blood loss, persistence of bleeding, haemodynamic status, the overall clinical condition of the patient and parity. It is important to have a discussion with the anaesthetist regarding the patient's ability to withstand possible further bleeding. This may help decide the feasibility of conservative surgical measures such as uterine massage, compression sutures and systematic pelvic devascularization. This is especially true in developing countries, where the patient might have lost a significant amount of blood by the time she reaches the referral centre. Radical measures (total or subtotal hysterectomy) may be required immediately in such cases to save the patient's life, albeit at the cost of her fertility.

Direct uterine massage

Direct uterine massage, which involves rubbing the myometrium between the surgeon's hands to stimulate contractions, may be tried initially. This is an extension of the bimanual compression as laparotomy enables direct myometrial compression. Intramyometrial injection of prostaglandins ($PGF_{2\alpha}$) may be tried at this stage. However, care should be taken to avoid systemic absorption and subsequent complications such as cardiac arrest, as mentioned earlier.

Compression sutures

The B-Lynch technique (Figure 15.1) is a suture that envelops and compresses the uterus and decreases bleeding [12]. Bimanual compression can be applied to the uterus to determine whether a compression suture is likely to be of value. The anterior and posterior walls are apposed by vertical brace sutures using a delayed absorbable suture material, resulting in continuous compression of the uterus. Various modifications have been made to this original technique. The Hayman technique uses two separate vertical compression sutures instead of one to increase the tension applied and, hence, the compression force [13]. This technique also alleviates the need for opening the uterus. It has the advantage of allowing blood to flow out from the uterine cavity and the possibility of two or three additional cervical sutures medial to the first two sutures. Horizontal full thickness compression sutures have also been tried, especially to control bleeding from the placental site in placenta praevia at the time of caesarean section [14]. These could also be applied in the lower segment, while taking care not to obliterate the cervical canal. The risk of damage to the bladder can be prevented by ensuring the bladder reflection is below the level of suture insertion. Placing sutures 2 cm medial to the lateral border of the uterus may help prevent ureteric injuries. A combination of multiple vertical compression sutures may be needed in some cases to arrest haemorrhage. Cho et al. [15] described a 'multiple square' suturing technique, which approximates anterior and posterior uterine walls at various points, virtually obliterating the uterine cavity. These vertical compression and multiple square sutures are easy to perform and less time-consuming. They can help junior obstetric trainees to arrest or reduce haemorrhage while awaiting senior help. These sutures can be placed well within the uterine body and do not involve areas traversed by uterine vessels or ureters.

Systematic pelvic devascularization

If the compression sutures fail to achieve haemostasis, ligation of blood vessels supplying the uterus could be tried in a systematic manner. These include ligation of both uterine arteries, followed by tubal branches of both ovarian arteries proximal to the ovarian ligament (called the 'quadruple ligation'). Uterine artery ligation is straightforward once the uterovesical fold of peritoneum is incised and the bladder is reflected down [5]. A window is made in the broad ligament just lateral to the uterine vessels and the needle is passed through this opening. A large, curved needle that is used for B-Lynch compression sutures (Figure 15.1) is preferable. Medially, the needle is passed

through the lower uterine myometrium, about 2 cm from the lateral margin, thus getting a good 'bite', and then tied. The same procedure is repeated on the other side. If bleeding continues, tubal branches of both ovarian arteries can be tied medial to the ovarian ligament. The needle should be passed through a 'clear' area of the mesosalpinx on either side of the blood vessels.

Internal iliac artery ligation is an option if bleeding persists. This requires an experienced surgeon who is familiar with the anatomy of the lateral pelvic wall. In many centres, it is a standard practice to involve the gynaecological oncologists, as they are more familiar with this procedure. Identification of the internal iliac vessels and the ureters during elective hysterectomies may help obstetricians to build up confidence when faced with an emergency [5]. The parietal peritoneum may be picked up divided at the lateral pelvic wall at the level of the pelvic brim after identifying the ureter, as it crosses the common iliac vessels. It may then be reflected medially along with the medial leaf of the broad ligament and the ureter held away from the internal iliac vessels by a loop. The internal iliac artery should then be traced from above downwards until it divides into the anterior and posterior divisions. The anterior division should be ligated with black silk or linen (permanent suture material). The procedure should be repeated on the opposite side. Alternatively, the broad ligament may be opened by clamping, cutting and ligating the round ligaments and the lateral pelvic wall approached through this route. Some obstetricians prefer this route as they are familiar with the same procedure during routine hysterectomy. Bilateral internal iliac artery ligation has been shown to reduce the pelvic blood flow by 49% and pulse pressure by 85% in arteries distal to the ligation. This translates to an acute reduction in the blood flow by about 50% in the distal vessels [16]. The reported success rate of this procedure has been between 40 and 100% [17], and the procedure averts hysterectomy in 50% of cases. Due to extensive collateral circulation within the pelvis, acute ischaemic necrosis of the uterus or other pelvic organs does not occur.

Potential complications of bilateral internal iliac artery ligation include haematoma formation in the lateral pelvic wall, injury to the ureters, laceration of the iliac vein and accidental ligation of the external iliac artery. Ligation of the main trunk of the internal iliac artery may result in intermittent claudication

(a)

(b)

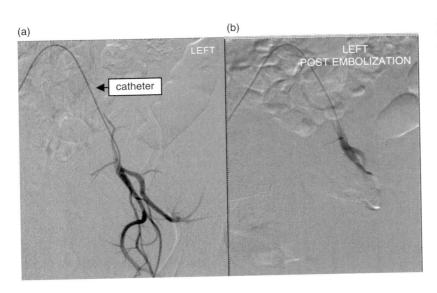

LEFT

LEFT
POST EMBOLIZATION

catheter

Figure 15.2 Uterine artery embolization. (a) Placement of the catheter prior to embolization, and (b) post-embolization

of the gluteal muscles due to ischaemia. Fortunately, these complications are rare and may be prevented by accurate identification of anatomical structures and ligating the anterior division of the internal iliac artery and by examining the femoral pulse prior to tightening the ligature to identify inadvertent ligation of the external iliac artery.

Interventional radiology: uterine artery catheterization

Interventional radiology can be considered in women who are not haemodynamically compromised and the clinical condition permits the placement of an uterine artery catheter. Recently, it has been recommended that all hospitals with delivery units should aim to provide an emergency interventional radiology service, as these have the potential to save lives of patients with catastrophic PPH [18]. Arterial embolization requires a radiologist with special skills in interventional radiology. The procedure involves placement of arterial catheter under a fluoroscopic guidance and injection of an 'embolus'. Embolic materials available for vascular occlusion include: gelfoam (gelatin), polyvinyl alcohol particles, steel coils and n-butyl-2-cyanoacrylate glue [19]. Most radiologists prefer gelfoam pletdgets, as these result in temporary distal occlusion of the uterine arterial bed for approximately 4 weeks duration. Figure 15.2 shows the cessation of uterine blood flow before and after uterine artery embolization. The vascular bed will eventually re-canalize, allowing the uterine vascularity to return to normal with full uterine function and reproductive potential. The reported success rate is approximately 90–95%. Menstruation typically returns within 3 months and subsequent pregnancies have been reported. Complications include vessel perforation, haematoma, infection, and bladder and rectal wall necrosis. Embolization can be used for bleeding that continues after hysterectomy [2].

Although the procedure has the potential of preserving future fertility, the need for specialized equipment, and the availability of experienced interventional radiologists and resources, preclude its widespread use [11].

Subtotal or total abdominal hysterectomy

Hysterectomy is a radical surgical option to save life when all other conservative measures have failed, or if the patient is haemodynamically very unstable. A senior obstetrician should take a decision to perform this procedure and the patient and her next of kin should be informed, if possible. If the bleeding is predominantly from the lower uterine segment (as in PPH following a major degree placenta praevia, accrete or rarely extension of uterine angles during caesarean section), a total abdominal hysterectomy is warranted. A subtotal hysterectomy may be performed if the bleeding is mainly from the upper segment and the aetiology is 'unresponsive' uterine atony. Subtotal hysterectomy has lower morbidity and mortality rates and requires less time to perform. The likelihood of ureteric or bladder injury is lower than for a total abdominal hysterectomy. It is important to realize that hysterectomy is the 'last resort' in the management of atonic PPH. However, as mentioned before, one may have to resort to hysterectomy much earlier if the haemodynamic condition is unstable, and if there is uncontrollable bleeding despite other medical and surgical measures.

It has been suggested that if hysterectomy is performed for uterine atony, there should be a clear and detailed documentation of the attempts at other measures to control bleeding [2]. Due to the anatomical changes of pregnancy, it is important to exercise the utmost care to prevent visceral trauma, especially of the bladder and ureters. It is also important to clamp the ovarian ligament medially to avoid non-intentional or inadvertent oophorectomy. Obstetric hysterectomy to control PPH should be performed by the senior-most obstetrician, as a 15-year experience of obstetric hysterectomy from a tertiary centre in Nigeria revealed a maternal mortality rate of 12.5% and urinary tract injury rate of 7.5% after this procedure [20].

Current concepts and new developments
The anti-shock garment

A new type of anti-shock garment has been developed (Figure 15.3), which reverses the effect of shock on the body's blood distribution. It is best described as a giant blood pressure cuff that applies external counter-pressure to the legs and abdomen. Based on the principle that the brain, heart and lungs of a person in shock incur a loss of oxygen because blood accumulates in the lower abdomen and legs, the anti-shock garment returns blood to the vital organs, thus stabilizing body pressure until a hospital can be reached.

A strap with a soft rugby ball goes over the uterine fundal area causing direct antero-posterior pressure and some aortic compression thus stopping or reducing the PPH in some cases.

The tamponade test

Condous *et al.* [21] described a 'tamponade test', which may help identify women with massive PPH who would require a laparotomy. In their prospective series, if the 'tamponade test' was positive (i.e. bleeding was arrested after uterine tamponade), 87.5% of the patients did not require a laparotomy [21]. Smaller uterine cavity in earlier gestations may not accommodate the standard balloons, and Foley's catheter balloon can be tried in these situations. Uterine tamponade works by exerting a counter-pressure on the placental bed, thereby arresting bleeding. This often helps to correct coagulation abnormalities by providing a window of opportunity to replace platelets and clotting factors.

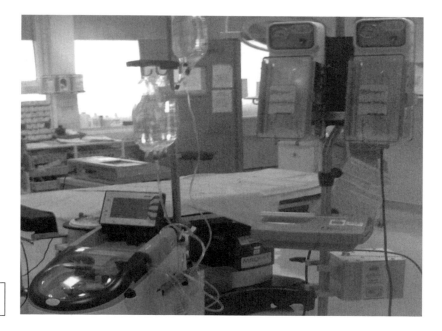

Figure 15.3 Cell salvaging equipment prior to caesarean section

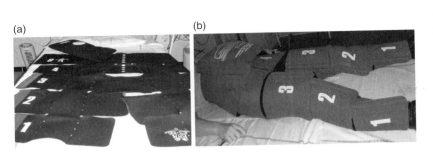

Figure 15.4 The anti-shock garment (a) layout (b) after application

Shock index

The shock index refers to the pulse rate divided by systolic blood pressure. It is based on the fact that in young healthy women, the systolic blood pressure may remain normal or near-normal until a critical point is reached, resulting in a rapid deterioration in clinical condition. The pulse rate increases well before such a fall in the systolic blood pressure is noted. The normal pulse index is between 0.5 and 0.7. It has been reported that a shock index (SI) of more than 0.9 is associated with a need for intensive therapy on admission [22]. A relative rise of the SI in that individual will help to identify the need for additional management, i.e. to detect or arrest haemorrhage or for adequate fluid replacement.

Activated factor VII

Intractable PPH may require human recombinant factor VIIa (rFVIIa), which has been shown to be effective in controlling severe, life-threatening haemorrhage by acting on the extrinsic pathway [2]. Intravenous doses may vary case by case. Generally the range is from 50 to 100 mcg/kg every 2 h until haemostasis is achieved. Cessation of bleeding ranges from 10 to 40 min after administration. Recently, it has been found to be useful in the management of major PPH [23]. It is estimated that it may avoid an emergency hysterectomy in about 76% of patients with massive PPH [24]. Concerns have been raised because of the apparent risk of subsequent thromboembolic events following rFVIIIa use. rFVIIIa may be considered as a treatment for life-threatening PPH, but should not be considered as a substitute for, nor should it delay, the performance of a life-saving procedure such as embolization or surgery, nor the transfer to a referring centre. It may not be widely available due to its cost, as a single treatment may cost up to £3500 [20].

Cell salvaging

Recovering, purifying and re-circulating the patient's blood is especially useful in patients who refuse blood and blood products, such as Jehovah's Witnesses. It is important to discuss this procedure during the antenatal consultation, prior to signing the 'Advance Directive'. Auto-transfusion, using the patient's own blood, using a cell salvaging mechanism (Figure 15.4), may be acceptable for some patients. If excessive blood loss is contemplated in these patients, as in placenta praevia, the use of recombinant erythropoiein and iron treatment to increase the haemoglobin concentration, if the patient is anaemic, and the prophylactic placement of uterine artery catheters with a view to embolization after delivery, if necessary, should be considered.

Conclusion

Postpartum haemorrhage is a leading cause of severe maternal morbidity and mortality. The confidential inquiries have re-emphasized that deaths caused by PPH are due to 'too little done too late'. Primary postpartum haemorrhage may be due to atonic uterus, genital tract trauma, coagulopathy or retained products of conception. Secondary postpartum haemorrhage occurs after the first 24 h of delivery and is due to infection, often secondary to retained products of conception. Morbidly adherent placenta (accreta, increta or percreta) may sometimes cause profuse haemorrhage after delivery that may necessitate a hysterectomy or methotrexate therapy. Rare complications of PPH include Sheehan's syndrome (pituitary necrosis secondary to massive PPH and resultant hypovolumia and hypoperfusion) that may present with panhypopituitarism. Dealing with ill, bleeding women requires a skilled multi disciplinary approach and may require anaesthetists, haematologists, vascular surgeons and radiologists in addition to obstetricians.

References

1. CEMACH. *Saving Mothers' Lives – Reviewing Maternal Deaths to Make Motherhood Safer 2003-2005*. London: CEMACH, 2007.

2. American College of Obstetricians and Gynaecologists. ACOG Practice Bulletin: Clinical Management Guidelines for Obstetrician–Gynaecologists Number 76, October 2006: Postpartum Haemorrhage. *Obstet Gynecol* 2006; **108**: 1039–47.

3. Chesley L C. Plasma and red cell volumes during pregnancy. *Am J Obstet Gynecol* 1972; **112**: 440–50.

4. Chandraharan E, Arulkumaran S. Massive postpartum haemorrhage and management of coagulopathy. *Obstet Gynaecol Reprod Med* 2007; **1794**: 119–22.

5. Chandraharan E, Arulkumaran S. Management algorithm for atonic postpartum haemorrhage. *J Paed Obstet Gynaecol* 2005; 106–12.

6. Hofmeyr G J, Mohlala B K. Hypovolumic shock. *Best Pract Res Clin Obstet Gynaecol* 2001; **15**: 645–62.

7. Santosa J T, Lin D W, Miller D S. Transfusion medicine in obstetrics and gynecology. *Obstet Gynecol Surv* 1995; **50**: 470–81.

8. Mousa H A, Wilkinshaw S. Major postpartum haemorrhage. *Curr Opin Obstet Gynecol* 2001; **13**: 593–603.

9. Chong Y C, Su L L, Arulkumaran S. Current strategies for the prevention of postpartum haemorrhage in the third stage of labour. *Curr Opin Obstet Gynecol* 2004; **16**: 143–50.

10. Takagi S, Yoshida T, Togo Y, *et al.* The effects of intramyometrial injection of prostaglandin F2 alpha on severe postpartum haemorrhage. *Prostaglandins* 1976; **12**: 565–79.

11. Doumouchtsis S K, Papageorghiou A T, Arulkumaran S. Systematic review of conservative management of postpartum hemorrhage: what to do when medical treatment fails. *Obstet Gynecol Surv* 2007; **62**: 540–7.

12. Price N, B-Lynch C. Technical description of the B-Lynch brace suture for the treatment of massive postpartum haemorrhage and review of published cases. *Int J Fertil Womens Med* 2005; **50**: 148–63.

13. Hayman R G, Arulkumaran S, Steer P J. Uterine compression sutures: surgical management of postpartum haemorrhage. *Obstet Gynecol* 2002; **99**: 502–6.

14. Tamizian O, Arulkumaran S. The surgical management of postpartum haemorrhage. *Best Pract Res Clin Obstet Gynaecol* 2002; **16**: 81–98.

15. Cho J H, Jun H S, Lee C N. Hemostatic suturing technique for uterine bleeding during caesarean delivery. *Obstet Gynecol* 2000; **96**: 129–31.

16. Burchell R C. Physiology of internal iliac artery ligation. *J Obstet Gynaecol Brit Cwlth* 1968; **75**: 642–51.

17. Vedantham S, Godwin S C, Mohr G. Uterine artery embolization: an underused method of controlling haemorrhage. *Am J Obstet Gynecol* 1997; **176**: 938–48.

18. Investigation into 10 maternal deaths at, or following delivery at, Northwick Park Hospital, North West London Hospitals NHS Trust, between April 2002 and April 2005. Commission for Healthcare, Audit and Inspection, 2006. Available at: www.healthcarecommission.org.uk/_db/_documents/Northwick_tagged.pdf

19. Corr P. Arterial embolization for haemorrhage in the obstetric patient *Best Pract Res Clin Obstet Gynaecol* 2001; **15**: 557–61.

20. Franchin M, Mauzato F, Salvaguno G L, Lipp G. Potential role for recombinant activated factor VII for the treatment of severe bleeding associated with DIC: a systematic review. *Blood Coagul Fibrinol.* 2007; **18**: 589–93.

21. Condous G S, Arulkumaran S, Symonds I, *et al.* The tamponade test for massive postpartum haemorrhage. *Obstet Gynecol* 2003; **104**: 767–72.

22. Rady M Y, Smithline H A, Blake H, Nowak R. A comparison of shock index and conventional vital signs to identify acute clinical illness in the emergency department. *Ann Emerg Med* 1994; **24**: 685–715.

23. Ahoren J, Jolela R, Korttila K. An open non-randomised study of recombinant activated factor VII in major PPH. *Acta Anaesthesiol Scand* 2007; **57**: 929–36.

24. Bouma L S, Bolte A C, Van Geijn H P. Use of recombinant activated factor VII in massive postpartum haemorrhage. *Eur J Obstet Gynecol Reprod* 2008; **137**: 172–7.

Chapter 16

Acute illness and maternal collapse in the postpartum period

Guy Jackson and Steve Yentis

Introduction

For most new mothers the postpartum period is a time of celebration and relief, but it can also represent a time of great danger, even in apparently straightforward cases.

For the purposes of this chapter we have defined 'acute illness' as onset of a new condition, or worsening of an existing one, within a few hours of delivery, that might present with maternal collapse or lead to it, and 'postpartum period' as the first 24 h after delivery.

Several aspects of this chapter may be also covered in other chapters in this book.

Incidence

The true incidence of postpartum collapse is impossible to estimate since the definitions and clinical presentations vary enormously and data collection is difficult. In 2005 the World Health Organization estimated that each year there are 529,000 maternal deaths worldwide during pregnancy, childbirth or in the postpartum period [1]. In the UK, the Confidential Enquiries into Maternal and Child Health (CEMACH) reports have estimated an incidence of 14 deaths per 100,000 maternities [2], but it is not possible to ascertain the proportion of women who die within the first 24 h of delivery or those who become acutely unwell during this time. Studies of obstetric morbidity are even more varied in their methodology and variability of definitions, but many of the conditions described may present or become more severe shortly after delivery [3–5].

Certain conditions with the potential to cause acute illness and/or death are common enough that every unit might expect to experience them regularly, whilst others might only occur once every few years.

It is important, therefore, that every unit is equipped to deal with both common and rare causes of postpartum collapse.

Causes

Acute postpartum illness can result from a wide range of underlying pathologies (Table 16.1). Although the incidences of different causes are difficult to determine, the leading causes of maternal death as reported by the CEMACH report for 2003–2005 are listed in Table 16.2.

Presentation

The timing, speed of onset and presentation depend on the underlying pathology and may even suggest the cause. However, conditions that typically develop relatively slowly in the non-obstetric setting may do so much faster in pregnancy or after delivery. For example, it is unusual for non-pregnant patients to suffer rapidly progressing, overwhelming sepsis, whereas the CEMACH reports describe many cases in which an apparently healthy woman becomes moribund and dies of sepsis within hours of the first symptoms [2,6]. This may be related to an impaired ability to withstand infection associated with pregnancy itself, or it may reflect the ability of young fit patients to compensate for physiological challenges very effectively until just before their compensatory mechanisms become overwhelmed. A classic example of this in obstetrics is the response to haemorrhage, in which the mother maintains blood pressure and perfusion relatively well until sudden, catastrophic collapse.

Since mothers may be discharged from the delivery suite to other wards or into the community soon after delivery, those who develop an acute illness may

Best Practice in Labour and Delivery, ed. R. Warren and S. Arulkumaran. Published by Cambridge University Press.
© Cambridge University Press 2009.

Table 16.1 Causes of acute illness and/or collapse in the postpartum period. The list is not exhaustive and there is some overlap, i.e. more than one may co-exist.

Obstetric	Hypertensive disorders	• Eclampsia, pre-eclampsia/HELLP syndrome with haemorrhage, liver rupture, stroke
	Postpartum haemorrhage	
	Genital tract/abdominal sepsis	
	Amniotic fluid embolism	
	Peripartum cardiomyopathy	
Non-obstetric	Thromboembolic disease	• Pulmonary embolism, cerebral vein thrombosis
	General anaesthesia	• Aspiration pneumonitis, atelectasis, respiratory depression, airway obstruction
	Regional anaesthesia	• Hypotension, high block, local anaesthetic toxicity, meningitis, spinal haematoma/abscess
	Cardiac disease	• Cardiac failure, myocardial infarction, aortic dissection, arrhythmias
	Respiratory disease	• Asthma, pneumonia
	Adverse drug reactions	• Anaphylaxtic/anaphylactiod reactions*, toxicity/side effects, drug withdrawal
	Metabolic	• Hypo/hyperglycaemia; hyponatraemia
	Primary neurological	• Epilepsy, stroke
	Other	• Air embolus, vasovagal syncope, splenic artery rupture, mesenteric infarction

Note: *remember latex allergy.

do so in a variety of locations. It is important, therefore, that staff who might encounter such cases (e.g. general practitioners, emergency department doctors and nurses) are aware of the immediate problems they may pose, and that the women themselves have ready access to clinical services if they are not in hospital.

Presentation ranges from non-specific mild symptoms to sudden collapse with loss of consciousness. It is important that all symptoms are taken seriously and, if appropriate, investigated and treated as early as possible, the aim being to prevent clinical deterioration leading to severe systemic collapse. Successive CEMACH reports abound with tales of women whose conditions' severity was not recognized until it was too late, and the latest report emphasizes the potential value of early warning systems, based on deviations from pre-determined physiological limits (e.g. heart rate, blood pressure, respiratory rate, temperature, urine output and neurological response), to alert staff

of clinical deterioration [2]. Although such systems, some of which include allocation of specific scores indicating severity of illness, are well described in the non-obstetric setting [7], there are few data supporting or validating their use in pregnant or recently pregnant women. CEMACH highlights research in this area as having a high priority [2].

Management

The basic principles of management are the same as for any patient presenting acutely, and can be divided into immediate and subsequent.

Immediate management

The two initial priorities are, first, resuscitation and stabilization of the patient and, second, assessment and immediate investigations to determine the differential diagnosis. In practice, a focused history and

Table 16.2 Leading causes of maternal death as reported by the CEMACH report for 2003–2005 [2].

Condition	Rate per 100,000 maternities
Direct causes	
Thromboembolism	1.94
Hypertensive disorders	0.85
Genital tract sepsis	0.85
Amniotic fluid embolism	0.80
Haemorrhage	0.66
Early pregnancy deaths	0.66
Other direct	0.19
Anaesthetic	0.28
Indirect causes	
Cardiac	2.27
Psychiatric	0.85
Other indirect	4.12

examination, in the context of any known specific issues relating to the recent pregnancy, can be undertaken during immediate resuscitation.

Resuscitation and stabilization

Guidelines for basic and advanced adult life support are now well established and all clinical staff should be familiar with them [8]. However, in the obstetric setting there are three factors that may make it more difficult to keep up both individual and team skills: (i) the physiological changes accompanying pregnancy and the particular aspects of resuscitation, especially in late pregnancy, many of which continue into the early postpartum period (Table 16.3) [9,10]; (ii) the rarity of cardiac arrest in this patient population; and (iii) a relatively high turnover of large numbers of staff (especially junior) that is typical of most delivery units.

Assessment

Assessment should be directed towards the most likely causes (see Table 16.1 and below). Level of consciousness is most usefully assessed using the Glasgow Coma Score (GCS), which although originally introduced for the assessment of patients with head injury, has been adopted as a convenient and useful tool in most clinical settings (Table 16.4).

After the immediate 'ABC' assessment, a systematic assessment is then required.

- *Obstetric:* see other chapters.
- *Respiratory:* breathlessness is a common feature of acute illness, but the degree may indicate the severity. Chest pain may suggest pulmonary embolism or pneumonia if pleuritic, or cardiac causes if central. Wheeze may indicate aspiration of gastric contents, anaphylaxis or pulmonary oedema; crepitations may indicate aspiration, pneumonia or pulmonary oedema. Tachypnoea is a relatively non-specific symptom and can occur in most illnesses; it is an important feature of early warning systems. Hypoxaemia (on saturation monitoring or blood gas) is also non-specific but important to detect, so early use of a pulse oximeter is vital. One potential problem with the pulse oximeter is that in hypoventilation, once oxygenation has been restored by administering oxygen, the saturation may be restored to near-normal even though the patient may only be taking a few breaths each minute. In such situations there may be severe hypercapnia despite reassuring oxygen saturation. Therefore, it is important to monitor respiratory rate and, if low, to monitor carbon dioxide tension by taking blood gas samples. A chest X-ray may be useful, although many conditions (e.g. amniotic or thromboembolism, bronchospasm) are typically not associated with early signs.
- *Cardiovascular:* breathlessness is a non-specific symptom, as discussed above. Cardiac pain is typically central and may indicate myocardial ischaemia or aortic dissection (classically severe and radiating through to the back). Hypertension may indicate pre-eclampsia or be related to pain/anxiety. Rarely it may indicate raised intracranial pressure. Hypotension may reflect loss of circulating volume, a pump problem (heart failure, pulmonary embolism) or a dilated vasculature, e.g. in sepsis. Tachycardia is relatively non-specific but, like tachypnoea, important. Bradycardia may suggest vasovagal syncope (which does not exclude other conditions), but it may also indicate severe hypovolaemia or hypoxaemia, in which sudden severe slowing of the heart rate may indicate imminent cardiac arrest. Heart murmurs can either reflect simple flow murmurs that often develop in pregnancy

Table 16.3 Main points of current resuscitation guidelines [8] with comments related to specific aspects relevant to pregnancy and the immediate postpartum period.

	General	Obstetric
A – Airway	• Open airway • Give high-flow oxygen • Call for help	• May be oedema, e.g. in pre-eclampsia • Risk of regurgitation/aspiration of gastric contents ever-present; cricoid pressure should be applied if unconscious • Incidence of difficult intubation in obstetrics is ~1:300–1:800.
B – Breathing	• Assess saturations, respiratory rate and auscultate	
C – Circulation	• Assess pulse – presence, rate and rhythm • Large-bore intravenous access and fluid resuscitation	• Aortocaval compression must be avoided with lateral tilt/uterine displacement. Even after delivery the uterus remains bulky • O negative blood should always be available in case of emergency
D – Disability	• Assess Glasgow Coma Score (see Table 16.4) • Blood glucose	
E – Exposure	• Ensure no obvious pathology missed	• Postpartum haemorrhage may be concealed
Reversible causes in cardiac arrest	• Hypovolaemia • Hypo/hyperkalaemia • Hypothermia • Hypoxia • Tension pneumothorax • Tamponade, cardiac • Toxins • Thrombosis – coronary or pulmonary	
Monitoring	• Electrocardiogram • Pulse oximeter • Non-invasive blood pressure	• Use appropriately sized cuff for obese patients
Investigations	• Basic blood tests including full blood count, urea/electrolytes, liver function tests, clotting studies and blood cultures • Arterial blood gas sample • Chest X-ray	

due to an increased cardiac output, or structural disease. If a cardiac condition is suspected, electrocardiography (ECG) is vital, and a cardiological referral and echocardiogram should be considered.

- *Neurological:* the GCS is a useful overall assessment tool, as discussed above. A reduced conscious level may result from a primary neurological disorder, such as stroke, or be secondary to other pathology, such as severe hypotension. Hypoglycaemia should always be sought as a cause of unconsciousness. Limb weakness may indicate stroke, although residual neuraxial blockade may confuse the clinical picture. Visual disturbances may be seen in primary hypertension, secondary to pre-eclampsia or due to raised intracranial pressure. A headache might be innocent in nature, but might also suggest postdural puncture headache, subarachnoid stroke, or severe

Table 16.4 Glasgow Coma Score.

	Response	Score
Eye opening	Spontaneous	4
	Eye opening to speech	3
	Eye opening to pain	2
	No eye opening	1
Verbal	Orientated, spontaneous speech	5
	Confused conversation	4
	Inappropriate words	3
	Incomprehensible sounds/grunts	2
	No verbal response	1
Motor	Obeys commands	6
	Localizes to pain	5
	Withdraws limb from painful stimuli	4
	Abnormal flexion or decorticate posture to pain	3
	Extensor response, decerebrate posture to pain	2
	No motor response	1

hypertension/pre-eclampsia. Convulsions may be due to previously diagnosed epilepsy, or result from eclampsia or local anaesthetic toxicity.

- *Other*: Bleeding may be obvious from operative site or vagina but may be concealed. Bleeding from puncture sites suggests a coagulopathy. Pyrexia may indicate an infective process. Skin rash may indicate allergic reaction or sepsis.

Subsequent management

Clearly, this will depend on the underlying cause and may involve further investigation and/or treatment that may involve other specialists and units. Labour wards are busy clinical areas, and this presents difficulties in coordinating care of the acutely unwell mother. It may be difficult to devote adequate attention to her whilst other priorities continue to present, and organising invasive procedures and investigations may take longer in an area unfamiliar to them. It is important that specialists from other acute areas, especially the critical care/high-dependency unit, be involved early, and that all staff appreciate that the patient does not physically have to be in the intensive care unit in order to receive high-level care.

Specific conditions
Hypertensive disorders

Pre-eclampsia can deteriorate after delivery leading to acute collapse with pulmonary oedema, cerebral haemorrhage, coagulopathy or convulsions. Oedema may also affect the airway leading to respiratory collapse. In the UK almost 40% of eclamptic fits occur after delivery [11].

This topic is covered in more detail in Chapter 24.

Postpartum haemorrhage

Acute blood loss is a major cause of collapse in the immediate and early postpartum period. It is defined as blood loss >500 ml after delivery of the placenta. The degree of blood loss is frequently underestimated and sometimes unnoticed when attention is focused on the baby. In addition, young patients are often able to compensate until hypovolaemia is severe.

Because of the tendency to underestimate hypovolaemia, it is important that administration of intravenous fluids is prompt and that appropriately sized cannulae are used. Below is an estimate of flow rates through different sizes of cannula:

- 20G = 40–80 ml/min
- 18G = 75–120 ml/min
- 16G = 130–220 ml/min
- 14G = 250–360 ml/min

Postpartum haemorrhage is covered in more detail in Chapter 15.

Genital tract/abdominal sepsis

'Sepsis' is a non-specific term that refers to the systemic inflammatory response to infection. Systemic inflammatory response syndrome (SIRS) is defined as a clinical state including two or more of the following:

- temperature >38°C or <36°C
- heart rate >90/min
- respiratory rate >20/min or $PaCO_2$ <4.3 kPa
- white cell count >12×10^9/l

The clinical condition defined as 'SIRS' is very non-specific and occurs commonly. Furthermore, it may be caused by many other conditions than infection alone.

In severe sepsis, organ dysfunction develops as a result of hypotension and hypoperfusion. 'Septic shock' is defined as severe sepsis with hypotension, despite adequate fluid resuscitation, along with perfusion abnormalities such as lactic acidosis, oliguria and mental disturbance.

The clinical presentation of sepsis is very variable and often insidious, with rapid clinical deterioration. Typically the patient presents with pyrexia >38°C, tachycardia and tachypnoea, progressing to hypotension and hypoxaemia. There may be other symptoms such as abdominal pain, nausea and vomiting.

A high index of suspicion should be maintained with early implementation of broad spectrum antibiotics after screening for sources of sepsis, and early referral to critical care services if severe.

Amniotic fluid embolus

The mortality rate from amniotic fluid embolism in the UK is estimated at 0.25–0.8 per 100,000 maternities [2]. Between 26 and 61% of diagnosed cases result in death [2,12].

The traditional explanation is that amniotic fluid enters the maternal circulation following forceful contractions, causing pulmonary vascular obstruction and thence right ventricular failure and cardiovascular collapse, although this has been questioned [13].

It is diagnosed by the presence of fetal squames and lanugo hair in the pulmonary vasculature at autopsy. In the case of survival, the diagnosis remains clinical.

Amniotic fluid embolus can present at any point from early labour until the early postpartum period. Classically, symptoms include sweating, cyanosis, cardiovascular collapse, confusion, convulsions and disseminated intravascular coagulation (DIC). These symptoms typically progress quickly with rapid deterioration in clinical condition [12,13].

Management remains supportive with early recognition, prompt resuscitation and early involvement of critical care. There are no specific therapies that have been shown to improve survival.

Peripartum cardiomyopathy

Peripartum cardiomyopathy (PPCM) develops between the last month of pregnancy and up to 5 months after delivery [14]. Typical symptoms include breathlessness, oedema and orthopnoea with tachycardia and tachypnoea. A wheeze is often mistaken for asthma but may result from heart failure.

Classically, PPCM results in a dilated cardiomyopathy with reduced cardiac contractility and raised right-sided pressures.

Treatment of PPCM includes inotropes (dobutamine or dopamine acutely) and reduction in afterload with diuretics and vasodilators. Anticoagulation is advised because of the risk of thromboembolic disease.

PPCM often recurs in subsequent pregnancies and carries significant maternal mortality.

Thromboembolic disease

There are many risk factors in pregnancy for thromboembolic disease and successive CEMACH reports have highlighted its importance [2,6].

Pulmonary embolism

Pulmonary emboli (PE) present in many ways, often depending on their size. Micro or small emboli might initially be asymptomatic but present subtle, increasing symptoms such as worsening exertional dyspnoea, tiredness or syncope. Small and medium emboli occlude segmental arteries causing pleuritic chest pain, haemoptysis and tachypnoea. Massive emboli become lodged in the proximal pulmonary arteries and chambers of the right heart, resulting in acute and massive reduction in cardiac output with hypotension, right heart failure and major disruption in pulmonary perfusion.

Arterial blood gas measurement classically, but not always, reveals hypoxaemia and hypocapnia. Metabolic acidosis may be present if there is shock. An ECG most often shows sinus tachycardia; however, other signs can be present. A chest radiograph should be performed, although only ~50% of confirmed PE exhibit signs. Most commonly, non-specific features are present such as cardiac enlargement, pleural effusions and localized infiltrates.

An echocardiogram is often useful, indicating right ventricular size and function, although it is poor at excluding PE. The choice for further imaging is usually between a ventilation–perfusion lung scan or computed tomography pulmonary angiogram depending on local availability and clinical condition.

Management should involve a multidisciplinary resuscitation team including senior physicians, obstetricians, radiologists and anaesthetists [15].

The management of PE depends on the patient's clinical state. Massive PE with clinical compromise justifies more immediate and invasive treatment including thrombolysis, which may be instituted on clinical grounds alone if cardiac arrest is imminent. Current recommendations suggest a 50 mg bolus of alteplase. Invasive approaches, such as thrombus fragmentation and placement of an inferior vena caval filter, can be considered where facilities and expertise are readily available. In non-massive PE, heparin at therapeutic dosage is recommended instead of thrombolysis, before any imaging is undertaken.

Cerebral vein thrombosis

Pregnancy predisposes to cerebral vein thrombosis. It is likely to present as either headache, focal neurological signs, or reduced consciousness (see below).

General anaesthesia

Aspiration pneumonitis

Pregnant patients present particular problems when undergoing general anaesthesia, in particular increased risk of difficult intubation and acid regurgitation. Often the anaesthetic is urgent. Aspiration of gastric contents might occur and present at induction, intraoperatively or postoperatively. Features include bronchospasm, hypoxaemia, raised airway pressure, tachypnoea, tachycardia and pyrexia. Management is largely supportive, as prophylactic antibiotics and steroids are no longer advocated. Chest radiographs may be useful to assess evidence of aspiration and monitor progression.

Atelectasis, respiratory depression and airway obstruction

During general anaesthesia, patients usually receive opioids for postoperative analgesia. Their potent respiratory depressant effects can be exacerbated by the anaesthetic agents during early recovery, leading to airway obstruction and respiratory depression. The situation is made worse if there is weakness caused by residual neuromuscular blockade. The development of special recovery areas with staff who are familiar with postoperative recovery care is important in preventing such complications. Simple airway manoeuvres can be tried and oxygen administered while anaesthetic help is summoned. Naloxone can be titrated to effect if respiratory depression is due to opioids.

Basal atelectasis commonly follows general anaesthesia and describes small airway collapse due to poor regional ventilation and/or mucous plugging. Patients typically are hypoxaemic with reduced tidal volumes and raised respiratory rates. Effective analgesia must be ensured to allow deep breathing and coughing. Physiotherapy may be useful in encouraging adequate lung expansion and effective removal of secretions.

Regional anaesthesia

The physiological effects of regional anaesthesia extend into the postpartum period and can present problems for both the anaesthetist and for those caring for the patient after the procedure.

A residual regional block can result in hypotension due to the sympathetic block that accompanies the sensory blockade. This is exacerbated by any hypovolaemia already present or that develops after delivery, and by bradycardia that may occur if the block extends up to the cardiac sympathetic fibres at thoracic spinal segments T2–T4. If the block extends to the cervical segments (C3–C5), there is risk of diaphragmatic weakness, leading to hypoventilation. There may also be inability to talk/swallow, weakness of the arms/hands, and sedation (which may be put down to simple tiredness). Any patient who has received a spinal or epidural anaesthetic must be monitored carefully to exclude a dangerously high block, which may develop 30–60 min after the procedure.

Following epidural anaesthesia, in which larger volumes of local anaesthetic are used than for spinal anaesthesia, local anaesthetic toxicity may be encountered. Typically the signs and symptoms progress from mild features such as circumoral tingling, tinnitus and visual disturbances, to cardiac arrhythmias, convulsions and reduced consciousness. Resuscitation in this circumstance is notoriously difficult. Recently, the use of lipid suspension has been advocated following experimental work, and anecdotal reports are encouraging [16].

Both trauma and infection may be caused during regional anaesthesia. Epidural/spinal haematomas can present acutely with acute cord compression. Investigation of any suspected lesion should be prompt with referral to an appropriate neurosurgical centre. Meningitis is a rare complication; classic signs include headache, neck stiffness, photophobia, vomiting, fever and leukocytosis. Lumbar puncture should be considered, and broad spectrum antibiotics started pending the result. Spinal abscesses and other rare neurological complications such as arachnoiditis are unlikely to present in the early postpartum period.

Cardiac disease

Cardiac disease is becoming more common due to increasing maternal age, improved survival of girls with complex congenital heart disease, and the influx of immigrant women with pre-existing uncorrected conditions. Risk factors associated with ischaemic heart disease include obesity, smoking, older age, higher parity, diabetes, pre-existing hypertension and a family history.

The early postpartum period is associated with large fluid shifts that potentially contribute to haemodynamic instability. Most cardiac disease is sensitive to these changes, hence this period can be associated with cardiac complications such as heart failure, arrhythmias and ischaemia [17]. Systolic 'flow' heart murmurs are common as are ECG changes such as axis deviation and abnormalities in the ST, T and Q waves, contributing to difficulties in diagnosis.

Myocardial infarction (MI)

MI in the postpartum period is rare. Typically, chest pain occurs at rest and is described as central, crushing or heavy, radiating to the arm or neck, although presentation is often 'atypical'. Early management includes aspirin 300 mg orally and cardiological referral. The choice between thrombolysis and primary coronary angioplasty will depend on local availability as well as other factors, such as risk of haemorrhage following delivery and surgical procedures.

Aortic dissection

Typically, severe sudden anterior chest pain radiates to the interscapular area, often associated with hypertension. Sudden death or profound shock is usually due to aortic rupture or cardiac tamponade. Patients can also present with other features including cardiac failure, stroke, acute limb ischaemia, paraplegia, MI, renal failure, or abdominal pain.

The ECG may be normal or show left ventricular hypertension or even acute MI. A chest radiograph may show a widened upper mediastinum with enlargement of the aortic knuckle. An echocardiogram may show aortic root dilatation or aortic regurgitation. CT or angiography may also be indicated.

Management will depend on the type of dissection. If the aortic arch is affected, surgical repair is usually required. If medical management is indicated, then control of blood pressure is the main goal of therapy to stop the spread of intramural haematoma and prevent rupture.

Arrhythmias

The incidence of cardiac arrhythmias is increased in the pregnant population, and presentation ranges from mild symptoms only to severe hypotension and even cardiac arrest. The most common rhythms include supraventricular tachycardia and atrial fibrillation. Evidence of deranged electrolytes or hypovolaemia should be sought and treated accordingly. Supraventricular tachycardias may respond to vagal manoeuvres, adenosine or amiodarone, but may require DC cardioversion in severe compromise.

Respiratory disease
Asthma

Acute exacerbations of asthma are uncommon in the peripartum period, but the physiological changes of pregnancy may potentially lead to misinterpretation of the signs and symptoms of disease severity – for example, hyperventilation. Asthma can be exacerbated by general anaesthesia and some drugs, such as non-steroidal anti-inflammatories. The classical symptoms include wheeze, breathlessness and cough, and patients can present with either gradually worsening symptoms or acute severe bronchospasm.

The severity of the attack should be assessed along with the cause of the exacerbation (drugs, infection). Immediate management includes oxygen, nebulized salbutamol (bronchodilator) and ipratropium bromide, hydration, antibiotics and steroids. Intravenous aminophylline, salbutamol and adrenaline can be considered in life-threatening attacks.

Pneumonia

Patients typically present with cough, fever, breathlessness, chest pain and abnormal chest radiograph. Appropriate broad spectrum antibiotics should be started along with oxygen, adequate hydration and chest physiotherapy.

Adverse drug reactions
Anaphylaxtic/anaphylactiod reactions

Anaphylactic reactions are IgE-mediated type-B hypersensitivity reactions to an antigen resulting in histamine and serotonin release from mast cells and basophils. Anaphylactoid reactions produce indistinguishable clinical features, but are IgG-mediated, with complement activation, and require no previous exposure to the stimulus.

Common causes include latex and drugs, such as antibiotics and some anaesthetic drugs, although there are many other possible causes including intravenous colloids and some foods. Reactions against blood or blood components must also be remembered.

Anaphylaxis typically presents with cardiovascular collapse, erythema, bronchospasm, angio-oedema and rash. However, skin lesions may not be present and features (which may include abdominal pain) may be confusing, especially against a background of recent delivery, and a high index of suspicion is required.

Management involves removal of the suspected antigen and immediate supportive care with adrenaline 0.5–1 mg boluses IM (or 50 μg increments IV if the doctor is familiar with this route of injection and there is ECG monitoring) repeated until symptoms improve. Antihistamines (chloramphenamine 10–20 mg IV) and corticosteroids (hydrocortisone 100–200 mg IV) should be given to lessen the subsequent inflammatory response. Bronchodilators may also be considered.

All patients with a suspected anaphylactic reaction should have blood taken 1 h following the start of the reaction followed by a further sample at 6 h. A raised tryptase level will confirm mast cell degranulation, although other measurements (e.g. complement) may also be useful. All patients should be followed up after the event and allergy testing arranged.

Toxicity/side effects

Most drugs have side effects, even at normal doses, while in overdose many have significant untoward effects. Opioids can cause respiratory depression, hypotension, bradycardia and reduced consciousness. Naloxone can be used to reverse the effects, but care should be taken to titrate to effect, and the antagonist's effect may be shorter than the duration of action of the original opioid so that repeated dosage or an infusion may be required.

Syntocinon® may cause profound hypotension and tachycardia, although this should not preclude its careful administration in a patient who is hypovolaemic from haemorrhage. Ergometrine may cause hypertension and severe vomiting. Antiemetics such as metoclopramide and cyclizine may cause severe tachycardia and rarely, dystonic reactions. Beta-adrenergic agonists used for tocolysis may cause tachycardia and pulmonary oedema. Early signs of magnesium toxicity include nausea, vomiting and flushing. Later signs include ECG changes, loss of tendon reflexes, respiratory depression, apnoea and cardiac arrest. Toxicity is reversed by intravenous calcium gluconate (10 ml of 10% solution IV).

Drug withdrawal

The proportion of pregnant women who abuse drugs is difficult to determine and varies depending on the socio-economic area. Whilst patients are unlikely to present with acute intoxication in the immediate postpartum period, symptoms of withdrawal may occur. Withdrawal from alcohol typically is worst about 24–36 h after cessation of intake, resulting in aggression, confusion and tremor. Opioid withdrawal occurs within 6–12 h of the last dose and may cause problems with postoperative analgesia as well as hypertension, tachycardia, sweating, abdominal pain and vomiting. Myocardial ischaemia, arrhythmias and convulsions can occur with both cocaine withdrawal and acute intoxication.

Metabolic

Diabetes can be particularly difficult to manage during pregnancy, with significant increases in insulin requirements. Following delivery, requirements fall dramatically, and hypoglycaemia can occur if the infusion rates of insulin are not reduced. Hypoglycaemia can present with symptoms ranging from mild (nausea, anxiety, tremor, pallor) to more severe (personality change, confusion, ataxia, coma). Any acute illness in a diabetic mother should prompt a glucose level check and treatment of hypoglycaemia. Initial treatment includes a glucose bolus (50 ml of 50% glucose IV). Hyperglycaemia in a poorly controlled diabetic can also present with a range of symptoms including ketoacidosis and coma. Treatment involves recognition and treatment with insulin.

The potential danger of hyponatraemia from excessive administration of hypotonic intravenous fluids is well described, and this may occur in the delivery suite [18]. Parturients may be at increased risk because of the dilution of oxytocics in hypotonic solutions and the antidiuretic action of oxytocin.

Rarely, there may be other, unexpected, metabolic causes of collapse or acute illness (e.g. severe abnormalities of potassium or calcium status) and the usefulness of routine electrolyte analysis should not be forgotten.

Primary neurological

Epilepsy

Convulsions due to epilepsy may present for the first time in the postpartum period or may occur in a patient with known epilepsy. Epilepsy tends towards poorer control in pregnancy due to altered pharmacokinetics and pharmacodynamics, as well as reduced compliance with and alteration of normal medication. In some epileptics, convulsions are triggered by pain, anxiety and hyperventilation, all of which may occur during or after delivery. There are, of course, other causes of seizures on the labour ward (particularly eclampsia), and other pathology should always be excluded. Typical treatment includes diazepam 5–10 mg followed by phenytoin 10–15 mg/h (with ECG monitoring) if seizures continue.

Stroke/cerebrovascular accident (CVA)

The most common cause of haemorrhagic CVA is subarachnoid haemorrhage. Typically, patients present with sudden onset severe headache with photophobia, neck stiffness, vomiting and sometimes reduced conscious level. Management involves early consultation with neurosurgeons regarding surgical intervention along with supportive treatment. There is usually underlying pathology, such as an arteriovenous malformation or berry aneurysm. Rarely, subarachnoid haemorrhage has followed dural puncture (spinal anaesthesia, diagnostic lumbar puncture or accidental dural tap during epidural analgesia/anaesthesia).

Patients may also present with focal neurological signs due to ischaemic or haemorrhagic stroke affecting the cortex. Again, this may be accompanied by reduced conscious level. Stroke is a common feature in deaths due to hypertensive diseases of pregnancy, and focal neurological features may be a presentation of cerebral venous thrombosis, so that these diagnoses must be considered.

Other non-obstetric

Air embolus

Air emboli may occur for a variety of reasons. Subclinical entry of air into the circulation has been shown to occur in caesarean sections, and this is more likely if the uterus is exteriorized and held above the level of the heart; positioning the patient head-up may reduce this [19]. In the postpartum period, the most likely mechanism of air embolism is entrainment into the circulation on insertion or manipulation of central venous catheters or peripheral cannulae where the pressure within the vein is negative relative to atmospheric pressure. Inadvertent injection of air into venous lines can also occur in the form of small bubbles, or as large boluses when pressure devices are used with air-containing bags of fluid.

The clinical features are usually non-specific (hypotension, tachycardia, reduced arterial saturation) and the diagnosis is not always clear. Chest pain with ST segment depression may suggest air in the coronary circulation. Larger volumes of air may cause reduced cardiac output due to obstruction of right ventricular output. If a patent foramen ovale is present (seen in about 30% of the population) air can pass into the arterial circulation and cause systemic lesions such as stroke or MI. In the case of massive air embolism, auscultation of the heart may reveal 'mill wheel' or churning noises.

Management includes prevention of further entrainment of air followed by supportive care. It has been suggested that aspiration of air from the right ventricle is possible, but in practice this is rarely successful or practical. Positioning the patient in the left lateral position may reduce right ventricle outflow obstruction.

Vasovagal syncope

Vasovagal syncope may be associated with chronic autonomic instability or occur de novo. Triggers include stress, prolonged standing, dehydration, painful or unpleasant procedures, and hyperthermia. Collapse is usually preceded by prodromal symptoms such as feeling faint, nausea, sweating and visual disturbance.

The underlying mechanism involves increased activity of the parasympathetic nervous system ± reduced sympathetic activity. The common feature is usually hypotension due to either a bradycardia (vagal effect) or vasodilatation (sympathetic effect).

Specific treatment is usually not required other than lying the patient down with legs elevated to increase venous return. In the postpartum period, dehydration as well as the other common triggers may be more prevalent.

Other vascular

CEMACH reports have contained cases of splenic artery rupture and mesenteric infarction; although rare, such conditions may be more common in pregnancy. Rare causes of postpartum collapse should always be considered during resuscitation, especially if the patient is unresponsive to initial management.

Other considerations

Finally, the effect of acute illness/collapse on the mother's partner/relatives and on other women around her should not be forgotten. The typical maternity suite is not an area where acute critical illness is commonly seen, and the psychological impact of a sudden deterioration, compounded by the lack of familiarity of the attending staff, may be considerable. If time permits it might be appropriate to transfer the patient to an area more familiar with acute medical management, such as the recovery area or even the labour ward operating theatre; alternatively, screens/curtains should be used and other patients even moved away from the area. Counselling for other patients, relatives and even staff may be appropriate after the event.

Summary

The causes of postpartum collapse are varied, but the initial approach to the management remains the same. A systematic approach (Airway, Breathing, Circulation) helps to address the immediate issues while helping to establish the underlying cause and therefore allowing appropriate treatment.

Large numbers of patients present with acute illness in the postpartum period although exact numbers are difficult to establish. Most of these patients have a good outcome, but a few remain severely unwell and require management by a combination of obstetric, anaesthetic and intensive care staff. Systems should be in place for the recognition, monitoring and referral of these patients, as well as for the training of staff who might be involved in their management.

References

1. World Health Organization. *The World Health Report 2005 – Make Every Mother and Child Count*. WHO 2005. Available from: http://www.who.int/whr/2005/en/index.html (accessed 13 February 2008).

2. Lewis, G, ed. *The Confidential Enquiries into Maternal and Child Health (CEMACH). Saving Mothers' Lives: Reviewing Maternal Deaths to Make Motherhood Safer – 2003–2005. The Seventh Report on Confidential Enquiries into Maternal Deaths in the United Kingdom*. London: CEMACH, 2007.

3. Hazelgrove J F, Price C, Pappachan V J, Smith G B. Multicenter study of obstetric admissions to 14 intensive care units in southern England. *Crit Care Med* 2001; **29**: 770–5.

4. Waterstone M, Bewley S, Wolfe C. Incidence and predictors of severe obstetric morbidity: case-control study. *Br Med J* 2001; **322**: 1089–93.

5. Brace V, Penney G, Hall M. Quantifying severe maternal morbidity: a Scottish population study. *Br J Obstet Gynaecol* 2004; **111**: 481–4.

6. Lewis G, ed. *Confidential Enquiries into Maternal and Child Health. Why Mothers Die. The Sixth Report of the United Kingdom Confidential Enquiries into Maternal Deaths in the United Kingdom*. London: RCOG Press, 2004.

7. McGaughey J, Alderdice F, Fowler R, Kapila A, Mayhew A, Moutray M. Outreach and Early Warning Systems (EWS) for the prevention of Intensive Care admission and death of critically ill adult patients on general hospital wards. *Cochrane Database Syst Rev* 2007; **3**: CD005529.

8. Resuscitation Council (UK). *The Resuscitation Guidelines 2005*. 5th edn. London: Resuscitation Council (UK), 2005.

9. Morris S, Stacey M. Resuscitation in pregnancy. *Br Med J* 2003; **327**: 1277–9.

10. Al-Shabibi N, Penna L. Postpartum collapse. *Curr Obstet Gynaecol* 2006; **16**: 72–8.

11. Knight M. Eclampsia in the United Kingdom 2005. *Br J Obstet Gynaecol* 2007; **114**: 1072–8.

12. Tuffnell D J. United Kingdom amniotic fluid embolism register. *Br J Obstet Gynaecol* 2005; **112**: 1625–9.

13. Clark S L. New concepts of amniotic fluid embolism: a review. *Obstet Gynecol Surv* 1990; **45**: 360–8.

14. Sliwa K, Fett J, Elkayam U. Peripartum cardiomyopathy. *Lancet* 2006; **368**: 687–93.

15. Greer I E, Thompson A J. *Thromboembolic Disease in Pregnancy and the Puerperium: Acute Management*. Green-Top Guideline No. 28. London: RCOG, 2007.

16. Picard J, Meek T. Lipid emulsion to treat overdose of local anaesthetic: the gift of the glob. *Anaesthesia* 2006; **61**: 107–9.

17. Dob D P, Yentis S M. Practical management of the parturient with congenital heart disease. *Int J Obstet Anesth* 2006; **15**: 137–44.

18. Ophir E, Solt I, Odeh M, Bornstein J. Water intoxication – a dangerous condition in labor and delivery rooms. *Obstet Gynecol Surv* 2007; **62**: 731–8.

19. Fong J, Gadalla F, Druzin M. Venous emboli occurring caesarean section: the effect of patient position. *Can J Anaesth* 1991; **38**: 191–5.

Episiotomy and obstetric perineal trauma

Ranee Thakar and Abdul H. Sultan

Perineal repair after childbirth affects millions of women worldwide. In the United Kingdom, approximately 85% of women sustain some form of perineal trauma during vaginal delivery, and of these, 69% will require stitches [1]. The prevalence of perineal trauma is dependent on variations in obstetric practice, including rates and types of episiotomies, which not only vary between countries but also between individual practitioners within hospitals. In the Netherlands, the rate of episiotomy is 8%, compared to 14% in England, 50% in the USA and 99% in East European countries. Rates also vary between hospitals in the same country; for example, in the United States, the rates of episiotomy vary between 20 and 70% in individual units [2].

The overall risk of obstetric anal sphincter injuries (OASIS) is 1% of all vaginal deliveries. However 'occult' anal sphincter injury (i.e. defects in the anal sphincter detected by anal endosonography) has been identified in 33% of primiparous women following vaginal delivery [3]. The most plausible explanation for an 'occult' injury is either an injury that has been missed, recognized but not reported, or wrongly classified as a second-degree tear [4,5]. With increased awareness and training, there appears to be an increase in detection of anal sphincter injuries [6]. In centres where mediolateral episiotomies are practised, the rate of OASIS occurs in 1.7% (2.9% in primiparae) compared to 12% (19% in primiparae) in centres practising midline episiotomy [7].

The majority of women experience some form of short-term discomfort or pain following perineal repair, and up to 20% will continue to have long-term problems, such as superficial dyspareunia. Short- and long-term morbidity associated with perineal repair can lead to major physical, psychological and social problems affecting the woman's ability to care for her newborn baby and other members of the family [8]. The morbidity associated with perineal trauma depends on the extent of perineal damage, the technique and materials used for suturing, and the skill of the person performing the procedure. It is important that practitioners ensure that routine procedures, such as perineal repair, are evidence-based in order to provide care which is effective, appropriate and cost-efficient.

Applied anatomy

An understanding of the anatomy of the pelvic floor, anal sphincters and perineum is essential for healthcare providers managing and suturing perineal trauma.

Anatomy of the perineum

The perineum corresponds to the outlet of the pelvis and is somewhat lozenge-shaped. The perineum can be divided into two triangular parts by drawing a line transversely between the ischial tuberosities. The anterior triangle, which contains the urogenital organs, is known as the *urogenital triangle*, and the posterior triangle, which contains the termination of the anal canal, is known as the *anal triangle* [9].

Urogenital triangle

The urogenital triangle has been divided into two compartments, the superficial and deep perineal spaces, separated by the perineal membrane, which spans the space between the ischiopubic rami. Just beneath the skin and subcutaneous fat lie the superficial perineal muscles: superficial transverse perineal, bulbospongiosus and ischiocavernosus. The superficial transverse perineal muscle is a narrow slip of muscle which arises from the inner and forepart of

Best Practice in Labour and Delivery, ed. R. Warren and S. Arulkumaran. Published by Cambridge University Press.

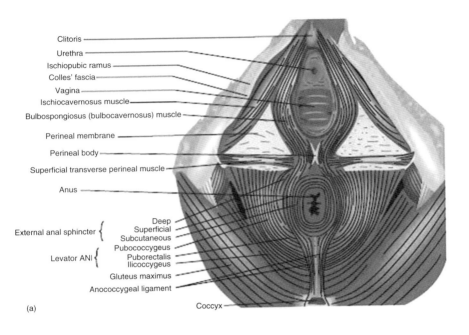

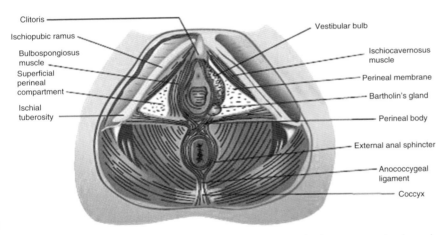

Figure 17.1 (a) The superficial muscles of the perineum; namely, the superficial transverse perineal muscle, the bulbospongiosus and the ischiocavernosus form a triangle on either side of the perineum. (b) The left bulbospongiosus muscle has been removed to demonstrate the vestibular bulb (with permission) [9]. (See colour plate section.)

the ischial tuberosity and is inserted into the central tendinous part of the perineal body. The bulbospongiosus muscle runs on either side of the vaginal orifice, covering the lateral aspects of the vestibular bulb anteriorly and the Bartholin's gland posteriorly. The ischiocavernosus muscle is situated on the side of the lateral boundary of the perineum. The deep transverse perineal muscle lies in the deep perineal space. It is thin and difficult to delineate, and hence some authors deny the existence of this muscle (Figure 17.1).

Anal triangle

The anal triangle includes the anal canal, the anal sphincters, and ischioanal fossae. The anal canal is approximately 3.5 cm long and is attached posteriorly to the coccyx by the anococcygeal ligament, a midline fibromuscular structure which runs between the posterior aspect of the EAS and the coccyx. The anus is surrounded laterally and posteriorly by loose adipose tissue within the ischioanal fossae. The pudendal nerves pass over the ischial spines and can be accessed

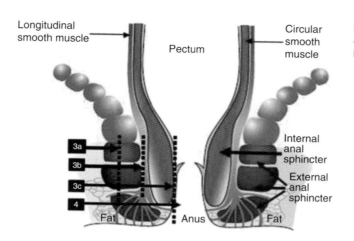

Figure 17.2 Classification of perineal trauma depicted in a schematic representation of the anal sphincters (with permission) [5]. (See colour plate section.)

digitally at this site for measurement of pudendal nerve terminal motor latency using a modified electrode. The perineum can also be anaesthetized by injection of local anaesthetic into the pudendal nerve at this site. Anteriorly, the perineal body separates the anal canal from the vagina. The anal canal is surrounded by an inner epithelial lining, a vascular subepithelium, and the anal sphincter complex. The lining of the anal canal varies along its length due to its embryologic derivation. The proximal anal canal is lined with rectal mucosa (columnar epithelium) and is separated by the dentate line from the distal anoderm, which consists of modified squamous epithelium. Since the epithelium in the lower canal is well supplied with sensory nerve endings, acute distension or invasive treatment of haemorrhoids in this area causes profuse discomfort, whereas treatment can be carried out with relatively few symptoms in the upper canal lined by insensate columnar epithelium. The anal sphincter complex consists of the external anal sphincter (EAS) and internal anal sphincter (IAS) separated by the conjoint longitudinal coat (Figure 17.2). The striated EAS is subdivided into subcutaneous, superficial and deep, and is responsible for voluntary squeeze and reflex contraction pressure. It is innervated by the pudendal nerve, which is a mixed sensory and motor nerve. However, these subdivisions are not easily demonstrable during anatomical dissection or surgery, but may be of relevance during imaging. To the naked eye, the EAS appears like red meat. The IAS, which is a thickened continuation of the circular smooth muscle of the bowel, contributes about 70% of the resting pressure and is under autonomic control. In contrast to the EAS, the IAS has a pale appearance to the naked eye. As shown in Figure 17.2, the subcutaneous EAS lies at a lower level than the IAS, but during regional or general anaesthesia the paralysed EAS lies at almost the same level as the IAS. The longitudinal layer is situated between the EAS and IAS and consists of a fibromuscular layer, the conjoint longitudinal coat and the intersphincteric space with its connective tissue components. Traced downwards, it separates opposite the lower border of the IAS, and the fibrous septae fan out to pass through the EAS and ultimately attach to the skin of the lower anal canal and perianal region. As a result of tonic circumferential contraction of the sphincter, the skin is arranged in radiating folds around the anus, and this is called the anal margin. These folds appear to be flat or ironed out when there is underlying sphincter damage [9].

Perineal body

The perineal body is the central point of the perineum and is situated between the urogenital and the anal triangles of the perineum. Its three-dimensional form has been likened to that of the cone of the red pine, with each 'petal' representing an interlocking structure, such as an insertion site of fascia or a muscle of the perineum. Within the perineal body there is interlacing of muscle fibres from the bulbospongiosus, superficial transverse perineal and EAS muscles. Above this level, there is a contribution from the longitudinal rectal muscle and the medial fibres of the puborectalis muscle.

Levator ani

The pelvic floor (pelvic diaphragm), is a musculotendineous sheet that spans the pelvic outlet and consists mainly of the symmetrically paired levator ani. The levator ani is a broad muscular sheet of variable thickness attached to the internal surface of the true pelvis and is subdivided into parts according to their attachments and pelvic viscera to which they are related, namely iliococcygeus, pubococcygeus, and ischiococcygeus. The pubococcygeus is often subdivided into separate parts according to the pelvic viscera to which they relate (i.e. pubourethralis and puborectalis in the male, pubovaginalis and puborectalis in the female). The most medial fibres of the pubococcygeus form a sling around the rectum and are named the puborectalis. The levator ani and the muscles of the perineum are supplied by the pudendal nerve.

Classification

Perineal trauma may occur spontaneously during vaginal birth, or intentionally when a surgical incision (episiotomy) is made to facilitate delivery. It is also possible to have both an episiotomy and a spontaneous tear either as an extension of the episiotomy or as a separate tear. Anterior perineal trauma is defined as injury to the labia, anterior vagina, urethra or clitoris. Posterior perineal trauma is defined as any injury to the posterior vaginal wall, perineal muscles or anal sphincters, and may include disruption of the anal sphincter.

In order to standardize the classification of perineal trauma (Figure 17.2), Sultan proposed the following classification that has been adopted by the Royal College of Obstetricians and Gynaecologists and also recommended by the International Consultation on Incontinence [6,10].

First degree: laceration of the vaginal epithelium or perineal skin only.
Second degree: involvement of the perineal muscles (bulbocavernosus, transverse perineal), but not the anal sphincter. If the trauma is very deep, the pubococcygeus muscle may be disrupted.
Third degree: disruption of the anal sphincter muscles, which should be further subdivided into:

3a: <50% thickness of external sphincter torn;
3b: >50% thickness of external sphincter torn;
3c: internal sphincter also torn.
Fourth degree: a third-degree tear with disruption of the anal epithelium as well.

If there is any doubt about the grade of a third-degree tear, it is advisable to classify it to the higher

degree to avoid underestimation [6]. Isolated tears of the anal epithelium (buttonhole) without involvement of the anal sphincters are rare. In order to avoid confusion, they are not included in the above classification.

Episiotomy

Episiotomy is a surgical incision made with scissors or a scalpel into the perineum in order to increase the diameter of the vulval outlet and facilitate delivery. There are two main types of episiotomy incision: midline and mediolateral. A midline episiotomy is an incision from the midpoint of the posterior fourchette directed vertically towards the anus, whilst with a mediolateral episiotomy the incision is directed 40–60 degrees away from the midline [6]. It is claimed that the midline incision is easier to repair and that it is associated with less blood loss, better healing, less pain, and earlier resumption of sexual intercourse. However, there is no reliable evidence to support these claims. It has been shown that there is a lower risk of anal sphincter disruption with a larger angle of episiotomy [6]. Limited evidence from one quasi-randomized trial suggested that the midline incision may increase the risk of third- and fourth-degree tears compared with the mediolateral incision. However, these data should be interpreted with caution, as there may be an increased risk of selection bias due to quasi-random treatment allocation, and also analysis was not by intention to treat [11].

Indications for episiotomy

Episiotomy is still performed routinely in many parts of the world in the belief that it protects the pelvic floor. However, evidence from randomized controlled trials (RCTs) suggests that routine episiotomy does not prevent severe posterior perineal tears. Carroli and Belizan have conducted the most recent systematic review of randomized clinical trials using the Cochrane Collaboration methodology to determine the possible benefits and risks of restrictive episiotomy versus routine episiotomy. Mediolateral episiotomy was the method of incision for the six trials included in the review, except for a North American trial where midline episiotomy was performed. The review revealed that there is a lower risk of posterior perineal trauma, need for suturing and healing complications associated with the restrictive use of episiotomy at 7 days postpartum. However, there is no difference in the incidence of major outcomes such as severe vaginal or perineal trauma, pain, dyspareunia or urinary incontinence between the restrictive and routine/liberal use of episiotomy. The only disadvantage shown in restrictive use of episiotomy is an increased risk of anterior perineal trauma. However, this is not of any clinical significance. This systematic review concluded that there is evidence to support the restrictive use of episiotomy compared to routine episiotomy (irrespective of the type of episiotomy performed). This finding applied to both primiparous and multiparous women [11].

There is currently an absence of clear, evidence-based clinical indications for the use of episiotomy. However, it is reasonable to suggest that an episiotomy should be performed to accelerate vaginal delivery in cases of fetal distress, to facilitate manoeuvres during shoulder dystocia, to minimize severe perineal trauma during a forceps delivery, to reduce the occurrence of multiple lacerations in the presence of a thick or rigid perineum, and in situations where prolonged 'bearing down' may be harmful for the mother (e.g. severe hypertensive or cardiac disease).

Diagnosis of perineal trauma

1. Before assessment for genital trauma, the healthcare professional should [12]:

   - explain to the woman what they plan to do and why;
   - offer inhalational analgesia or ensure that epidural analgesia is effective;
   - ensure good lighting;
   - position the woman so that she is comfortable and the genital structures can be seen clearly, and if this is not possible then the woman should be placed in lithotomy.

2. Informed consent should be obtained for a vaginal and rectal examination.

3. If the examination is restricted because of pain, adequate analgesia must be given prior to examination.

4. Following a visual examination of the genitalia, the labia should be parted and a vaginal examination should be performed to establish the full extent of the vaginal tear. When multiple or deep tears are present it is best to examine and repair in lithotomy. The apex of the vaginal laceration should always be identified.

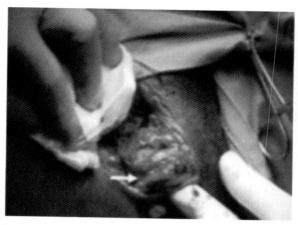

Figure 17.3 A partial tear (arrow) along the length of the external anal sphincter (with permission) [5]. (See colour plate section.)

5. A rectal examination should then be performed to exclude OASIS. Figure 17.3 shows a partial tear along the EAS which would have been missed if a rectal examination was not performed. The vagina should be exposed by parting the labia with the index and middle fingers of the other hand. Every woman should have a rectal examination prior to suturing in order to avoid missing isolated tears such as 'button hole' of the rectal mucosa [12]. Furthermore, a third- or fourth-degree tear may be present beneath apparently intact perineal skin, highlighting the need to perform a rectal examination in order to exclude OASIS following every vaginal delivery [5]. Following diagnosis of the tear, it should be graded according to the recommended classification [6].

6. In order to diagnose OASIS, clear visualization is necessary, and the injury should be confirmed by palpation. By inserting the index finger in the anal canal and the thumb in the vagina, the anal sphincter can be palpated by performing a pill-rolling motion. If there is still uncertainty, the woman should be asked to contract her anal sphincter and if the anal sphincter is disrupted, there will be a distinct gap felt anteriorly. If the perineal skin is intact there will be an absence of puckering on the perianal skin anteriorly. This may not be evident under regional or general anaesthesia. As the EAS is in a state of tonic contraction, disruption results in retraction of the sphincter ends. Therefore the sphincter ends need to be grasped and retrieved prior to repair [5].

7. The IAS is a circular smooth muscle that appears paler (similar to raw fish) than the striated EAS (similar to raw red meat). If the IAS or anal epithelium is torn, the EAS will invariably be torn.

Management and repair of perineal trauma

Basic principles prior to repairing perineal trauma include [5–7] the following.

- The skills and knowledge of the operator are important factors in achieving a successful repair. The woman should be referred to a more experienced healthcare professional if uncertainty exists as to the nature or extent of trauma sustained.
- Repair of the perineum should be undertaken as soon as possible to minimize the risk of bleeding and oedematous swelling of the perineum, as this makes it more difficult to recognize tissue structures and planes when the repair eventually takes place.
- Perineal trauma should be repaired using aseptic techniques.
- Equipment should be checked and swabs and needles counted before and after the procedure.
- Good lighting is essential to visualize and identify the structures involved.
- A repair undertaken on a non-cooperative patient, due to pain, is likely to result in a poor repair. Ensure that the wound is adequately anaesthetized prior to commencing the repair. It is recommended that 10–20 ml of Lignocaine 1% is injected evenly into the perineal wound. If the woman has an epidural it may be 'topped-up' and used to block perineal pain during suturing instead of injecting local anaesthetic [12]. Repair of obstetric anal sphincter trauma should be undertaken in theatre, under general or regional anaesthesia. In addition to providing pain relief, this provides the added advantage of relaxing the muscles, enabling the operator to retrieve the ends of the torn sphincter while performing an overlap repair [6,13].
- An indwelling catheter should be inserted for at least 12 h to avoid urinary retention.

First-degree tears and labial lacerations

Women should be advised that in the case of first-degree trauma, the wound should be sutured in order to improve healing, unless the skin edges are well opposed [12]. If the tear is left unsutured, the midwife or doctor must discuss the implications with the woman and obtain her informed consent. Details regarding the discussion and consent must be fully documented in the woman's case notes.

Labial lacerations are usually very superficial but may be very painful. Some practitioners do not recommend suturing, but if the trauma is bilateral the lacerations can sometimes adhere together over the urethra and the woman may present with voiding difficulties. It is important to advise the woman to part the labia daily during bathing to prevent adhesions from occurring.

Episiotomy and second-degree tears

Women should be advised that in the case of second-degree trauma, the muscle should be sutured in order to improve healing [2,12].

In a recent Cochrane review which included seven studies, Kettle *et al.* showed that the three-layered continuous suturing technique for perineal closure, compared to the interrupted method, was associated with less short-term pain. Moreover, if the continuous technique was used for all layers (vagina, perineal muscles and skin) compared to perineal skin only, the reduction in pain was even greater [8]. There was an overall reduction in the need for analgesia use, dyspareunia and the need for suture removal in the group of women who had continuous suturing compared to interrupted sutures. However, the use of a two-layer procedure for perineal repair, where the skin is apposed but not sutured, is associated with an increase in wound gaping up to 10 days following birth, but less dyspareunia at 3 months postpartum than a three-layer technique involving skin closure [2]. With second-degree tears there is no need to suture the skin if it is adequately opposed following suturing of the muscle [12].

It has been shown that the use of a more rapidly absorbed form of polyglactin 910 for repair of perineal trauma is associated with a significant reduction in pain and a reduction in suture removal when compared with standard absorbable synthetic material [6]. It can be concluded from current robust research evidence that perineal trauma should be repaired using the continuous non-locking technique to re-approximate all layers (vagina, perineal muscles and skin) with absorbable polyglactin 910 material (Vicryl rapide®) [2,11,12].

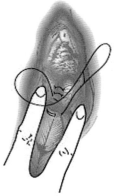
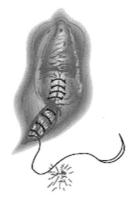
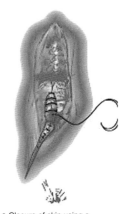
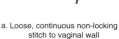

Figure 17.4 Continuous suturing technique for mediolateral episiotomy (with permission) [14]. (See colour plate section.)

a. Loose, continuous non-locking stitch to vaginal wall

b. Loose, continuous non-locking stitch to perineal muscles

c. Closure of skin using a loose subcutaneous stitch

The following steps should be followed [14] (Figure 17.4).

(1) *Suturing the vagina.*

The first stitch is inserted above the apex of the vaginal trauma to secure any bleeding points that might not be visible. Close the vaginal trauma with a loose, continuous, non-locking technique, making sure that each stitch is inserted not too wide otherwise the vagina may be narrowed. Continue to suture down to the hymenal remnants and insert the needle through the skin at the fourchette to emerge in the centre of the perineal wound.

(2) *Suturing the muscle layer.*

Check the depth of the trauma and close the perineal muscle (deep and superficial) with continuous non-locking stitches. If the trauma is deep, the perineal muscles can be closed using two layers of continuous stitches. Realign the muscle so that the skin edges can be re-approximated without tension, ensuring that the stitches are not inserted through the rectum or anal canal.

(3) *Suturing the perineal skin.*

At the inferior end of the wound, bring the needle out just under the skin surface reversing the stitching direction. The skin sutures are placed below the skin surface in the subcutaneous tissue thus avoiding the profusion of nerve endings. Continue to take bites of tissue from each side of the wound edges until the hymenal remnants are reached. Secure the finished repair with a loop or Aberdeen knot placed in the vagina behind the hymenal remnants. Once the vaginal mucosa has been closed

to the hymenal ring, the needle is passed from the midline to the perineal body and a crown stitch is inserted to re-approximate the bulbocavernosus muscles. A subcuticular stitch is carried from the inferior perineal margin to the hymen and tied.

Third- and fourth-degree tears

1. Repair should be conducted in the operating theatre where there is access to good lighting, appropriate equipment and aseptic conditions. In our unit we have a specially prepared instrument tray containing a Weislander self-retaining retractor, four Allis tissue forceps, McIndoe scissors, tooth forceps, four artery forceps, stitch scissors and a needle holder (www.perineum.net). In addition, deep retractors (e.g. Deavers) are useful when there are associated paravaginal tears.

2. On rare occasions an isolated 'buttonhole' type tear can occur in the rectum without disrupting the anal sphincter or perineum (Figure 17.5). This is best repaired transvaginally using interrupted Vicryl (polyglactin) sutures. To minimize the risk of a persistent rectovaginal fistula, a second layer of tissue should be interposed between the rectum and vagina by approximating the rectovaginal fascia. A colostomy is rarely indicated unless there is a large tear extending above the pelvic floor or there is gross faecal contamination of the wound.

3. In the presence of a fourth-degree tear, the torn anal epithelium is repaired with interrupted Vicryl 3/0 sutures with the knots tied in the anal lumen. This technique has been widely described and

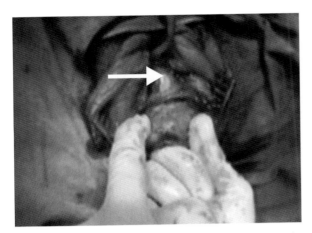

Figure 17.5 A buttonhole tear of the rectal mucosa (arrow) with an intact external anal sphincter demonstrated during a digital rectal examination (with permission) [5]. (See colour plate section.)

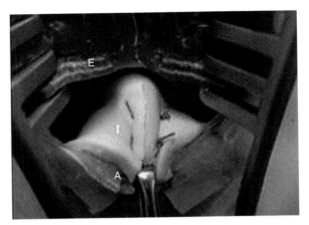

Figure 17.6 Internal anal sphincter (I) repair using mattress sutures demonstrated on a model (E, external sphincter; A, anal epithelium) (with permission) [7]. (See colour plate section.)

proponents of this technique argue that by tying the knots outside, the quantity of foreign body within the tissue would be reduced, and hence the risk of infection reduced. However, this concern probably applies to the use of catgut that dissolves by proteolysis as opposed to the newer synthetic material, such as Vicryl or Dexon (polygylcolic acid) that dissolve by hydrolysis. A subcuticular repair of the anal epithelium via the transvaginal approach has also been described, and could be equally effective provided the terminal knots are secure [15].

4. The sphincter muscles are repaired with either monofilament fine sutures such as 3-0 PDS (Polydioxanone) or modern braided sutures such as 2-0 Vicryl (polyglactin – Vicryl®), as these may cause less irritation and discomfort with equivalent outcome. To minimize suture migration, care should be taken to cut suture ends short and ensure that they are covered by the overlying superficial perineal muscles. Women should be warned of the possibility of knot migration to the skin surface, with the long-acting and non-absorbable suture materials [6].

5. The IAS should be identified and, if torn, repaired separately from the EAS. The ends of the torn muscle are grasped with Allis forceps and an end-to-end repair is performed with interrupted sutures (3-0 PDS or 2-0 Vicryl) [7] (Figure 17.6). There is some evidence that repair of an isolated IAS defect is beneficial in patients with established anal incontinence.

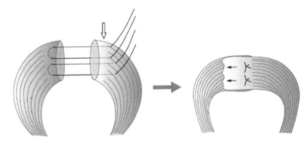

Figure 17.7 Repair of a fourth-degree tear using the overlap repair technique for the external anal sphincter

6. As the EAS is normally under tonic contraction, it tends to retract when torn. The torn ends of the EAS therefore need to be identified and grasped with Allis tissue forceps. When the EAS is only partially torn (Grade 3a and some 3b), then an end-to-end repair should be performed using two or three mattress sutures instead of haemostatic 'figure of eight' sutures. If there is a full thickness EAS tear (some 3b, 3c or fourth-degree), either an overlapping (Figure 17.7) or end-to-end method can be used with equivalent outcome [6]. The limited data available from the Cochrane review on the topic showed that compared to immediate primary end-to-end repair of OASIS, early primary overlap repair appears to be associated with lower risks of faecal urgency and anal incontinence symptoms and deterioration of anal incontinence over time. Four women need to be treated with the overlap technique to prevent one woman developing faecal incontinence. However,

189

as the experience of the surgeon was addressed in only one of the three studies reviewed, it would be inappropriate to recommend one type of repair over the other [16].

7. After repair of the sphincter, the perineal muscles should be sutured to reconstruct the perineal body in order to provide support to the repaired anal sphincter. Furthermore, a short, deficient perineum would make the anal sphincter more vulnerable to trauma during a subsequent vaginal delivery. Finally, the vaginal skin should be sutured and the perineal skin approximated with a Vicryl 2-0 subcuticular suture [7].

8. Basic principles after repair of perineal tears [6,7,12]:

   - Check that complete haemostasis is achieved and confirm that the finished repair is anatomically correct.
   - A rectal and vaginal examination should be performed to confirm adequate repair so as to ensure that no other tears have been missed, and that a suture is not inadvertently placed through the rectal mucosa.
   - Confirm that all tampons or swabs have been removed.
   - Detailed notes should be made of the findings and repair. Completion of a pre-designed proforma and a pictorial representation of the tears prove very useful when notes are being reviewed following complications, audit or litigation.
   - An accurate detailed account of the repair should be documented in the woman's case notes following completion of the procedure, including details of the suture method and materials used. It is also useful to include a simple diagram illustrating the structures involved.
   - The woman should be informed regarding the use of appropriate analgesia, hygiene, and the importance of a good diet and daily pelvic floor exercises.
   - It is important that the woman is given a full explanation of the injury sustained and contact details if she has any problems during the postnatal period. Special designated clinics should be available for women with perineal problems to ensure that they receive appropriate, sensitive and effective treatment.

- Women should be advised that the prognosis following EAS repair is good, with 60–80% asymptomatic at 12 months. Most women who remain symptomatic describe incontinence of flatus or faecal urgency [6].

Postoperative care

There are no randomized trials to substantiate the benefits of intraoperative and postoperative antibiotics following repair of OASIS. However, intraoperative and postoperative broad spectrum antibiotics are recommended following obstetric anal sphincter injury repair to reduce the incidence of infection and wound breakdown that could jeopardize the outcome of repair and lead to incontinence or fistula formation. Inclusion of metronidazole is advisable to cover possible anaerobic contamination from faecal material [6,7].

Severe perineal discomfort, particularly following instrumental delivery, is a known cause of urinary retention, and following regional anaesthesia it can take up to 12 h before bladder sensation returns. A Foley catheter should be inserted for about 24 h unless medical staff can ensure that spontaneous voiding occurs at least every 3–4 h without undue bladder overdistension.

The degree of pain following perineal trauma is related to the extent of the injury, and OASIS are frequently associated with other, more extensive injuries, such as paravaginal tears. In a systematic review, Hedayati et al. [17] found that rectal analgesia such as Diclofenac is effective in reducing pain from perineal trauma within the first 24 h after birth, and women used less additional analgesia within the first 48 h after birth. Diclofenac is almost completely protein-bound and therefore excretion in breast milk is negligible [18]. In women who had a repair of a fourth-degree tear, Diclofenac should be administered orally, as insertion of suppositories may be uncomfortable and there is a theoretical risk of poor healing associated with local anti-inflammatory agents. Codeine-based preparations are best avoided, as they may cause constipation leading to excessive straining and possible disruption of the repair.

It is of utmost importance that constipation is avoided, as passage of constipated stool or indeed faecal impaction may disrupt the repair. The use of postoperative laxatives is recommended [6]. Stool softeners (Lactulose 15 ml bd) for 10–14 days are recommended.

It is recommended that women with OASIS be called by a healthcare provider 24 or 48 h after hospital discharge to ensure bowel evacuation has occurred.

Follow-up

All women who sustain OASIS should be assessed by a senior obstetrician at 6–12 weeks after delivery [6]. If facilities are available, follow-up of women with obstetric anal sphincter injuries should be in a dedicated clinic with access to endoanal ultrasonography and anal manometry, as this can aid decision on future mode of delivery [6,19].

In the clinic, a genital examination should be performed, looking specifically for scarring, residual granulation tissue, and tenderness. All women should undergo anal manometry and endosonography. The women are advised to continue pelvic floor exercises, while others with minimal sphincter contractility may need electrical stimulation.

If a perineal clinic is not available, women with OASIS should be given clear instructions, preferably in writing, before leaving the hospital. In the first 6 weeks following delivery, they should look for signs of infection or wound dehiscence. They should contact the clinic if there is increase in pain or swelling, rectal bleeding, or purulent discharge. Any incontinence of stool or flatus should also be reported. Under such circumstances, referral to a specialist gynaecologist or colorectal surgeon for endoanal ultrasound and manometry should be considered [6].

Management of subsequent pregnancy

There are no randomized studies to determine the most appropriate mode of delivery following a third- or fourth-degree tear. In order to counsel women with previous third- or fourth-degree tears appropriately, it is useful to have a symptom questionnaire along with anal ultrasound and manometry results. Tests should be performed during the current pregnancy unless performed previously and found to be abnormal. Figure 17.8 provides a flow diagram demonstrating the management of subsequent pregnancy following OASIS.

If there are no facilities for anal manometry and endosonography, then the management will depend on symptoms and clinical evaluation. Asymptomatic women without any clinical evidence of sphincter compromise as determined by assessment of anal tone could be allowed a vaginal delivery. All women who are symptomatic should be referred to a centre with facilities for anorectal assessment, and should be counselled for caesarean section (CS). Current evidence suggests that if a large sonographic defect (>one quadrant) is present, or if the squeeze pressure increment is less than 20 mmHg, then the risk of impaired continence is increased after a subsequent delivery. These women should be counselled and, particularly those who have mild symptoms, offered a CS. There is evidence that when this protocol is followed, there is no deterioration in symptoms in both the vaginal delivery and CS group. Figure 17.9 demonstrates the four-layered ultrasound appearance of an intact anal sphincter, in contrast to Figure 17.10, which demonstrates endosonography of an extensive tear following vaginal delivery involving both the internal and external sphincters between 9 and 2 o'clock. Mild incontinence (faecal urgency or flatus incontinence) may be controlled with dietary advice, constipating agents (loperamide or codeine phosphate), physiotherapy or biofeedback. Asymptomatic women who do not have compromised anal sphincter function can be allowed a normal delivery by an experienced accoucher [7]. If an episiotomy is considered necessary, e.g. because of a thick, inelastic or scarred perineum, a mediolateral episiotomy should be performed. There is no evidence that routine episiotomies prevent recurrence of OASIS [6]. The threshold at which these women may be considered for a CS may be lowered if a traumatic delivery is anticipated, e.g. in the presence of one or more additional relative risk factors, e.g. big baby, shoulder dystocia, prolonged labour, difficult instrumental delivery. However, in deciding the mode of delivery, counselling (and its clear documentation) is extremely important. Some of these women who have sustained OASIS may be scarred both physically and emotionally and may find it difficult to cope with the thought of another vaginal delivery. These women will require sympathy, psychological support and consideration to their request for CS [7].

Women who sustained a previous third- or fourth-degree tear with subsequent severe incontinence should be offered secondary sphincter repair by a colorectal surgeon, and all subsequent deliveries should be by CS. Some women with faecal incontinence may chose to complete their family before embarking on anal sphincter surgery. It remains to be established whether these women should be allowed a vaginal delivery, as it could be argued that

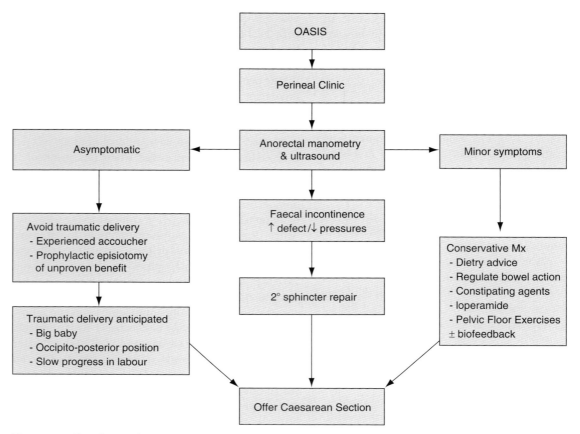

Figure 17.8 Flow diagram demonstrating the management of subsequent pregnancy following OASIS (with permission) [7]

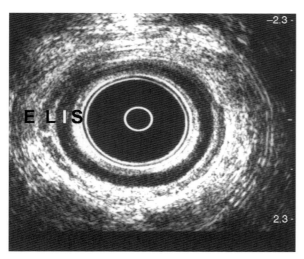

Figure 17.9 The normal four-layer pattern of the anal canal on axial endosonography in the normal orientation. The subepithelium (S) is moderately reflective; the internal sphincter (I) a well-defined, low reflective ring; the longitudinal layer a mixture of muscle (L) and fibroelastic tissue so of varying reflectivity; and the external sphincter (E) of low reflectivity

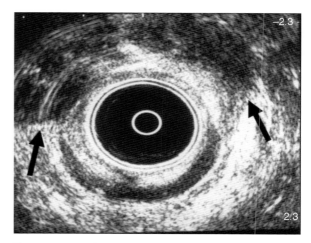

Figure 17.10 Endosonography of an extensive tear following vaginal delivery involving both the internal and external sphincters between 9 and 2 o'clock (arrows)

damage has already occurred and risk of further damage is minimal and possibly insignificant in terms of outcome of surgery. The benefit, if any, should be weighed against the risks associated with CS for all subsequent pregnancies. Women who have had a previous successful secondary sphincter repair for faecal incontinence should be delivered by CS [7].

Medico-legal considerations

Although creating a third- or fourth-degree tear is seldom found to be culpable, missing a tear is considered to be negligent. It is essential that a rectal examination is performed before and after any perineal repair and findings are carefully documented in the notes. Delay in repairing in theatre, poor note keeping, repair by untrained personnel, poor lighting and inadequate exposure, inadequate anaesthesia, failure to recognize the extent of the tear, use of the wrong suture material, a forgotten swab in the vagina, deviation from recommended safe practice, failure to inform and counsel the woman, failure to inform the general practitioner, and inappropriate follow-up and advice regarding subsequent pregnancy are common issues raised at litigation [7,13].

Training

As more than two-thirds of doctors practising obstetrics feel inadequately trained, it is important that focused and intensive training is available. In this regard, Sultan and Thakar have introduced an ongoing course using video presentations, specially designed models and fresh animal specimens to demonstrate anatomy and techniques of repair (www. perineum.net). The feedback from attendees is that this type of training has resulted in a change in practice and should become an essential part of the modular training for specialist registrars.

Prevention

The case for prevention of perineal trauma and its consequences is compelling. How to achieve this is less than clear. The incidence of perineal trauma can be reduced by modifying some of the risk factors, such as episiotomy and instrumental delivery. Episiotomy should only be performed when indicated, and a mediolateral episiotomy is preferable to a midline episiotomy [11]. Fewer women with vacuum delivery have anal sphincter trauma compared to forceps

delivery [20], and the Royal College of Obstetricians and Gynaecologists supports the recommendation that the vacuum extractor should be the instrument of choice for operative vaginal delivery [21]. A recent Cochrane review has concluded that antenatal perineal massage reduces the likelihood of perineal trauma (mainly episiotomies) and the reporting of ongoing perineal pain and is generally well-accepted by women. As such, women should be made aware of the likely benefit of perineal massage and provided with information on how to do it [22]. Other interventions such as waterbirth, position during labour and birth, delayed pushing with an epidural, second stage pushing advice, perineal stretching massage during second stage, and perineal support at delivery have not been shown to reduce the risk of perineal trauma in randomized studies. Increased perineal trauma with epidural analgesia is due to the increased associated risk of an instrumental delivery [23].

Conclusions

The majority of women undergoing vaginal delivery sustain perineal trauma. While CS is the only alternative available to bypass vaginal delivery, it is associated with increased morbidity and mortality. It is therefore mandatory that every effort is made to minimize injury and make vaginal delivery safer. In this chapter we have endeavoured to highlight safe obstetric practice and preventative measures in the light of the best available evidence to minimize perineal and anal sphincter trauma.

References

1. McCandlish R, Bowler U, van Asten H, et al. A randomised controlled trial of care of the perineum during second stage of normal labour. Br J Obstet Gynaecol 1998; 105: 1262–72.

2. Royal College of Obstetricians and Gynaecologists. Methods and Materials used in Perineal Repair. Guideline No. 23. London: RCOG Press, 2004.

3. Sultan A H, Kamm M A, Hudson C N, Thomas J M, Bartram C I. Anal sphincter disruption during vaginal delivery. New Engl J Med 1993; 329: 1905–11.

4. Andrews V, Thakar R, Sultan A H. Occult anal sphincter injuries – myth or reality. Br J Obstet Gynaecol 2006; 113: 195–200.

5. Sultan A H, Kettle C. Diagnosis of perineal trauma. In: Sultan A H, Thakar R, Fenner D, eds. Perineal and Anal Sphincter Trauma. London: Springer-Verlag, 2007; 13–9.

6. Royal College of Obstetricians and Gynaecologists. *Management of Third and Fourth Degree Perineal Tears Following Vaginal Delivery.* Guideline No. 29. London: RCOG Press, 2007.

7. Sultan A H, Thakar R. Third and fourth degree tears. In: Sultan A H, Thakar R, Fenner D, eds. *Perineal and Anal Sphincter Trauma.* London: Springer-Verlag, 2007; 33–51.

8. Kettle C, Hills R K, Ismail K M. Continuous versus interrupted sutures for repair of episiotomy or second degree tears. *Cochrane Database Syst Rev* 2007; **4**: CD000947.

9. Thakar R, Fenner D E. Anatomy of the perineum and the anal sphincter. In: Sultan A H, Thakar R, Fenner D E, eds. *Perineal and Anal Sphincter Trauma.* London: Springer-Verlag, 2007; 1–12.

10. Norton C, Christensen J, Butler U, *et al. Anal Incontinence.* 2nd edn. Plymouth: Health Publication Ltd, 2005; 985–1044.

11. Carroli G, Belizan J. Episiotomy for vaginal birth. *Cochrane Database Syst Rev* 1999; **3**: CD00081.

12. Intrapartum Care. NICE Clinical Guideline. Guideline 55, 2007. Available from: URL: www.nice.org.uk/CG055 (accessed 1 January 2008).

13. Jaiyesimi R A K. Pitfalls in the management of perineal trauma. *Clin Risk* 2007; **13**: 89–91.

14. Kettle C, Fenner D. Repair of episiotomy, first and second degree tears. In: Sultan A H, Thakar R, Fenner D, eds. *Perineal and Anal Sphincter Trauma.* London: Springer, 2007; 20–32.

15. Sultan A H, Thakar R. Lower genital tract and anal sphincter trauma. *Best Pract & Res – Clin Obstet Gynaecol* 2002; **16**: 99–116.

16. Fernando R, Sultan A H, Kettle C, Thakar R, Radley S. Methods of repair for obstetric anal sphincter injury. *Cochrane Database Syst Rev* 2006; **3**: CD002866.

17. Hedayati H, Parsons J, Crowther C A. Rectal analgesia for pain from perineal trauma following childbirth. *Cochrane Database Syst Rev* 2003; **3**: CD003931.

18. Kettle C, Hills R K, Jones P, Darby L, Gray R, Johanson R. Continuous versus interrupted perineal repair with standard or rapidly absorbed sutures after spontaneous vaginal birth: a randomised controlled trial. *Lancet* 2002; **359**: 2217–23.

19. Thakar R, Sultan A. Postpartum problems and the role of a perineal clinic. In: Sultan A H, Thakar R, Fenner D, eds. *Perineal and Anal Sphincter Trauma.* London: Springer-Verlag, 2007; 65–79.

20. Johanson R B, Menon V. Vacuum extraction versus forceps for assisted vaginal delivery. *Cochrane Database Syst Rev* 1999; **2**: CD000224.

21. Royal College of Obstetricians and Gynaecologists. *Operative Vaginal Delivery.* Guideline No. 26. London: RCOG Press, 2005.

22. Beckmann M M, Garrett A J. Antenatal perineal massage for reducing perineal trauma. *Cochrane Database Syst Rev* 2006; **1**: CD005123.

23. Thakar R, Eason E. Prevention of perineal trauma. In: Sultan A H, Thakar R, Fenner D, eds. *Perineal and Anal Sphincter Trauma.* London: Springer-Verlag, 2007; 52–64.

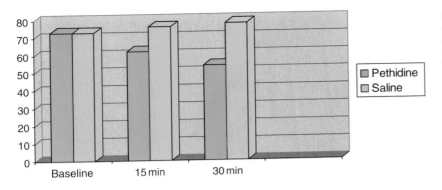

Figure 3.1 Pethidine vs saline for analgesia in labour. At 30 min the median visual analogue pain score (VAS) was lower in the pethidine compared with the saline group (0 = no pain, 100 = worst pain imaginable)

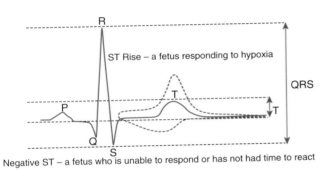

Figure 4.1 Principles of how to calculate the T/QRS ratio and the physiology behind different ST patterns

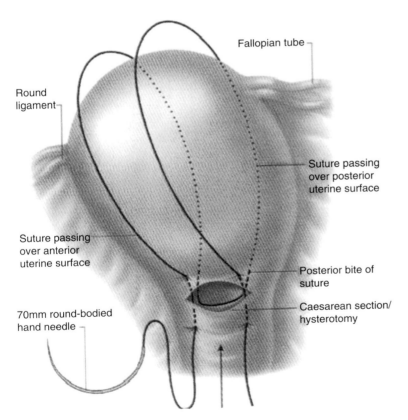

Figure 15.1 B-Lynch compression suture. (Reproduced with permission: Sapiens Publishing, 2006)

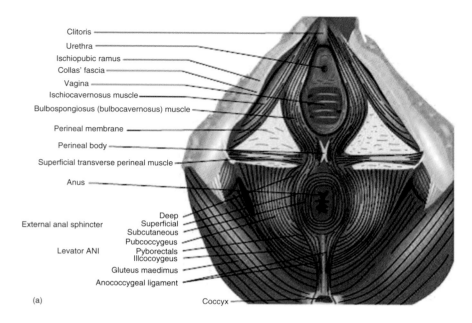

Clitoris
Urethra
Ischiopubic ramus
Collas' fascia
Vagina
Ischiocavernosus muscle
Bulbospongiosus (bulbocavernosus) muscle
Perineal membrane
Perineal body
Superficial transverse perineal muscle
Anus

External anal sphincter

Levator ANI

Deep
Superficial
Subcutaneous
Pubcoccygeus
Pyborectals
Illcocoygeus
Gluteus maedimus
Anococcygeal ligament

(a)

Coccyx

Figure 17.1 (a) The superficial muscles of the perineum; namely, the superficial transverse perineal muscle, the bulbospongiosus and the ischiocavernosus form a triangle on either side of the perineum. (b) The left bulbospongiosus muscle has been removed to demonstrate the vestibular bulb (with permission) [9]

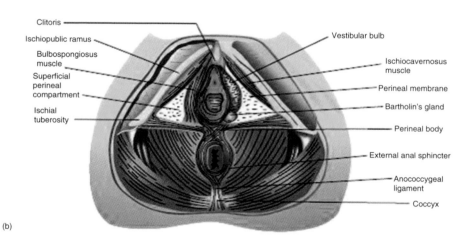

Clitoris
Ischiopublic ramus
Bulbospongiosus muscle
Superficial perineal compartment
Ischial tuberosity

Vestibular bulb

Ischiocavernosus muscle
Perineal membrane
Bartholin's gland
Perineal body
External anal sphincter
Anococcygeal ligament
Coccyx

(b)

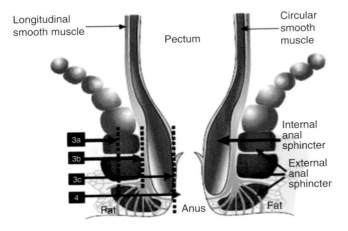

Longitudinal smooth muscle

Pectum

Circular smooth muscle

Internal anal sphincter

External anal sphincter

3a

3b

3c

4

Fat

Anus

Fat

Figure 17.2 Classification of perineal trauma depicted in a schematic representation of the anal sphincters (with permission) [5]

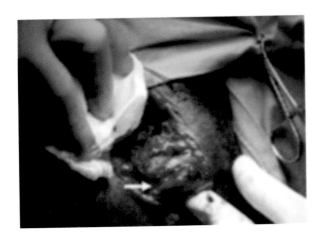

Figure 17.3 A partial tear (arrow) along the length of the external anal sphincter (with permission) [5]

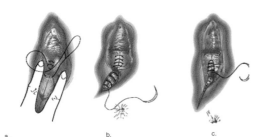

a.
Loose, continuous non-locking stitch to vaginal wall

b.
Loose, continuous non-locking stitch to perineal muscles

c.
Closure of skin using a loose subcutaneous stitch

Figure 17.4 Continuous suturing technique for mediolateral episiotomy (with permission) [14]

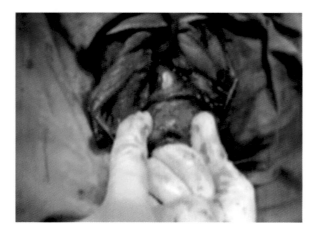

Figure 17.5 A buttonhole tear of the rectal mucosa (arrow) with an intact external anal sphincter demonstrated during a digital rectal examination (with permission) [5]

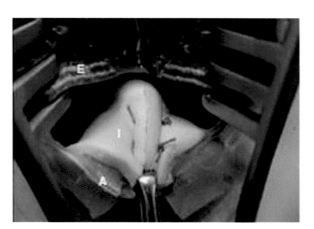

Figure 17.6 Internal anal sphincter (I) repair using mattress sutures demonstrated on a model (E, external sphincter; A, anal epithelium) (with permission) [7]

Induction of labour

Devi Subramanian and Leonie Penna

Induction of labour is one of the most common interventions practised in modern obstetrics. It describes the process of artificially ripening the cervix and stimulating uterine contractions with the intention of precipitating the active phase of labour, thus leading to progressive dilation and effacement of the cervix with the intention of achieving a vaginal delivery. In the developed world, the ability to induce labour has contributed to the reduction in maternal and perinatal mortality and morbidity.

Induction of labour should only be considered in situations when the balance of risks are such that the mother and baby will be safer if delivery occurs than if the pregnancy is allowed to continue, and when vaginal birth is thought to be the appropriate route of delivery. In general, this limits induction to pregnancies of gestation greater than the legal limits of viability (usually 24 weeks' gestation). Induction of labour prior to 24 weeks may be necessary for maternal reasons (for example, evidence of maternal sepsis following ruptured membranes), but in the absence of any expectation of fetal survival or intention to resuscitate the fetus, this type of induction should be considered a termination of pregnancy and the appropriate legal processes should be followed.

As one of the potential complications of induction is a failure to initiate labour, a decision to induce labour should equate with a decision to perform delivery by caesarean section (CS) if labour induction fails. This is particularly important when induction is undertaken in the absence of a medical indication.

Methods of induction of labour
Non-pharmacological methods

Non-medical approaches to cervical ripening and labour induction have included herbal compounds, castor oil, hot baths, enemas, sexual intercourse, breast stimulation, acupuncture, acupressure and transcutaneous nerve stimulation. For some women (especially with a prolonged pregnancy), a medical induction of labour is perceived as interfering in the natural process of pregnancy and represents a 'drastic' change to their birth plan. The reasons why many pregnant women are interested in using complementary therapies to ripen the cervix and induce labour are important, but have not been proven to be effective.

Membrane 'sweeping'

A membrane sweep is a commonly used procedure by midwives and obstetricians. It causes release of endogenous prostaglandins from the membranes and the decidua. This can stimulate uterine contractions as well as ripening the cervix.

Membrane sweeping is associated with a shorter time between treatment and spontaneous labour, a reduction in the incidence of prolonged pregnancy and the need for the use of formal induction. To avoid one formal induction of labour, membrane sweeping must be performed in eight women. Discomfort during the vaginal examination and procedure is virtually inevitable if a proper sweep is performed, and other adverse effects (such as bleeding and irregular contractions) are reported more frequently by women having sweeps. Sweeps should be offered to women who may benefit from the reduction in the need for formal induction, but this must be balanced against discomfort and other adverse effects; the ultimate decision as to whether to have a sweep is up to the woman involved.

Mechanical methods

Mechanical devices for induction include various types of catheters and laminaria tents; these are

Best Practice in Labour and Delivery, ed. R. Warren and S. Arulkumaran. Published by Cambridge University Press.
© Cambridge University Press 2009.

introduced into the cervical canal or into the extra-amniotic space via the cervix. This causes mechanical stretching of the cervical canal and also release of endogenous prostaglandins and oxytocin. A Foley catheter can be used, as well as a specially developed 'Atad' double-balloon catheter. A modified catheter based on the Atad catheter is now available in the UK, but data regarding its safety and efficacy are awaited.

Cervical dilators made from sterile seaweed or synthetic hydrophilic materials (®Lamicel and Dilapam) can be introduced into the cervical canal, where they increase in diameter because of their hydrophilic properties, achieving a gradual stretching of the cervix. These dilators are commonly used for cervical preparation prior to late termination of pregnancy, but are not widely used in obstetrics, and thus the safety and efficacy is poorly documented.

Artificial rupture of membranes (ARM, or amniotomy)

Amniotomy (deliberate rupture of the membranes) is a simple procedure, which can be used alone for induction of labour if the membranes are accessible, sometimes avoiding the need for pharmacological intervention. Amniotomy releases endogenous prostaglandins that can initiate labour. However, the time interval from amniotomy to established labour may not be acceptable to clinicians and women, and in a number of cases labour may not ensue at all. Current practice reflects this, with amniotomy being recommended 6 h after the last prostaglandin used for induction and with the intention of commencing oxytocin either immediately or after a short interval of 2–4 h. There are clinical situations where amniotomy alone may be considered, such as in grand-multiparous women and women with previous CS, where the risk of scar rupture with prostaglandins and oxytocin are higher than if labour starts spontaneously. In these women amniotomy can be performed with a long time interval planned before further intervention is considered. This management is not appropriate in HIV-positive women with a low viral load planning vaginal delivery that require induction, or in other women at high risk of infection (group B streptococcus positive). In HIV-positive women, amniotomy should be avoided, with induction methods that allow the membranes to remain intact for as long as possible preferred.

Pharmacological methods
Oxytocin

Oxytocin is a neurohormone secreted by the posterior pituitary. It stimulates the myometrium to contract, and also causes decidual prostaglandin production. The sensitivity of the uterus to oxytocin increases as pregnancy progresses, following rupture of the membranes and after prostaglandins. For induction, oxytocin (®Syntocinon and Pitocin) is given intravenously to allow the dose to be titrated against contractions. Oxytocin can be used alone, in combination with amniotomy, or following cervical ripening with other pharmacological or non-pharmacological methods. Prior to the introduction of prostaglandins, oxytocin was used for cervical ripening as well. In developed countries, oxytocin alone is more commonly used in the presence of ruptured membranes, whether spontaneous or artificial. In developing countries where the incidence of HIV is high, delaying amniotomy in labour reduces vertical transmission rates, and oxytocin is more commonly used with intact membranes.

Amniotomy combined with oxytocin results in more vaginal deliveries and fewer instrumental deliveries, but is associated with an increase in the rate of postpartum haemorrhage compared to prostaglandin [1]. Also, more women report dissatisfaction with the induction process when amniotomy and oxytocin are used compared to women receiving prostaglandins.

In women with prelabour rupture of membranes requiring induction, oxytocin and vaginal prostaglandins are equally efficacious. Term women with prelabour rupture of membranes induced with prostaglandins have a lower rate of epidural analgesia usage and a lower rate of fetal heart rate monitoring [1]. This is likely to be an effect of the increased mobility that can be maintained during induction with prostaglandins, especially as many local protocols allow such women to have intermittent auscultation until they are in active labour (fetal monitoring guidelines are rarely specific on this point, but the risk of fetal hypoxia is low prior to the onset of regular contractions unless hyperstimulation occurs), whereas women having oxytocin will be on continuous monitoring as soon as the infusion is commenced (as this is a recommendation in all fetal monitoring guidelines). There is an increased risk of chorioamnionitis and neonatal infections with prostaglandin induction compared to oxytocin.

Table 18.1 Recommended high-volume syntocinon regimens [1].

Time	milliU/min	30 IU/500 ml* ml/h	10 IU/500 ml* ml/h
0	1	1	3
30	2	2	6
60	4	4	12
90	4	8	24
120	12	12	36
150	16	16	48
180	20	20	60
210	24	24	72
240	28	28	84
270	32	32	96

Low-volume syntocinon regimen used in King's College Hospital

Time	ml/h	Primigravida 8 IU in 50 ml* = 160 milliU/ml milliU/min	Multigravida 4 IU in 50 ml* = 80 milliU/ml milliU/min
0	1.5	4	2
15	3	8	4
30	4.5	12	6
45	6	16	8
60	7.5	20	10
75	9	24	12
		Discuss further increase with senior obstetrician	
90	10.5	28	14
105	12	32	16

Note: *Normal saline.

There are a number of regimens for oxytocin infusions with different incremental rises, interval of rise and maximum doses (see Table 18.1). The 'low-dose' regimens currently recommended are not associated with increased operative deliveries, hypercontractility or precipitate labour compared to 'high-dose regimens'. Oxytocin should be delivered in a syringe drive or infusion pump to avoid fluid overload and give accurate dosage.

Dinoprostone

Dinoprostone is a synthetic analogue of PGE2 (®Prostin). It is available as a number of different formulations, all licensed for induction of labour (see Table 18.2). Intravenous, oral and extra-amniotic administration has previously been used, but has now been replaced by vaginal formulations. One dose of prostaglandins is recommended for all women undergoing induction even if the cervix is unfavourable, as the use of prostaglandins is associated with an increase in the successful delivery within 24 h in all women when compared to oxytocin induction [1].

Misoprostol

Misoprostol, a synthetic prostaglandin E1 (®Cytotec) that was developed for the prevention of gastric ulcers, is less expensive and easier to store than other prostaglandin analogues. It is commonly used in obstetrics for medical abortion, cervical priming, induction of labour, and the management of postpartum haemorrhage. It can be given orally, vaginally or rectally, with higher plasma levels occurring with oral administration. Misoprostol has been used for the induction of labour since 1987. In early studies with large misoprostol doses (e.g. 200 μcg) there were high rates of uterine hyperstimulation. Misoprostol shortened the induction-to-delivery interval, but is associated with a higher incidence of fetal heart rate abnormality than PGE2, and this has limited its use.

Table 18.2

Prostaglandin formulation	Recommended dose	Timing and maximum dose	UK cost*
Intravaginal dinoprostone tablets	3 mg	6 hourly/2 doses	£26.58
Intravaginal dinoprostone gel	1 and 2 mg	6 hourly/2 doses	£26.58
Sustained release dinoprostone vaginal insert	10 mg	24 h single application	£30.00
Misoprostol	25–50 μg (not licensed in UK)	3–4 hourly (see text)	£0.18

Note: *UK cost based on maximum recommended dose.

Table 18.3

Score	0	1	2	3
Bishop's score [4]				
Dilatation (cm)	0	1–2	3–4	5–6
Effacement (%)	0–30	40–60	60–70	80+
Station (cm)	−3	−2	−1/0	+1/+2
Consistency	Firm	Medium	Soft	
Position	Posterior	Mid-position	Anterior	
Modified Bishop's score [5]				
Dilatation (cm)	<1	1–2	2–4	>4
Effacement (cm)	>4	2–4	1–2	<1
Station (cm)	−3	−2	−1/0	+1/+2
Consistency	Firm	Average	Soft	−
Position	Posterior	Mid-anterior	−	−

The risk of hyperstimulation is dose-dependent, and so lower doses should be associated with fewer problems. In a recent randomized trial comparing 50 μg doses of vaginal misoprostol with 3 mg doses of prostaglandin tablets, misoprostol was associated with a reduced induction to delivery interval and reduced use of oxytocin [2]. There was more tachysystole in the misoprostol group, but no difference in the abnormal fetal heart pattern, mode of delivery and the need for neonatal resuscitation.

When used in low doses, misoprostol is as effective as vaginal dinoprostone, with no increased hyperstimulation [2]. Twenty-five micrograms of vaginal misoprostol 4-hourly, 50 μg oral misoprostol 4-hourly or 20 μg oral misoprostol solution 2-hourly are regimens that have been recommended as safe and effective. Only scored 100 μg and 200 μg tablets are currently available in the UK, therefore giving very low doses accurately is difficult.

Misoprostol is not currently licensed for induction of labour in the UK, although this position is likely to change in the future. The RCOG has recommended that as there are safety aspects of misoprostol that have not been fully evaluated, its use should be restricted to clinical trials only [1]. A product licence for use in pregnancy was approved in the USA in 2003, and even prior to this the American College of Obstetricians and Gynaecologists (ACOG) has been more positive regarding its use for induction [3].

Assessing suitability for induction of labour

Bishop score (see Table 18.3)

Success of labour induction is related to the state of the cervix, and therefore it is very important to assess the cervical status prior to induction of labour. In 1964, Bishop devised a 13-point cervical scoring system to predict the responsiveness of a patient to induction [4]. It has undergone several modifications over the years, and the most widely used is Calder's modified Bishop's score [5]. There is an inverse relationship between the Bishop score and failure of labour induction, with scores below 6 associated with high failure rate, prolonged labour, and caesarean section.

The Bishop scoring system remains the most cost-effective method of evaluating the cervix before labour induction, and most evidence suggests that newer and more expensive techniques do not significantly improve accuracy.

Cervical length measurement by ultrasound

Recently, there have been several studies that have assessed the predictive accuracy of ultrasound for successful labour induction. A study comparing the performance of the Bishop score and transvaginal ultrasonography in predicting successful labour induction suggested that cervical length is a better predictor than the Bishop score [6]. A further study found that transvaginal measurement of cervical length measurement is better tolerated than digital examination for Bishop score assessment [7]. Both cervical length and Bishop score seem to be useful predictors of the need for CS delivery following labour induction, with a cervical length of more than 20 mm at labour induction an independent predictor of caesarean delivery.

Fetal fibronectin

Fibronectin is a basement membrane glycoprotein present in high concentrations in amniotic fluid. It leaks into the vaginal fluid before labour, and studies have suggested that the presence of fetal fibronectin can predict successful labour induction. A prospective comparison of clinical history, digital examination, cervical ultrasound and fetal fibronectin assay in predicting successful labour induction at term found that only history and digital examination predicted vaginal delivery within 24 h accurately and were independently associated with labour duration [8]. Fetal fibronectin and ultrasound measurements failed to predict accurately the outcome of induced labour.

Indications for induction of labour

Prolonged pregnancy

A pregnancy that exceeds 42 complete weeks (294 days) after last menstrual period (LMP) is considered a prolonged pregnancy, and it is associated with increased perinatal mortality and morbidity.

Population studies indicate that risk of stillbirth increases from 1 per 3000 ongoing pregnancies at 37 weeks to 3 per 3000 (a threefold increase) ongoing pregnancies at 42 weeks to 6 per 3000 (a sixfold increase) ongoing pregnancies at 43 weeks. The increased morbidity is due to macrosomia, birth trauma, meconium aspiration, and placental insufficiency, which increase with advancing gestation. This increase in risk has led to a policy of recommending induction of labour to women who reach 41 weeks gestation, on the basis that this will reduce perinatal mortality. As the actual risk to the fetus is still low, this has to be balanced against the possible increased risk of labour complications related to induction. Evidence suggests that the policy of offering routine induction of labour after 41 weeks does not increase the chances of delivery by CS and might even lead to a reduction in the CS risk [9].

Thus the decision to offer induction of labour for post-dates will be based on local considerations (such as the ability to provide surveillance), and should only occur after appropriate discussion with the woman. It is essential that gestation is reviewed; ideally, this should include measurements from ultrasound prior to 20 weeks of gestation, as this has been shown to reduce the need for induction for perceived post-term pregnancy.

Prelabour rupture of membranes (PROM)

Prelabour rupture of membranes occurs in 6–19% of term pregnancies. Epidemiological data on time interval from PROM to spontaneous labour suggest that 86% of women will go into labour within 24 h of rupture of membranes. The rate of spontaneous labour after this is about 5% per day. Six percent of women will not be in spontaneous labour at 96 h after PROM. As time between the rupture of membranes and the onset of labour increases, so do the risks of maternal and fetal infection. A risk of about 1% of serious neonatal infection exists in women presenting with PROM, and this risk is likely to increase with the passage of time; this statistic has to be compared to the 0.5% risk of infection in labour with intact membranes. A number of systematic reviews have examined the outcomes of pregnancies with PROM at term, comparing a policy of no intervention (expectant management) with induction. These show no change in the operative delivery or CS rate, but show a reduction in the infective sequelae in both mother and baby. Thus, in the UK, guidelines now recommend that women are offered induction at no later than 24 h post-PROM [10]. It is not unreasonable to discuss the option of immediate induction, as this may reduce the severity of a neonatal infection if a fetal infection exists; although this policy appears to have no effect on the mode of delivery, it does remove the chance of the woman labouring spontaneously. Previous guidance in the UK had suggested that induction could be deferred for up to 96 h [1]. As the evidence regarding the escalation of infective risks to the neonate with increasing time post-PROM is poor, some units may prefer to continue with this policy, but this should be done in full consultation with the woman about the balance of risks.

Both prostaglandin and oxytocin can be used as induction agents in PROM; however, although commonly used, prostaglandin preparations are not licensed for this purpose. In general, prostaglandin is preferred initially as it allows the woman to be more mobile (although continuous electronic fetal monitoring is recommended). Meta-analysis shows that prostaglandins have clinical advantages compared to oxytocin, as they are associated with an increase in successful vaginal delivery within 24 h and a reduction in the use of epidural [1]. However, as oxytocin is not associated with any increase in the rate of CS or of satisfaction with the method from the woman's perspective, it can be used particularly in women where the control offered by gradually increasing oxytocin may be preferred to a less controllable response to prostaglandins, such as grand multi parous women or women with a scar on their uterus. The only significant risk with prostaglandins is an increase in the rate of chorioamnionitis, and oxytocin is preferred if a woman with PROM has clinical signs suggestive of possible sepsis. For the same reason, induction of labour with oxytocin may be preferable for group B streptococci-positive women with prelabour rupture of membranes at term, due to the serious risk of perinatal morbidity associated with neonatal infection.

Fetal growth restriction

Suspected fetal growth restriction is a common reason for induction of labour, as babies with growth restriction have a higher incidence of perinatal mortality and morbidity. Ultrasound allows the identification of fetuses that are at risk and where early delivery is likely to be beneficial. Beyond 34 weeks' gestation, induction of labour should be considered, but it must be remembered that the fetus may have a lower reserve than normal and thus is at increased risk of intrapartum hypoxia. If delivery is necessary in a fetus below 34 weeks' gestation or at any gestation due to abnormalities of fetal dopplers (absent end-diastolic flow in the umbilical arteries or abnormal ductus venosus waveform), induction is unlikely to be successful, as the fetal reserve will be insufficient to tolerate anything other than a rapid onset quick labour. The results of a cervical assessment should be included in the decision to induce as the option of elective CS should be considered in primigravid women with an unfavourable cervix at all gestations and in multigravid women below 34 weeks. Electronic fetal monitoring is mandatory throughout induction and ensuing labour. The higher rate of fetal heart rate

abnormalities will result in more instrumental deliveries and caesarean sections in this group.

Hypertension

Hypertensive disorders, pregnancy-induced hypertension (PIH) and pre-eclampsia (PET), complicate 10–15% of all pregnancies at term, and are a significant cause of maternal and perinatal morbidity and mortality. As the only definitive treatment is delivery, it is one of the commonest indications for induction of labour. In preterm pregnancies (below 34 weeks) complicated by pre-eclampsia, expectant monitoring is advocated to increase the chance of fetal maturity, as long as the risks for the mother remain acceptable. Labour induction is a reasonable option for patients with severe pre-eclampsia from 34 weeks' gestation (depending on fetal condition), as evidence shows that 48% of hypertensive women given the chance will deliver vaginally. The Bishop score on admission is the best predictor of success, and the chance of successful labour induction increases with advancing gestational age.

There is little consensus on how to manage mild hypertensive disease in pregnancies at term. It is unclear whether in this situation expectant management is beneficial for the mother and her baby, since evidence is lacking. Despite the lack of evidence to justify intervention, many obstetricians induce labour in women after 37 weeks with PIH/PET because of the known unpredictability of the hypertensive disease. Induction of labour might prevent maternal and neonatal complications at the expense of increased instrumental vaginal delivery rates and CS rates.

Isolated oligohydramnios at term

Oligohydramnios in the absence of maternal and fetal complications (such as growth restriction) creates a dilemma in management. The increased use of ultrasound in antenatal surveillance has resulted in the detection of abnormalities in amniotic fluid volume. In the absence of good evidence regarding the implications of this finding, obstetricians chose to 'play it safe' and recommend induction of labour. However, evidence to support the practice is lacking, with small studies showing no overall benefit and an increase in operative vaginal delivery and CS rates. Larger studies are unlikely to occur, but a commonsense approach suggests that regardless of when labour happens there will be a high incidence of fetal heart rate abnormalities due to cord compression, and that early induction is unlikely to worsen outcome.

Diabetes

In women with diabetes there is a four- to fivefold increase in perinatal mortality and an increase in birth trauma including shoulder dystocia due to macrosomia. Reasons given for inducing labour at term in pregnancies complicated by diabetes include the avoidance of fetal demise and the prevention of excessive fetal growth (and its associated complications, particularly shoulder dystocia and caesarean delivery).

Induction of labour at term in women with diabetes reduces the risk of macrosomia, and does not increase the CS rate or neonatal morbidity. The RCOG recommends that women with diabetes should be offered induction prior to the estimated date of delivery [11].

Macrosomia

Many obstetricians favour induction of labour in cases of suspected fetal macrosomia in non-diabetic mothers. The rationale for this is that the policy will reduce the risk of CS and birth trauma associated with further increase in birthweight that will happen with expectant management.

However, evidence does not support this view, showing that induction for fetal macrosomia alone does not improve fetal outcome and is associated with significantly higher emergency CS rate. As the methods available for estimating fetal weight, symphysio-fundal height and ultrasound have poor predictive values, unnecessary intervention is likely to occur in some pregnancies.

Twin pregnancy

The risk of stillbirth in twins between 37 and 42 weeks is 6–9 per 1000 as compared to 2.7 per 1000 in singleton pregnancy. This has led many obstetricians to recommend induction at 38 weeks. There are no good studies to confirm the benefits of this policy in an uncomplicated twin [1].

Social/maternal (non-medical indication) request

Some women request induction prior to 41 weeks for reasons such as problematic pregnancy symptoms or a desire to shorten the duration of their pregnancy for domestic reasons. There is insufficient evidence to be certain of the risks associated with elective induction without a medical reason, but extrapolation of other evidence would suggest an increase in instrumental delivery, CS and respiratory distress in the baby. There would also be a huge resource implication if this is routinely practised, and it is never justified prior to 39 weeks' gestation due to the increased risk of neonatal respiratory morbidity at earlier gestations.

In developed countries, induction for maternal request is usually allowed where there are convincing psychological or social reasons and a cervical assessment is favourable [1].

Intrauterine fetal demise (IUD)

Induction of labour is recommended after fetal demise, as spontaneous labour may not occur for several weeks, with resulting maternal distress. The theoretical risk of disseminated intravascular coagulation (DIC) has been overexaggerated and is likely to be the result from the conservative management of women with IUD due to abruption and pre-eclampsia. It is therefore important that any woman presenting with intrauterine death is reviewed carefully with a full history, examination and blood clotting investigations.

Induction of labour in women with a previous caesarean section

In the UK, the RCOG recommends that women with previous caesarean delivery should be actively encouraged to consider attempting vaginal delivery in subsequent pregnancies [12]. However, when induction is required with previous caesarean section, the recommendations are less clear. In the USA, the ACOG recommendations state that the use of prostaglandins for induction of labour in women with previous CS should be discouraged [13].

The UK guidance makes less-explicit recommendations, but concludes that observational data suggest that vaginal prostaglandins are safe in women with a previous caesarean section. The available evidence is contradictory, with all evidence based on retrospective cohort studies.

The largest study in 2004 showed an increased risk of uterine rupture in women induced with prostaglandins. The study concluded a risk of 1 in 71 for women who had never given birth vaginally before (compared with a 1 in 210 risk in similar non-induced women) and 1 in 175 for women who had delivered vaginally in a previous pregnancy (compared with a risk of 1 in 514 for similar non-induced women) [14].

A more recent study showed no significant difference in the risk of uterine dehiscence in a woman with a uterine scar compared to an unscarred uterus, but the authors suggested that guidelines with strict intervention criteria should be used in women with uterine scars [15].

Yet another study in 2005 concluded that in women with previous caesarean section and no vaginal deliveries, induction of labour carries a high risk of uterine rupture (1 in 51 risk) and that this was regardless of the use of intrauterine pressure catheters [16].

There are few data regarding the safety of misoprostol, and both the RCOG and the ACOG advise against its use for induction of labour in women with uterine scars [1,13].

Induction of labour in women with a uterine scar using amniotomy and oxytocin is also associated with an increase in the risk of scar dehiscence, but the magnitude of risk appears to be less than for prostaglandins. A cohort analysis from the USA concluded that the risk of scar dehiscence was 1 in 192 for spontaneous labour, 1 in 129 for non-prostaglandin-induced labour, and 1 in 41 for prostaglandin-induced labour [17].

Mechanical cervical dilatation may be an option for consideration in women with a uterine scar. Only small studies exist, but the largest concluded that the method appeared safe, and reported a 78% vaginal delivery rate in a small group of women induced with a double-balloon device.

Elective repeat CS or induction of labour for women with a uterine scar both have risks and benefits; modern obstetric practice should aim to explain these risks based on the best available evidence, and allow her to choose how she wishes to be managed.

On the basis of the available evidence:

- the decision to induce and the method chosen should be discussed with the woman by a senior obstetrician;
- women should be informed that there is an increased risk of scar dehiscence associated with induction of labour with prostaglandins. This risk is greater in women who have not given birth vaginally before;
- the risk is likely to be reduced if good local guidelines are in place and these are strictly adhered to (particularly regarding the maximum dose of prostaglandin, management of hyperstimulation and the management of slow progress in labour); and

- healthcare professionals should be aware of the increased risk of uterine rupture and offer support to the woman accordingly.

Risks associated with induction of labour

Side effects of prostaglandins

Prostaglandins are very well tolerated as induction agents. Documented side effects include nausea, vomiting and diarrhoea, but in practice these are rarely troublesome. Vaginal discomfort may occur, with a feeling of warmth or irritation described. Allergic reactions are very rare, but cases of bronchospasm have been reported in women with asthma. A rise in temperature may be seen (especially with misoprostol) and a slight increase in the leukocyte count [18].

Increased analgesia requirements and operative delivery

Induction of labour leads to more epidural usage, instrumental delivery and caesarean section. This is especially true in nulliparous women. The higher CS rate is attributed to failure to progress in the first stage due to lack of cervical favourability during the start of induction, failed induction and fetal distress due to uterine hypercontractility and prolonged labour. The high rate of instrumental delivery is attributed to the increased usage of epidural analgesia in women undergoing induction. The effect of induction is confounded by the indication for induction, as this independently increases the risk of assisted delivery for many indications.

Hyperstimulation

Uterine hyperstimulation can occur with administration of prostaglandins and/or oxytocin. The incidence of hypercontractility with or without fetal heart rate changes on cardiotocography (CTG) ranges from 1 to 5%.

Signs and symptoms of hyperstimulation include:

- five contractions or more in 10 min (or more than 10 contractions in 20 min) without CTG changes;
- hypertonus, contractions lasting more than 120 s without CTG changes; and
- uterine hyperstimulation syndrome – excessive uterine activity (>4 contractions in 10 min) with a non-reassuring CTG.

If prostaglandins have been administered, then removal of the remainder of the agent will help alleviate the symptoms. If the uterine hypercontractility is due to oxytocin, then the infusion should be reduced or stopped. An abnormal CTG (non-reassuring or pathological) associated with uterine hypercontractility not resolving after the infusion is stopped (or where prostaglandin has all been absorbed) means that immediate tocolysis with 0.25 mg of subcutaneous terbutaline should be considered [19].

In case of acute fetal compromise (prolonged deceleration or other pathological FHR pattern), delivery should be expedited if recovery does not happen rapidly following tocolysis.

Fetal heart rate abnormalities

Uterine hyperstimulation will result in an increased incidence of cord compression and may cause recurrent or prolonged deceleration. As amniotomy is often used as part of the induction process, this further increases the incidence of cord compression decelerations.

Encouraging the mother to change position (avoiding the dorsal position) will help reduce the incidence of CTG abnormalities and routine amniotomy should be avoided, reserving it for women who are not progressing following prostaglandin.

Uterine rupture

Induction of labour in women with high parity or uterine scars (previous CS or myomectomy) is associated with an increased risk of uterine rupture. It is advisable to limit the amount of prostaglandin administered to such women, with amniotomy performed as soon as the Bishop score is above 6. Mobilization for 4 h (if the indication allows this) following amniotomy may reduce the number of women requiring syntocinon.

Failed induction

There is the risk of failure to initiate labour with prostaglandins and oxytocin. In such a situation, the initial indication for the decision to induce has to be reviewed, and either postpone a further attempt for a few days or offer delivery by CS.

Care during induction of labour

Organization of induction of labour

The exact timing of induction will depend on local considerations, but should be planned to ensure that examinations are likely to be able to occur in a timely fashion, and so that the minimum number of women labour overnight. Thus administration of the first dose of dinoprostone to primigravid women and multigravid women with an unfavourable cervix late on the evening of day 1 with examination early the next morning is practised in many units. Multigravid women with a favourable cervix should receive a dose of dinoprostone as early as possible in the morning with the intention of performing amniotomy 6 h later, still allowing a chance of delivery on the first day.

The prostaglandin can be administered by an appropriately trained midwife or doctor. The baseline Bishop score should be recorded. It is essential that the prostaglandin is administered high into the posterior fornix and that the woman is advised to remain recumbent for 30–60 min postadministration to ensure that the prostaglandin is administered to the cervix. It is also important that inadvertent intracervical administration is avoided, as this will increase the chances of uterine hyperstimulation occurring.

Induction of labour should follow informed consent by the woman. This should include an explanation of the reason for induction, the recommended method to be used and the risks associated with the process. Women should be given access to evidence-based information to ensure that they are fully informed about the process [1].

Prostaglandin induction of labour can be carried out in the antenatal ward until the start of the active first stage of labour for low-risk cases, such as postdates and those performed on maternal request at term inductions.

The procedure for high-risk prostaglandin inductions, such as for pre-eclampsia or growth restriction and where oxytocin is to be used, should occur in the labour ward with continuous CTG monitoring [19].

The capacity pressures in many maternity units has led to the consideration of outpatient induction protocols, especially with the sustained release prostaglandin agents. There is currently a paucity of data to confirm the safety of this, and thus it can only be recommended as part of ongoing research with careful selection and supervision of the women involved.

Due to 1–5% incidence of hypercontractility associated with induction with prostaglandins, continuous electronic monitoring should be recommended, with reassuring monitoring a requirement prior to commencing induction [1]. The decision to undertake induction in the presence of a non-reassuring fetal heart rate trace requires the input of an experienced obstetrician, but if there is any suspicion of fetal compromise the option of delivery by CS should be considered, as induction and labour is likely to cause further stress on the already compromised fetus.

Women should be advised to have continuous electronic monitoring for 30 min after prostaglandin administration. As the response to prostaglandins is rarely idiosyncratic, the need for repeat monitoring pre- and post-repeat prostaglandins could be questioned, as if there is no adverse response to the initial dose, the chance of a future adverse response is low. However, limited evidence is available, and thus most induction protocols continue to recommend monitoring after each new dose. When contractions become established, continuous electronic monitoring is recommended [19]. Ultimately, the strength of this recommendation depends on the indication for induction; for example, a woman having induction for symphysis pubis dysfunction at 40 weeks who labours after one dose of prostaglandin has a completely different risk profile to a woman being induced due to pre-eclampsia at 37 weeks' gestation requiring a long induction procedure. A review and discussion of the need for monitoring may be required for women who wish to remain mobile or use water for pain relief in their labour.

Oxytocin should not be used for 6 h after prostaglandin administration, and when oxytocin is used, continuous uterine contractions and fetal heart rate monitoring should be used [1].

When uterine hypercontractility occurs following prostaglandin administration, removal of remainder of the drug may help, but this is only practical with sustained release preparations, as the active agent is rapidly absorbed from the delivery matrix in both gels and tablets. In hypercontractility due to oxytocin, reducing or stopping the infusion usually reduces the uterine activity and should occur in any woman contracting more than 5 in 10 min, even if the fetal heart rate pattern is normal. If the fetal heart rate is abnormal, then tocolysis with terbutaline should be considered unless the fetal heart rate normalizes rapidly.

Pain relief should be discussed with women who are undergoing induction of labour. Prostaglandins may be associated with significant discomfort before the onset of proper labour (so-called 'prostin' pains). Simple analgesia may suffice, but some women will require stronger opiate analgesia. If an oxytocin infusion is to be commenced, women should be offered the option of epidural anaesthesia prior to commencing the infusion [10].

Options on failed induction

There is no standard agreement of what constitutes a failed induction. A cervix where the Bishop score remains below 6 (so that amniotomy is not possible) after prostaglandin administration would be one definition, but even then there is variation in the number of doses of prostaglandin that are administered before reaching this conclusion. Administration of more than two doses of prostaglandin is outside the product licence for most prostaglandin preparations, and published UK guidelines [1] recommend administration of a maximum of two doses.

Local guidelines should allow the administration of no more than two doses of prostaglandin to any woman before a senior medical review occurs to plan further management. The options include:

- epidural anaesthesia to allow a difficult amniotomy to be performed,
- consideration of administering syntocinon prior to amniotomy,
- delivery by caesarean section,
- administration of further prostaglandins, and
- awaiting events as an inpatient or an outpatient (delaying induction).

Ultimately the decision will require a review of the urgency of the need for delivery, whether there are any other factors that mitigate against success, and the wishes of the woman and her partner.

Management of induction of labour in intrauterine death

Vaginal gemeprost, a synthetic analogue of PGE1 (®Cervagem) was previously widely used for induction in women with IUD before 28 weeks. A regimen of a 1 mg pessary given vaginally every 3 h for 5 doses, with the option of giving a second course 24 h after the start of treatment if delivery had not occurred. This has now been superseded by the use of regimens including misoprostol.

Misoprostol can be used for all gestations, but dinoprostone induction is often recommended for intrauterine death at later gestations due to the concerns about using misoprostol at term [1]. Various dose regimens have been recommended, but the most

Table 18.4 Induction regimen for intrauterine fetal death.

Gestation (weeks)	Initial vaginal dose	Further oral doses
<24	Misoprostol 800 µg	Misoprostol 400 µg 3 hourly (maximum 5 doses)
24–34	Misoprostol 200 µg	Misoprostol 200 µg 3 hourly (maximum 4 doses)
34–37	Misoprostol 100 µg	Misoprostol 100 µg 3 hourly (maximum 4 doses)
37–39	As above or below	As above or below
>39	Dinoprostone	

common give a vaginal dose followed by oral (see Table 18.4).

Misoprostol induction can be considered in women with previous uterine surgery, especially at earlier gestations where the risk of uterine dehiscence in labour should be lower due to the small fetal size and where the risks of a surgical procedure to deliver the dead fetus (hysterotomy or classical caesarean section) carry significant risks in future pregnancy. In women at gestations above 34 weeks with one previous CS, the option of induction should be offered, as although there is an increase in the risk of uterine dehiscence related to induction, it is normally the fetal risk of this that makes women opt for repeat caesarean as the maternal risks with careful management are less serious. However, care is required during the labour, as a major indicator of uterine dehiscence (fetal heart rate change) is absent, so diagnosis will be more difficult.

It is now standard practice in modern obstetrics to give oral mifepristone, which acts as an anti-progesterone, 'down-regulating' the placenta and increasing the cervical and uterine sensitivity to prostaglandins. The combination of mifepristone and misoprostol for induction of labour following late fetal death has been shown to be both effective and safe, reducing the induction–delivery interval when compared to either agent used alone.

Early studies used 600 mg of mifepristone, but subsequent practice has shown that a dose of 200 mg is equally effective in shortening induction-to-delivery intervals.

Mifepristone is ideally given 48–72 h prior to labour induction using a prostaglandin, and this should be the recommendation given to women. However, sometimes they do not wish to wait following oral mifepristone, or there may be medical reasons why the induction should begin immediately. On the basis that some effect will be likely even in the first few hours after administration, oral mifepristone can still be administered, with misoprostol being commenced simultaneously. Mifepristone will also be active if the labour is not induced by the first course of misoprostol. As studies have shown that pretreatment with mifepristone is more effective at earlier gestations, it is less important to delay induction beyond 28 weeks' gestation.

If labour progress is slow, a syntocinon oxytocin infusion may be required; this can be done either after spontaneous rupture of membranes, or with the membranes intact (the risk of amniotic fluid embolus may be more theoretical). The membranes should be left intact for as long as possible, as this reduces the chances of ascending infection (which is more likely with a dead fetus) and maintains the forewaters, which may be a better cervical dilator than a fetal head with significant overlapping of the skull bones that happens after IUD. However, as syntocinon is less effective in the presence of intact membranes, if labour progress remains slow, amniotomy may be unavoidable. This decision should be made at a senior level, intravenous antibiotics should be commenced, and a strict time limit imposed on the length of the labour after amniotomy.

Women undergoing induction for IUD should be offered parenteral pain relief at an early stage in the process. The full range of obstetric anaesthesia including epidural should be offered, but patient-controlled analgesia with a pump containing diamorphine can also be offered, as the neonatal side effects are not a concern. This method has the advantage of offering good pain relief whilst maintaining full mobility and wearing off quickly after delivery to allow early discharge.

If delivery does not occur after the first course of misoprostol, the following options can be considered.

- Surgical uterine evacuation (for gestations below 24 week where appropriate expertise is available).
- Repeat course of misoprostol, 24 h or more after commencing treatment.
- Oxytocin infusion on intact membranes (to avoid infection, or if amniotomy is not possible).

- Amniotomy and oxytocin.
- Hysterotomy or caesarean section (if the maternal condition is deteriorating).

Conclusion

Induction of labour is an obstetric intervention that has become established. The misuse and mismanagement of the process is likely to cause compromise to the mother and the fetus/newborn. The decision to induce should not be taken lightly. Considerable thought on the part of the obstetrician with due consideration to indication, parity, cervical score and other medical issues (e.g. caesarean scar) should help in the appropriate decision-making. Counselling the patient should include the explanation of indication and the process of induction, and the pros and cons.

References

1. RCOG. *Clinical Effectiveness Support Unit Induction of Labour* London: RCOG Press, 2001.

2. Sifakis S, Angelakis E, Avgoustinakis E, *et al.* Cochrane meta-analysis on misoprostol. A randomised comparison between intravaginal misoprostol and prostaglandin E2 for labor induction. *Arch Gynecol Obstet* 2007; **275**(4): 263–7.

3. ACOG. Committee Opinion Number 283. New U.S. Food and Drug Administration labeling on Cytotec (misoprostol) use and pregnancy. *Obstet Gynecol* 2003; **101** (5 Pt 1): 1049–50.

4. Bishop E H. Pelvic scoring for elective induction of labour. *Obstet Gynecol* 1964; **24**: 266–8.

5. Calder A A, Emprey M P, Hillier K. Extra-amniotic prostaglandin E2 for induction of labour at term. *J Obstet Gynaecol Br Commonw* 1974; **81**: 39–44.

6. Gabriel R, Darnaud T, Chalot F, Gonzalez N, Leymarie F, Quereux C. Transvaginal sonography of the uterine cervix prior to labour induction. *Ultrasound Obstet Gynecol* 2002; **19**(3): 254–7.

7. Tan P C, Vallikkannu N, Suguna S, Quek K F, Hassan J. Transvaginal sonographic measurement of cervical length vs. Bishop score in labor induction at term: tolerability and prediction of Cesarean delivery. *Ultrasound Obstet Gynecol* 2007; **29**(5): 568–73.

8. Reis F M, Gervasi M T, Florio P, *et al.* Prediction of successful induction of labor at term: role of clinical history, digital assessment of the cervix and fetal fibronectin assay. *Am J Obstet Gynecol* 2003; **189**(5): 1361–7.

9. Crowley P. Interventions for preventing or improving the outcome of delivery at or beyond term (Cochrane Review) In: *The Cochrane Library* 2002; **3**. Oxford: Update Software.

10. National Collaborating Centre for Women's and Children's Health. *Intrapartum Care. Care of Healthy Women and their Babies during Childbirth. Clinical guideline.* London: RCOG Press, 2007.

11. National Collaborating Centre for Women's and Children's Health.*Diabetes in Pregnancy – Management of Diabetes and its Complications from Preconception to the Postnatal Period.* London: RCOG Press, 2008.

12. National Collaborating Centre for Women's and Children's Health. *Caesarean Section – Clinical Guideline.* London: RCOG Press, 2004.

13. American College of Obstetricians and Gynecologists Committee on Obstetric Practice. COG previous CS and IOL ACOG committee opinion No. 342: Induction of labor for vaginal birth after cesarean delivery. *Obstet Gynecol* 2006; **108**(2): 465–8.

14. Smith G C, Pell J P, Pasupathy D, Dobbie R. Factors predisposing to perinatal death related to uterine rupture during attempted vaginal birth after caesarean section: retrospective cohort study. *Br Med J* 2004; **14**: 375.

15. Locatelli A, Ghidini A, Ciriello E, Incerti M, Bonardi C, Regalia A L. Induction of labor: comparison of a cohort with uterine scar from previous cesarean section vs. a cohort with intact uterus. *J Matern Fetal Neonatal Med* 2006; **19**(8): 471–5.

16. Kayani S I, Alfirevic Z. Uterine rupture after induction of labour in women with previous caesarean section. *Br J Obstet Gynaecol* 2005; **112**(4): 451–5.

17. Lyndon-Rochell M, Holt V L, Easterling T R, Martin D P. Risk of uterine rupture during labour among women with a prior cesarean delivery. *N Engl J Med* 2001; **345**(1): 3–8.

18. British Medical Association and the Royal Pharmaceutical Society of Great Britain. *British National Formulary* 54. British Medical Association, 2007.

19. RCOG Clinical Effectiveness Support Unit. *The Use of Electronic Fetal Monitoring.* London: RCOG Press, 2001.

Preterm prelabour rupture of membranes (pPROM)

Austin Ugwumadu

Introduction

Preterm prelabour rupture of membranes (pPROM) is defined as the spontaneous rupture of fetal membranes at least an hour prior to the onset of labour, and before 37 completed weeks of gestation. It complicates 2–3% of all pregnancies, thus affecting some 14,000 pregnancies in the UK and 140,000 in the USA. Preterm prelabour rupture of membranes accounts for 30–40% of preterm deliveries, and is an independent risk factor for neonatal morbidity and mortality from prematurity, sepsis and pulmonary hypoplasia. Infants born after prolonged periods of pPROM have an excess risk of long-term neurological and pulmonary deficits. Subclinical intrauterine infection has been implicated as a major aetiological factor in the pathogenesis of pPROM and its associated feto-maternal morbidity. Studies of transabdominal amniocentesis following pPROM show that the frequency of positive culture for infection of the amniotic fluid is 25–40%. The risk of a positive culture is inversely related to the gestational age at which pPROM occurred. Women with intrauterine infection have shorter latency than non-infected women, and infants born with sepsis have a fourfold increase in mortality compared to infants born without sepsis [1]. These findings have fuelled interest in the use of antibiotics to prevent pPROM in women at risk, to increase latency after pPROM, and as prophylaxis against neonatal morbidity such as oxygen dependency, intraventricular haemorrhage, necrotizing enterocolitis, neonatal sepsis, and mortality. In one study, women with a prior history of pPROM had a 13.5% risk of subsequent preterm birth due to pPROM compared to 4.1% risk amongst their peers without such a history (RR 3.3, $p<0.01$) [2]. These women also had a 14-fold higher risk of pPROM at less than 28 weeks in the subsequent pregnancy (1.8% versus 0.13%, $p<0.01$), raising the question of whether antibiotics may reduce this risk of pPROM. McGregor and colleagues showed that in women who are at increased risk of pPROM, prophylactic antibiotics significantly reduced the incidence of pPROM in the subsequent pregnancy [3].

Aetiology and pathophysiology

The tensile strength of the membranes is resident mostly in the amnion, an avascular structure consisting of five distinct histological layers. The amniotic epithelial cells secrete types III and IV collagen, and non-collagenenous glycoproteins including fibronectins [4]. The chorion, on the other hand, provides the feto-maternal interface through the interaction between the cytotrophoblasts and the maternal decidua. In recent years, our understanding of the cellular and molecular factors that govern the structural integrity of fetal membranes and their regulation has increased, and it is now clear that only a proportion of pPROM cases are infection-driven. Evidence is accumulating that other pathologic processes unrelated to infection may play a role, and they include choriodecidual fusion defects [5], fetal growth dysregulation [6], activation of membrane apoptosis [7], up-regulation of matrix metalloproteinases, and inhibition of tissue inhibitors of matrix metalloproteinases [8], nutritional factors [9] and smoking [10] may be important in a significant proportion of cases of pPROM. A detailed review of these factors and processes is outside the scope of this chapter, but these observations raise the question that routine antibiotics for the treatment of pPROM may be an oversimplistic response to a very complex problem.

Best Practice in Labour and Delivery, ed. R. Warren and S. Arulkumaran. Published by Cambridge University Press.
© Cambridge University Press 2009.

Diagnosis and initial assessment

The diagnosis of pPROM is made by clinical suspicion, maternal history, speculum examination and simple bedside tests. Although maternal history has an accuracy of 90% for the diagnosis of pPROM [11], the management and prognosis of a pregnancy complicated by pPROM is so drastically different from the one without that it is good practice to confirm the diagnosis before applying the label of pPROM. The presence of a pool of amniotic fluid in the posterior fornix on speculum examination is confirmatory of pPROM. Whether this fluid needs to be tested for confirmation is debatable. There may be a role for nitrazine pH paper testing when there is a very small amount of fluid in the posterior fornix and the observer is uncertain. However, the nitrazine test is not specific, and has a false positive rate of 17% [11]. The pH of vaginal fluid changes towards the alkaline range in the presence of bacterial vaginosis, other vaginitis, contamination with cervical secretion, blood, semen or urine. In doubtful cases, the clinician may display the cervix with a Cusco's speculum to visualize the external os, and ask the patient to cough gently. Amniotic fluid can be observed to trickle down through the external cervical os. An extended pad test is also useful. A panel of newer tests have been evaluated for pPROM, including fetal fibronectins and raised insulin-like growth factor binding protein-1 (IGFBP-1) in cervico-vaginal secretions. These have sensitivities of 94 and 75%, respectively, and specificities of 97% [12,13]. Spontaneous rupture of membranes during the second and early third trimesters is usually associated with a near total loss of the entire amniotic fluid pool. Therefore, an ultrasound scan evidence of marked oligohydramnios or anhydramnios is highly suggestive of a diagnosis of pPROM in this context [14]. Such an ultrasound examination should be extended to evaluate the fetal growth and development, and the estimated fetal weight and presentation.

A digital vaginal examination should be avoided following a diagnosis of pPROM unless there is a strong suspicion of labour or imminent delivery. Recent studies have shown that two or fewer digital vaginal examinations were associated with a shorter latency period but no increase in fetal or maternal infectious morbidity [15,16]. Thus, if one or two digital vaginal examinations were done after pPROM, this should not constitute an indication to abandon conservative management or pursue an immediate induction of labour for fear of increased risk of feto-maternal infectious morbidity.

Current state of the management of pPROM

In many units, women with a diagnosis of pPROM are admitted into hospital and managed conservatively until 37 completed weeks of gestation in an attempt to increase fetal maturity. Conservative management involves nursing in a Trendelenburg (head-down tilt) position, four-hourly measurements of maternal temperature, heart rate, respiratory rate, and blood pressure, daily cardiotocographs (CTG), weekly, twice or thrice weekly maternal white cell counts, C-reactive protein assays, and culture of vaginal swabs, all in an effort to detect intrauterine infection or chorioamnionitis. However, chorioamnionitis is a fetal disease, not maternal, and maternal inflammatory markers are raised in only 10–15% of cases of proven histological chorioamnionitis [17], suggesting that maternal markers are not sufficiently sensitive to guide clinical decisions. The intrauterine compartment is sequestrated and not necessarily contiguous with the maternal systemic circulation. Furthermore, the bacterial species that commonly participate in chorioamnionitis are frequently subpathogenic, non-pyrogenic, and are often not detected on routine microbiological culture methods. For prognosis, it is fetal rather than maternal evidence of inflammation that is predictive of adverse neonatal outcome. However, the search for evidence of fetal inflammation by amniocentesis and/or cordocentesis is not routinely done, and indeed its role in reducing the risk of neonatal complications has not been adequately evaluated.

Appropriate setting for management

The value of inpatient management beyond 5 days is dubious. The majority of women with infection-driven pPROM will deliver within this time frame. Outpatient care with instruction for the patient to take her own temperature and be reviewed once or twice weekly in hospital is reasonable. She should, however, be discouraged from vaginal intercourse, protected or not, and any form of intravaginal cleansing. Immersion in bath water is not associated with an increase in infectious morbidity. A one-off vaginal swab for pathogens and specifically for group B streptococcus will suffice. There is little or no correlation between the organisms that cause amniotic fluid infection/chorioamnionitis and those isolated from the lower genital tract. Nursing women with pPROM in a head-down tilt position is unnecessary, and may encourage a stagnant pool of amniotic fluid and cervico-vaginal secretions with a potential for encouraging bacterial growth and multiplication. Although fetal CTG is recommended as part of the surveillance, there are no specific or reliable CTG patterns that are predictive of fetal inflammation or sepsis until very late, and neurological injuries may occur without significant CTG changes. Clinical chorioamnionitis defined as maternal fever (temperature $\geq 38°C$) and the presence of any two or more of the following – maternal or fetal tachycardia, uterine tenderness, foul-smelling or purulent vaginal discharge, maternal leukocytosis or raised C – reactive protein – is poorly predictive of histologic chorioamnionitis, which has been shown to be more predictive of abnormal neonatal cerebral outcomes including periventricular echodensity/echolucency, ventriculomegaly, intraventricular haemorrhage and seizures [18].

Biophysical profile scores have been proposed and in some centres used for the prediction of intrauterine infection. There is conflicting evidence that abnormal biophysical profile scores or Doppler studies of the placenta or fetal circulation provided accurate distinction between infected and non-infected fetuses [14,19,20].

Timing of delivery

The practice of expectant management until 37 completed weeks of gestation to improve fetal maturity is historical and based on the assumption that the prolongation of pregnancy automatically translates to better fetal maturity and neonatal outcome. The risks of cord events including acute cord compression, cord prolapse, or ascending infection are not insignificant. It is now well-established that the risks of prematurity-related morbidity including respiratory distress syndrome, necrotizing enterocolitis, and high-grade intraventricular haemorrhage and mortality, diminish significantly beyond 32–34 weeks, and that neonatal survival at 34 weeks in tertiary units is similar to 37–40 weeks. The increase in survival per additional week of conservative management is less than 1%. Furthermore, studies evaluating the risk–benefit analysis of induction of labour at 34 weeks found similar vaginal delivery rates, and no increase in the risk of obstetric intervention such as instrumental vaginal or caesarean delivery [21]. On the other hand, these studies documented an excess incidence of ascending infection, neonatal sepsis, cord prolapse or compression, fetal demise and longer hospital stay in cases managed conservatively [21,22]. They concluded that the benefits of delivery at 34 weeks' gestation outweigh the risks of conservative management without increasing obstetric intervention. This balance, however, is in favour of expectant management prior to 32 completed weeks. Delivery before 32 weeks' gestation is associated with a significant risk of gestational age-related morbidity and mortality. Therefore, unless there are concerns regarding fetal well-being, clinical or biochemical evidence of infection, women with pPROM remote from term should be managed conservatively to prolong gestation and reduce the risk of gestational age-dependent morbidity and mortality in the newborn. Even with conservative management, 70–80% of women with preterm prelabour rupture of membranes deliver within 1 week of membrane rupture, leaving a smaller subset of fetuses to remain and mature in utero. The potential benefit has to be balanced against the risk of amnionitis, abruption, umbilical cord compression or prolapse, and fetal demise.

Antibiotic therapy to prolong latency and prevent neonatal morbidity after pPROM

Evidence from meta-analysis of randomized trials suggests that antibiotic therapy (ampicillin and/or erythromycin) delayed preterm delivery, and reduced maternal and neonatal morbidity after a diagnosis of pPROM [23,24]. Routine antibiotics are therefore recommended for women with pPROM. However, questions have persisted regarding the methodology and interpretation of the primary studies from which these conclusions were drawn. Initial studies of antibiotic therapy in pPROM to treat/prevent ascending infection, prolong pregnancy, and reduce neonatal infectious and gestational age-dependent morbidity [25–26] showed significant increase in latency but an inconsistent effect on morbidity and mortality. A significant number of women enrolled in these studies were near term and would not have benefited from pregnancy prolongation.

The National Institute of Child Health and Human Development Maternal–Fetal Medicine Units Network conducted a randomized, placebo-controlled trial to determine whether intravenous antibiotic therapy (ampicillin 2 g and erythromycin 250 mg 6 hourly) for 48 h followed by oral amoxycillin 250 mg + erythromycin 333 mg 8 hourly, reduced perinatal morbidity and mortality in 614 women with pPROM between 24 and 32 weeks' gestation [24]. The primary outcome was a 'composite' morbidity, including any of: fetal or postnatal death, respiratory distress syndrome (RDS), sepsis within 72 h, grade 3 or 4 intraventricular haemorrhage (IVH), or stage 2 or 3 necrotizing enterocolitis. Corticosteroid or tocolytic therapy was not permitted in the trial. The study showed significant reductions in the rate of composite morbidity (44 vs. 53%, RR 0.84, $p=0.037$); RDS (41 vs. 49%, RR 0.83, $p=0.037$) and stage 2–3 necrotizing enterocolitis (2 vs. 6%, RR 0.40, $p=0.030$) in the antibiotic group [24]. The antibiotic group had a lower incidence of clinical amnionitis (23 vs. 33%, $p=0.010$). By prohibiting corticosteroid administration in the trial, the authors demonstrated a direct correlation between antibiotic therapy and a reduced frequency of RDS, an effect most likely related to the significant prolongation of pregnancy. Since corticosteroid administration is associated with reductions in gestational age-related morbidities and is routinely given between 24 and 32 weeks' gestation in current practice, it raises the question of whether there are any additional benefits from antibiotic therapy.

This trial was followed by the larger, multi-arm, multicentre placebo-controlled ORACLE (Overview of the Role of Antibiotics in Curtailing Labour and Early delivery) trial [27]. It aimed to determine whether a composite neonatal outcome (defined as one or more of: death before discharge, oxygen dependency at 28 days of postnatal age, or major cerebral abnormality on ultrasound) was improved with antibiotic therapy in women with pPROM. A total of 4809 women with pPROM (ORACLE 1) and 6241 women in spontaneous labour with intact membranes (ORACLE II) [28] were initially randomized to receive oral erythromycin, amoxycillin–clavulonic acid (Augmentin), both, or placebo for up to 10 days. Oral erythromycin led to a brief prolongation of pregnancy (not significant at 7 days), decreased oxygen dependency (31 vs. 36%, $p=0.02$), less positive blood cultures (6 vs. 8%, $p=0.02$), but no significant reduction in composite morbidity (13 vs.

15%, $p=0.08$) [27]. Secondary analysis of singleton gestations revealed a reduction in oxygen dependency at 28 days (7 vs. 9%, $p=0.03$), positive blood cultures (5 vs. 7%, $p=0.04$) abnormal cerebral ultrasonography (3 vs. 5%, $p=0.04$) and composite morbidity (11 vs. 14%, $p=0.02$) with erythromycin. Augmentin increased latency and reduced supplemental oxygen need, but was associated with increased necrotizing enterocolitis without reducing other morbidities. The combination of Augmentin and erythromycin yielded similar results. The authors concluded that oral erythromycin reduced perinatal morbidity in pPROM prior to 37 weeks' gestation. However, given the small differences in the actual incidences of morbidity in the study groups, many women would need to be treated to prevent one adverse outcome.

Within 6 months of publication, 50% of obstetric units in the UK had adopted the findings of the ORACLE trial [29]. However, its methodology and the interpretation of the findings remained controversial. The biochemical processes that drive preterm labour and pPROM are likely to be irreversibly established by the time women present with symptoms, and antibiotic intervention at this stage may be too late. Although the role of bacterial vaginosis in spontaneous preterm delivery was known at the time, none of the antibiotics used (co-amoxiclav and erythromycin) is sufficiently effective against bacterial vaginosis organisms. The investigators were reported to have performed over 400 statistical analyses, each analysis with a 5% chance of a spurious finding. When all randomized women are included in the analyses, there were no statistically significant reductions in the primary outcome, or any of its components, for any of the comparisons, in either trial [30], and the key findings derived from a previously unspecified subgroup analysis of women with pPROM may be due to chance [30].

Widespread use of broad-spectrum antibacterial drugs may lead to the emergence of antibiotic-resistant organisms. There had been an increase in erythromycin-resistant organisms even in the years leading up to the publication of the ORACLE trial [31–33]. This trend was attributed to increased use of erythromycin for prophylaxis against Group B streptococcus for women who were allergic to penicillin, and is likely to escalate with its increased use for pPROM. Broad-spectrum antibiotics may eliminate protective commensal flora, especially in the gut, encourage antimicrobial resistance and the emergence of unusual and more pathogenic species. Furthermore, early-life exposures are recognized as an important factor in the immunological health of children. It has been suggested that the significant rise in childhood allergy in developed countries may be related to abnormal initial gut colonization of infants as a result of obstetric and neonatal practices including antibiotic exposure [34].

Routine antibiotic therapy presumes an infectious aetiology, lacks guidance from microbiological cultures and sensitivity, and is based on the belief that antibiotics somehow prevent or reverse fetal damage. A significant number of fetus–mother pairs whose pPROM were unrelated to infection may be exposed to broad-spectrum antibiotics. At present, no studies have yet examined the risk versus benefit equation of mass antibiotic therapy for pPROM.

Tocolysis

Tocolysis may be applied prophylactically to prevent the onset of uterine contractions and labour in women with pPROM, or used therapeutically to abolish uterine contractions and labour after pPROM. Randomized trials of prophylactic administration of tocolysis did not show a prolongation of pregnancy in women with pPROM nor a reduction in perinatal morbidity and mortality [35,36]. Randomized trials [37,38] and case control studies [39] of therapeutic tocolysis consistently show that this approach did not prolong pregnancy or reduce perinatal morbidity or mortality. Therefore, the use of tocolysis should be individualized and restricted to those situations where there is no clinical or biochemical evidence of infection and a course of corticosteroids needed to be completed, or to allow the transfer of the woman to a tertiary centre. The choice of a tocolytic agent in this setting is a matter for local guidelines. The efficacies of the available agents on the market are broadly similar. The β-adrenoceptor agonists have become less popular because of their marked cardiovascular side effects.

Antenatal corticosteroids administration

Initial concerns that corticosteroids may increase the risks of chorioamnionitis, postpartum endometritis, and neonatal sepsis are not supported by current evidence. A meta-analysis of 15 randomized controlled trials including over 1400 women with pPROM showed that antenatal steroids did not increase the risk of maternal RR 0.86; 95% CI (0.61–1.20) or neonatal infectious morbidity, RR 1.05; 95% CI (0.66–1.68) [40]. On the other hand, it showed that antenatal steroids reduced the risks of respiratory distress syndrome, RR 0.56; 95% CI (0.46–0.70), intraventricular haemorrhage, RR 0.47; 95% CI (0.31–0.70), and necrotizing enterocolitis RR 0.21; 95% CI (0.05–0.82) [40]. Taken together, these substantial reductions in the risk of major gestational age-related morbidity translate to a significant reduction in neonatal mortality. The data are scanty on whether when using the same dose of corticosteroid, this magnitude of benefit may also accrue for twins and other higher-order pregnancies with pPROM, because of greater maternal volume of distribution. In diabetic women, the administration of corticosteroids may result in the loss of glycaemic control. The risk of this has to be carefully balanced with the potential benefit. Therefore, the value of steroid administration is questionable for women with pPROM near term, for example ≥32–34 weeks, or in whom fetal lung maturation can be demonstrated. Below 32 completed weeks of gestation, consideration should be given for sliding scale insulin/glucose infusion for 48–96 h during the course of antenatal prophylactic steroid. Intramuscular betamethasone 12 mg, 24 h apart is preferable to dexamethasone 12 mg, 12 h apart. Betamethasone has a stronger evidence base and, unlike dexamethasone, it is not associated with necrotizing enterocolitis.

Group B streptococcal colonization and pPROM

Approximately 20–30% of pregnant women are group B streptococcus (GBS) carriers, with higher rates of colonization in Black compared to White or Asian women [41]. It is fairly common for women with pPROM to be colonized by GBS. Their babies are at risk of ascending or established intrauterine GBS infection, sepsis, death, or intrapartum fetal distress. Very rarely, GBS may be vertically transmitted to the fetus from the mother via the haematogenous route. In this setting, the mother is usually very unwell with GBS sepsis, which may be isolated from her blood cultures. Histopathological examination of the placenta will show villitis rather than the predominant polymorphonuclear cell infiltration of the extraplacental membranes observed in the case of GBS ascending infection. Regardless of whether the fetal infection is of the ascending or haematogenous type, the risk of perinatal death or long-term sequelae is inversely related to gestational age. For optimal detection of GBS, a recto-vaginal or vagino-perineal swab inoculated into a selective medium should be obtained [42]. If conservative management is planned following pPROM and the woman is colonized by GBS, consideration should be given to eradication of the GBS with benzyl penicillin for 24–48 h if appropriate sampling and selective subculture techniques can be applied; otherwise treat for 5 days. Within 5–6 weeks there is a 5–10% chance of recolonization, and the treatment may be reconsidered. For women who are allergic to penicillin, clindamycin or erythromycin should be used, but sensitivity studies should be undertaken, as GBS strains displaying resistance to these antibiotics are on the increase. During labour intrapartum, antibiotic prophylaxis should be offered.

The role of amniocentesis

Studies of amniocentesis in pPROM women show that up to 40% will have positive amniotic fluid cultures at presentation, with the proportion increasing with latency. More recent studies using DNA amplification techniques have shown higher rates of amniotic fluid colonization by a variety of organisms. Women with established intrauterine infection deliver soon after pPROM and before amniocentesis can be performed, weakening the accuracy of prevalence studies of intra-amniotic fluid infection and pPROM. Other studies have defined intra-amniotic infection using low glucose levels, elevated polymorphs, inflammatory cytokines including IL-6, IL-8 or TNF-α, and viral proteins and footprints. Amniocentesis and/or cordocentesis are powerful tools in distinguishing pPROM cases with intra-amniotic infection from non-infected cases. However, the isolation of micro-organisms from the amniotic fluid does not equate infection. It is fetal host inflammatory response rather than mere amniotic fluid colonization or maternal response that is correlated with adverse neonatal outcome. The characterization of cases complicated by infection is critically important because amniotic fluid infection is associated with a shorter latency and a higher risk of adverse neonatal and childhood outcomes, including respiratory distress syndrome, neonatal sepsis, chronic lung disease, periventricular leukomalacia, intraventricular haemorrhage and mortality.

Amniocentesis, culture of amniotic fluid and determination of the presence or absence of fetal host response may allow clinicians to select and triage cases for conservative or aggressive management. There is no evidence, however, that characterization of the amniotic fluid inflammatory status to guide management improved perinatal outcome. The timing of fetal injury is unknown, and it is plausible that by the time women present with pPROM, it is already too late to reverse established inflammatory cascade. Although ampicillin and/or erythromycin therapy delayed preterm delivery, and reduced maternal and neonatal morbidity, the exact mechanism(s) through which antibiotics exerted these beneficial effects are unknown. Candidate mechanistic hypotheses include the eradication of intrauterine infection, reduction/prevention of host inflammatory response, or prevention of ascending infection from the lower genital tract. Gomez and colleagues addressed the question of whether antibiotic administration to the mother eradicated intra-amniotic infection and/or reduced the frequency of intrauterine inflammation [43]. The authors studied the microbiologic and inflammatory profiles of the amniotic fluid of 541 women with pPROM admitted to their institution over a period of just under 5 years. Of the 541 women, 481 (88.9%) delivered within 5 days. Antibiotics (ceftriaxone, clindamycin and erythromycin for 10–14 days {iv. for 48 h and oral thereafter}) and corticosteroid therapy were initiated from 24 weeks' gestation if there was evidence of microbial invasion of the amniotic cavity (MIAC) or inflammation. Antibiotic therapy was initiated before 24 weeks' gestation if there was evidence of MIAC, but without steroid administration. If there was no evidence of MIAC or inflammation, ampicillin and erythromycin were administered for 7 days (iv. for 48 h and oral thereafter). Tocolysis was not used in patient management. Of the 60 women who remained undelivered, 46 had a second amniocentesis after 5 days. Patients with intra-amniotic inflammation had a lower median gestational age at admission and at delivery than those without intra-amniotic inflammation. The prevalence of intra-amniotic inflammation was 39% (18/46) before antibiotic treatment and increased to 53% (24/45) after antibiotic therapy. The prevalence of a positive amniotic fluid culture was 15% (7/46) at the first amniocentesis, increasing to 28% (13/46) at the second amniocentesis, after completion of antibiotic therapy. Of 7 patients with positive amniotic fluid culture for micro-organisms at first amniocentesis, 6 (86%) had persistent positive amniotic fluid culture after antibiotic treatment, while a positive amniotic fluid culture was found in 18% (7/39) of cases with negative amniotic fluid culture at admission. Of 18 patients with intra-amniotic inflammation, 3 (17%) did not have evidence of inflammation after antibiotic therapy. Among 28 patients without intra-amniotic inflammation at admission, 9 (32%) developed inflammation, despite antibiotic treatment. Five of these women also had positive amniotic fluid culture [43].

This study showed that antibiotic treatment very rarely eradicated MIAC in patients with pPROM. An overwhelming 86% of pPROM patients with positive amniotic fluid culture and 83% with intra-amniotic inflammation maintained the same microbiologic/inflammatory profile, respectively, despite aggressive antibiotic therapy for 10–14 days. This is consistent with data that showed poor transplacental transfer of macrolide antibiotics [44]. Therefore, if antibiotic therapy genuinely reduced neonatal complications in pregnancies with pPROM, it is unlikely to be as a result of the eradication of MIAC or attenuation of the host inflammatory response. Also disturbing is the study's findings that women with negative amniotic fluid culture or inflammation at admission developed MIAC despite antibiotic therapy. The authors speculated that routine antibiotic therapy currently recommended for pPROM patients may be exerting its beneficial effects by preventing ascending infection or the development of fetal systemic inflammatory syndrome (FSIRS). Both of these suggestions are unlikely. Firstly, their data suggested that almost 90% of women admitted with pPROM delivered within the first 5 days, suggesting that in the majority of cases infection/inflammation may be so established that delivery was imminent. In the undelivered group, the infection may be localized within the choriodecidual interface, where it may provoke pPROM but give a false negative amniocentesis, which might explain, at least in part, the higher prevalence of positive amniotic fluid culture and inflammation at the second amniocentesis. Secondly, although both clindamycin and erythromycin exhibit anti-inflammatory properties, there is no evidence that these antibiotics reach the fetal compartment in sufficient amounts to alter its host inflammatory response. The

timing of initiation of antibiotic therapy may be important in determining the outcome. In a rabbit model of ascending intrauterine infection, antibiotic administration within 12 h of inoculation, but not after 18 h, reduced the rate of preterm delivery and increased neonatal survival [45]. Such a near precise timing of the onset of intrauterine infection is impossible in human pregnancy. Neither our group [46] nor others [47] demonstrated a reduction in the frequency of histologic chorioamnionitis in randomized trials of antibiotic administration early in the second trimester in women at risk of chorioamnionitis, suggesting that even a pre-emptive antibiotic therapy earlier in pregnancy does not prevent histologic chorioamnionitis.

Conclusions

- Preterm prelabour rupture of membranes accounts for over a third of preterm deliveries and is an independent risk factor for adverse fetal and neonatal outcome.
- Erythromycin and/or ampicillin is currently recommended for pPROM, although a significant proportion of pPROM cases are unrelated to infection, and antibiotic therapy may be raising their risks.
- Further research is needed to define the natural history of intrauterine infection and what subset of fetuses benefit from the use of antibiotic therapy.
- Conservative management should be adopted if pPROM occurred prior to 34 weeks and delivery undertaken at or greater than 34 weeks' gestation.

References

1. Cotton D B, Hill L M, Strassner H T, Platt L D, Ledger W J. Use of amniocentesis in preterm gestation with ruptured membranes. *Obstet Gynecol* 1984; **63**: 38–43.

2. Mercer B M, Goldenberg R L, Moawad A H, *et al.* The preterm prediction study: effect of gestational age and cause of preterm birth on subsequent obstetric outcome. *Am J Obstet Gynecol* 1999; **181**: 1216–21.

3. McGregor J A, Schoonmaker J N, Lunt B D, Lawellin D W. Antibiotic inhibition of bacterially induced fetal membrane weakening. *Obstet Gynecol* 1990; **76**: 124–8.

4. Parry S, Strauss J F, III. Premature rupture of the fetal membranes. *N Engl J Med* 1998; **338**: 663–70.

5. Bryant-Greenwood G D, Millar L K. Human fetal membranes: their preterm premature rupture. *Biol Reprod* 2000; **63**: 1575–9.

6. Cooperstock M S, Tummaru R, Bakewell J, Schramm W. Twin birth weight discordance and risk of preterm birth. *Am J Obstet Gynecol* 2000; **183**: 63–7.

7. Fortunato S J, Menon R, Bryant C, Lombardi S J. Programmed cell death (apoptosis) as a possible pathway to metalloproteinase activation and fetal membrane degradation in premature rupture of membranes. *Am J Obstet Gynecol* 2000; **182**: 1468–76.

8. Fortunato S J, Menon R, Lombardi S J. MMP/TIMP imbalance in amniotic fluid during PROM: an indirect support for endogenous pathway to membrane rupture. *J Perinat Med* 1999; **27**: 362–8.

9. Barrett B M, Sowell A, Gunter E, Wang M. Potential role of ascorbic acid and beta-carotene in the prevention of preterm rupture of fetal membranes. *Int J Vitam Nutr Res* 1994; **64**: 192–7.

10. Barrett B, Gunter E, Jenkins J, Wang M. Ascorbic acid concentration in amniotic fluid in late pregnancy. *Biol Neonate* 1991; **60**: 333–5.

11. Friedman M L, McElin T W. Diagnosis of ruptured fetal membranes. Clinical study and review of the literature. *Am J Obstet Gynecol* 1969; **104**: 544–50.

12. Gaucherand P, Guibaud S, Awada A, Rudigoz R C. Comparative study of three amniotic fluid markers in premature rupture of membranes: fetal fibronectin, alpha-fetoprotein, diamino-oxydase. *Acta Obstet Gynecol Scand* 1995; **74**: 118–21.

13. Rutanen E M, Pekonen F, Karkkainen T. Measurement of insulin-like growth factor binding protein-1 in cervical/vaginal secretions: comparison with the ROM-check Membrane Immunoassay in the diagnosis of ruptured fetal membranes. *Clin Chim Acta* 1993; **214**: 73–81.

14. Carroll S G, Papaioannou S, Nicolaides K H. Assessment of fetal activity and amniotic fluid volume in the prediction of intrauterine infection in preterm prelabor amniorrhexis. *Am J Obstet Gynecol* 1995; **175**: 1427–35.

15. Alexander J M, Mercer B M, Miodovnik M, *et al.* The impact of digital cervical examination on expectantly managed preterm rupture of membranes. *Am J Obstet Gynecol* 2000; **183**: 1003–7.

16. Lewis D F, Major C A, Towers C V, Asrat T, Harding J A, Garite T J. Effects of digital vaginal examinations on latency period in preterm premature rupture of membranes. *Obstet Gynecol* 1992; **80**: 630–4.

17. Romero R, Sirtori M, Oyarzun E, *et al.* Infection and labor. V. Prevalence, microbiology, and clinical significance of intraamniotic infection in women with preterm labor and intact membranes. *Am J Obstet Gynecol* 1989; **161**: 817–24.

18. De Felice C, Toti P, Laurini R N, *et al.* Early neonatal brain injury in histologic chorioamnionitis. *J Pediatr* 2001; **138**: 101–4.

19. Carroll S G, Papaioannou S, Nicolaides K H. Doppler studies of the placental and fetal circulation in pregnancies with preterm prelabor amniorrhexis. *Ultrasound Obstet Gynecol* 1995; **5**: 184–8.

20. Lewis D F, Adair C D, Weeks J W, Barrilleaux P S, Edwards M S, Garite T J. A randomized clinical trial of daily nonstress testing versus biophysical profile in the management of preterm premature rupture of membranes. *Am J Obstet Gynecol* 1999; **181**: 1495–9.

21. Naef R W, III, Allbert J R, Ross E L, Weber B M, Martin R W, Morrison J C. Premature rupture of membranes at 34 to 37 weeks' gestation: aggressive versus conservative management. *Am J Obstet Gynecol* 1998; **178**: 126–30.

22. Grable I A. Cost-effectiveness of induction after preterm premature rupture of the membranes. *Am J Obstet Gynecol* 2002; **187**: 1153–8.

23. Kenyon S, Boulvain M, Neilson J. Antibiotics for preterm rupture of the membranes: a systematic review. *Obstet Gynecol* 2004; **104**: 1051–7.

24. Mercer B M, Miodovnik M, Thurnau G R, *et al.* Antibiotic therapy for reduction of infant morbidity after preterm premature rupture of the membranes. A randomized controlled trial. *J Am Med Assoc* 1997; **278**: 989–95.

25. Egarter C, Leitich H, Karas H, *et al.* Antibiotic treatment in preterm premature rupture of membranes and neonatal morbidity: a metaanalysis. *Am J Obstet Gynecol* 1996; **174**: 589–97.

26. Mercer B M. Antibiotic therapy for preterm premature rupture of membranes. *Clin Obstet Gynecol* 1998; **41**: 461–8.

27. Kenyon S L, Taylor D J, Tarnow-Mordi W. Broad-spectrum antibiotics for preterm, prelabour rupture of fetal membranes: the ORACLE I randomised trial. ORACLE Collaborative Group. *Lancet* 2001; **357**: 979–88.

28. Kenyon S L, Taylor D J, Tarnow M. Broad-spectrum antibiotics for spontaneous preterm labour: the ORACLE II randomised trial. ORACLE Collaborative Group. *Lancet* 2001; **357**: 989–94.

29. Kenyon S, Taylor D J. The effect of the publication of a major clinical trial in a high impact journal on clinical practise: the ORACLE Trial experience. *Br J Obstet Gynaecol* 2002; **109**: 1341–3.

30. Hannah M. Antibiotics for preterm prelabour rupture of membranes and preterm labour? *Lancet* 2001; **357**: 973–4.

31. Manning S D, Foxman B, Pierson C L, Tallman P, Baker C J, Pearlman M D. Correlates of antibiotic-resistant group B streptococcus isolated from pregnant women. *Obstet Gynecol* 2003; **101**: 74–9.

32. Manning S D, Pearlman M D, Tallman P, Pierson C L, Foxman B. Frequency of antibiotic resistance among group B Streptococcus isolated from healthy college students. *Clin Infect Dis* 2001; **33**: E137–9.

33. Pearlman M D, Pierson C L, Faix R G. Frequent resistance of clinical group B streptococci isolates to clindamycin and erythromycin. *Obstet Gynecol* 1998; **92**: 258–61.

34. Murch S H. Toll of allergy reduced by probiotics. *Lancet* 2001; **375**: 1057–9.

35. How H Y, Cook V D, Miles D E, Spinnato J A. Preterm prelabour rupture of membranes: aggressive tocolysis versus expectant management. *J Mat Fetal Med* 1998; **7**: 8–12.

36. Levy D L, Warsof S L. Oral ritodrine and preterm premature rupture of membranes. *Obstet Gynecol* 1985; **66**: 621–3.

37. Weiner C P, Renk K, Klugman M. The therapeutic efficacy and cost-effectiveness of aggressive tocolysis for premature labor associated with premature rupture of the membranes. *Am J Obstet Gynecol* 1988; **159**: 216–22.

38. Garite T J, Keegan K A, Freeman R K, Nageotte M P. A randomized trial of ritodrine tocolysis versus expectant management in patients with premature rupture of membranes at 25 to 30 weeks of gestation. *Am J Obstet Gynecol* 1987; **157**: 388–93.

39. Combs, McCiene M, Clark R, Fishman A. Aggressive tocolysis does not prolong pregnancy or reduce neonatal morbidity after preterm premature rupture of membranes. *Am J Obstet Gynecol* 2004; **190**: 1723–8.

40. Harding J E, Pang J, Knight D B, Liggins G C. Do antenatal corticosteroids help in the setting of preterm rupture of membranes? *Am J Obstet Gynecol* 2001; **184**: 131–9.

41. Regan J A, Klebanoff M A, Nugent R P. The epidemiology of group B streptococcal colonization in pregnancy. Vaginal Infections and Prematurity Study Group. *Obstet Gynecol* 1991; **77**: 604–10.

42. Jamie W E, Edwards R K, Duff P. Vaginal–perianal compared with vaginal–rectal cultures for identification of group B streptococci. *Obstet Gynecol* 2004; **104**: 1058–61.

43. Gomez R, Romero R, Nien J K, et al. Antibiotic administration to patients with preterm premature rupture of membranes does not eradicate intra-amniotic infection. *J Matern Fetal Neonatal Med* 2007; **20**: 167–73.

44. Witt A, Sommer E, Cichna M, et al. Placental passage of clarithromycin surpasses other macrolide antibiotics. *Am J Obstet Gynecol* 2003; **188**: 816–9.

45. Fidel P, Ghezzi F, Romero R, et al. The effect of antibiotic therapy on intrauterine infection-induced preterm parturition in rabbits. *J Matern Fetal Neonatal Med* 2003; **14**: 57–64.

46. Ugwumadu A, Reid F, Hay P, Manyonda I, Jeffrey I. Oral clindamycin and histologic chorioamnionitis in women with abnormal vaginal flora. *Obstet Gynecol* 2006; **107**: 863–8.

47. Goldenberg R L, Mwatha A, Read J S, et al. The HPTN 024 Study: the efficacy of antibiotics to prevent chorioamnionitis and preterm birth. *Am J Obstet Gynecol* 2006; **194**: 650–61.

Chapter 20

Preterm labour and delivery

Sarah L. Bell and Jane E. Norman

Introduction

Preterm birth is the single most important factor affecting perinatal outcomes in terms of morbidity and mortality. Preterm labour is defined by WHO [1] as the onset of regular uterine contractions, between viability and 37 weeks' gestation, associated with cervical effacement and dilatation. Current guidelines from the British Association of Perinatal Medicine [2] describe a 'threshold of viability' between 22 and 26 weeks; thus preterm birth occurs between 22–26 weeks and 37 weeks' gestation. Up to 30–40% of cases of preterm birth are iatrogenic due to deliberate induction of labour or prelabour caesarean section for conditions causing maternal or fetal compromise. Some of these conditions are listed in Table 20.1 [3].

The remainder of the cases of preterm birth follow spontaneous preterm labour, with or without preterm prelabour membrane rupture, and the initiating factors are the subject of much scientific interest and debate. In this chapter we will discuss the important aspects of preterm labour and highlight areas of scientific interest.

Epidemiology

The incidence of preterm birth in the developed world is thought to have increased over the past decade, with an estimated annual incidence of 10–15% of all live births [4]. There are a number of possible explanations for this. Rates of multiple births have risen in recent years due to advances in assisted conception techniques such as IVF. There have also been increased rates of obstetric intervention at very early gestations and major developments in the resuscitation and care of very premature babies in specialist neonatal intensive care. Furthermore, changes in the registration of

births will have an effect on the rates of preterm birth, as those babies that would have been previously classified as stillborn are now often classified as live births.

However, there are some discrepancies in the current statistics provided on preterm birth. A study by Balchin et al. [5] showed that many hospitals in London had inaccurately recorded the gestation at birth by rounding up the gestational age to the nearest week, therefore resulting in up to 10% of babies being incorrectly classified. The most recent statistics for preterm birth in England and Wales are from the National Office of Statistics [6]. In 2005 there were 626,924 recorded singleton live births, with 38,593 singleton births (6.2%) between 22 and 36 weeks. In addition, there were 18,776 multiple births with 9876 (53%) born between 22 and 36 weeks (Table 20.2). These statistics show that 6.2% of singleton births in England and Wales were premature, which is similar to the rates of premature delivery in other developed countries. Statistics showing the rates of preterm birth in the UK prior to 2005 are limited. A recent population-based study from Denmark [7] showed a 22% increase in the rates of preterm birth between 1995 and 2004. Low-risk primiparous women in 2004 were found to have double the risk of preterm birth than those in 1995. The incidence of risk factors such as IVF and multiple pregnancy were also found to have increased. Scottish data collated from the same period have also shown an 11% increase in rates of preterm birth [8].

Sequelae of preterm birth

Rates of perinatal morbidity and mortality increase with decreased gestational age at birth, although there is considerable variation between gestations. Perinatal outcomes between 32 weeks and term are quite similar, whereas those infants born before 32 weeks have

Table 20.1 Maternal and fetal conditions resulting in iatrogenic preterm birth.

Mother	Fetus
Severe pre-eclampsia	Fetal distress
Eclampsia	Severe IUGR
Antepartum haemorrhage	
Placenta praevia (Grade 3/4)	

Table 20.2 Number of live births registered in England and Wales in 2005 (with percentage of all live single and multiple births shown in brackets). Adapted from National Office of Statistics data.

Gestational age (weeks)	Singleton births	Multiple births
<22	279 (0.0%)	51 (0.3%)
22–27	2,307 (0.4%)	648 (3.5%)
28–36	36,286 (5.8%)	9,228 (49.5%)
37–41	556,136 (89.3%)	8,676 (46.5%)
42+	27,730 (4.5%)	40 (0.2%)
Unknown	4,186	133

a poorer outcome. The EPICure study [9] looked at survival trends and health outcomes of very premature infants born under 26 weeks in the UK and Ireland. This study showed increased survival and lower rates of severe or moderate disability with each additional week of gestation. The more recent Trent health region study [10] also produced similar results on survival rates and rates of discharge home, but did not investigate the long-term sequelae. The EPICure 2 study, which began in 2006, should provide even more up-to-date information on the survival of very premature babies and the outcomes of neonatal facilities. Adverse outcomes in terms of morbidity include respiratory distress syndrome, necrotizing enterocolitis, jaundice, retinopathy of prematurity, and neonatal hypoglycaemia [11]. These problems often lead to profound long-term disabilities, which have many social and psychological implications on the child and their family. Long-term problems include cerebral palsy, deafness, visual impairment, developmental delay, and bronchopulmonary dysplasia [12]. It is therefore paramount that preterm labour is diagnosed early in order to allow time for management interventions, such as antenatal corticosteroids, to reduce the incidence of perinatal problems.

Current concepts in the pathophysiology of preterm labour

The exact initiating factors in preterm birth are the subject of much scientific interest and debate. Developing adequate strategies to prevent preterm birth requires thorough understanding of the mechanisms which cause it. Unfortunately, these exact mechanisms remain a mystery. It is possible that the causes of preterm labour are similar to those in term labour, but initiated earlier; an alternative explanation is that some or all cases of preterm birth arise from specific mechanisms, such as intrauterine infection and inflammation.

The onset of both term and preterm labour is preceded by cervical ripening, uterine contractions and occasionally rupture of the membranes. Current evidence suggests that mediators of the inflammatory cascade such as cytokines are important in initiating all three of these processes [13]. Cytokines are small, extracellular proteins involved in cellular communication and help mediate the immune response to infection and inflammation. Interleukin-6 (IL-6), IL-8 and tumour necrosis factor alpha (TNF-α) induce cervical ripening and effacement by activating elastinases and matrix metalloproteinases. They also increase production of cyclooxygenase (COX) 2 and prostaglandin E2 (PGE$_2$), which are both potent stimulators of cervical dilatation. These cytokines increase the production of enzymes responsible for collagen degradation, which results in rupture of the fetal membranes. IL-6 also increases the expression of oxytocin receptors in the myometrium. Co-ordination of cytokine regulation and production is thought to be by transmembrane Toll-like receptors expressed at the materno-fetal interface [14].

The hypothalamic–pituitary–adrenal (HPA) axis is important in the regulation and maintenance of pregnancy. In animal models, withdrawal of progesterone during pregnancy results in the onset of labour. This theory provides the rationale behind the current therapeutic use of progesterone to prevent preterm labour. Around the time of onset of labour, the fetal pituitary increases production of corticotrophin-releasing hormone (CRH). This, coupled with a decrease in placental production of 15-OH prostaglandin dehydrogenase, results in raised levels of cortisol, which stimulates intrauterine prostaglandin production and promotes cervical effacement and myometrial contractility [15].

It is likely that there are many other factors important in the initiation of preterm labour. Genetics

217

may also play a role in preterm labour and delivery, and some women may have a genetic predisposition which increases their likelihood of early delivery [16].

Risk factors for preterm labour

There have been a number of factors identified which increase the risk of spontaneous preterm birth. Identification of these risk factors during pregnancy may help to find those women at risk of preterm labour, and allow increased surveillance and early management of complications.

Obstetric history

The most important factor increasing the risk of preterm birth is a previous preterm delivery. This is thought to be due to underlying cervical insufficiency. The Preterm Prediction Study [17] showed that the risk of preterm birth increases twofold with every subsequent preterm delivery. A more recent study in 2007 [18] showed that women with a previous second-trimester loss were 10 times more likely to deliver preterm than those with a previous full-term delivery. This means that the outcome of the last pregnancy is important in predicting the success of the next. Other factors which can affect cervical competence, which leads to preterm birth, include previous cervical trauma such as cone biopsy, or cervical instrumentation and forced dilatation, such as after termination of pregnancy.

Uterine overdistension as a result of multiple pregnancy or polyhydramnios also increases the risk of preterm labour. The rates of IVF are increasing, and this accounts for the rise in multiple pregnancies; however, even with correction for multiple pregnancies, women who have undergone IVF are still at an increased risk of preterm labour compared with the rest of the population.

Infection

Genital tract infections such as bacterial vaginosis and chlamydia trachomatis have been shown to increase the rates of preterm labour. Bacterial vaginosis results from repopulation of the normal vaginal flora with *Gardnerella vaginalis*, *Mobiluncus*, *Bacteroides* and *Mycoplasma*. Chlamydia is caused by the bacterium *Chlamydia trachomatis* and is often asymptomatic. Women infected with chlamydia are at three times the risk of preterm labour compared with the normal population [19]. Women with bacterial vaginosis in early pregnancy are also at a much higher risk of preterm delivery. In particular, women diagnosed with bacterial vaginosis before 16 weeks' gestation are at seven times the risk than those without the infection [20]. Ascending infection from the genital tract can result in intrauterine infection and chorioamnionitis. This is one of the most likely mechanisms. Other modes of infection include transplacental and transfallopian infection from the peritoneal cavity. Causative organisms of ascending infection include *Chlamydia* species, Group B streptococcus, mycoplasmas and gonnorrhoea. Chorioamnionitis is thought to cause preterm premature rupture of the membranes (pPROM) by stimulating the production of bacterial byproducts, such as proteases and collagenases, which degrade the fetal membranes causing them to rupture. This causes preterm premature membrane rupture, itself an antecedent of preterm labour in approximately 40% of babies born preterm. The resulting inflammation can initiate a cascade which may result in myometrial contractions and subsequent preterm birth.

Other maternal infections resulting in a systemic inflammatory response may also be responsible for initiating preterm labour, including pyelonephritis and pneumonia. In the developing world, malaria is an important cause of preterm labour and accounts for 200,000 preterm births per year, along with HIV and tuberculosis [21].

Demographics

There are a number of demographic factors which increase the likelihood of preterm birth. The Preterm Prediction Study in 1998 showed that women with a prepregnancy Body Mass Index (BMI) of lower than 19 are at a higher risk of preterm birth than those with a normal prepregnancy BMI [22]. The reasons for this are unclear and may be related to maternal nutritional status affecting fetal nutrition and growth. The same study showed that race also plays a role in increasing the risk of preterm labour. Women from African or Caribbean origin are at a higher risk of preterm birth than Caucasian women.

Psychosocial factors

Socioeconomic factors play a significant role in increasing the risk of preterm delivery. Studies have shown that factors such as low social class, social isolation and poverty all affect the rates of preterm delivery, along with alcohol and drug abuse [23,24]. These lifestyle factors coupled with other psychological strains, such as stress, domestic abuse and depression, contribute to the increased risk.

Long-term prediction of preterm labour

Fetal fibronectins

Fetal fibronectins are extracellular matrix proteins located at the choriodecidual junction and are secreted by the trophoblast to facilitate adhesion of fetal membranes to the decidua [25]. Fetal fibronectins are detectable in the cervico-vaginal secretions up to 22 weeks, and are also detectable just prior to the onset of labour. They are rarely detectable between 24 and 34 weeks unless there has been disruption to the decidua or inflammation of the chorion.

A positive fetal fibronectin test is considered to be greater than 50 ng/ml [26]. Current bedside testing involves the use of an immunoassay technique where a sample of cervico-vaginal secretions is obtained via speculum examination and placed into a tube containing extraction buffer. The test strip is then placed into the buffer. This strip contains polyclonal antifetal fibronectin antibody. This antibody, also known as FDC-6, recognizes a specific region (III-CS) on the fetal fibronectin isoform. Therefore if fetal fibronectin is present in the sample, the antibody will bind to it, and produce a visible positive result on the test strip.

Many studies have evaluated the role of fetal fibronectin testing in predicting preterm birth both in asymptomatic and symptomatic populations. A positive fetal fibronectin (FfN) test is associated with an increased likelihood of birth before 34 weeks' gestation within 14 days of the test [27,28]. However, the positive predictive value of the test is only 16%. Fetal fibronectin testing appears to be most useful in symptomatic women with intact membranes as a negative predictive test to exclude a diagnosis of preterm labour. Large multicentre trials have shown that if the test is negative, less than 1% of women will deliver within the next 14 days [29,30]. Therefore, fetal fibronectin testing has been used in many obstetric centres to aid in the diagnosis of preterm labour and avoid unnecessary admission and treatment. The test has also been shown to be useful in excluding preterm

labour in symptomatic twin gestations with a negative predictive value of 97% [31]. As for singleton pregnancies, the positive predictive value is low.

The test appears to be most useful at 24–34 weeks' gestation in women with intact membranes, cervical dilatation less than 3 cm and access to a rapid result. A recent study in New Zealand evaluated the routine use of FfN testing in clinical practice. A negative result was associated with lower rates of admission, fewer healthcare-associated costs, and less use of corticosteroids and tocolytics [32]. However, studies in other environments have been less convincing, and further work is required in this area.

Cervical length

Shortening and effacement of the cervix is diagnostic of preterm labour. In the past, digital vaginal examination was relied on to assess the degree of activity in the cervix and to diagnose preterm labour. Cervical length can be accurately measured using transvaginal ultrasound scanning, which is preferable to transabdominal scanning where measurements are limited by bladder size and false elongation of the cervix.

There is considerable evidence that in asymptomatic populations, the shorter the cervical length measurement, the higher the risk of preterm birth. Cervical length appears to follow a bell curve distribution with biological variation in cervical length. The 50th percentile at 24–28 weeks' gestation is approximately 35 mm. A cervical length of less than 25 mm, which equates to the 10th percentile, is associated with a sixfold increase in the rate of preterm birth when detected at 22–24 weeks' gestation [33]. In low-risk populations, cervical length measurement at 24–28 weeks' gestation has a low sensitivity for predicting preterm birth. Like FfN testing, the value of the test is in its negative predictive value. In twin pregnancies at 24 weeks where the cervical length measurement is over 35 mm, only a small number of women will deliver before 35 weeks [34].

Inflammatory markers

There is no doubt that women with bacterial vaginosis have a higher chance of preterm delivery. Women at high risk of preterm birth treated for bacterial vaginosis with antibiotics are less likely to have preterm prelabour rupture of the membranes and to deliver preterm [35]. What is unclear is the value of screening and treating populations which are at low risk, i.e. asymptomatic, during early pregnancy. Recent studies treating low-risk populations screened for bacterial vaginosis with metronidazole or clindamycin failed to show a reduction in rates of preterm birth [36,37]. In addition, treatment of low-risk populations with metronidazole in early pregnancy may increase the rates of preterm delivery. In the PREMET study, the trial was stopped early because 62% of women treated with metronidazole delivered before 37 weeks compared to 39% of women in the placebo group [38].

Risk scoring systems

Risk scoring systems aim to identify those at high risk of preterm labour. They use primary predictors, i.e. variables which are present prepregnancy, such as previous obstetric history, socioeconomic and demographic factors, or secondary predictors which only become apparent during the pregnancy, such as those described above. Unfortunately, many studies to date have failed to demonstrate the value of risk scoring systems in clinical practice. For example, the Preterm Prediction Study [14] assessed multiple risk factors for preterm labour in 2929 women at 23–24 weeks' gestation. This risk assessment only identified a minority of women who delivered preterm, and the positive predictive value of the test was only 28.6% in nulliparous and 33% in multiparous women. The combined use of FfN testing and ultrasound assessment of the cervix is more accurate in predicting preterm labour, and these tests will be discussed later.

Management of preterm labour

When preterm labour is suspected, accurate fetal and maternal assessment is essential. There are a number of plausable interventions, including antibiotics, tocolysis and steroids, which are indicated in certain cases of preterm labour. Ultimately, the aim is to reduce neonatal adverse outcomes associated with early delivery without increasing risks to the mother. Clinical assessment involves a full history, including risk factors for preterm labour, previous obstetric history and clinical examination. Vaginal examination is contra-indicated if preterm prelabour rupture of membranes (pPROM) is suspected to reduce the risk of intrauterine infection [39]. Fetal assessment of well-being includes methods such as cardiotogography and biophysical profiling.

Tocolysis

Treatment of preterm labour aims to reduce the high perinatal morbidity and mortality rates associated with early delivery. Tocolytic drugs aim to suppress uterine contractions and prolong the duration of pregnancy. Unfortunately, trials are yet to prove that tocolysis can have a major effect on the incidence of preterm birth or the incidence of adverse neonatal outcomes.

There are many tocolytic drugs currently in use worldwide, including ritodrine, nifedipine, atosiban, magnesium sulphate and indometacin. Current guidelines from the Royal College of Obstetricians and Gynaecologists [40] state that there is little evidence to advocate the use of tocolytic drugs, and therefore it is reasonable not to use them in clinical practice. However, they may be used to allow the administration of antenatal corticosteroids or to facilitate in-utero transfer to a specialist neonatal facility. There are four drugs licensed for tocolytic use in the UK [41]: atosiban, an oxytocin receptor antagonist; and ritodrine, salbutamol and turbutaline – all beta$_2$ agonists. Ritodrine is the most widely used drug, and in a meta-analysis of all randomized trials looking at tocolytic drugs versus placebo it has been shown to be effective in prolonging pregnancy at 24 h, 48 h and 7 days [42]. However, these trials failed to show a significant effect on rates of birth or overall outcome. In a more recent Cochrane review [43], trials comparing only betamimetics against placebo were assessed. Again, there was a reduction in the number of births at 48 h and 7 days, but there was no significant reduction in births before 37 weeks. There was also no significant reduction in perinatal death or rates of necrotizing enterocolitis. Ritodrine and other betamimetics are known to cause a number of troublesome and sometimes life-threatening adverse maternal side effects including nausea, tachycardia, tremor, headache, chest pain and pulmonary oedema [44]. Therefore current RCOG guidelines suggest using atosiban or nifedipine over beta-agonist alternatives. Atosiban has been shown to have a comparable effect to ritodrine, in terms of prolongation of pregnancy, without the maternal adverse effects [45]. Disadvantages include its mode of administration via intravenous infusion and its expensive cost, with one course of treatment retailing at approximately £240.

At present, nifedipine is unlicensed for use in the UK. To date there have been no placebo-controlled

Table 20.3 Number of deliveries at 24 h, 48 h, 7 days and 14 days postadministration of tocolytic agent ritodrine or nifedipine [46].

	24 h	48 h	7 days	14 days
Ritodrine group	22	29	45	52
Nifedipine group	11	21	36	43
P-value	0.006	0.03	0.009	0.005

trials assessing its efficacy. However, in 1997, a randomized trial comparing nifedipine and ritodrine showed improved neonatal outcome and delay in delivery with nifedipine [46]. In this study, 185 singleton pregnancies were randomized to receive either intravenous ritodrine or oral nifedipine. Outcomes measured were rates of delivery, maternal side effects and admission rates to neonatal intensive care. Delivery rates at 24 h, 48 h, 7 days and 14 days were significantly lower in the nifedipine group with fewer maternal side effects recorded (Table 20.3).

There were also fewer admissions to NICU in the nifedipine group (68.4%) compared to 82.1% of the ritodrine group. However, further studies comparing these two agents have been criticized regarding their research design and methodology.

Use of corticosteroids

Administration of corticosteroids during preterm labour was first introduced in the 1970s. Since then, a number of large, randomized controlled trials (RCTs) have shown that steroids reduce the rates of respiratory distress, intraventricular haemorrhage and necrotizing enterocolitis in premature neonates if administered antenatally.

Corticosteroids work by increasing neonatal production of surfactant by type 2 pneumocytes and improve the morphological structure of lung tissue by thinning the walls of the alveoli to improve gas exchange [47].

Crowley's analysis in 1995 [48] showed a significant reduction in rates of respiratory distress syndrome before 34 weeks gestation with equivocal evidence after 34 weeks and before 28 weeks. In terms of numbers needed to treat, 94 women at over 34 weeks gestation need to be treated to prevent 1 case of RDS, whereas at less than 34 weeks, 5 women need to be treated to prevent 1 case. Roberts and Dalziel's analysis from 2006 [42] reconfirmed the beneficial effects of antenatal corticosteroids, and showed a significant reduction in rates of RDS up to and including 36 weeks.

Corticosteroids are indicated between 24 and 36 weeks in women presenting with preterm labour, antepartum haemorrhage, pPROM, or elective preterm delivery. The value of corticosteroids is limited in the treatment of choriamnionitis and maternal systemic infection, as it is often inappropriate to delay delivery. The optimal administration time is between 24 h and 7 days before delivery. Current recommendations from the RCOG are 2 doses of 12 mg betamethasone given IM 24 h apart [49]. Betamethasone has a lower risk of periventricular leukomalacia compared to dexamethasone [50]. The IM route is also recommended, as oral dosing has shown higher rates of neonatal sepsis and intraventricular haemorrhage. At present, multiple courses are not recommended due to concerns over adverse effects, such as growth problems and metabolic effects. At present, there is controversy regarding repeat administration of antenatal corticosteroids and long-term neurological effects. The current RCOG guidelines advise entering any patients being considered for repeated therapy into a randomized trial. A recently published trial[51] followed up 556 children after weekly IM administration of antenatal steroids between 23 and 31 weeks' gestation versus one repeat dose at 24 h. There was no significant difference in the physical outcomes of the children in both groups at 2 years. However, there were six cases of cerebral palsy in the weekly treatment group. A Cochrane review from 2003 also showed a reduction in the occurrence (RR 0.82) and severity (RR 0.60) of RDS with repeated doses of corticosteroids [52] (Table 20.4). Long-term follow-up showed lower rates of developmental delay and a trend towards lower rates of cerebral palsy in those treated with multiple courses of steroids. Further studies are warranted to assess the long-term outcomes of repeated administration of corticosteroids.

Antibiotics

Routine antibiotic use in preterm labour with intact membranes is not recommended. In the ORACLE I trial, 6295 women were randomized to receive erythromycin, co-amoxiclav or both in the treatment arm versus placebo [53]. Results showed there was no significant difference in the rates of neonatal death or lung disease, but antibiotic administration does prolong pregnancy and reduce maternal infection.

Table 20.4 Effects of corticosteroids on neonatal outcomes in terms of morbidity and mortality – a summary of all meta-analyses [60].

Neonatal outcomes	Relative risk	95% Confidence intervals
Neonatal death	0.69	0.58–0.81
Respiratory distress	0.66	0.59–0.73
Cerebroventricular haemorrhage	0.54	0.43–0.69
Necrotizing enterocolitis	0.46	0.29–0.74
Intensive care admissions	0.80	0.65–0.99
Systemic infection	0.56	0.38–0.85

Antibiotics are only indicated in women with preterm prelabour rupture of membranes to prevent neonatal and maternal infection, preterm delivery and chorioamnionitis. The Royal College of Obstetricians and Gynaecologists [34] currently recommend treating women with PPROM with 250 mg of Erythromycin 6 hourly for 10 days. Co-amoxiclav is not recommended, as the ORACLE trial showed increased rates of necrotizing enterocolitis in the babies of those women treated with it.

At 7- year follow-up, the ORACLE study showed an increased risk of functional impairment and cerebral palsy in those children whose mothers were given antibiotics with intact membranes.

Prevention of preterm labour

Progesterone

Progesterone is an essential hormone for the maintenance of early pregnancy by promoting uterine quiescence. Animal studies have shown that a reduction in circulating progesterone may be important in the initiation of labour. Whilst these findings have not been confirmed in women, there is still an interest in the role of progesterone in preventing preterm labour in humans. 17-Alpha-hydroxyprogesterone has been used in clinical trials since the 1970s to prevent preterm labour. Early meta-analyses had promising results with a reduction in the rates of preterm delivery; however, there was controversy surrounding the trial populations and outcomes. More recently, a large, multicentre trial by Meis *et al.* [54] administered progesterone or placebo to 463 women with a history of previous preterm birth. Results showed a reduction in delivery from 54.9% in the placebo group to 36.3% in the treatment group at 37 weeks with a similar reduction in delivery rates at 35 and 30 weeks. There was also a trend towards a reduction in adverse neonatal outcomes.

A Cochrane review from 2006 [55] looked at all trials where women were administered progesterone, and found a reduction in the risk of preterm birth in those women who were treated (RR at less than 37 weeks 0.65, RR at less than 34 weeks 0.15). There were also fewer babies born with a birth weight of less than 2500 kg; however, there was no significant reduction in perinatal death rates. Until a reduction in perinatal morbidity (and ideally mortality) is confirmed in randomized trials, the routine use of progesterone in clinical practice cannot be recommended.

At present, there is no evidence in the current literature to suggest any adverse effects from antenatal administration of progesterone. However, the results of further trials are awaited for further information on the efficacy of progesterone and the best mode of administration and dosage. We are involved in two such trials: STOPPIT (study of progesterone for the prevention of preterm birth in twins) and OPPTIMUM, which is a study of progesterone for the prevention of preterm birth in high-risk singletons, with follow up to the neonatal period.

Cervical cerclage

Cervical cerclage is often used in cases of cervical insufficiency where a suture is placed around the cervix to prevent dilatation. The exact mechanism of action in preventing cervical dilatation is unclear. There may be a mechanical effect preventing the cervical os opening, or cerclage may help to maintain a critical cervical length, therefore preventing ascending infection and activation of an inflammatory cascade which initiates labour. There are two approaches to placing the suture – transabdominal and transvaginal. There have been no randomized trials carried out which compare the two approaches. Transabdominal sutures are associated with more trauma to the mother and are usually reserved for cases were transvaginal cerclage is not possible. Transvaginal methods include the McDonald purse-string suture and the Shirodkar suture, which is more technically difficult to place and involves dissection of the vaginal mucosa. There appears to be no difference in the efficacy of both these techniques; however, the McDonald suture is often preferred, as it is technically easier to place. Cerclage is usually carried out between 12 and 14 weeks' gestation. Complications include bleeding, infection, initiation of contractions, pPROM and cervical scarring.

Unfortunately, the evidence for or against cerclage is unclear. The benefits of cerclage are well documented if there is a clear history of cervical incompetence, such as previous preterm births or mid trimester pregnancy losses, and an ultrasound examination documenting short cervical length. In 1993, the Medical Research Council and RCOG carried out a large, multicentre randomized trial where 1292 women with a history of pregnancy loss or cervical trauma where the indications for a stitch were unclear were randomized to either cerclage or watchful waiting [56]. Results of the study showed a reduction in deliveries at less than 33 weeks' gestation in those with a history of greater than three mid trimester pregnancy losses. In a more recent meta-analysis of ultrasound-indicated cerclage [57], the authors found that women with a history of previous preterm birth and documented cervical length of less than 25 mm on transvaginal ultrasound would benefit from cerclage before 24 weeks' gestation. At present there is not enough evidence to suggest those women with other risk factors for preterm birth such as previous cone biopsy or multiple pregnancy would benefit.

The difficulty comes with those women with ultrasound findings but no clear-cut history. To *et al.* [58] screened 47,123 cases at the second trimester scan with no history of incompetence. Women with a cervical length measurement less than 15 mm on ultrasound examination were randomized to either undergo cervical cerclage or be monitored. Results showed there was no significant difference in the rates of PTB at less than 33 weeks. Therefore there is little evidence to support screening and cerclage in women at low risk.

From the current body of evidence available, it appears that cervical cerclage may be indicated in women with a significant history of preterm delivery or mid trimester pregnancy loss with documented short cervical length during the current pregnancy, although, again, evidence of a reduction in perinatal morbidity is lacking.

Obstetric issues in preterm labour
Mode of delivery

At present there is insufficient evidence to suggest the most appropriate mode of delivery for preterm infants. As with term pregnancies, vaginal delivery is associated with lower maternal morbidity and mortality and is therefore the preferred method unless there are indications for CS. The type of CS incision is important, as at <26 weeks' gestation the lower uterine segment is not formed. However, classical vertical incisions carry greater risks for the mother and have implications for future deliveries. CS is rarely justifiable at <25 weeks' gestation given the poor outcome for the fetus.

Care of the premature neonate

There have been public concerns regarding staffing levels in UK obstetric departments. With premature deliveries it is paramount that there are experienced staff available during the delivery, including paediatricians with appropriate neonatal advanced resuscitation experience. The Safer Childbirth report describes the importance of teamwork between obstetricians, anaesthetists, paediatricians and midwives to provide optimum care for women with high-risk deliveries[59]. This report also highlights the importance of maintaining good clinical practice by providing regular staff training in managing high-risk deliveries, development of clear clinical guidelines for the multidisciplinary management of preterm delivery, and regular audit of departmental practice.

Good communication with the mother is essential when dealing with preterm labour and delivery, especially with very premature babies when the outcome is often poor. NICE guidelines on intrapartum care recommend women with preterm labour or preterm prelabour rupture of the membranes or a condition requiring elective preterm birth should be managed in a dedicated obstetric unit [60].

Conclusions

Preterm labour is the single most important factor affecting perinatal morbidity and mortality. The rates of preterm birth in the developed world appear to be increasing. With the exception of antenatal corticosteroids, no other treatment has been shown to significantly improve perinatal outcome. Further research is urgently required to help identify women at risk of preterm labour and to develop new management strategies.

References

1. World Health Organization. Managing complications in pregnancy and childbirth – abdominal pain in later pregnancy. 2003. Available at: www.who.int/reproductive-health/impac/Symptoms/Abdominal_pain_later_S119_S123.html#S122%20Preterm (accessed November 2007).

2. British Association of Perinatal Medicine Executive Committee. Memorandum – Fetuses and newborn infants at the threshold of viability a framework for practice. 2000. Available at: www.bapm.org/documents/publications/threshold.pdf (accessed November 2007).

3. Svigos J M, Robinson S. Threatened and actual preterm labour including mode of delivery. In: James D K, Steer P J, Weiner C P, eds. *High Risk Pregnancy Management Options*. Oxford: WB Saunders, 1999; Chapter 56.

4. Ananth C V, Joseph K S, Oyelese Y, Demissie K. Trends in preterm birth and perinatal mortality among singletons: United States 1989–2000. *Am J Obstet Gynecol* 2005; **105**: 1084–91.

5. Balchin I, Whittacker J C, Steer P J, Lamont R F. Are reported preterm birth rates reliable? An analysis of interhospital differences in the calculation of gestation at delivery and preterm birth rate. *Br J Obstet Gynaecol* 2004; **111**: 160–3.

6. National Office of Statistics. Preterm Birth in England and Wales. 2005. Available at: http://www.statistics.gov.uk/pdfdir/preterm0507.pdf (accessed October 2007).

7. Langhoff R J, Kesmodel U, Jacobsson, *et al.* Spontaneous preterm delivery in primiparous women at low risk in Denmark: a population based study. *Br Med J* 2006; **332**: 937–9.

8. Chalmers J W, Shanks E, Stott A, Paton C. Preterm deliveries in Scotland. 2006. Available at: bmj.com/cgi/eletters/332/7547/937 (accessed December 2007).

9. Costeloe K, Gibson A T, Marlow N, Wilkinson A R. The EPICure Study: outcome to discharge from hospital for babies born at the threshold of viability. *Paediatrics* 2000; **106**(4): 659–71.

10. Draper E S, Manktelow B, Field D, James D. Prediction of survival for preterm births by weight and gestational age: retrospective population based study. *Br Med J* 1999; **319**: 1093–7.

11. Ward R M, Beachy J C. Neonatal complications following preterm birth. *Br J Obstet Gynaecol* 2003; **111**(s20): 8–16.

12. Marlow N, Wolke D, Bracewell M, Samara M, for the EPICure Study Group. Neurologic and developmental disability at six years of age after extremely preterm birth. *N Engl J Med* 2005; **352**: 9–19.

13. Keelan J A, Blumenstein M, Helliwell R J, *et al.* Cytokines, prostaglandins and parturition – a review. *Placenta* 2003; **24**(A): 33–46.

14. Patni S, Flynn P, Wynen L P, *et al.* An introduction to Toll-like receptors and their possible role in the initiation of labour. *Br J Obstet Gynaecol* 1997; **114**(11): 1326–34.

15. Bernal A L. Preterm labour: mechanisms and management. *BMC Pregn Childbirth* 2007; **5**: S2–5.

16. Esplin M S, Varner M W. Genetics in preterm birth – the future. *Br J Obstet Gynaecol* 2005; **112**(s1): 97–102.

17. Mercer B M, Goldenberg R I, Das A, *et al.* The Preterm Prediction Study: a clinical risk assessment system. *Am J Obstet Gynecol* 1996; **174**: 1885–93.

18. Edlow A G, Srinivas S K, Elovitz M A. Second trimester loss and subsequent pregnancy outcomes: what is the real risk? *Am J Obset Gynecol.* 2007; **197**(6): 581–6.

19. Andrews W W, Goldenberg R L, Mercer B, *et al.* The Preterm Prediction Study: association of second-trimester genitourinary chlamydia infection with subsequent spontaneous preterm birth. *Am J Obstet Gynecol* 2000; **183**(3): 662–8.

20. Leitich H, Bodner-Adler B, Brunbauer M, *et al.* Bacterial vaginosis as a risk factor for preterm delivery: a meta-analysis. *Am J Obstet Gynecol* 2003; **189**: 139–47.

21. Steer P. The epidemiology of preterm labour. *Br J Obstet Gynaecol* 2000; **112**(s1): 1–3.

22. Goldenberg R L, Iams J D, Mercer B M, *et al.* The preterm prediction study: the value of new vs. standard risk factors in predicting early and all spontaneous preterm births. NICHD MFMU Network. *Am J Publ Hlth* 1998; **88**: 233–8.

23. Peacock J L, Bland J M, Ross H R. Preterm delivery: effects of socioeconomic risk factors, psychological stress, smoking, alcohol and caffeine. *Br Med J* 1995; **311**: 531–5.

24. Kramer M S, Galet L, Lydon J, *et al.* Socioeconomic disparities in preterm birth: causal pathways and mechanisms. *Paediat Perinat Epidemiol* 2001; **15**(s2): 104–23.

25. Goffinet F. Primary predictors of preterm labour. *Br J Obstet Gynaecol* 2005; **112**(s1): 38–47.

26. Lockwood C J, Sonyei A E, Dische M R, *et al.* Fetal fibronectin in cervical and vaginal secretions as a predictor of preterm delivery. *N Engl J Med* 1991; **325**: 669–74.

27. Honest H, Bachmann L M, Gupta J K, Kleijnen J, Khan K S. Accuracy of cervicovaginal fetal fibronectin test in predicting risk of spontaneous preterm birth: systematic review. *Br Med J* 2001; **325**: 301–10.

28. Iams J D, Casal D, McGregor J A, *et al*. Fetal fibronectin improves the accuracy of diagnosis of preterm labor. *Am J Obstet Gynecol* 1995; **173**: 141–5.

29. Goldenberg R L, Mercer B M, Meis P J, Copper R L, Das A, McNellis D. The preterm prediction study: fetal fibronectin testing and spontaneous preterm birth. NICHD Maternal Fetal Medicine Units Network. *Obstet Gynecol* 1996; **87**(5): 643–8.

30. Leitich H, Egarter C, Kaider A, Hohlagschwandtner M, Berghammer P, Husslein P. Cervicovaginal fetal fibronectin as a marker for preterm delivery: a meta-analysis. *Am J Obstet Gynecol* 1999; **180**: 1169–76.

31. Singer E, Pilpel S, Bsat F, *et al*. Accuracy of fetal fibronectin to predict preterm birth in twin gestations with symptoms of labour. *Obstet Gynaecol* 2007; **109**(5): 1083–7.

32. Groom K M, Liu E, Atlenby K. The impact of fetal fibronectin testing for women with symptoms of preterm labour in routine clinical practice within a New Zealand population. *Austr NZ J Obstet Gynaecol* 2006; **177**: 13–8.

33. Iams J D, Goldenberg R L, Meis P J, *et al*. The length of the cervix and the risk of spontaneous preterm delivery. *N Engl J Med* 1996; **334**: 567–72.

34. Goldenberg R L, Iams J D, Miodovnik M, *et al*. The preterm prediction study: risk factors in twin gestations. *Am J Obstet Gynaecol* 1996; **175**: 1047–53.

35. McDonald H, Brodehurst P, Parsons J, *et al*. Antibiotics for treatment of bacterial vaginosis in pregnancy. *Cochrane Database System Rev* 2003; **2**: CD000262.

36. Carey J C, Klebanoff M A, Hauth J C, *et al*. Metronidazole to prevent preterm delivery in pregnant women with asymptomatic bacterial vaginosis. *N Engl J Med* 2000; **342**: 534–40.

37. Ugwumadu A, Mayonda I, Reid F, Hay P. Effect of early oral clindamycin on late miscarriage and preterm delivery in asymptomatic women with abnormal vaginal flora and bacterial vaginosis: a randomised controlled trial. *Lancet* 2003; **361**: 983–8.

38. Shennan A, Crawshaw S, Briley A, *et al*. A randomised controlled trial of metronidazole for the prevention of preterm birth in women positive for cervicovaginal fetal fibronectin: the PREMET study. *Br J Obstet Gynaecol* 2006; **113**(1): 65–74.

39. Carroll S G M. RCOG Clinical Guideline No. 44: Preterm prelabour rupture of membranes. 2006.

40. Duley L M M. RCOG Clinical Guideline 1B: Tocolytic drugs for women in preterm labour. 2002. Available at: www.rcog.org.uk/resources/Public/pdf/Tocolytic_Drugs_No1(B).pdf (accessed October 2007).

41. British National Formulary. *Section 7.3.1 Myometrial Relaxants. In BNF 54*. Wallingford: Pharmaceutical Press, 2007.

42. Gyetvai K, Hannah M E, Hodnett E D, Ohlsson A. Tocolytics for preterm labour: a systematic review. *Obstet Gynaecol* 1999; **94**: 869–77.

43. Anotayanonth S, Subhedar N V, Neilson J P, Harigopal S. Betamimetics for inhibiting preterm labour. *Cochrane Database System Rev*. 2004; **4**: CD004352.

44. King J F. Tocolysis and preterm labour. *Curr Opin Obstet Gynaecol* 2004; **16**: 459–63.

45. Worldwide Atosiban versus Beta-agonists Study Group. Effectiveness and safety of the oxytocin antagonist atosiban versus beta-adrenergic agonists in the treatment of preterm labour. *Br J Obstet Gynaecol* 2001; **108**: 133–42.

46. Papatsonis D N, van Geijin H P, Ader H J, *et al*. Nifedipine and ritodrine in the management of preterm labour: a randomised multicentre trial. *Obstet Gynaecol* 1997; **90**: 230–4.

47. Ogueh O, Johnson M R. The metabolic effect of antenatal corticosteroid therapy. *Human Reprod Update* 2000; **6**(2): 169–76.

48. Crowley P A. Antenatal corticosteroid therapy: a meta-analysis of the randomised trials 1972–1994. *Am J Obstet Gynecol* 2005; **173**: 322–55.

49. Penney G C. RCOG Clinical Guideline No. 7: Antenatal corticosteroids to prevent respiratory distress syndrome. 2004. Available at: www.rcog.org.uk/resources/Public/pdf/Antenatal_corticosteroids_No7.pdf (accessed October 2007).

50. Baud O, Foix-L'Helias L, Kaminski M, *et al*. Antenatal glucocorticoid treatment and cystic periventricular leukomalacia in very premature infants. *N Engl J Med* 1999; **341**: 1190–6.

51. Wapner R J, Sardan Y, Johnson F, *et al*. Long term outcomes after repeat doses of antenatal corticosteroids. *N Engl J Med* 2007; **357**(12): 1190–8.

52. Crowther C, Harding J E. Repeat doses of prenatal corticosteroids for women at risk of preterm birth for preventing neonatal respiratory disease. *Cochrane Database System Rev* 2003; **3**: CD003935.

53. Kenyon S L, Taylor D J, Mordi W, ORACLE Collaborative Group. Broad spectrum antibiotics for spontaneous preterm labour: the ORACLE I randomised trial. *Lancet* 2001; **357**: 979–88.

Available at: www.rcog.org.uk/resources/Public/pdf/green_top44_preterm.pdf (accessed October 2007).

54. Meis P J, Klebanoff M, Thom E, *et al.* Prevention of recurrent preterm delivery by 17 alpha-hydroxyprogesterone caproate. *N Engl J Med* 2003; **348**: 2379–85.

55. Dodd J M, Flenady V, Cincotta R, Crowther O A. Prenatal administration of progesterone for preventing preterm birth. *Cochrane Database System Rev* 2006; **3**: CD004947.

56. MRC/RCOG Working Party of Cervical Cerclage. Final report of the MRC/RCOG multicentre randomised trial of cervical cerclage. *Br J Obstet Gynaecol* 1993; **100**: 516–23.

57. Berghella V, Obido A O, To M S, *et al.* Cerclage for a short cervix on ultrasound: meta-analysis of trials using individual patient-level data. *Obstet Gynaecol* 2005; **106**: 181–9.

58. To M S, Alfirevic Z, Heath V C F, *et al.* Cervical cerclage for prevention of preterm delivery in women with short cervix: randomised controlled trial. *Lancet* 2004; **363**: 1849–53.

59. Safer Childbirth Working Party. *Safer Childbirth – Minimum Standards for the Organisation and Delivery of Care in Labour.* London: RCOG Press, 2007.

60. National Institute of Clinical Excellence. *Intrapartum Care: Care of Healthy Women and their Babies during Childbirth.* Clinical Guideline No. 55. London: NICE, 2007.

Chapter 21

Labour in women with medical disorders

Mandish Dhanjal and Catherine Nelson-Piercy

Introduction

The process of labour and delivery affects the maternal physiology in a number of ways which are important to consider when managing women with medical disorders. Cardiac output greatly increases, and the pain of labour causes extreme stress and increases catecholamine release. Extra energy is required to push in the second stage, and the rise in arterial and venous pressure may raise concerns in those with vulnerable coronary and cerebral circulations. Bowel transit time is reduced, and this and gastric stasis leads to delayed drug absorption such that many drugs will need to be administered parenterally to be effective.

There is an increased tendency for obstetricians to induce labour or to perform a caesarean section in women with medical disorders, often to ensure the availability of suitable personnel or to adjust anticoagulation. However, induction is more likely to lead to prolonged labour and an increase in instrumental delivery and caesarean section. These operative procedures carry inherent risks of thrombosis and infection, which may compound a pre-existing tendency of these risks in conditions such as previous venothromboembolism and those on immunosuppressive agents or steroids.

Some conditions may deteriorate around labour and delivery, such as sickle cell disease, diabetes, epilepsy, critical heart disease and restrictive lung disease. Others, such as asthma and arrhythmias, are not affected by labour.

Some drugs which are commonly used in labour and delivery, such as ergometrine, boluses of syntocinon and carboprost may cause deterioration in certain forms of heart disease. Clearly documented plans for suitable alternatives should be made prior to labour in the event of postpartum haemorrhage.

Key conditions which require multidisciplinary management plans prior to labour and delivery will be discussed.

Heart disease

The key concerns in labour and delivery in a woman with heart disease are:

- reducing the effect of tachycardia and increased cardiac output in labour,
- managing anticoagulation,
- timing and mode of delivery,
- ensuring effective analgesia,
- bacterial endocarditis prophylaxis, and
- management of postpartum haemorrhage.

By term, the cardiac output will have increased by 25% due mainly to an increase in stroke volume, but also a 10–20 beat per minute increase in the resting heart rate. In labour, the cardiac output increases further, by 15% in the first stage and 50% in the second stage, to a mean of 10.6 l/minute. The sympathetic response to uncontrolled pain in labour is likely to contribute significantly to this increased cardiac output. There are similar but less marked increases in cardiac output during caesarean section. Following delivery of the placenta, there is up to a litre autotransfusion of blood necessitating a further rise in cardiac output by 60–80%. This is followed by a rapid decline back to prelabour values within an hour of delivery. These dramatic cardiovascular changes may be poorly tolerated by women with heart disease. Avoidance of tachycardia is possible through effective analgesia, limited exertion in the second stage of

Best Practice in Labour and Delivery, ed. R. Warren and S. Arulkumaran. Published by Cambridge University Press.
© Cambridge University Press 2009.

labour and cautious use of syntocinon for the third stage.

Managing anticoagulation

See section below on intrapartum management of anticoagulation.

Timing of delivery

This is usually dependent on the severity of maternal disease and any associated maternal compromise. In women with cyanotic heart disease, there may be significant intrauterine growth restriction which may warrant preterm delivery. A judgement needs to be made as to the gestation of delivery, taking into consideration the neonatal morbidity and mortality associated with preterm birth. If delivery is to occur before 34 weeks' gestation, antenatal steroids should be administered for fetal lung maturity. In a woman at risk of pulmonary oedema, due care and monitoring should occur for 24–48 h following steroid administration which can result in fluid retention and cardiac decompensation responsive to diuretics.

Delivery in a tertiary unit is recommended for those with moderate or severe cardiac disease. Induction of labour may be considered in those on anticoagulation or those with complex or severe heart disease to allow for adjustment of anticoagulation, insertion of lines, and availability of relevant senior staff to be present for the delivery. Prostaglandin E_2 can be used for induction of labour, as can syntocinon. The doses of syntocinon used for induction and augmentation of labour are not sufficient to cause concern about maternal tachycardia; however, prolonged use can result in fluid retention through its antidiuretic effect, which may precipitate pulmonary oedema. To prevent this, it is sensible to administer the oxytocin through a syringe driver in a small volume of normal saline, e.g. 50 ml rather than 1 litre.

Mode of delivery

In general, vaginal delivery should be the aim unless there is an obstetric indication for caesarean section. There are few conditions where caesarean section is recommended (see Box A). Consideration should be given to sterilization at the same time as caesarean section in non-reversible severe conditions, such as pulmonary hypertension. This should be discussed with the patient antenatally. The caesarean section

> **Box A.** Cardiac indications for caesarean section
> - Aortic root dilatation: progressive enlargement or >4.5 cm
> - Severe peripartum cardiomyopathy/severe left ventricular dysfunction
> - Aortic dissection

should be performed in operating theatres that have access to cardiothoracic facilities.

Lithotomy and supine positions should be avoided. Lithotomy results in increased venous return, which may not be tolerated in those with severe stenotic heart lesions or those at risk of heart failure. The supine position reduces venous return and can reduce cardiac output by 25%, resulting in fetal compromise. The delivery position best tolerated is with the woman sitting upright with her legs lower than her abdomen and her feet supported on foot rests or on reversed lithotomy poles.

The active second stage may need to be shortened or avoided in those with severe heart disease who would not tolerate the increased cardiac output associated with pushing, such as those with ischaemic heart disease, critical mitral or aortic stenosis. In such cases, one should wait for the head to descend through the pelvis in the passive second stage followed by an instrumental delivery of the baby.

A dilute infusion of 5 units of syntocinon in 20 ml normal saline over 30 min is recommended for the third stage in women with moderate or severe heart disease. Ergometrine can be used in women with peripartum cardiomyopathy, but should not be used in patients who will decompensate with the resulting peripheral vasoconstriction and coronary vasospasm and tachycardia, i.e. those with stenotic valvular lesions, pulmonary hypertension, ischaemic heart disease or hypertension.

Effective regional analgesia

This is an important element in the management of delivery in women with severe heart disease. The advantages are that of minimization of pain and hence a reduced heart rate and blood pressure, peripheral vasodilatation, reducing preload and effective analgesia so that procedures such as assisted vaginal delivery and caesarean section can be performed. Consultant anaesthetic involvement is imperative.

Monitoring

Invasive monitoring in labour is recommended with arterial and central venous lines for those with severe heart disease. Pulmonary wedge pressure readings are not usually necessary.

Infective endocarditis

Bacterial endocarditis prophylaxis prevents propagation of bacteria on a diseased heart valve, mural endocardium or on implanted prosthetic material in the heart during times of bacteraemia. Indications for prophylaxis are given in Table 21.1

Prophylaxis against bacterial endocarditis should be given before any obstetric procedure is performed in the presence of infection, i.e. in the presence of ruptured membranes, during urinary catheterization, at the onset of the second stage of labour, or before caesarean section. It is mandatory for women with artificial heart valves and those with a previous episode of endocarditis.

The current recommendations are amoxycillin 2 g i.v. plus gentamicin 1.5 mg/kg i.v. at the onset of labour or ruptured membranes or 30 min to 1 h prior to caesarean section, followed by amoxycillin 1 g orally 6 h later. For women who are penicillin-allergic, vancomycin 1 g i.v. over 1–2 h can be used instead of the initial i.v. amoxycillin dose.

Postpartum haemorrhage (PPH)

Syntocinon may be given cautiously in women with severe heart disease, as long as it is given slowly in low doses. Ergometrine should be avoided in the conditions described previously. Carboprost, a synthetic prostaglandin F2α, causes bronchospasm and is generally avoided in cardiac patients. Misoprostol, a synthetic prostaglandin analogue, is given rectally and can cause diarrhoea and shivering, but is otherwise well tolerated and is an effective agent at stopping PPH due to uterine atony.

Intrauterine tamponade using hydrostatic balloons such as the Rusch balloon can be used in cases of uterine atony. Antibiotic cover should be given whilst the balloon is in situ. Mechanical compression sutures, such as the B-Lynch brace suture, can be used prophylactically in a woman with severe heart disease having a caesarean section as an adjunct to medical treatment.

Table 21.1 Indications for bacterial endocarditis prophylaxis.

Antibiotic prophylaxis required	Cardiac condition
Definitely	Previous bacterial endocarditis
	Artificial heart valves or other foreign material
Possibly	Surgically created systemic or pulmonary conduits
	Congenital heart disease (except secundum-type ASD)
	Acquired valvular heart disease
	Mitral valve prolapse with mitral regurgitation
	Hypertrophic cardiomyopathy
No	Isolated ostium secundum or sinus venosus ASD
	Surgically repaired ASD, ventricular septal defect, or patent ductal arteriosus (providing no left valve abnormalities)
	Mitral valve prolapse without mitral regurgitation
	Physiological heart murmurs
	Cardiac pacemakers
	Pulmonary stenosis
	Total anomalous pulmonary drainage
	Repaired tetralogy of Fallot with no shunts, aortic regurgitation or valve grafts
	Arrhythmias

Note: ASD = atrial septal defect.

Thrombosis

Women with a venous thromboembolism (VTE) in pregnancy will be on treatment doses of low molecular weight heparin (LMWH). Induction of labour and caesarean section should be for obstetric indications. Operative delivery increases the risk of further thrombosis and should be avoided if possible. LMWH should be stopped as described in the intrapartum management of anticoagulation section below. During labour, graduated elastic compression stockings should be worn. If flowtron boots are available,

Table 21.2 Therapeutic doses of LMWH.

	Early pregnancy weight (kg)	Enoxaparin	Dalteparin	Tinzaparin
Antenatally		1 mg/kg bd	100 units/kg bd	175 units/kg daily for all weights
	<50	40 mg bd	5,000 iu bd	
	50–69	60 mg bd	6,000 iu bd	
	70–89	80 mg bd	8,000 iu bd	
	>90	100 mg bd	10,000 iu bd	
Postnatally		1.5 mg/kg od or 0.75 mg/kg bd	70 units/kg bd	175 units/kg daily

Table 21.3 Cautionary use of regional analgesia techniques in pregnant women on LMWH.

Regional analgesia in pregnant women on LMWH		Timing to avoid epidural haematoma
Regional analgesia can be given	On prophylactic LMWH	≥12 h after last dose
	On therapeutic LMWH	≥24 h after last dose
Epidural catheter removal	On LMWH	10–12 h after last dose
	Next dose LMWH	≥3 h after removal

these should be used. The woman should be kept well hydrated and remain mobile if possible.

Intrapartum management of anticoagulation

Women may present for delivery on prophylactic (e.g. 40 mg enoxaparin), high prophylactic (e.g. 40 mg 12 hourly enoxaparin) or fully anticoagulant doses of LMWH (see Table 21.2), or occasionally fully anticoagulated on warfarin. The approach to the management of anticoagulation for labour and delivery is dependent on the indication for anticoagulation, and therefore the importance of maintaining a given antithrombotic or anticoagulant effect.

For women receiving prophylactic doses of LMWH, this is usually because of previous thromboembolic events or because of a perceived risk of venous thromboembolism in, for example, obese women admitted with pre-eclampsia. Some women may be receiving prophylactic LMWH for recurrent miscarriage, sickle cell disease or previous adverse pregnancy outcome with or without documented thrombophilia.

In all the situations described below, it is imperative that joint protocols are developed, agreed and documented between obstetricians and obstetric anaesthetists such that women may be informed prior to delivery of the issues and likely plan for discontinuation of anticoagulants, delivery and analgesia and anaesthesia. In some circumstances including the fully anticoagulated woman, individual referral to an obstetric anaesthetist is appropriate. Epidural haematoma is a very rare complication of regional anaesthesia in patients receiving LMWH; however, caution is recommended. There is national consensus regarding the desired intervals between LMWH doses and insertion or removal of regional analgesia catheters (see Table 21.3).

If analgesia is required for labour before it is considered safe to administer a regional block, fentanyl patient-controlled analgesia may be used with senior anaesthetic involvement.

Intrapartum anticoagulation management in specific situations

Women receiving prophylactic low-dose LMWH for recurrent miscarriage or previous adverse pregnancy outcome

In these circumstances, LMWH can be discontinued at 37 weeks. If there are risk factors for VTE, it can be discontinued 12 h prior to planned induction, caesarean section, or at the onset of labour.

There is no need to restart LMWH postpartum unless there is a thrombophilia or other identified risk factors for VTE.

Women receiving prophylactic low-dose LMWH for VTE prophylaxis because of previous VTE or other identified risk factors for VTE

These women may be advised to discontinue LMWH 12 h prior to planned induction, caesarean section, or at the onset of labour. This ensures that for planned delivery there is at least a 12 h window to allow siting of regional anaesthesia or analgesia.

There is a possibility that with this strategy, particularly in a multiparous woman in whom the plan is to await the spontaneous onset of labour, that she may request (and be declined) an epidural within 12 h of her last dose of LMWH. This is also more likely in women receiving high-dose prophylaxis (e.g. enoxaparin 40 mg twice daily). This possibility should be discussed with the individual patient and a risk assessment made of the relative merits of earlier discontinuation of LMWH versus a possible delay in receiving pain relief via an epidural.

If a caesarean section is required less than 12 h after the last dose of LMWH, this will need to be performed under general anaesthetic. Alternatively, it may be appropriate to request an anti-Xa level and proceed with a regional block if this is very low.

LMWH should be restarted within 12 h postpartum and continued for 6 weeks in the case of previous VTE, hereditary thrombophilia or sickle cell disease.

Women fully anticoagulated with LMWH

The main indications for full anticoagulation in pregnancy are:

- VTE in the current pregnancy, and
- metal heart valves.

VTE in the current pregnancy

The highest risk of further thrombosis or a pulmonary embolus following a deep venous thrombosis is in the first few weeks after the index event. This provides a very strong rationale for delaying delivery if possible in women who develop VTE at or near term. This allows for a longer period of full anticoagulation before the necessary temporary interruption for delivery. These women can be managed in a similar way to women on prophylactic LMWH, but with cessation of LMWH 24 h prior to planned induction, caesarean section, or at the onset of labour. For a caesarean section, spinal and/or epidural anaesthesia can then be safely employed. For women in labour or undergoing induction of labour, several strategies are possible starting from 24 h after the last therapeutic dose of LMWH.

(a) Withhold heparin until after delivery (facilitating use of regional analgesia if required); not suitable if VTE less than 1 week before delivery.

(b) Give further prophylactic dose of LMWH every 24 h in labour (considering/offering siting of an epidural prior to each dose).

(c) Give doses of subcutaneous prophylactic unfractionated heparin (7500 iu) every 12 h (allowing siting of an epidural after 2 h).

(d) Elective placement of an epidural catheter that may be used if required (allowing a further dose of LMWH to be given 3 h after).

(e) Use intravenous unfractionated heparin (UFH). The dose of intravenous heparin used is designed to provide prophylactic levels (about 1000 units/h). The infusion is discontinued at onset of the second stage of labour, or interrupted 1–2 h prior to regional anaesthesia or analgesia.

All strategies should include use of grade II elastic compression stockings. Whichever option is employed, the implications should be carefully explained to the woman. Full anticoagulant doses of LMWH should be recommended after delivery, remembering that the correct therapeutic dose for enoxaparin and dalteparin falls to the normal nonpregnant dose, i.e. 1.5 mg/kg daily. This can be divided into a bd regimen if there is concern about giving a large bolus dose. If there is concern about postpartum haemorrhage, the dose can be kept at high prophylactic levels until this concern passes. It is important to remember that postpartum haemorrhage and blood transfusion are independent risk factors for VTE.

Metal heart valves

Women with metal heart valves may be on warfarin or full therapeutic doses of LMWH antenatally to prevent valve thrombosis. Warfarin should be stopped 10 days to 2 weeks prior to delivery to allow clearance of warfarin by the fetus. Anticoagulation should then be continued with full anticoagulant doses of LMWH, which does not cross the placenta. When LMWH is used, low-dose aspirin (75 mg/day) should be added as adjunctive antithrombotic therapy.

Many clinicians prefer to plan delivery in women with mechanical heart valves. The risk of thrombosis is high in these women and for those maintained on warfarin antenatally. Stopping this at 36 weeks and inducing labour or performing a caesarean section at 38 weeks minimizes the time spent off warfarin. In women where the risk of thrombosis is lower (large aortic new-generation valves, e.g. Carbomedics) in whom the decision was taken to convert to LMWH for the entire pregnancy, it would seem reasonable to await spontaneous labour unless there is an obstetric reason for earlier delivery.

LMWH should be stopped as soon as contractions start. If labour is to be induced, LMWH should be stopped 24 h before induction. Regional analgesia can be administered 24 h after the last dose of therapeutic LMWH.

As a general rule, some form of anticoagulation should be administered within 24 h of the last dose of therapeutic LMWH. Thus option (a) above is not appropriate for women with metal valves. Options (b)–(d) may be employed but some clinicians prefer to use option (e). The latter is labour-intensive, requires admission to hospital and careful monitoring of APTT levels, which can be very problematic and often leads to under-or overanticoagulation.

For women with VTE in the index pregnancy or those with mechanical valves, full anticoagulant doses of heparin should be resumed after delivery. This can be with subcutaneous LMWH. Conversion back to warfarin should be delayed for at least 3–7 days to minimize the risk of secondary PPH. It is important to continue LMWH until the INR is ≥ 2 for VTE or ≥ 2.5 with mechanical valves.

Women presenting in labour or needing urgent delivery fully anticoagulated on warfarin or heparin

In the event of an urgent need to deliver a fully anticoagulated patient, warfarin may be reversed with fresh frozen plasma (FFP) and vitamin K (1 mg intravenously is usually sufficient), and UFH with protamine sulphate. UFH has a short half-life and reversal is not usually required (especially not with doses of 1000 units per hour as suggested above). LMWH is partially reversed with protamine sulphate. However, bleeding complications are very uncommon with

LMWH. There is a 2% chance of wound haematoma with both LMWH and UFH. If a fully anticoagulated patient requires a caesarean section, this should be performed under general anaesthesia with consideration given to insertion of wound drains and use of staples or interrupted skin sutures.

If vitamin K has been given, anticoagulation with warfarin postpartum becomes very difficult. Both warfarin and LMWH are safe to use in a mother who is breast feeding or who intends to breast feed.

Thrombocytopenia (Table 21.4)

The key concerns in labour and delivery in a woman with thrombocytopenia are:

- administering a regional anaesthetic,
- surgical bleeding,
- postpartum haemorrhage, and
- fetal intracranial haemorrhage in a thrombocytopenic fetus.

Anaesthetists will usually not site a regional anaesthetic if the platelet count is $<80 \times 10^9/l$ due to concerns around epidural haematoma. Surgical incisions can, however, be made safely with counts of $>50 \times 10^9/l$. The aim predelivery is to keep the platelet count above $50 \times 10^9/l$.

Delivery is the time of maximum concern for the thrombocytopenic mother. The risk of maternal and fetal haemorrhage is not reduced with caesarean section compared with an uncomplicated vaginal delivery. Casarean section should therefore only be

Table 21.4 Action for treatment and delivery according to platelet count.

Platelet count $\times 10^9/l$	Action
<20	Treat*
>20	Treat if symptomatic*
30	Possibly safe for vaginal delivery
>50	Safe for vaginal delivery and caesarean section
>80#	Considered safe for regional analgesia

Notes: *Treatment may be with steroids, intravenous human IgG (IVIG), anti-D or platelet transfusion depending on aetiology of thrombocytopenia.
#Thromboelastography may be helpful.

performed for obstetric reasons. Ventouse delivery should be avoided, but the use of outlet forceps should be considered if there is a delay in the second stage.

If the third stage is managed actively using oxytocin, there is seldom excessive bleeding from the placental bed. However, there is a risk of bleeding from surgical incisions, soft tissue injuries and tears. An umbilical platelet count should be performed.

Imminent delivery with a platelet count $<50 \times 10^9/l$

Management of a patient with a platelet count of $<50 \times 10^9/l$ who is soon to deliver will depend on the aetiology of the thrombocytopenia. It is important to increase the platelet count above $50 \times 10^9/l$ to prevent maternal bleeding. Close liaison with the consultant haematologist should occur. If the diagnosis is idiopathic thrombocytopenic purpura (ITP), a condition caused by antiplatelet antibodies, platelet transfusion will only help transiently, as the antibodies will destroy the platelets transfused. Platelets should only be transfused in this instance if delivery is imminent, or if an invasive procedure such as central venous line insertion is required. If delivery is not imminent, treatment should be with intavenous human IgG (IVIG), which can raise the count within 48–72 h. Anti-D can be used as an alternative if the woman is Rhesus-positive. Steroids take longer to elevate the platelet count.

If the thrombocytopenia is not due to antiplatelet antibodies, then platelets can be transfused to elevate the count. Platelet transfusion will also be beneficial where there are abnormally functioning platelets. In conditions where the patient may require recurrent platelet transfusions in the future, HLA-matched platelets should be ordered if time permits.

Inherited coagulation deficiencies
Haemophilia and von Willebrands Disease (VWD)

Haemophilia A and B are sex-linked recessive disorders with a deficiency of coagulation factors VIII (FVIII) and IX (FIX), respectively. Heterozygous female carriers usually have FVIII and FIX levels 50% of normal, but are usually asymptomatic. There is a 50% chance that any male offspring will have haemophilia A or B.

> **Box B. Prophylactic treatment will be required with:**
> - any clotting factor level of <50 IU/dl prior to insertion of a regional block (which should be performed by a senior anaesthetist), and for all types of delivery;
> - type 2 VWD for operative delivery or perineal trauma;
> - type 3 VWD for all types of delivery.
>
> Regional anaesthesia is generally not recommended for those with type 2 or 3 VWD.

VWD is a quantitative or qualitative deficiency of von Willebrand factor. Deficiency of VWF results in FVIII deficiency and abnormal platelet function. Types 1 and 2 are autosomal-dominant and type 3 is autosomal-recessive.

Treatment

Maternal FVIII levels and VWF increase with gestation and may be normal by the time of labour and delivery. Maternal FIX levels do not rise significantly in pregnancy. A plan for delivery should be made with the haematologist, obstetrician and anaesthetist before delivery.

Treatment should be given with haematological advice (see Box B). Recombinant factors VIII or IX may be used as well as Desmopressin (DDAVP). DDAVP is a synthetic analogue of vasopressin which increases the levels of endogenous VWF and FVIII in patients with mild haemophilia A, in carriers of haemophilia A, and in most patients with VWD. It increases the level of VWF and FVIII three- to fivefold within half an hour. The increased levels are maintained for 6–8 h. Close monitoring for water retention should accompany its use. It should be used only with caution in women who also have pre-eclampsia.

Delivery

Women with hereditary coagulation deficiencies who are pregnant with an affected fetus and women with severe VWD should deliver at a unit where the necessary expertise in the management of these disorders and resources for laboratory testing and clotting factor treatments are readily available. Blood should be group and saved.

The male fetus of a haemophilia A or B carrier and the male or female fetus of a woman with VWD

233

types 1 and 2 have a 50% chance of being affected. Vaginal delivery carries a small risk of serious fetal or neonatal bleeding, which is not eliminated by caesarean section. Fetal scalp electrodes, scalp fetal blood sampling, ventouse extraction and rotational forceps delivery should not be performed in an affected or potentially affected fetus. Lift-out forceps may be used if required. A prolonged second stage should be avoided. The third stage should be actively managed. Cord blood should be sent for clotting factor assay in all male offspring of haemophilia carriers. VWF is elevated in the neonate, and testing should be delayed.

Postnatally

The gestation-related rise in FVIII and VWF reverts postnatally. Prophylactic recombinant clotting factor or DDAVP may be required to keep clotting factor levels >50 IU/dl for 3–5 days following delivery. Tranexamic acid may help controlling prolonged and/or intermittent secondary PPH. The affected neonate should be given oral vitamin K.

Sickle cell disease

Preterm birth is common in those with sickle cell disease. The increase is due to spontaneous preterm labour as well as iatrogenic due to complications including pre-eclampsia, recurrent crises, and placental insufficiency from placental infarcts leading to fetal growth restriction. Labour may need to be induced. Operative delivery increases the risk of infection, sickle cell crises, acute chest syndrome and thromboembolism in women with sickle cell disease, and hence caesarean section should only be performed for obstetric reasons. There should be close involvement with the haematology consultant. Before a planned delivery in a woman with recurrent crises or acute chest syndrome, it may be necessary to perform an exchange transfusion particularly if the percentage of sickle cells is high.

Sickle cell crises can be precipitated by dehydration, infection and the increased catecholamine response to pain, all of which may occur in labour. Women should be kept well hydrated and receive 2 l/min oxygen via nasal prongs or mask. Epidural analgesia is recommended for pain control. Blood should be grouped and saved. Broad-spectrum antibiotics should be administered if there is any suspicion of infection, and routinely after operative delivery.

The fetus is often growth-restricted and hence continuous fetal monitoring should be performed.

Continuous positive airway pressure (CPAP) may be advocated postnatally to reduce the incidence of acute chest syndrome (ACS), particularly in postoperative patients. ACS is the most common cause of postoperative death among patients with sickle cell disease. Women should use graduated elastic compression stockings and be given prophylactic LMWH for 6 weeks postnatally to prevent thromboses.

Diabetes

Women with diabetes should be delivered in a consultant-led maternity unit with access to senior medical, obstetric and neonatal staff.

Pre-existing diabetes

The key concerns in labour and delivery in a diabetic pregnancy are:

- timing of delivery to avoid stillbirth and shoulder dystocia,
- mode of delivery to avoid shoulder dystocia, and
- diabetic control in labour to prevent maternal diabetic ketoacidosis and neonatal hypoglycaemia.

Delivery

Delivery of a woman with pre-existing diabetes before term (38–39 weeks' gestation) is recommended in uncomplicated pregnancies with normal growth to avoid the increased risk of stillbirth, reduce the prevalence of macrosomia and reduce the risk of shoulder dystocia. If diabetic control has been excellent, and there are no fetal or maternal complications in the pregnancy, consideration can be given to delivery at term (40 weeks). Vaginal delivery is preferable, hence many diabetic women are induced. However, a caesarean section should be recommended if the estimated fetal weight at delivery is >4.25 kg to reduce the risk of shoulder dystocia. In diabetic pregnancies 80% of cases of shoulder dystocia occur above this birthweight.

Diabetic control in labour and delivery

Diabetic control throughout active labour and delivery is best achieved with a sliding scale of short-acting intravenous insulin and dextrose, as the dietary intake in labour is reduced and metabolism is varied (see Box C).

Box C. Setting up a sliding scale of insulin

50 units of short-acting insulin, e.g. actrapid or Humulin S, in 50 ml of 0.9% sodium chloride at a rate determined by capillary blood glucose

Fluid regimen

5% dextrose infusion 1 l per 8 h if blood glucose <12mmol/l, 0.9% sodium chloride 1 l in 8 h if blood glucose >12 mmol/l, switch to 5% glucose when blood glucose falls to <12mmol/l

Add 20–40 mmol of KCl to each 1 l bag of dextrose or sodium chloride

Table 21.5 Sliding scale regimen for type 1 diabetes once in established labour.

Capillary blood glucose (BM) (mmol/l)	Rate of insulin infusion (ml/h)
<3	0 *treat for hypoglycaemia and recheck in 20 mins*
3.1–5	1
5.1–10	2
10.1–15	3
15.1–20	4 *check for urinary ketones*
>20	5 *call for assistance*

Note: If having elective caesarean section, give one-third of normal dose of long-acting insulin the night before and put first on the list.

The sliding scale used will depend on whether they have type 1 or type 2 diabetes and the individual daily insulin requirements. Examples of such scales are shown in Tables 21.5 and 21.6. The capillary blood glucose (BM) is estimated each hour and the insulin infusion rate adjusted accordingly. The usual insulin dose range is 2–6 units per hour. The aim is to maintain glucose levels of between 4–6 mmol/l during labour and delivery, avoiding hypoglycaemia and preventing ketoacidosis. This may be difficult and most centres will aim for 4–8 mmol/l. Separate giving sets should be used for the insulin and dextrose so that in the event of hypoglycaemia, the glucose infusion can be increased and insulin infusion can be stopped. Women with type 1 diabetes are at particular risk of diabetic ketoacidosis, which has a high mortality rate. Urinary ketones should be checked each time urine is passed and particularly if the BM>15.

Insulin drives extracellular potassium into the cells. Therefore, it is important to include a potassium replacement with the intravenous dextrose to avoid hypokalaemia, which may otherwise result, especially if glucose levels are high.

Diabetic control postpartum

Insulin requirements in women with type 1 diabetes drop significantly following delivery of the placenta. The rate of infusion of insulin should therefore be

Table 21.6 Different sliding scale regimens for type 2 diabetes depending on total daily insulin requirement once in established labour.

Total daily insulin dose Capillary blood glucose mmol/l (BM)	A <60 units	B 60–120 units	C >120 units	If target still not achieved With sliding scale C each 2 h increase sliding scale by following no. of units until target achieved
≤3.0	0[#]	0[#]	0[#]	0[#]
3.1–5.0	1	2	3	1
5.1–8.0	2	3	4	2
8.1–11.0	3	4	6	2
11.1–15.0	4	6	8	2
15.1–20.0*	5	8	10	2
>20.0*	6	10	12	2

Notes: [#]Treat for hypoglycaemia and recheck in 20 mins.
*Call for assistance from obstetric medicine/diabetic team; check for ketonuria.
Select initial sliding scale (A–C) from table depending on final pregnancy total insulin dose. If target not achieved in 2 h, move to next sliding scale. If hypoglycaemia occurs, move to previous sliding scale.
If having elective caesarean section, give half normal dose of long-acting insulin the night before and put first on the list.

halved to prevent hypoglycaemia. Postpartum, insulin requirements return rapidly to prepregnancy levels. Once women with type 1 diabetes are eating normally, subcutaneous insulin should be recommenced at either the prepregnancy dose, or at a 25% lower dose if the women intends to breastfeed, which is associated with increased energy expenditure. Most women with established diabetes are capable of adjusting their own insulin doses and can be advised that tight glycaemic control is not as important during the postpartum period.

Women with type 2 diabetes who were diet-controlled prepregnancy can discontinue insulin immediately after delivery, even if they were on high doses in pregnancy. Those previously on oral hypoglycaemic drugs who are not intending to breastfeed can switch to their prepregnancy therapy. Those previously on oral hypoglycaemic drugs intending to breastfeed could continue with half-dose insulin to avoid the theoretical risk of neonatal hypoglycaemia with oral hypoglycaemic agents. There are few data on oral hypoglycaemic drugs and breastfeeding. Metformin is excreted into breast milk, but the amounts seem to be insignificant. In small case series there have been no neonatal detrimental effects of metformin. Glipizide is not detected in breast milk.

Neonate

Paediatricians do not need to be at the delivery of a diabetic mother routinely, but should see the baby as soon as possible after birth. The baby should be fed early. Neonatal capillary blood glucose should be checked at 2, 4 and 8 h if there are no signs of hypoglycaemia.

Gestational diabetes (GDM)

Delivery

Delivery of a woman with gestational diabetes who has an otherwise uncomplicated pregnancy should be at term. GDM requiring insulin treatment and co-morbidities such as pre-eclampsia, previous adverse outcome such as stillbirth or shoulder dystocia, poor diabetic control or fetal macrosomia may justify earlier delivery. Vaginal delivery is preferable unless there is an obstetric contra-indication or if the fetal weight at delivery is estimated to be >4.25 kg.

Diabetic control

Women with diet-controlled GDM and those on small amounts of insulin (<20 units/day) do not usually require a sliding scale in active labour due to the reduced oral intake in labour. If taking >20 units insulin/day, they should be started on a sliding scale as described for type 2 diabetes (Table 21.6).

Following delivery of the placenta, the insulin infusion should be discontinued as insulin resistance falls quickly. Monitoring of blood glucose should continue for 24 h following resumption of oral intake, as some women diagnosed with GDM will actually have type 2 diabetes.

All women with GDM should undergo formal 75 g OGTT 6 weeks following delivery to exclude impaired glucose tolerance or pre-existing diabetes. Women with GDM should be counselled that the risks of future diabetes may be as high as 80%. They should be made aware of diabetic symptoms and should receive lifestyle advice concerning exercise and diet, particularly reduced fat intake. Obese women should be encouraged to lose weight postpartum and all should be advised to avoid obesity.

Addison's disease

Adrenal insufficiency requires daily hydrocortisone and fludrocortisone (mineralocorticoid) supplementation. Clinical well-being and blood pressure together provide a good index of the adequacy of steroid replacement.

In labour and other situations of acute stress such as infection, there is normally an increased output of endogenous steroids from the adrenal gland. Those with Addison's disease cannot mount such a response and need increased doses of steroid. Labour should be managed with parenteral hydrocortisone 100 mg, intramuscularly, 6 hourly.

The physiological diuresis that occurs following delivery may cause profound hypotension in women with Addison's disease. This can be treated with i.v. saline. Alternatively, the higher dose of steroids to cover labour could be weaned gradually over a number of days rather than over 24 h to prevent hypotension.

Asthma

Asthma attacks are very rare in labour because of endogenous steroid production. Women should continue to use all their inhalers during labour. There is no evidence that inhaled β_2-agonists delay the onset of labour or impair uterine contractions. Women taking oral steroids (prednisolone ≥7.5 mg/day for

Table 21.7 Steroid support in labour for women on prednisolone >7.5 mg/day for >2 weeks.

Dose of prednisolone per day	Dose of i.v. hydrocortisone to cover labour (and until drinking)
≥7.5 to ≤20 mg	50 mg tds
>20 mg	100 mg tds

>2 weeks prior to delivery) should receive parenteral hydrocortisone to cover the stress of labour, and until oral medication is restarted (Table 21.7).

Caesarean section is only indicated for obstetric reasons. Induction of labour with prostaglandin E_2 is safe, as this is a bronchodilator. Syntocinon can be used safely for augmentation of labour, the third stage and for treatment of PPH. Misoprostol is preferable to prostaglandin F2α for the treatment of PPH. Prostaglandin F2α can cause bronchospasm and should be avoided if possible. It may be used with caution, and only after informing the anaesthetist, to treat life-threatening PPH. Ergometrine has been reported to cause bronchospasm, in particular in association with general anaesthesia, but this does not seem to be a practical problem when Syntometrine (oxytocin and ergometrine) is used for the prophylaxis of PPH.

All forms of pain relief in labour, including Entonox, opiates and regional analgesia, can be used safely by women with controlled asthma. In the unlikely event of an acute severe asthmatic attack, opiates for pain relief should be avoided. Epidural, rather than general anaesthesia, is preferable if caesarean section is required because of the decreased risk of chest infection and atelectasis. General anaesthesia should particularly be avoided in those with brittle asthma and, if required, should be supervised by a consultant anaesthetist.

Cystic fibrosis

Most women with cystic fibrosis (CF) deliver vaginally at term. Some may be inpatients by the end of pregnancy because of a resting hypoxia or fetal growth restriction, necessitating bed rest, oxygen therapy and nutritional supplements. Early delivery may be necessary if there is a significant deterioration in maternal or fetal well-being. Caesarean section is only necessary for obstetric indications and general anaesthesia should be avoided if possible.

Patients with CF are particularly prone to pneumothoraces, which may be precipitated by prolonged attempts at pushing and repeated Valsalva manoeuvres in the second stage of labour. Instrumental delivery may be indicated to avoid a prolonged second stage.

Breastfeeding should usually be encouraged, although the mother may continue to require nutritional supplements in the puerperium, especially if she is breastfeeding. Most of the drugs used will be secreted into the breast milk, but this is rarely a contra-indication to breastfeeding. Analysis of breast milk of women with CF has shown normal content of sodium and protein.

Epilepsy

Women with major convulsive seizures should deliver in hospital as the risk of seizures increases around the time of delivery. Of women with epilepsy, 1–2% will have a seizure during labour, and 1–2% will have one in the first 24 h postpartum. This is because fitting is more likely with stress, tiredness and sleep deprivation, all of which occur in labour and postpartum. Additionally, there is reduced absorption of anti-epileptic medication due to reduced gastric motility. Anti-epileptic drugs (AEDs) may be inadvertently omitted.

Women should not be left unattended in labour or for the first 24 h postpartum. They should continue their regular AEDs in labour. Consideration should be given to giving AEDs in suppository form. To limit the risk of precipitating a seizure due to pain and anxiety, early epidural analgesia should be considered.

If seizures that are not rapidly self-limiting occur in labour, give oxygen and either:

- intravenous lorazepam 4 mg over 2 min or
- diazepam 10–20 mg (rectal gel) or
- 10–20 mg intravenously at 2 mg/min.

Most women with epilepsy have normal vaginal deliveries and caesarean section is only required if there are recurrent generalized seizures in late pregnancy or in labour. Epileptic women should not use the birth pool to labour or have a water birth.

For women who have had seizures during previous deliveries, an option is to use rectal carbamezepine or intravenous sodium valproate or phenytoin to replace the usual oral therapy and ensure adequate absorption in labour. Alternatively, clobazam can be started prior to labour and discontinued 48 h after delivery.

Myaesthenia gravis

Myasthenia gravis (MG) is an autoimmune neuro-muscular disorder causing fatigable weakness of the skeletal muscles following repetetive activity. It results in ptosis, diplopia, difficulty speaking, and occasionally respiratory distress due to fatigue of the intercostal muscles. It does not affect the smooth muscle of the myometrium, therefore contractions and uterine involution are not impaired.

A vaginal delivery should be the aim, although instrumental delivery may be required to prevent maternal exhaustion. Postpartum haemorrhage is not increased in myasthenics. Caesarean section should only be performed for obstetric indications.

The key concerns in labour and delivery in a woman with myasthenia gravis are:

- drug use and drug interactions,
- neonatal myasthenia gravis, and
- puerperal infection.

Drug use and drug interactions in MG

Treatment of MG includes anticholinesterase inhibitors such as pyridostigmine. These should be administered parenterally in labour. Postnatally, shorter dose intervals should be used, as large doses can cause gastrointestinal upset in breastfed newborns.

Pregnant women with myasthenia should see an experienced obstetric anaesthetist, preferably prior to delivery to make appropriate plans for safe analgesic and anaesthetic use in labour.

- Regional analgesia is safe, but if the mother is being treated with anticholinesterases avoid the ester type of local anaesthetics (e.g. chlorprocaine, tetracaine). These depend on maternal plasma cholinesterase for their metabolism. Bupivacaine and lignocaine, the amide type of local anaesthetics, are metabolized by a different pathway and are therefore safe for use in labour and delivery.
- General anaesthesia: if an inhalational anaesthetic is required, ether and halothane should be avoided. Myasthenics are also particularly sensitive to non-depolarizing muscle relaxants, such as curare and suxamethonium, which may have an exaggerated or prolonged effect.

Other drugs that may exacerbate or cause muscle fatigue include aminoglycosides (e.g. gentamicin) and β-adrenergics (salbutamol, terbutaline and ritodrine). Narcotics should be used with caution, as they can reduce respiratory drive.

Although magnesium sulphate is the drug of choice for seizure prophylaxis in eclampsia and pre-eclampsia (see Chapter 24), it should be avoided in women with MG since it may precipitate a myasthenic crisis.

Myasthenics on immunosuppression should continue these drugs during labour. If on steroids, they will need i.v. hydrocortisone in labour: see Table 21.7.

Neonatal myasthenia gravis

Transient neonatal myasthenia gravis (TNMG) presents with poor sucking and generalized hypotonia usually by 4 days (but up to one week) of life. It is due to transplacental transfer of anticholinesterase receptor (AChR) antibodies. Respiratory distress is usually mild, but may be severe and life-threatening, requiring ventilation. Neonates of women with MG should be monitored with an apnoea monitor. Treatment is with anticholinesterase inhibitors. Breastfeeding should be avoided in babies with TNMG, as AChR antibodies are present in breast milk.

Puerperal infection

This is not more common in myasthenics, but if it occurs can result in severe deterioration and should therefore be treated promptly.

Berry aneurysms and cerebral arteriovenous malformations

There is an increased tendency for untreated cerebral aneurysms and arteriovenous malformations (AVM) to rupture in pregnancy. Berry aneurysms rarely bleed for the first time in labour, although rebleeding can occur if they have not been surgically treated or clipped. Caesarean section is therefore recommended. The risk of rupture is considered to be related to the increased intracranial pressure that occurs with pushing. Vaginal delivery is possible with a passive second stage and a forceps delivery without maternal effort, but should probably be reserved for the informed multiparous woman, who should have an epidural in labour. Elective caesarean section is recommended for those with a large AVM close to term.

If a woman has had a previous AVM which has been excised, or a Berry aneurysm which has been clipped, she can be delivered vaginally without any special precautions even if her surgery occurred in pregnancy following an intracerebral bleed.

Infectious diseases

HIV

The key concerns in labour and delivery in a woman with HIV are:

- prevention of vertical transmission, and
- avoidance of maternal infection/sepsis.

Vertical transmission of HIV without any intervention is around 25%. This risk is reduced to 1% using antiretroviral treatment antenatally, during delivery and for the neonate postnatally, performing a caesarean section, and avoiding breastfeeding.

Mode of delivery

The mode of delivery should be discussed by a multidisciplinary team including the HIV physician, the obstetrician and the woman.

A prelabour caesarean section should be offered to HIV-positive women with either a detectable viral load, or those who are not taking highly active antiretroviral treatment (HAART), as this will reduce vertical transmission. Caesarean section is less effective at reducing transmission when performed in labour or after membrane rupture. Transmission increases with increasing duration of membrane rupture.

It is unknown whether prelabour caesarean section is protective in women who have been on HAART and who have very low viral load levels of <50/ml. Such women may opt for a vaginal delivery. Transmission has been shown to be <1% in women with a viral load of <1000 copies/ml.

If a vaginal delivery is considered, membranes should not be ruptured artificially. Fetal trauma with fetal scalp electrodes, fetal scalp blood sampling and ventouse delivery should be avoided. Forceps may be used if necessary.

If a caesarean section is to be performed, this should be planned at 38–39 weeks, as those on retroviral treatment often labour earlier. Prophylactic antibiotics are imperative, as these will reduce postoperative morbidity from infection.

A maternal sample for plasma viral load should be taken at delivery. The umbilical cord should be clamped as quickly as possible after delivery, and the baby should be bathed immediately to remove maternal blood.

Antiretroviral treatment

Antiretroviral therapy should be continued up to delivery. Intravenous zidovudine should be given at delivery to women on monotherapy or with viral loads >50/ml. This should be started 4 h before caesarean section, or at the onset of labour. It should continue until the cord is clamped.

Hepatitis B

Hepatitis B can be vertically transmitted to the fetus if the mother has acute hepatitis B infection in the third trimester, or if she is a chronic hepatitis B antigen carrier. Caesarean section is not protective. Neonatal infection is prevented by administering hepatitis B vaccine to all neonates of women who are hepatitis B surface antigen (HepBsAg) positive at birth, 4 weeks and 1 year. Additional hepatitis B immune globulin is administered in a different site to the vaccine within 12 h of birth if the mother is hepatitis Be antigen (HepBe) positive.

Hepatitis C

Current evidence does not show that elective caesarean section is protective in women with hepatitis C unless they are co-infected with HIV.

Genital herpes (Table 21.8)

Caesarean section should be recommended to all women who have a primary episode of genital herpes at or within 6 weeks of delivery to prevent risks of neonatal herpes. If the woman opts for a vaginal birth, the membranes should not be artificially ruptured, and consideration should be given to treatment with intravenous aciclovir to the mother and subsequently to the neonate. The neonatologist should be informed.

Women with recurrent genital herpes at the onset of labour have a small risk of neonatal herpes. If their membranes rupture, delivery should be expedited, usually by augmentation of labour. Invasive procedures in labour should be avoided. The neonatologist should be informed during labour.

Renal disease

Renal function, blood pressure and fluid balance should be monitored in women with renal disease during labour and delivery. Treatment should be continued and parenteral steroids should be administered

Table 21.8 Neonatal risks of maternal genital herpes at delivery.

Maternal genital herpes	Risk of neonatal herpes (%)	Elective CS recommended
Primary episode >6 weeks before delivery	0	No
Primary episode <6 weeks before delivery	41	Yes
Recurrent episode at the onset of labour	1–3	No

to those on prednisolone as with any woman on maintenance steroids (see Table 21.7). Those who are immunosuppressed will be at increased risk of infection and should be given prophylactic antibiotics to cover any surgical procedure, including episiotomy.

Caesarean section is only required for obstetric indications, although the overall rate is increased (25%) compared to background rates. The renal allograft in the pelvis does not obstruct vaginal delivery.

Obstetric cholestasis (OC)

Labour should be induced at 37–38 weeks gestation in cases where the bile acids are greater than 40 to avoid the increased risk of stillbirth. There is a higher risk of fetal distress in OC, therefore close monitoring is required throughout induction and labour. Ursodeoxycholic acid can be discontinued postnatally.

The neonate should receive i.m. vitamin K.

Further readings

Adamson D L, Dhanjal M K, Nelson-Piercy C. Heart disease and its management in obstetrics. In: Greer I A, Nelson-Piercy C, Walters B, eds. *Maternal Medicine: Medical Problems in Pregnancy* Elsevier Ltd., 2007.

Task Force on Infective Endocarditis of the European Society of Cardiology. Guidelines on prevention, diagnosis and treatment of infective endocarditis. *Eur Heart J* 2004; **25**: 267–76.

Chan W S, Anand S, Ginsberg J S. Anticoagulation of pregnant women with mechanical heart valves. *Arch Int Med* 2000; **160**: 191–6.

RCOG. Guideline No. 28. *Thromboembolic Disease in Pregnancy and the Puerperium: Acute Management.* London: RCOG, 2007.

Greer I A, Nelson-Piercy C. Low-molecular-weight heparins for thromboprophylaxis and treatment of venous thromboembolism in pregnancy: a systematic review of safety and efficacy. *Blood* 2005; **106**(2): 401–7.

British Committee for Standards in Haematology, General Haematology Task Force. Guidelines for the investigation and management of idiopathic thrombocytopenic purpura in adults, children and in pregnancy. *Br J Haematol* 2003; **120**: 574–96.

Lee C A, Chi C, Pavord S R, *et al.* UK Haemophilia Centre Doctors' Organization. The obstetric and gynaecological management of women with inherited bleeding disorders – review with guidelines produced by a taskforce of UK Haemophilia Centre Doctors' Organization. *Haemophilia* 2006; **12**(4): 301–36.

ACOG. Practice Bulletin No. 78: Haemoglobinopathies in pregnancy. ACOG Committee on Obstetrics. *Obstet Gynecol* 2007; **109**(1): 229–37.

Confidential Enquiry in Maternal and Child Health. *Diabetes in Pregnancy: Are We Providing the Best Care? Findings of a National Enquiry.* London: CEMACH, 2007.

Crowther C A, Hiller J E, Moss J R, McPhee A J, Jeffries W S, Robinson J S. Effect of treatment of gestational diabetes mellitus on pregnancy outcomes. *N Engl J Med* 2005; **352**: 2477–86.

Rey E, Boulet L P. Asthma in pregnancy. *Br Med J* 2007; **334**(7593): 582–5.

Tonelli M R, Aitken M L. Pregnancy in cystic fibrosis. *Curr Opin Pulm Med* 2007; **13**(6): 537–40.

Tomson T, Hiilesmaa V. Epilepsy in pregnancy. *Br Med J* 2007; **335**(7623): 769–73.

Téllez-Zenteno J F, Hernández-Ronquillo L, Salinas V, Estanol B, da Silva O. Myasthenia gravis and pregnancy: clinical implications and neonatal outcome. *BMC Musculoskelet Disord* 2004; **5**: 42.

Kittner S J, Stern B J, Feeser B R, *et al.* Pregnancy and the risk of stroke. *N Engl J Med* 1996; **335**(11): 768–74.

RCOG. Guideline No. 39. *Management of HIV in Pregnancy.* London: RCOG, 2004

McIntyre P G, Tosh K, McGuire W. Caesarean section versus vaginal delivery for preventing mother to infant hepatitis C virus transmission. *Cochrane Database Syst Rev* 2006; **4**: CD005546.

RCOG. Guideline No. 30. *Management of Genital Herpes in Pregnancy.* London: RCOG, 2007.

RCOG. Guideline No. 43. *Obstetric Cholestasis.* London: RCOG, 2006.

Chapter 22

Management of women with previous caesarean section

Rajesh Varma and Gordon C. S. Smith

Introduction

There is widespread public and professional concern about the increasing proportion of births by caesarean section [1,2]. Increasing rates of primary caesarean section have led to an increased proportion of the obstetric population who have a history of prior caesarean delivery. Labour and delivery represent a particularly high-risk time for such women. This chapter provides a guide to their care, with emphasis on their intrapartum management.

Antenatal clinics and delivery suites are recommended to develop their own guidelines for managing the antenatal counselling and intrapartum management of women with prior caesarean delivery [3–5]. Ideally, this guidance should involve multidisciplinary input (health professionals and consumers), consider national guidelines (RCOG [2], NICE [1,4]) and acknowledge the need for specific resources to be readily available (e.g. access to theatres, anaesthetists, paediatricians, and haematological support).

Limitations of data

Presently, there are no published randomized controlled trials (RCTs) comparing planned vaginal birth after caesarean section (VBAC) against planned elective repeat caesarean section (ERCS). Evidence for these interventions is obtained mainly from retrospective non-randomized studies [2], making their conclusions less reliable. However, a study by the National Institute of Child Health and Human Development (NICHD) Maternal–Fetal Medicine Units Network [6] has overcome some of the shortcomings of previous studies by combining a large sample size, a prospective cohort design and utilization of standardized definitions for assessing outcomes. Where

possible, data on various risks and benefits of VBAC and ERCS reported in this chapter originate from this study. Further robust data on maternal and infant health outcomes will become available following completion of the BAC trial (Birth After Caesarean) [7].

Definitions

Key terms used in this chapter are defined in Table 22.1.

Options for delivery: VBAC or ERCS

Pregnant women with a history of previous caesarean section may be offered either planned VBAC or ERCS for their delivery. Such women would have consultant-led antenatal care and typically would follow an antenatal strategy that is depicted in Figure 22.1.

Determining the mode of delivery

Multiparous women with a single previous lower segment caesarean delivery, with or without a history of vaginal delivery, compose the vast majority of pregnant women referred to obstetricians due to their history of previous caesarean delivery. Provided there are no other complicating factors in the current pregnancy (e.g. multiple pregnancy, placenta not low lying at midtrimester scan) or previous caesarean delivery, and the pregnancy is otherwise low-risk, such women may be counselled by consultant midwives and a preferred mode of delivery determined and documented. A suggested optimal time for this counselling review is 16 to 28 weeks gestation. This visit should incorporate an individualised risk benefit assessment of VBAC and ERCS, examination of the previous obstetric medical case record in relation to the caesarean delivery and provision of a patient information

---

Best Practice in Labour and Delivery, ed. R. Warren and S. Arulkumaran. Published by Cambridge University Press.
© Cambridge University Press 2009.

Table 22.1 Definition of terms [2].

Planned VBAC	Planned VBAC (vaginal birth after caesarean) refers to any woman who has experienced a prior caesarean birth who plans to deliver vaginally rather than by elective repeat caesarean section (ERCS).
Successful and unsuccessful planned VBAC	A vaginal delivery (spontaneous or assisted) in a woman undergoing planned VBAC indicates a *successful* VBAC. Delivery by emergency caesarean section during the labour indicates an *unsuccessful* VBAC.
Uterine rupture	Disruption of the uterine muscle extending to and involving the uterine serosa or disruption of the uterine muscle with extension to the bladder or broad ligament.
Uterine dehiscence	Disruption of the uterine muscle with intact uterine serosa
Term perinatal mortality	Combined number of stillbirths (antepartum and intrapartum) and neonatal deaths (death of a live born infant from birth to age 28 days) per 10,000 live births and stillbirths at or beyond 37 weeks' gestation. Term perinatal mortality rates exclude deaths due to fetal malformation unless otherwise stated.
Term delivery-related perinatal death	Combined number of intrapartum stillbirths and neonatal deaths per 10,000 live births and stillbirths at or beyond 37 weeks' gestation. Delivery-related perinatal mortality rates exclude antepartum stillbirths and deaths due to fetal malformation unless otherwise stated.
Neonatal respiratory morbidity	Combined rate of transient tachypnoea of the newborn (TTN) and respiratory distress syndrome (RDS).

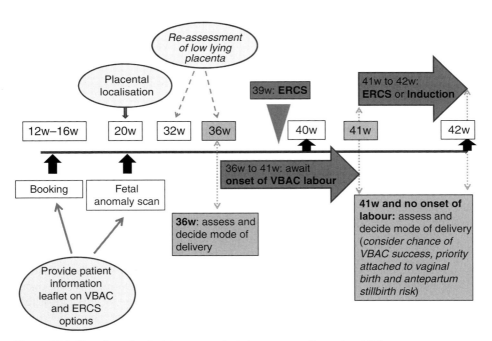

Figure 22.1 Plan of care for singleton uncomplicated pregnancy with previous LSCS

leaflet (such as that produced by the RCOG-see additional resources). Items that should be discussed and documented during the consultation are listed in Table 22.2 and are expanded on below. Decision

aids and specific patient information literature may facilitate this process [8].

Assuming a decision for planned VBAC is confirmed at the consultant midwife review, antenatal

Table 22.2 Items to be discussed when determining mode of delivery.

Items	Special considerations
1. Her understanding of the maternal and perinatal risks and benefits of VBAC compared to ERCS	Particularly her attitude towards the risk of rare but serious adverse outcomes.
2. Any contra-indications to VBAC	Any complicating obstetric factors, e.g. placenta praevia, fetal malpresentation, obstructing cervical fibroid, maternal medical disorders. Assessment of previous caesarean delivery and any perioperative complications. A classical scar or more than two previous lower segment incisions or previous uterine rupture would be absolute contra-indications to VBAC.
3. The likelihood of a successful VBAC	Particularly if she has had a previous vaginal birth or successful VBAC.
4. Her plans for future pregnancies	
5. Her personal preference and motivation to achieve vaginal birth or ERCS	

care may continue in the usual manner for low risk pregnancies (i.e. shared between GP and midwife) and a consultant obstetrician review organised for 41 weeks. For all other women, the final decision on mode of delivery should be established at a consultant-led review at 36 weeks. This group would include women who opted for ERCS or were undecided at the consultant midwife review, or have complicating medical or obstetric risk factors that may preclude VBAC as a delivery option.

Decision-making should be a shared process between the woman and her obstetrician. Items that should be discussed and documented during the consultation are listed in Table 22.2 and are expanded on below. Decision aids and specific patient information literature may facilitate this process [8].

Maternal and perinatal risks and benefits of VBAC compared to ERCS

The trade-off between risks and benefits for VBAC and ERCS is highly individualized. Women differ in the magnitude of risks they are willing to expose either themselves or their unborn child to during delivery [9]. For example, women who wish to minimize the risk of rare but severe adverse outcome for their child may choose ERCS in preference to VBAC. Conversely, there are many reasons why a woman might prefer to attempt vaginal birth, and these may lead them to accept a small degree of risk to both themselves and their infant during labour and to choose VBAC in preference to ERCS.

In the NICHD study [6], maternal morbidity and perinatal mortality at term were significantly greater among women opting for VBAC than ERCS (Table 22.3).

- The increased maternal morbidity was due to the higher prevalence of complications in those 27% of women with unsuccessful VBAC. This group, compared to successful VBAC, experienced higher risks of uterine rupture (231 per 10,000 vs. 11 per 10,000), uterine dehiscence (210 per 10,000 vs. 14.5 per 10,000), hysterectomy (46 per 10,000 vs. 14.5 per 10,000), transfusion (319 per 10,000 vs. 116 per 10,000) and endometritis (767 per 10,000 vs. 116 per 10,000).

- The increased perinatal mortality was largely attributable to the combined risks of antepartum stillbirth beyond 37 weeks and delivery-related perinatal death in the planned VBAC cohort. Essentially, women who opt for planned VBAC experience a 50 per 10,000 (0.5%) risk of uterine scar rupture, 10 per 10,000 risk of antepartum stillbirth beyond 39 weeks and a 4 per 10,000 risk of delivery-related perinatal death (if conducted in a large centre) [2]. It is likely that these risks are significantly reduced, if not eliminated, for women who opt for ERCS at the start of the 39th week; however, direct evidence to support this is lacking. Furthermore, women considering ERCS

243

Table 22.3 Risks and benefits of opting for VBAC or ERCS.

	Planned VBAC[†]	ERCS at 39 weeks
Mother benefits	72–76% chance of successful VBAC	Able to plan to known delivery date
	If successful, shorter hospital stay and convalescence	**Lower risk of blood transfusion (1%) and endometritis (1.8%)
	Increases likelihood that future pregnancies may be delivered vaginally	*Essentially zero risk of uterine scar rupture
		No risk of vaginal tears and no worsening of pelvic floor support and continence mechanisms
		Able to be surgically sterilized at the same time
Mother risks	*Around 50 per 10,000 (0.5%) risk of uterine scar rupture – if occurs associated with maternal morbidity and fetal morbidity/mortality	0.1–2% risk of serious surgical complications such as injury to bladder
	24–28% chance of emergency caesarean	Longer stay and convalescence
	10–15% chance of instrumental delivery and/or perineal tear requiring suturing	Future pregnancies would require caesarean delivery
	**Higher risk of blood transfusion (1.7%) and endometritis (2.9%)	Increased risk of surgical complications with each subsequent caesarean delivery due to adhesions, placental praevia/accreta
Infant benefits	1% risk of transient respiratory morbidity	Avoids the 10 per 10,000 prospective risk of antepartum stillbirth as delivery is undertaken at commencement of 39th week
		1 per 10,000 (0.01%) risk of delivery-related perinatal death or hypoxic ischaemic encephalopathy (HIE) at delivery
Infant risks	10 per 10,000 (0.1%) prospective risk of antepartum stillbirth beyond 39 weeks whilst awaiting spontaneous labour	1–3% risk of transient respiratory morbidity [6% risk if delivery performed at 38 instead of 39 weeks]
	4 per 10,000 (0.04%) risk of delivery-related perinatal death	
	[§]8 per 10,000 (0.08%) risk of hypoxic ischaemic encephalopathy (HIE) during labour	

Note: [†]The estimates of risk for adverse maternal or fetal events in VBAC are based on women receiving continuous electronic monitoring during their labour. The relative and absolute risks of such events in the absence of continuous electronic fetal monitoring are unknown.
*Uterine rupture in an unscarred uterus is extremely rare at 0.5 to 2 per 10,000 deliveries, and this risk is mainly confined to multiparous women in labour [37].
**In the NICHD study there was no statistically significant difference between planned VBAC and ERCS groups in relation to hysterectomy (23 per 10,000 vs. 30 per 10,000), thromboembolic disease (4 per 10,000 vs. 6 per 10,000) or maternal death (17 per 100,000 vs. 44 per 100,000) [6].
[§]Approximately half of the increased risk of HIE in planned VBAC arises due to the additional risk of HIE caused by uterine rupture (4.6 per 10,000) [6].

should be counselled that delaying delivery by one week from 38 to 39 weeks enables about a 5% reduction in the incidence of respiratory morbidity, but this delay may be associated with a 5 per 10,000 increase in the risk of antepartum stillbirth [10,11].

Contra-indications to VBAC

Contra-indications to VBAC may be considered in two main categories.

Obstetric complications. Assessment at 36 weeks' gestation aims to identify any obstetric complications that may preclude vaginal delivery should spontaneous labour ensue thereafter. An exception is women who have a low-lying placenta identified at their mid-pregnancy anomaly scan. These women should be re-scanned and reviewed at 32 weeks to assess the placenta and to plan delivery should there be placenta praevia. The reasoning for a 32 week rather than 36 week scan is discussed in the 'Placenta praevia and accreta' section below.

Previous uterine incision. A review of the operative notes of the previous caesarean delivery is important to identify women who may have an increased risk of uterine scar rupture. Thus, on this basis, planned VBAC is contra-indicated in women with:

- previous uterine rupture – risk of recurrent rupture is unknown;
- previous high vertical classical caesarean section (200–900 per 10,000 risk of uterine rupture) – where the uterine incision has involved the whole length of the uterine corpus [2]; and
- more than two previous caesarean deliveries (reliable estimate of risks of uterine rupture risk are unknown).

However, it is recognized that in certain extreme circumstances (e.g. miscarriage, intrauterine fetal death), for some women in the above groups, the vaginal route (although risky) may not necessarily be contra-indicated. A number of other variants are associated with an increased risk of uterine rupture. These include: women with a prior inverted T or J incision (190 per 10,000 rupture risk) and women with prior low vertical incision (200 per 10,000 rupture risk) [6]. There is insufficient and conflicting information on whether the risk of uterine rupture is increased in women with previous myomectomy or prior complex uterine surgery [2].

Analysis of the NICHD study showed that there was no significant difference in the rates of uterine rupture in VBAC with two or more previous caesarean sections (9/975, 92 per 10,000) compared to women with a single previous caesarean section (115/16,915, 68 per 10,000) [12]. However, the rates of hysterectomy (60 per 10,000 vs. 20 per 10,000) and transfusion (3.2% vs. 1.6%) were increased in the former group [12]. These findings concur with other observational studies, which, overall, have shown similar rates of VBAC success with two previous caesarean deliveries (VBAC success rates of 62–75%) and single prior caesarean delivery [2]. Therefore, planned VBAC is permissible in women with two previous low transverse caesarean deliveries provided they have been carefully assessed and counselled. However, this should be applied very cautiously to women with any other unfavourable factors, such as obesity, advanced age, no previous vaginal births, and previous caesarean sections for dystocia.

Likelihood of successful VBAC

Several pre-admission- and admission-based multivariate models have been developed to predict the likelihood of VBAC success [13,14] or uterine rupture [15] in planned VBAC. However, their usefulness in assisting health professionals or pregnant women in decision-making to minimize adverse outcome has not been established. Individual studies report success rates of 72–76% for planned VBAC after a single previous caesarean, which concurs with pooled rates derived by systematic and summative reviews [2].

Successful VBAC. Previous vaginal delivery, particularly previous VBAC, is the single best predictor for successful VBAC and is associated with an approximately 85–90% planned VBAC success rate [16]. Women with previous caesarean delivery for multiple pregnancy or fetal malpresentation also have higher than average VBAC success rates [16,17].

Unsuccessful VBAC. Induced labour, no previous vaginal delivery, BMI greater than 30 and previous caesarean for dystocia are associated with unsuccessful VBAC [16]. If all of these factors are present, successful VBAC is achieved in only 40% of cases [16]. Other factors associated with failed VBAC include: VBAC at or after 41 weeks' gestation; birthweight >4000 g; no epidural anaesthesia; previous preterm caesarean delivery; cervical dilatation at admission less than 4 cm; less than 2 years from previous caesarean delivery; advanced maternal age; non-Caucasian ethnicity; short stature; and a male infant. There is limited and conflicting evidence on whether the cervical dilatation achieved at the primary caesarean for dystocia impacts on the subsequent VBAC success rate [2].

Intrapartum care during planned VBAC

Even though most women would have received antenatal counselling on their planned VBAC, it is important that the health professional reconfirms that the woman understands and consents to these risks at the beginning of her admission to the labour ward. This reaffirmation should be documented in the notes: forming part of the informed consent process. Many of the priorities stated in National Institute of Clinical Excellence's guideline on intrapartum care [4] are applicable to managing VBAC labour, and the key ones are emphasized below.

Delivery setting

Planned VBAC should be conducted in a suitably staffed and equipped delivery suite, with continuous intrapartum care and monitoring, and available resources for immediate caesarean section and neonatal resuscitation [2,3,5]. There is evidence to suggest that larger-sized delivery units are better at minimizing adverse outcomes with planned VBAC such as uterine rupture and perinatal death due to uterine rupture [18,19].

Epidural anaesthesia is not contra-indicated in planned VBAC

Concerns that epidural analgesia might mask the signs and symptoms associated with uterine rupture have not been proven. In fact, epidural analgesia leads to comparable, if not better, rates of successful VBAC compared to those women not receiving epidural analgesia [16]. None the less, women considering epidural analgesia should be advised of an increased risk of a longer second stage of labour and an increased chance of vaginal instrumental birth.

Monitoring in labour

In women without scarred uteri, continuous monitoring is necessary to enable prompt identification and management of fetal compromise and labour

Table 22.4 Clinical features associated with uterine scar rupture.

Abnormal CTG
Severe abdominal pain, especially if persisting between contractions
Acute onset scar tenderness
Abnormal vaginal bleeding or haematuria
Cessation of previously efficient uterine activity
Maternal tachycardia, hypotension or shock
Loss of station of the presenting part

Note: An abnormal CTG is the most consistent finding in uterine scar rupture and is present in 55–87% of these events [38].

dystocia. However, in women with scarred uteri, there should also be extra vigilance for clinical features associated with uterine scar rupture (Table 22.4). Early diagnosis of both uterine scar rupture and labour dystocia (which itself could predispose to uterine rupture) is essential to reduce associated morbidity and mortality to mother and infant. Approximately half of the increased risk of hypoxic ischaemic encephalopathy (HIE) in planned VBAC arises due to the additional risk of HIE caused by uterine rupture (4.6 per 10,000) [6]. Consequently, all women in established VBAC labour should receive:

- supportive one-to-one care,
- continuous electronic fetal monitoring (Table 22.4),
- continuous monitoring of maternal symptoms and signs (Table 22.4), and
- regular (no less than 4 hourly) assessment of their cervicometric progress in labour.

Observational studies, with varying methodology and case mix, have shown intrauterine pressure catheters may not always be reliable and are unlikely to add significant additional ability to predict uterine rupture over clinical and CTG surveillance [2].

Induction and augmentation

The risk of adverse maternal and perinatal outcomes are lower among women in spontaneous VBAC labour not requiring induction or augmentation (Table 22.5). Although augmentation and induction are not contra-indicated in women with prior caesarean delivery, there remains considerable disagreement amongst clinicians on their use. Induction

Table 22.5 Risks of planned VBAC labours from NICHD study (N=17,898 planned VBACs) [6,16].

	Induced	Augmented	Spontaneous	Overall planned VBACs
Uterine rupture	*Overall*	87 per 10,000	36 per 10,000	69 per 10,000
	102 per 10,000	0.9%	0.4%	0.7%
	1.0%			
	PG method			
	140 per 10,000			
	1.4%			
	Non-PG method			
	89 per 10,000			
	0.9%			
Caesarean section	33%	26%	19%	27%

(particularly women with an unfavourable cervix or by prostaglandin method) or augmentation of VBAC labour are associated with a two- to threefold increased risk of uterine rupture and around a 1.5-fold increased risk of caesarean section compared to spontaneous VBAC labour (Table 22.5) [6,16,20]. In the NICHD study, the increased risk of uterine rupture after labour induction was found only in women with no prior vaginal delivery [20].

Given the increased risk of adverse outcome, it is imperative that the decision to induce or augment should be determined following careful obstetric assessment and be consultant-led. Women should be involved in the decision-making process for induction or augmentation, and provided with clear information on the potential risks and benefits of such a decision and how this may impact on their long-term health. For example, women who are contemplating many future pregnancies may be prepared to accept the short-term additional risks associated with induction and/or augmentation in view of the reduced risk of serious complications in future pregnancies if they have a successful VBAC.

Prostaglandin vs. non-prostaglandin induction methods

Analysis of a data set from Scotland showed that prostaglandin (PG) induction compared to non-PG induction was associated with a higher uterine rupture risk (87 per 10,000 vs. 29 per 10,000) and a higher risk of perinatal death due to uterine rupture (11.2 per 10,000 vs. 4.5 per 10,000) [19]. This compares to 6 per 10,000 risk of perinatal death in women with an unscarred uterus induced by prostaglandin identified by a Cochrane review [21]. Therefore, it is important not to exceed the safe recommended limit for prostaglandin priming in women with prior caesarean delivery (6 mg PGE_2 tablets or 3 mg PGE_2 gel) [22]. Moreover, due consideration should be given to restricting the dosaging and adopting a lower threshold of total PG dose exposure and/or considering non-PG methods of induction, such as intracervical Foley catheter.

Postdates induction

The RCOG induction of labour guideline suggests induction for postdates be offered from 41 weeks, as this reduces perinatal mortality without an increase in caesarean section rates. There are no adequate data which directly address this issue among women with a previous caesarean section. However, there are some specific issues about women with a previous caesarean delivery which may influence the decision-making process. First, these women are at increased risk of antepartum stillbirth [11,23]. Hence, the reduction in risk of perinatal death associated with postdates elective delivery may be even greater among women with a previous caesarean. However, it is also possible that the effect of routine postdates induction on the risk of emergency caesarean section may be different among women with a previous caesarean delivery. These women have a higher background

Table 22.6 Management of augmentation in established VBAC labour.

Clinical management issues
1 The decision for augmentation should follow careful obstetric assessment, maternal counselling, and should be consultant-led.
2 Oxytocin augmentation should be titrated such that it should not exceed the maximum rate of contractions of 4 in 10 minutes. Particular caution is necessary when using high oxytocin augmentation doses as there is a 'dose response' for maximum oxytocin amount and uterine rupture.
3 Careful serial cervical assessments, preferably by the same person, are necessary to show adequate cervicometric progress, thereby allowing augmentation to continue. These intervals should not exceed 4 h.
4 If there was less than 2 cm progress after 4 h of oxytocin, then caesarean section should be considered. A more conservative threshold of inadequate progress after 2 h of augmentation may also justify consideration for caesarean section depending on the woman's individual circumstances.
5 If there was 2 cm or more progress, augmentation could be continued and vaginal examinations performed 4-hourly.

risk of emergency intrapartum caesarean section, and the risk of a failed VBAC is increased both post-dates and with induction of labour. These issues lead some women to decide to attempt VBAC if they labour spontaneously prior to 41 weeks, but to have a planned caesarean section if their pregnancy proceeds postdates. The choice about the method of elective delivery postdates will also be informed by other factors determining the likelihood of a successful VBAC (favourable cervix and previous vaginal birth), and by the priority attached to achieving vaginal birth (such as plans for many future pregnancies).

Augmentation and labour dystocia

There is no direct evidence to recommend what is acceptable or unacceptable cervicometric progress in women with spontaneous or augmented VBAC labour [2]. Amongst women with unscarred uteri, the NICE intrapartum guideline defines delay in the established first stage of labour as cervical dilatation of less than 2 cm in 4 h [4]. For women with intact membranes, an amniotomy would then be recommended and repeat vaginal examination performed 2 h later: if progress was still less than 1 cm, then diagnosis of delay would be confirmed. If there was less than 2 cm progress after 4 h of oxytocin, further obstetric review would be required to consider caesarean section. If there was 2 cm or more progress, augmentation could be continued and vaginal examinations performed 4-hourly.

If, in the presence of adequate (strength and frequency) uterine contractions, there is a slowing down of a previously normally progressing labour, augmentation may increase the risk of uterine rupture. A small-sized retrospective study suggested that early recognition and intervention for labour dystocia (specifically, not exceeding 2 h of static cervicometric progress) may have prevented a proportion of uterine ruptures among women attempting VBAC [24]. Awareness of the increased risk of uterine rupture in scarred uteri, particularly if there is labour dystocia, implies that a more conservative threshold to the upper time limit (such as 2 h instead of 4 h) of oxytocin augmentation without progress may be justified. Furthermore, a retrospective multicentre study showed a 'dose response' for maximum oxytocin amount and uterine rupture, with a uterine rupture rate of 2.07% at the highest dosages [25]. Therefore, particular caution is necessary when using high oxytocin augmentation doses. A summary of the key management issues relating to augmented VBAC is shown in Table 22.6.

Intrapartum care at ERCS
Timing of ERCS

ERCS should be performed at commencement of the 39th week of gestation, as this represents the optimum time to minimize the risks of respiratory morbidity [10,11].

Mode of delivery and the outcome of future pregnanies

When considering mode of delivery, women should be advised about the effect of their decision on future pregnancies. The following risks significantly increase with increasing number of previous caesarean deliveries [2].

- *Placenta praevia.* Overall, placenta praevia occurs in 0.5% of deliveries. However, praevia is present in 0.38, 0.63 and 0.72% after single vaginal delivery, single caesarean, and two consecutive caesareans, respectively [26].
- *Placenta accreta.* Overall, placenta accreta is between 0.25 and 2 per 1000 deliveries [27]. However, accreta is present in 0.24, 0.31, 0.57, 2.13, 2.33 and 6.74% of women undergoing their first, second, third, fourth, fifth, and sixth or more caesarean deliveries, respectively [28]. The risk that placenta accreta co-exists with placenta praevia is 3, 11, 40, 61 and 67% for first, second, third, fourth, and fifth or more repeat caesarean deliveries, diagnosed to have placenta praevia [28].
- *Placental abruption.* Overall, placenta abruption occurs in 1% of deliveries. However, abruption is present in 0.74, 0.95 and 1.06% after single vaginal delivery, single caesarean, and two consecutive caesareans, respectively [26].
- *Injury to bladder, bowel or ureter.* A retrospective study of approximately 3000 women from Saudi Arabia showed a linear increase in the risk of bladder injury (0.3, 0.8, 2.4%), with a history of two, three and five caesarean sections, respectively [29].
- *Ileus.*
- *Need for postoperative ventilation.*
- *Intensive care unit admission.*
- *Hysterectomy* – required in 0.65, 0.42, 0.90, 2.41, 3.49 and 8.99% of women undergoing their first, second, third, fourth, fifth, and sixth or more caesarean deliveries, respectively.
- *Blood transfusion* (requiring 4 or more units).
- *Duration* of operative time and hospital stay.

Given the high absolute risks of serious complications, caesarean delivery of women with high numbers of previous caesarean sections requires the immediate availability of senior surgical staff.

Placenta praevia and accreta: pre-operative investigations

It is widespread practice in the UK, and endorsed by a RCOG guideline [30], that women identified to have low-lying placentas at the routine mid-pregnancy fetal anomaly scan should be rescanned in the third trimester. Provided the woman is asymptomatic (not bled), it is suggested that rescan be conducted at 32 or 36 weeks' gestation, depending on whether the mid-pregnancy scan suggested major or minor praevia, respectively [30]. However, given the strong association between placenta praevia, placenta accreta and prior caesarean birth, and the importance of their pre-operative identification, then rescan and placental localization assessment should commence at 32 weeks (and be repeated at 36 weeks) for women with prior caesarean delivery. Furthermore, those women identified to have praevia (especially anterior placenta praevia) should undergo further antenatal imaging (such as power amplitude ultrasonic angiography, MRI, or colour flow Doppler) to help clarify the risk of accreta [3,30].

Identification of placenta accreta prior to delivery enables instigation of specific management strategies to minimize adverse outcome at delivery. These include: consultant anaesthetist and obstetrician conducting the delivery; access to cross-matched blood; colleagues from other specialities/subspecialities to be on standby to attend as needed; and discussing the risk of haemorrhage, transfusion and hysterectomy with the women as part of the consent procedure. In addition, advance planning and consideration could be given to: prophylactic or therapeutic uterine artery embolization; internal iliac artery ligation at the same time as initial surgery; methotrexate treatment following delivery; and expectant management (placenta left in place at the end of the caesarean section) [3,30].

Planned VBAC in special circumstances

A cautious approach should be adopted when considering planned VBAC in women with preterm VBAC, twin gestation, fetal macrosomia and short interdelivery interval, as there is uncertainty in the safety and efficacy of planned VBAC in such situations.

Preterm VBAC

The NICHD study showed planned VBAC success rates for preterm and term pregnancies were similar (72.8 vs. 73.3%); however, the rates of uterine rupture (34 per 10,000 vs. 74 per 10,000, respectively) and dehiscence (26 per 10,000 vs. 67 per 10,000, respectively) were significantly lower in preterm compared with term VBAC [31]. Perinatal outcomes were similar with preterm VBAC and preterm ERCS [31].

Twin gestation

The NICHD study [32] (n=186 twins), US retrospective study [33] (n=535 twins) and a review [34] (7 studies, n=233 twins) have reported similar successful rates of VBAC in twin pregnancies to that in singleton pregnancies (65–84%).

Fetal macrosomia

A review [34] of four retrospective studies, and the NICHD study [16], has reported a significantly decreased likelihood of successful trial of VBAC for pregnancies with infants weighing 4000 g or more (55–67%) compared to smaller infants (75–83%). A subgroup analysis of the NICHD study showed that women with previous caesarean delivery for dystocia, and greater birth weight in the subsequent planned VBAC labour relative to the first birthweight decreased the likelihood of VBAC success [35].

Short interdelivery interval

A short interdelivery interval (below 12 months) from the previous caesarean delivery is associated with a two- to threefold increased risk of uterine rupture, major maternal morbidity and blood transfusion [2,16,36]. Furthermore, irrespective of the method of delivery in the first pregnancy, a short interdelivery interval increases risks of both placenta praevia and placental abruption [26]. Although this information is useful antenatally, it should also be shared with women postnatally to enable them to plan their preferred spacing intervals for subsequent pregnancies.

Conclusion and future directions

There should be documented discussion of risks and benefits of VBAC and ERCS and shared decision making when determining the mode of delivery. There should be consultant-led antenatal care (Figure 22.1) and consultant involvement when establishing a plan for induction or augmentation.

Planned VBAC compared to ERCS increases the risks of maternal morbidity, perinatal morbidity and perinatal mortality, particularly if the VBAC is unsuccessful. The principle risk associated with VBAC labour is uterine rupture.

The NICHD study showed that the additional attributable risk for experiencing a serious adverse perinatal outcome (antepartum stillbirth, delivery-related perinatal death or HIE) at term for planned VBAC, compared to ERCS, appears to be approximately 1 in 400 (or 0.25%). It is likely that this risk is significantly reduced, or even eliminated, for women who opt for ERCS at the start of the 39th week, however, direct evidence to support this is lacking.

References

1. NICE. *National Institute of Clinical Excellence, RCOG Caesarean Section.* Guideline No. 13. Available at: www.nice.org.uk/CG013NICEguideline. 2004.

2. RCOG. *Birth after Previous Caesarean Birth.* RCOG Green top guideline No. 45. London: RCOG Press, 2007.

3. The Confidential Enquiry into Maternal and Child Health (CEMACH). *Saving Mothers' Lives: Reviewing Maternal Deaths to Make Motherhood Safer – 2003–2005. The Seventh Report on Confidential Enquiries into Maternal Deaths in the United Kingdom.* London: CEMACH, 2007.

4. National Insititute of Clinical Excellence. *Intrapartum Care: Care of Healthy Women and their Babies during Childbirth.* NICE Clinical Guideline 55. London: NICE, 2007.

5. RCOG. *Safer Childbirth: Minimum Standards for the Organisation and Delivery of Care in Labour.* Royal College of Anaesthetists, Royal College of Midwives, Royal College of Obstetricians and Gynaecologists, Royal College of Paediatrics and Child Health. London: RCOG Press, 2007.

6. Landon M B, Hauth J C, Leveno K J, *et al.* Maternal and perinatal outcomes associated with a trial of labor after prior cesarean delivery. *N Engl J Med* 2004; **351:** 2581–9.

7. Dodd J M, Crowther C A, Hiller J E, *et al.* Birth after caesarean study – planned vaginal birth or planned elective repeat caesarean for women at term with a single previous caesarean birth: protocol for a patient preference study and randomised trial. *BMC Pregn Childbirth* 2007; **7:** 17.

8. Montgomery A A, Emmett C L, Fahey T, *et al.* Two decision aids for mode of delivery among women with previous caesarean section: randomised controlled trial. *Br Med J* 2007; **334:** 1305.

9. Lyerly A D, Mitchell L M, Armstrong E M, *et al.* Risks, values, and decision making surrounding pregnancy. *Obstet Gynecol* 2007; **109:** 979–84.

10. Smith G C S. Life-table analysis of the risk of perinatal death at term and post term in singleton pregnancies. *Am J Obstet Gynecol* 2001; **184:** 489–96.

11. Smith G C S, Pell J P, Dobbie R. Caesarean section and risk of unexplained stillbirth in subsequent pregnancy. *Lancet* 2003; **362:** 1779–84.

12. Landon M B, Spong C Y, Thom E, *et al.* Risk of uterine rupture with a trial of labor in women with multiple and single prior cesarean delivery. *Obstet Gynecol* 2006; **108**: 12–20.

13. Grobman W A, Lai Y, Landon M B, *et al.* Development of a nomogram for prediction of vaginal birth after cesarean delivery. *Obstet Gynecol* 2007; **109**: 806–12.

14. Smith G C S, White I R, Pell J P, *et al.* Predicting cesarean section and uterine rupture among women attempting vaginal birth after prior cesarean section. *PLoS Med* 2005; **2**: 871–8.

15. Macones G A, Cahill A G, Stamilio D M, *et al.* Can uterine rupture in patients attempting vaginal birth after cesarean delivery be predicted? *Am J Obstet Gynecol* 2006; **195**: 1148–52.

16. Landon M B, Leindecker S, Spong C Y, *et al.* The MFMU Cesarean Registry: factors affecting the success of trial of labor after previous cesarean delivery. *Am J Obstet Gynecol* 2005; **193**: 1016–23.

17. Varner M W, Thom E, Spong C Y, *et al.* Trial of labor after one previous cesarean delivery for multifetal gestation. *Obstet Gynecol* 2007; **110**: 814–9.

18. DeFranco E A, Rampersad R, Atkins K L, *et al.* Do vaginal birth after cesarean outcomes differ based on hospital setting? *Am J Obstet Gynecol* 2007; **197**: 400–6.

19. Smith G C S, Pell J P, Pasupathy D, *et al.* Factors predisposing to perinatal death related to uterine rupture during attempted vaginal birth after caesarean section: retrospective cohort study. *Br Med J* 2004; **329**: 375.

20. Grobman W A, Gilbert S, Landon M B, *et al.* Outcomes of induction of labor after one prior cesarean. *Obstet Gynecol* 2007; **109**: t-9.

21. Kelly A J, Kavanagh J, Thomas J. Vaginal prostaglandin (PGE2 and PGF2a) for induction of labour at term. *Cochrane Database Syst Rev* 2006; CD003101.

22. NICE. National Institute of Clinical Excellence. *RCOG Induction of Labour. Evidence-based Clinical Guideline Number 9.* London: National Institute of Clinical Excellence, 2001.

23. Gray R, Quigley M A, Hockley C, *et al.* Caesarean delivery and risk of stillbirth in subsequent pregnancy: a retrospective cohort study in an English population. *Br J Obstet Gynaecol* 2007; **114**: 264–70.

24. Hamilton E F, Bujold E, McNamara H, *et al.* Dystocia among women with symptomatic uterine rupture. *Am J Obstet Gynecol* 2001; **184**: 620–4.

25. Cahill A G, Stamilio D M, Odibo A O, *et al.* Does a maximum dose of oxytocin affect risk for uterine rupture in candidates for vaginal birth after cesarean delivery? *Am J Obstet Gynecol* 2007; **197**: 495.

26. Getahun D, Oyelese Y, Salihu H M, *et al.* Previous cesarean delivery and risks of placenta previa and placental abruption. *Obstet Gynecol* 2006; **107**: 771–8.

27. Faiz A S, Ananth C V. Etiology and risk factors for placenta previa: an overview and meta-analysis of observational studies. *J Matern Fetal Neonatal Med* 2003; **13**: 175–90.

28. Silver R M, Landon M B, Rouse D J, *et al.* Maternal morbidity associated with multiple repeat cesarean deliveries. *Obstet Gynecol* 2006; **107**: 1226–32.

29. Makoha F W, Felimban H M, Fathuddien M A, *et al.* Multiple cesarean section morbidity. *Int J Gynaecol Obstet* Guideline No. 27 2004; **87**: 227–32.

30. RCOG. *Placenta Praevia and Placenta Praevia Accreta: Diagnosis and Management* London: RCOG, 2005.

31. Durnwald C P, Rouse D J, Leveno K J, *et al.* The Maternal–Fetal Medicine Units Cesarean Registry: safety and efficacy of a trial of labor in preterm pregnancy after a prior cesarean delivery. *Am J Obstet Gynecol* 2006; **195**: 1119–26.

32. Varner M W, Leindecker S, Spong C Y, *et al.* The Maternal–Fetal Medicine Unit cesarean registry: trial of labor with a twin gestation. *Am J Obstet Gynecol* 2005; **193**: 135–40.

33. Cahill A, Stamilio D M, Pare E, *et al.* Vaginal birth after cesarean (VBAC) attempt in twin pregnancies: is it safe? *Am J Obstet Gynecol* 2005; **193**: 1050–55.

34. Guise J M, Hashima J, Osterweil P. Evidence-based vaginal birth after Caesarean section. *Best Pract Res Clin Obstet Gynaecol* 2005; **19**: 117–30.

35. Peaceman A M, Gersnoviez R, Landon M B, *et al.* The MFMU Cesarean Registry: impact of fetal size on trial of labor success for patients with previous cesarean for dystocia. *Am J Obstet Gynecol* 2006; **195**: 1127–31.

36. Stamilio D M, DeFranco E, Pare E, *et al.* Short interpregnancy interval: risk of uterine rupture and complications of vaginal birth after cesarean delivery. *Obstet Gynecol* 2007; **110**: 1075–82.

37. Ofir K, Sheiner E, Levy A, *et al.* Uterine rupture: risk factors and pregnancy outcome. *Am J Obstet Gynecol* 2003; **189**: 1042–6.

38. Guise J M, McDonagh M S, Osterweil P, *et al.* Systematic review of the incidence and consequences of uterine rupture in women with previous caesarean section. *Br Med J* 2004; **329**: 19–25.

251

Chapter

23

Rupture of the uterus

Nutan Mishra and Edwin Chandraharan

Introduction

Uterine rupture is an obstetric emergency character-ized by tearing (disruption/dehiscence) of the uterine wall during pregnancy or delivery. It is a catastrophic obstetric complication, associated with high rates of perinatal as well as maternal morbidity and mortality. The consequences of uterine rupture apply not only to the index pregnancy or to its immediate aftermath, but it impacts future fertility prospects, which may be hampered due to irreparable damage to the uterus that may necessitate a hysterectomy. Even if the uterus is conserved after uterine rupture, the course and outcome of any future pregnancy may be altered.

Fortunately, uterine rupture is rare in modern obstetric practice, despite the increase in caesarean section rates. Serious complications like maternal deaths are even rarer. Although the uterus can rup-ture in the antenatal period, especially in a patient with a previous classical (upper segment) caesarean section, it ruptures most commonly during labour. Uterine rupture can occur in both the scarred and unscarred uterus, but more often it occurs with the former in developed countries. In some parts of the developing world with poor healthcare delivery systems, rupture of the unscarred uterus does take place and is often due to 'grand' multiparity (due to poor availability of family planning services), coupled with intrapartum adverse factors like prolonged or obstructed labour, associated with cephalopelvic disproportion.

Epidemiology

Uterine rupture is a rare event. In a World Health Organization (WHO)-commissioned systematic review [1], prevalence figures were determined for groups of women, mainly hospital-based, from secondary and tertiary institutions. For community-based unselected pregnant women, the prevalence rates of uterine rup-ture were considerably lower (median 0.053, range 0.016–0.30%) than for facility-based studies (0.31, 0.012–2.9%). The prevalence tended to be lower for countries defined by the United Nations as developed than the less or least developed countries. For women with previous caesarean section, the prevalence of uterine rupture reported was in the region of 1%. The prevalence for women without previous caesar-ean section from a developed country was extremely low (0.006%).

Although there are case reports of rupture of the primigravid uterus [2], it is a very rare event. Gardiel et al. [3] found no case of primigravid uterine rupture over 10 years, representing 21,998 first pregnancies. Similar results were reported by Cahill et al. [4], who examined primigravid term deliveries over a 13-year period in an institution, where high-dose oxytocin augmentation was standard management for primi-gravid labour. There were no cases of uterine rupture for 30,874 deliveries.

The reported incidence of spontaneous rupture of the unscarred uterus ranges from 1 in 8000 to 1 in 15,000 deliveries [5].

Classification (Table 23.1)

There are two types of uterine rupture. Complete rupture involves the full thickness of the uterine wall (Figure 23.1a). Incomplete rupture occurs, when the visceral peritoneum remains intact (Figure 23.1b). It is important to make this distinction, because there are differences between the two in terms of clinical presentation and rates of complications. Complete rupture presents usually as a dramatic emergency,

Best Practice in Labour and Delivery, ed. R. Warren and S. Arulkumaran. Published by Cambridge University Press.
© Cambridge University Press 2009.

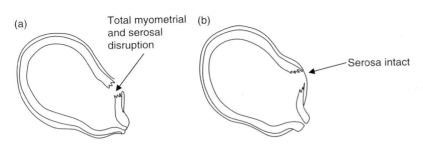

(a) Total myometrial and serosal disruption

(b) Serosa intact

Figure 23.1 Types of scar rupture.
(a) Complete rupture. (b) Scar dehiscence

Table 23.1 Classification of causes of uterine rupture.

Uterine injury or anomaly sustained before current pregnancy	Uterine injury or abnormality during current pregnancy
1. *Surgery involving the myometrium*	1. *Before delivery*
Caesarean section or hysterotomy	Labour stimulation
Previously repaired uterine rupture	External trauma
Myomectomy	External cephalic version (ECV)
Deep cornual resection	
Metroplasty	
2. Coincidental uterine trauma	2. *During delivery*
Abortion	Internal version
Sharp or blunt trauma	Difficult forceps
	Breech extraction
3. Congenital anomaly	3. *Acquired in pregnancy*
Pregnancy in undeveloped uterine horn	Placenta increta or percreta
	Adenomyosis
	Sacculation of entrapped retroverted uterus

which is potentially life-threatening for both the mother and the baby. Incomplete rupture presents typically as an asymptomatic dehiscence of a previous uterine scar found at the time of caesarean section. It is usually uncomplicated (Figure 23.1) [6].

Risk factors

The single most important factor in determining the risk of uterine rupture is whether the uterus has a previous scar or not. Rupture of an unscarred uterus is less frequent and usually traumatic in origin.

Previous caesarean section

A prospective 4-year observational study of over 33,000 women with a singleton pregnancy and a prior caesarean delivery has provided robust information on maternal and perinatal outcomes associated with a trial of labour [7]. Symptomatic uterine rupture occurred in 0.7% of women and hypoxic ischaemic encephalopathy occurred in 0.46 per 1000 infants of women undergoing trial of labour versus no cases of uterine rupture or hypoxic ischaemic encephalopathy, when delivered by elective caesarean delivery. A systematic review showed that compared with elective repeat caesarean delivery, trial of labour increased the risk of uterine rupture by 2.7 per 1000 cases.

Women who have not previously given birth vaginally and those whose labour is induced with prostaglandins are at increased risk of uterine rupture when attempting vaginal birth after caesarean section [8].

Previous uterine surgery

Although there is a well-documented association between abdominal myomectomy and uterine rupture during subsequent pregnancy, the reported incidence of this shows a wide variation. Location of the fibroid, depth of the required incision, surgical technique and presence of postoperative infection are thought to influence the likelihood of scar rupture in subsequent pregnancy [5].

Forty-seven pregnancies in 40 patients were reviewed after laparoscopic myomectomy. Vaginal birth was attempted in 72%, and this was achieved in 83% of these women with no case of uterine rupture. The authors advised that vaginal birth could be safely achieved after laparoscopic myomectomy, provided that delivery is managed in the same manner as for a vaginal birth after caesarean section (VBAC). A detailed review of literature confirms that risk of uterine rupture is very low when the myometrium is repaired appropriately [9].

Advances in fetal medicine have resulted in intra-uterine fetal surgery to improve perinatal outcome. Fetoscopic procedures involve injury to a pregnant uterus, with a subsequent risk of uterine rupture. The reproductive outcomes for women who have experienced a pregnancy complicated by maternal–fetal surgery were explored in a retrospective review of 83 women. The pregnancy rate was 62% and complications were reported in 12 of 34 pregnancies, including uterine rupture (6%) and dehiscence (12%) [10].

Uterine rupture has also been documented following myolysis, wherein uterine fibroids are coagulated laparoscopically [11].

Obstructed labour

This is an important cause of spontaneous rupture in the developing world, especially when a woman labours outside a hospital. Black African women have a high incidence of contracted pelvis and prolonged and obstructed labour. This leads to cephalo-pelvic disproportion, with an increased risk of uterine rupture. Multiparity is an independent risk factor for uterine rupture, as the uterus of a multiparous woman consists of a relatively greater proportion of collagen, as compared to smooth muscle. Hence, in the presence of an obstruction or a relative cephalo-pelvic disproportion, the uterus may rupture.

Administration of agents for induction of labour and termination of pregnancy

Artificial initiation or augmentation of uterine contractions have an inherent risk of causing uterine hyperstimulation, leading to uterine rupture. Such a risk increases in the presence of a uterine scar or multiparity.

The risk of uterine rupture after use of misoprostol for labour induction at term in women with history of uterine scar has been well documented. Misoprostol use in the second trimester in women with a uterine scar can trigger severe contractions that can lead to uterine rupture.

Congenital uterine malformation

Congenital uterine malformations complicate 1 in 594 pregnancies. The walls of congenitally abnormal uteri are likely to be thinner than those of normal uteri. Their myometrium tends to diminish in thickness as gestation advances and can be inconsistent over different aspects of the uterus. Additional wall thinning can occur as a result of uterine contractions [12]. All these factors could increase the risk of uterine rupture, the greatest risk being during labour.

Trauma

Uterine rupture complicates only a minority of trauma cases during pregnancy. It usually occurs in association with an automobile accident in which pregnant women were not restrained. Maternal and fetal outcomes were analysed in a retrospective cohort study. It was found that women delivering at the time of hospitalization had severe adverse outcomes compared with non-trauma controls, with a marked increase in uterine rupture. The study highlighted the need to optimize education in trauma prevention in pregnancy [13].

A further study on the same cohort focused on pregnancy outcomes among women hospitalized for assault. The incidence of uterine rupture was markedly increased compared with women with no history of assault [14]. Hence, it is vital to exclude uterine rupture in cases where domestic violence is suspected.

Connective tissue disorders

The uterus is a muscular organ with a connective tissue matrix. Disorders of connective tissues can affect the structure (i.e. integrity) as well as the function of the uterus. The Ehlers–Danlos syndrome has been reported to be a rare cause of uterine rupture in pregnancy [5].

Mechanisms

The underlying pathophysiology behind rupture of the uterus has received little attention to date. The increased risk of uterine rupture for women labouring with a uterine scar is exacerbated by the use of prostaglandins for induction of labour. Apart from increasing uterine contractility, there is also a possibility of biochemical changes within the collagen component of the scar by prostaglandins. Examination of the site of scar rupture was carried out in 26 women with a prior caesarean section who experienced uterine rupture in active labour to determine whether prostaglandins induced biochemical changes in the uterine scar, similar to the cervix. Women treated with prostaglandins experienced rupture at the site of the old scar more frequently than those in the oxytocin-only group, whose rupture tended to be remote from the old scar [15]. Hence, prostaglandins may induce changes in the collagen and the glycosaminoglycans of the uterine scar, similar to their effect on the cervix during induction of labour. This may predispose to an increased incidence of scar dehiscence or rupture.

Clinical features

The clinical findings may vary from mild and non-specific symptoms and signs to an obvious abdominal catastrophe. Classical symptoms and signs include abdominal pain (typically 'continuous and persisting in between the contractions'), vaginal bleeding, lower abdominal tenderness ('scar tenderness') and receding of the presenting part on vaginal examination. It is rare for all the classical features to be present in a single patient. Prior to the development of frank haemorrhagic shock, the symptoms and physical findings may appear 'non-specific' or at times 'bizarre', and therefore may be missed unless the possibility of uterine rupture is kept in mind. Abnormal patterns may be observed on a cardiotocograph (CTG). These include total loss of uterine contractions often preceded by tachysystole or hypertonus, reduced baseline variability of the FHR, variable or late decelerations, or a prolonged deceleration or a baseline bradycardia. Pathophysiological mechanisms responsible for the

CTG changes include cord prolapse through the ruptured scar (variable decelerations), partial or total placental separation and the resultant hypoxia (late decelerations or prolonged decelerations). Uterine rupture may present during the antepartum, intrapartum or postpartum period.

Antepartum rupture

In antepartum rupture, abdominal pain is the most important clinical symptom. Vaginal bleeding may occur, but haemorrhage may be entirely intra-abdominal. Haemoperitoneum from a ruptured uterus may result in irritation of the diaphragm and pain referred to the chest or to the shoulder ('shoulder tip' pain). There may be history of abdominal trauma, and the possibility of domestic violence should be kept in mind. Patients with a previous scar in the upper uterine segment may present early in pregnancy and may not experience uterine contractions before rupture [6].

On examination, the woman may have the clinical signs of shock, which is mainly hypovolumic, but also may have a 'neurogenic component'. There may be abdominal tenderness, especially if the contents of the uterus have been released into the abdominal cavity. Tenderness over a previous uterine scar is not a reliable sign of uterine rupture. The shape of the uterus may be distorted and the fetal parts easily palpable. Finally, there may be evidence of fetal distress or demise.

Intrapartum rupture

This is more common in current obstetric practice, as classical ('upper segment') caesarean section is rarely performed. The widespread use of electronic fetal monitoring (EFM) in high-risk labour (e.g. previous caesarean section) has enabled clinicians to rely on fetal heart rate abnormalities to diagnose scar dehiscence or rupture.

Abdominal pain is also a common presentation of intrapartum uterine rupture, and the development of constant pain should raise the suspicion of either rupture or placental separation. In labour, the symptom of abdominal pain due to rupture is difficult to interpret in the presence of uterine contractions. A few studies found abdominal pain to be a poor predictor of uterine rupture, and there was no association with the extrusion of the fetus in the abdominal cavity and the degree of abdominal pain.

The development of 'scar tenderness', changes in uterine shape and 'easy' palpation of fetal parts are suggestive of uterine rupture. However, these signs are unreliable. Overreliance on these parameters is likely to result in the overdiagnosis of scar rupture. Vaginal bleeding may or may not occur. Haematuria may be present in a small number of cases, especially if the trauma involves the bladder.

Continuous electronic monitoring is recommended for women with a previous caesarean section, as this may prove useful in warning about imminent rupture. Two recent studies report on fetal heart changes associated with uterine rupture. One compared 36 cases of uterine rupture with 100 controls. Fetal bradycardia in the first and second stage of labour was the only finding to differentiate uterine rupture from successful vaginal birth after caesarean section (VBAC) patients [16]. A second study compared tracings from 50 women with uterine rupture with 601 controls. Uterine tachysystole and reduced baseline variability were found to be independent patterns preceding uterine rupture in the first and second stages of labour [17]. Although variable and/or late decelerations precede fetal bradycardia, no specific fetal heart rate or uterine activity pattern is diagnostic of uterine rupture [18].

Loss of uterine pressure or cessation of labour (uterine activity) are thought to be associated with uterine rupture. However, this has been recently disputed. Rodriguez *et al.* reported the data from 39 of 76 women with uterine rupture in whom there was an intrauterine pressure catheter [19]. Loss of intrauterine pressure or cessation of labour was noted in none of these patients.

In situations where the fetal presenting part had already entered the pelvis with labour, there may be 'loss of station' (i.e. receding presenting part) that may be detected by abdominal and/or pelvic examination. If the fetus is partly or totally extruded, abdominal palpation or vaginal examination is helpful in identifying the presenting part lying away from the pelvic inlet. A firm, contracted uterus may at times be felt alongside the fetus. Often, fetal parts are more easily palpated than usual.

Postpartum rupture

This is a very rare complication and usually presents with abdominal pain and tenderness, and/or postpartum haemorrhage. On vaginal examination, it is sometimes possible to palpate a 'tear' in the uterine wall through which the fingers can be passed into the peritoneal cavity. However, routine palpation of the uterine scar after delivery by performing a vaginal examination, to exclude scar dehiscence, is not recommended. Such an examination may have a risk of inadvertently perforating the scar.

Findings at the time of laparotomy

The lower uterine segment is the most commonly involved part in rupture. In one study of the cases of rupture, the lower segment was ruptured in 92.6% and 92.3% of cases in the unscarred group and the scarred uterus group, respectively [20]. Other studies have also reported high rates of involvement of the lower segment of the uterus [21], probably caused by distension and elongation of the muscle fibres, thus leading to reduced thickness. However, other parts of the uterus may also be involved. There were four cases of rupture of the fundus in one series [22]. Involvement of the uterine cervix was found to be higher among patients without previous uterine scarring.

The rupture of the lower segment may extend anteriorly towards the back of the bladder, laterally towards the uterine arteries or into the broad ligament plexus of veins, causing extensive haemorrhage and damage. It is, therefore, important not only to examine the uterus properly in its entirety, but also to carry out a thorough examination of other pelvic organs as well.

Posterior rupture is uncommon, but it can occur and is usually associated with intrauterine malformations. However, it may also occur in association with an obstructed labour or rotational forceps delivery in patients who have had a previous CS. External cephalic version (ECV) done for breech presentation may also cause rupture of the uterus at any site.

Diagnosis
Prediction of uterine scar rupture

Attempts have been made to assess the integrity of the lower uterine segment of patients with a prior caesarean section using ultrasound antenatally [6]. A prospective observational study of 642 patients found that the risk of scar rupture and dehiscence was directly related to the degree of thinning of the lower segment at around 37 weeks of pregnancy [23]. Using a thickness value of 3.5 mm or greater, the sensitivity was 88% and the specificity 73.2%. However, the positive predictive value was only 11.8%, although the negative predictive value was 99.3%. While the finding of a thick lower segment on ultrasound may reassure the clinicians, there is no evidence that such measurements are superior to careful clinical practice in the prevention of rupture.

Ultrasound examination was performed in 102 pregnant women with history of one or more previous caesarean sections, between 36 and 38 weeks' gestation, to assess the thickness of the lower uterine segment and to assess the usefulness of this measurement in predicting the risk of uterine rupture [24]. The mean lower segment thickness was 1.8 mm (standard deviation 1.1 mm). These measurements were significantly lower in patients who had uterine dehiscence, although none of them developed uterine rupture. A lower segment thickness of 1.5 mm had a sensitivity of 89%, a specificity of 60%, a positive predictive value of 96% for dehiscence or a 'paper-thin' lower segment. It appears that there is currently some evidence to suggest that ultrasound assessment of the lower segment may be useful in predicting the risk of uterine rupture, but further research is needed prior to implementing this in clinical practice. It is likely that the use of arbitrary cut-off limits for the thickness of the lower segment using an ultrasound scan may increase the number of repeat elective caesarean sections, as there is insufficient evidence to suggest that it is superior to clinical evaluation.

The use of magnetic resonance imaging has been described as an alternative approach when ultrasound findings of dehiscence are still inconclusive, but expertise in this approach is still limited [25]. Clinical parameters that may be used to predict the possibility of uterine rupture include extension of uterine incision to the upper segment, uterine tears, and very preterm caesarean section (i.e. poor or no formation of the lower segment).

Management

Once the diagnosis of complete uterine rupture is suspected, immediate delivery is indicated to improve maternal and perinatal outcome. If the woman is clinically shocked, she needs to be resuscitated first, and this usually will include blood transfusion. Uterine rupture is an obstetric emergency that poses a threat to the life of both mother and fetus. Because the gravid uterus receives 12% of the cardiac output, when uterine rupture occurs, haemorrhage can be extremely rapid. Rupture of the uterus presents the anaesthetist with a unique challenge of maintaining haemodynamic status before haemostasis is secured, as the patient is often in hypovolumic shock.

With urgent need to control haemorrhage, anaesthesia may have to be induced in patients, who are hypovolumic and hypotensive.

Immediate laparotomy, delivery of fetus within 15 min by lower segment caesarean section (LSCS), (if still inside the uterus) and repair of the ruptured site is the main aim. Leung et al. undertook a retrospective review of 106 cases of uterine rupture [26]. They found a higher incidence of perinatal morbidity and at times mortality, associated with complete fetal extrusion, and significant mortality occurred when more than 18 min elapsed between the onset of prolonged decelerations and delivery. In another series, rapid intervention (<18 min) between prolonged deceleration and birth did not always prevent severe metabolic acidosis and serious neonatal outcome, but it probably reduced the incidence of neonatal death [27].

Once the baby and placenta are delivered, control of haemorrhage is a priority. The anatomy needs to be carefully identified, and this can be distorted, especially where the uterus ruptures into the bladder or broad ligament. A multidisciplinary approach with involvement of general, vascular, and urological surgeons may be necessary if extension occurs into ureters, bladder, broad ligament, or pelvic vessels.

The choice of operative procedure depends on a number of factors, including the patient's general condition, type and extent of rupture, facilities available, previous obstetric history, and experience of the surgeon.

Rupture of a previous caesarean delivery scar can often be managed by revision of the edges of the prior incision followed by primary closure.

In addition to the myometrial disruption, consideration must be given to the neighbouring structures, such as the broad ligament, parametrial vessels, ureters, and bladder. Hysterectomy may be necessary in a life-threatening situation to achieve haemostasis, especially if the patient is haemodynamically unstable and it is not possible to achieve haemostasis without hysterectomy. Such patients may also develop coagulopathy and, hence, would require blood and blood products. An experienced obstetrician and an anaesthetist should be present. The possibility of ureteric involvement should be borne in mind and if there are concerns after the surgery, a postnatal renal ultra-sound or intravenous urogram may need to be done.

The option of a subtotal hysterectomy may be considered based on the clinical situation. This may be associated with less risk of bladder and ureteric injuries as compared to a total hysterectomy. Giwa-Osagie *et al.* [28] reported a series of emergency obstetric hysterectomies in 61 patients, of whom 37 had a ruptured uterus. The lowest mortality (4%) followed subtotal hysterectomy in booked patients, while the mortality was higher (50%) in unbooked patients who had hysterectomy. Ligation of hypogastric (internal iliac) artery was found useful for attaining adequate haemostasis in five cases in one series [21]. Uterine artery embolization may not be feasible in an emergency situation. Facilities and expertise for immediate neonatal resuscitation is essential, as the neonate is often born in a poor condition. Cord blood gases are useful to evaluate the condition of the newborn.

Careful and clear documentation of operative findings and the procedures that are performed are essential to offer explanation and to counsel women of their future management. It would also be helpful in addressing medico-legal implications in the future. An adverse incident reporting form should be completed to alert the obstetric risk management team. In developed countries, uterine rupture is among the four most common clinical causes of medical litigation in obstetrics and gynaecology. Litigation raised in most cases is driven by bad outcomes and not by malpractice. High standards of clinical care, clear communication and careful documentation are of paramount importance if obstetricians are to be in a position to offer a balanced approach to patient care without fear of litigation.

Differential diagnosis

A number of conditions can present with abdominal pain, hypovolumia, and fetal compromise. Most commonly, this constellation of findings occurs with placental abruption, which may be concealed in the absence of vaginal bleeding. Other less-common conditions to be considered include subcapsular liver haematoma with or without rupture, rupture of broad ligament, splenic rupture, uterine torsion and uterine vein rupture. All of these conditions will require surgical intervention, and swift recourse to laparotomy is generally indicated for a patient presenting with these symptoms [5].

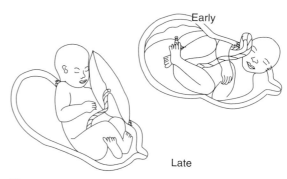

Figure 23.2 Uterine rupture with the prolapse of the cord (early) and expulsion of the fetus and the placenta (late)

Complications
Perinatal

Disruption of utero-placental circulation, secondary to stretching and tearing of uterine vessels, cord compression or placental separation may result in fetal hypoxia and metabolic acidosis. This may result in neurological sequelae, including cerebral palsy and, if severe, in perinatal death. It has been reported that severe metabolic acidosis was present in 9 (39%) of 23 neonates of women with uterine ruptures [27]. The median umbilical blood pH was 6.80, the median base deficit was 22, and the median 5 min Apgar score was 4. Hypoxic ischaemic encephalopathy (HIE) characterized by seizures and multiple organ failure is the immediate complication that may necessitate intubation and ventilation, and babies may need admission to the neonatal intensive care unit. Impaired motor development, learning difficulties and cerebral palsy are possible long-term problems. These complications are more likely to occur with placental or fetal extrusion outside the uterine cavity, as the degree of metabolic acidosis in this situation is severe [27].

Figure 23.2 shows the prolapse of the cord through the uterine incision in the early phases of the rupture, and this may produce 'variable decelerations' and complete occlusion may show prolonged deceleration in the CTG. As shown in Figure 23.2, the fetus and the placenta may be expelled into the peritoneal cavity and this is likely to result in prolonged deceleration.

Maternal

Haemoperitoneum and the resultant haemorrhagic shock as well as the interventions and their inherent complications are largely responsible for maternal morbidity and mortality. In less developed countries, uterine rupture is an important cause of maternal mortality, accounting for as many as 9.3% of maternal deaths in one Indian study [1]. In the Second Report on Confidential Enquiries into maternal deaths in South Africa 1999–2001, rupture of the uterus caused 6.2% of deaths due to direct causes and 3.7% of all deaths [1]. Difficulties in transport, access to health-care, availability of resources to deal with massive obstetric haemorrhage, cultural and organizational factors contribute to increased mortality.

In developed countries, uterine rupture rarely results in maternal death in modern obstetric prac-tice, but may result in significant maternal morbidity. Complications of massive blood transfusion, acute renal failure due to hypovolumia, interventions including unintended damage to adjacent structures during peripartum hysterectomy, and postoperative complications such as infections and thromboembo-lism may contribute to maternal morbidity. Women may also suffer from psychological disorders like depression or 'post-traumatic stress disorders', and these are likely to be severe if there is a poor perinatal outcome or hysterectomy.

In addition to haemorrhage, uterine rupture may result in urologic injury, and an incidence of 4.1% has been reported [29]. These were all iatrogenic urologi-cal injuries, sustained in the course of the operation and not caused by the rupture of the uterus. Patients who have massive haemorrhage may develop adult respiratory distress syndrome (ARDS), renal, liver or pituitary failure, and will generally require transfer to intensive care setting.

The long-term sequelae may be renal failure and Sheehan Syndrome (avascular necrosis of the pituitary gland characterized by failure of lactation followed by amenorrhoea, hypothyroidism and adrenal cortical insufficiency).

Maternal deaths are rare in the developed world and may be due to haemorrhage, shock, sepsis, dis-seminated intravascular coagulation and pulmonary embolism [30]. Often, they are likely due to 'too little done too late' with regard to the management of massive obstetric haemorrhage. Failure to appreciate the clinical condition, failure to institute timely and appropriate intervention, failure to seek timely senior help, and failure in effective multidisciplinary com-munication are some of the factors that may increase the likelihood of maternal mortality.

Subsequent reproductive outcome

Pregnancy after uterine rupture can be successful with good antenatal, intrapartum and postpartum care in the subsequent pregnancy. No clear evidence exists on the course of action that should be taken when a woman who previously had a uterine rupture presents with a new pregnancy. There seems to be a general agreement that the risk of a recurrent rupture would be too high to recommend a trial of vaginal delivery and that an elective caesarean delivery is the safest option [31]. The timing of delivery should be indi-vidualized based on data about gestational age at which the women went into labour in previous preg-nancies, type of scar, and gestational age at which the previous rupture occurred. Ideally a planned caesarean delivery should not be performed before 38 completed weeks to avoid the complications of iatrogenic prematurity. However, if the presumed risk of subsequent scar rupture is deemed to be very high beyond 38 weeks, then a decision may be made for a caesarean section prior to 37 weeks. This has to be clearly discussed with the patient, and the risks of possible complications of preterm delivery should be explained.

There are reports of vaginal birth after previous uterine rupture. In a study of 18 pregnancies in 15 women who had repair of a uterine rupture, 17 babies were delivered by caesarean and 1 baby delivered vaginally at 28 weeks' gestation. There was no case of recurrent uterine rupture [32]. There is a suggestion that patients with previous ruptured classical scars should be delivered by 35 weeks and those with previ-ous ruptured lower segment scars by 37 weeks' gesta-tion [33]. Some would advocate earlier hospitalization for patients with classical scars. As uterine rupture is a rare event, the basis of these recommendations is often based on 'expert opinion' or personal experience, rather than on any firm scientific evidence.

It is important to remember that uterine rupture and dehiscence after a previous classical caesarean section are neither predictable nor preventable. One in four patients will experience some form of maternal morbidity with uterine rupture, and although infre-quent, it can be fatal to the fetus. Uterine dehiscence, however, does not increase neonatal or peripartum maternal morbidity [34].

Recurrent uterine ruptures are associated with a high maternal and perinatal morbidity. It has been reported that although repair of uterine ruptures is possible, recurrences are frequent, especially after longitudinal ruptures and short intervals between rupture and subsequent pregnancy [35].

Conclusion

Uterine rupture may occur at any stage of pregnancy. In developed countries, the uterine rupture usually follows caesarean sections. It may be possible to minimize this catastrophic complication by careful selection of patients for vaginal birth after caesarean section (VBAC) and judicious administration of oxytocin, if required. Continuous electronic fetal monitoring during labour, recognizing fetal heart rate changes' and taking appropriate and timely action may reduce unfavourable fetal outcome [36].

In less developed countries, uterine rupture is more prevalent and the consequences are more serious. Strategies should be aimed at health education, improving the access to healthcare services and provision of resources to deal with obstetric emergencies. Although it is not currently possible to predict the occurrence of uterine rupture, timely diagnosis and institution of swift and appropriate interventions would help save the lives of mothers and their babies.

References

1. Hoffmeyr G J, Say L, Gulmezoglu A M. WHO systematic review of maternal mortality and morbidity; the prevalence of uterine rupture. *Br J Obstet Gynaecol* 2005; **112**: 1221–8.

2. Catanzarite V, Cousins L, Dowling D, Daneshmand S. Oxytocin – associated rupture of an unscarred uterus in a primigravida. *Obstet Gynecol* 2006; **108**: 723–5.

3. Gardiel F, Daly S, Turner M J. Uterine rupture in pregnancy reviewed. *Eur J Obstet Gynecol Reprod Biol* 1994; **56**: 107–10.

4. Cahill D J, Boylan P C, O'Herlihy C. Does oxytocin augmentation increase perinatal risk in primigravid labour? *Am J Obstet Gynecol* 1992; **166**: 847–50.

5. Walsh C A, Baxi L V. Rupture of the primigravid uterus: a review of the literature. *Obstet Gynecol Surv* 2007 May; **62**(5): 327–34.

6. Turner M J Uterine rupture [review]. *Best Pract Res Clin Obstet Gynaecol* 2002; **16**: 69–79.

7. Landon M B, Hauth J C, Levano K J, *et al.* Maternal and perinatal outcomes associated with a trial of labour after prior caesarean delivery. *N Engl J Med* 2004; **351**: 2581–9.

8. Smith G C, Pell J P, Pasupathy D, Dobbie R. Factors predisposing to perinatal death related to uterine rupture during attempted vaginal birth after caesarean section: retrospective cohort study. *Br Med J* 2004; **329**: 375.

9. Hurst B S, Matthews M L, Marshburn P B. Laparoscopic myomectomy for symptomatic uterine myomas. *Fertil Steril* 2005; **12**: 241–6.

10. Wilson R D, Johnson M P, Flake A W, *et al.* Reproductive outcomes after pregnancy complicated by maternal–fetal surgery. *Am J Obstet Gynecol* 2004; **19**: 1430–6.

11. Arcangeli S, Pasquarette M M. Gravid uterine rupture after myolysis. *Obstet Gynecol* 1997; **89**: 857.

12. Nahum G G. Uterine anomalies, induction of labour, and uterine rupture. *Obstet Gynecol* 2005 Nov; **106** (5 Pt 2): 1150–2.

13. El-Kady D, Gilbert W M, Anderson J, *et al.* Trauma during pregnancy: an analysis of maternal and fetal outcomes in a large population. *Am J Obstet Gynecol* 2004; **190**: 1661–8.

14. El-Kady D, Gilbert W M, Xing G, Smith L H. Maternal and neonatal outcomes of assaults during pregnancy. *Obstet Gynecol* 2005; **105**: 357–63.

15. Buhimschi C S, Buhimschi I A, Patel S, Malinow A M, Weiner C P. Rupture of the uterine scar during term labour: contractility or biochemistry? *Br J Obstet Gynaecol* 2005; **112**(1): 38–42.

16. Ridgeway J R, Weyrich D L, Benedetti T J. Fetal heart rate changes associated with uterine rupture. *Obstet Gynecol* 2004; **103**: 506–12.

17. Sheiner E, Levy A, Ofir K, *et al.* Changes in fetal heart rate pattern and uterine patterns associated with uterine rupture. *J Reprod Med* 2004; **49**: 373–8.

18. Menihan C A. Uterine rupture in women attempting a vaginal birth following caesarean birth. *J Perinatol* 1998; **18**: 440–3.

19. Rodriguez M H, Masaki D I, Phelan J P, Diaz F G. Uterine rupture: are intrauterine pressure catheters useful in diagnosis? *Am J Obstet Gynecol* 1989; **161**: 666.

20. Ofir K, Sheiner E, Levy A, Katz M, Mazor M. Uterine rupture: differences between a scarred and an unscarred uterus. *Am J Obstet Gynecol* 2004; **191**(2): 425–9.

21. Al Sakka M, Hamsho A, Khan L. Rupture of the pregnant uterus – a 21-year review. *Int J Gynaecol Obstet* 1998; **63**: 105–8.

22. Wang Y L, Su T H. Obstetric uterine rupture of the unscarred uterus: a twenty-year clinical analysis. *Gynecol Obstet Invest* 2006; **62**(3): 131–5.

23. Rozenberg P, Goffinet F, Philippe H J, Nisand I. Ultrasonographic measurement of lower uterine

segment to assess risk of defects of a scarred uterus. *Lancet* 1996; **347**: 281–4.

24. Cheung V Y. Sonographic measurement of the lower uterine segment thickness in women with previous caesarean section. *J Obstet Gynaecol Can* 2005; **27**: 674–81.

25. Murphy D J. Uterine rupture. *Curr Opin Obstet Gynecol* 2006; **18**(2): 135–40.

26. Leung A S, Leung E K, Paul R H. Uterine rupture after previous caesarean delivery: maternal and fetal consequences. *Am J Obstet Gynecol* 1993; **168**: 1358–63.

27. Bujold E, Gauthier R J. Neonatal morbidity associated with uterine rupture: what are the risk factors? *Am J Obstet Gynecol* 2002; **186**: 311–4.

28. Giwa-Osagie O F, Uguru V, Akinla O. Mortality and morbidity of emergency obstetric hysterectomy. *J Obstet Gynecol* 1983; **4**: 94–6.

29. Kwee A, Bots M L, Visser G H, Bruinse H W. Uterine rupture and its complications in the Netherlands: a prospective study. *Eur J Obstet Gynecol Reprod Biol* 2006; **128**(1–2): 257–61.

30. Nagarkatti R S, Ambiye V R, Vaidya P R. Rupture uterus: changing trends in etiology and management. *J Postgrad Med* 1991; **37**(3): 136–9.

31. Lim A C, Kwee A, Bruinse H E. Pregnancy after uterine rupture; a report of 5 cases and a review of the literature. *Obstet Gynecol Surv* 2005; **60**(9): 613–7.

32. Al Sakka M, Dauleh W, Al Hassani I. Case series of uterine rupture and subsequent pregnancy outcome. *Int J Fertil Womens Med* 1999; **44**: 297–300.

33. O'Connor R A, Gaughan B. Pregnancy following simple repair of the ruptured gravid uterus. *Br J Obstet Gynaecol* 1989; **96**: 942–4.

34. Chauhan S P, Magann E F, Wiggs C D, Barrilleaux P S, Martin J N, Jr. Pregnancy after classic caesarean delivery. *Obstet Gynecol* 2002; **100**(5 Pt 1): 946–50.

35. Usta I M, Hamdi M A, Musa A A, Nassar A H. Pregnancy outcome in patients with previous uterine rupture. *Acta Obstet Gynecol Scand* 2007; **86**(2): 172–6.

36. Chandraharan E, Arulkumaran S. Prevention of birth asphyxia: responding appropriately to cardiotocograph (CTG) traces. *Best Pract Res Clin Obstet Gynecol* 2007; **21**(4): 609–24.

Management of severe pre-eclampsia/eclampsia

James J. Walker

Introduction

Although pre-eclampsia is recognized as a placental disease which leads to varied systemic manifestations, it is the systemic signs and symptoms that bring it to the attention of the clinician [1]. The placental pathology is responsible for the fetal growth restriction, but is benign to the mother. However, the clinical disease of severe pre-eclampsia and eclampsia are, along with haemorrhage and sepsis, one of the three major killers of pregnant women worldwide. Within the UK, the incidence of maternal death for both pre-eclampsia and eclampsia has fallen dramatically over the last 50 years [2] (Figures 24.1 and 24.2), but its continuing potential dangers cannot be understated. Much of the reduction in death was before the advent of modern methods of care and was due to the increasing health of society, vigilant antenatal care, admission to hospital and expedited delivery. In recent years, the further reductions in death and morbidity have been helped by evidence-based guidelines [3], trials [4,5], reviews [6–10] and large case studies [11–15]. Despite this, the Confidential Enquiries into Maternal Deaths persistently show substandard care in a significant percentage of the deaths that do occur [2,16]. The aim of this chapter is to give guidance on the diagnosis and management of severe pre-eclampsia and eclampsia in the immediate pre- and postdelivery interval, and is based on established evidence-based guidelines and extensive experience.

Presentation and diagnosis

The diagnosis of pre-eclampsia has been greatly improved by vigilant antenatal care, but only around 60% of cases are picked up in this way, with many still presenting acutely with varied signs and symptoms.

Although the primary diagnosis is based on hypertension and proteinuria (Table 24.1), these are only signs of the underlying disease, and other wide-ranging complications can be present and virtually any organ system may be affected (Table 24.1). Although these complications can be given other labels such as HELLP (haemolysis, elevated liver enzymes and low platelet count) syndrome, they are all variations of the same underlying disease process and point to severity rather than a different diagnosis [13]. These variations contribute greatly to the complications found with this condition, with up to 35% of women having significant morbidities.

Definitions (Table 24.1)

However, it is high blood pressure that is the biggest immediate risk to mother, and it is this sign that is the most common presentation. Even in women who present with other symptoms, such as headache or abdominal pain, it is the elevation of blood pressure that makes the diagnosis and initiates intervention. There is now general agreement that severe hypertension is present if the systolic blood pressure is over 160 mmHg or the diastolic blood pressure is over 110 mmHg on three occasions within a space of 15 min [14]. Moderate hypertension is present if the systolic blood pressure is between 140 and 159 mmHg and the diastolic blood pressure between 100 and 109 mmHg on three occasions. This is classified as severe if it is present with significant proteinuria and/or at least two other significant signs or symptoms (Table 24.1). Eclampsia is defined as the occurrence of one or more convulsions superimposed on pre-eclampsia. Up to 40% of women presenting with eclampsia may have no obvious prodromal signs or symptoms, but have a clear diagnosis of pre-eclampsia after the convulsion has occurred [11].

Best Practice in Labour and Delivery, ed. R. Warren and S. Arulkumaran. Published by Cambridge University Press.
© Cambridge University Press 2009.

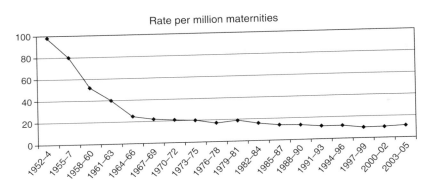

Rate per million maternities

Figure 24.1 Maternal mortality from eclampsia and pre-eclampsia: England and Wales 1952–84; United Kingdom 1985–2005

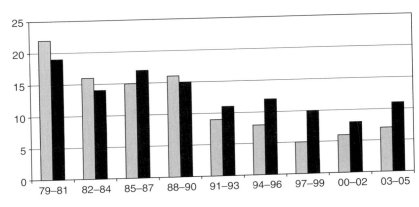

Figure 24.2 Maternal mortality from eclampsia (grey) and pre-eclampsia (black) in the United Kingdom

The problem

Although the classification of pre-eclampsia and its severity is primarily based on the level of blood pressure and the presence of proteinuria, clinicians should be aware of the potential involvement of other organs when assessing maternal risk and the degree of placental disease causing fetal manifestations. It is important that any presenting woman is managed on clinical grounds and not on any perceived presence or absence of a given diagnosis. Many of the maternal deaths and severe morbidity that occur are in women who do not fit the strict criteria of pre-eclampsia. Therefore clinical signs should not be ignored simply because the precise diagnosis is in doubt.

In the UK, the majority of the deaths have been due to cerebral causes, with cardiorespiratory complications being the next most common cause (Table 24.2). Renal failure, a perceived risk in pre-eclampsia, is a rare cause of death largely due to the fact that it is not that common, is generally due to acute tubular necrosis which is recoverable, and can be relatively easily managed with dialysis support if required. This has led to the establishment of guidelines that concentrate on the control of hypertension

and the management of fluid balance [3]. Using this form of standardized care package for pre-eclampsia, the Yorkshire series had no maternal deaths in over 1000 cases of severe pre-eclampsia and eclampsia with reduced maternal and neonatal morbidity [15].

Although the main disease morbidity for the baby is placental insufficiency and its consequences, the main cause of death is iatrogenic prematurity due to the need to end the pregnancy because of disease severity. The fact that growth restriction is more common in early onset disease means that these problems are additive.

Therefore, the approach on admission should be to assess the severity of the disease and the risk to both the mother and the baby. Blood pressure control should be the first line of management, as it is easy and life-saving. Convulsions, if present, need to be controlled, but the use of prophylactic anticonvulsive therapy is more controversial. Fluid management is more of a problem for intra- and postpartum care, but antenatally, judicious fluid replacement is necessary if delivery is planned. As far as the baby is concerned, emergency delivery on admission is rarely necessary in the absence of placental abruption, but

263

Table 24.1 Classification of pre-eclampsia/eclampsia.

1. Eclampsia	The occurrence of one or more convulsions superimposed on pre-eclampsia
2. Severe pre-eclampsia	Systolic blood pressure over 160 mmHg
	or diastolic blood pressure over 110 mmHg (**3 blood pressure readings in a 15 min period**) with at least proteinuria of a + + or >0.3 g in 24 h
3. Moderate pre-eclampsia	Systolic blood pressure over 140 mmHg
	or diastolic blood pressure over 90 mmHg (**3 blood pressure readings in a 45 min period**) with at least proteinuria ++ or >0.3 g in 24 h
and any of the following	symptoms of headache
	visual disturbance
	epigastric pain
	signs of clonus
	papilloedema
	liver tenderness
	platelet count falling to below $100 \times 10^9/l$
	Alanine amino transferase (ALT) above 50 iu/l

careful assessment of fetal well-being and the likelihood of prolonging the pregnancy needs to be assessed as part of the decision-making process.

How should women be assessed at initial presentation?

Many women with severe disease may have few if any symptoms and the problem is discovered as part of routine antenatal care. Others will present with convulsions, abdominal pain or general malaise. As in all medical situations, a clear history and examination should be carried out, and pre-eclampsia should always be considered as a potential diagnosis. The presence or absence of symptoms, particularly headache and abdominal pain, is important, as their presence implies systemic involvement, worsening disease and the increased risk of morbidity. Increasing oedema is a common presenting feature, but is not in itself a sign that should determine management. Enquiry about fetal movement should not be forgotten as an immediate assessment of fetal well-being.

Examination should start with the diagnostic signs of blood pressure measurement and urine analysis. Abdominal examination should be carried out to assess uterine size and liquor volume, presence of uterine tenderness suggestive of concomitant placental abruption, or upper abdominal tenderness suggestive of liver tenderness and HELLP syndrome. Maternal tendon reflexes, although useful to assess magnesium toxicity, are not of value in assessing the risk of convulsion, although the presence of clonus may be. If the woman is extremely unwell, particularly in the postpartum period, she should be assessed for signs of pulmonary oedema and continuous oxygen saturation monitoring with a pulse oximeter can be invaluable. Auscultation of the fetal heart and commencing of electronic fetal heart monitoring allows further fetal assessment.

An important consideration is the early involvement of senior obstetric and anaesthetic staff and experienced midwives in the assessment and management of women with severe pre-eclampsia and eclampsia. Repeatedly, the Confidential Enquiry into Maternal Deaths associates the absence of senior involvement with the occurrence of substandard care [2,16].

How should the blood pressure be taken?

It is important to take the blood pressure with a cuff of the appropriate size. If in doubt, it is better to use a larger cuff, as this will result in less error than a smaller cuff in an overweight women. At least three readings should be carried out and averaged to confirm the diagnosis because of natural variation (Table 24.1). Korotkoff phase 5 is the appropriate measurement of diastolic blood pressure [17]. Whatever method is used, it should be consistent and documented. Automated methods need to be used with caution, as they systematically underestimate blood pressure readings in pre-eclampsia, especially at higher blood pressure levels. Validation using a mercury sphygmomanometer or other validated device should be carried out if there is concern.

Table 24.2 The causes of maternal death from pre-eclampsia/eclampsia in the UK over the last 35 years.

Year	Cerebral	Pulmonary	Hepatic	Renal	Other	Total
70–72	25	8	5	3	6	47
73–75	23	7	14	1	4	49
76–78	21	4	5	0	3	33
79–81	17	8	8	0	3	36
82–84	21	3	0	0	1	25
85–87	11	11	1	1	2	26
88–90	14	10	1	0	2	27
91–93	5	11	0	1	3	20
94–96	7	8	3	0	2	20
97–99	7	2	2	0	5	16
00–02	9	1	0	0	4	14
03–05	12	0	2	0	4	18
Total	172	73	41	6	39	331

The blood pressure should be checked every 15 min in the acute phase until the woman is stabilized, and then less often depending on the clinical situation.

High blood pressure is the main maternal risk and commencement of antihypertensive therapy if the blood pressure is above 160/100 mmHg is recommended without requiring further assessment. Using the recommended drugs and doses has been shown to be beneficial to the mother and carry no increased risk to the baby [6].

How should proteinuria be measured?

The presence of proteinuria confirms the diagnosis of pre-eclampsia and systemic involvement, but the level does not differentiate severity [12]. Its presence is particularly associated with increased risk to the baby.

The usual screening test for proteinuria is visual dipstick assessment. While it is accepted that there is a poor predictive value from urine dipstick testing [18], an approximate equivalence is 1+ = 0.3 g/l, 2+ = 1 g/l and 3+ = 3 g/l. Therefore, generally, a 2+ dipstick measurement can be taken as evidence of proteinuria for clinical management. If a more accurate test is required, this should be a 24-h urine collection, the 'gold standard', or a spot protein creatinine ratio where a level of 0.03 g/mmol appears to be equivalent to 0.3 g/24 h, the accepted threshold diagnostic level.

Therefore, the immediate presumptive diagnosis and presumed severity can be assessed at the bedside: blood pressure and proteinuria measurement along with clinical history and examination. Initial treatment can be instigated without waiting for biochemical, haematological and ultrasound examination.

How should the woman be monitored [3]?

Once a woman has been assessed clinically and any high blood pressure or convulsion managed, a fuller assessment of her and her disease can be made. This requires a full blood count, liver and renal function tests. These should be repeated as required to assess clinical stability or deterioration. Generally, clotting studies are not required if the platelet count is over $100 \times 10^6/l$.

Uric acid

In pre-eclampsia, there is a rise in uric acid in most cases which helps to confirm the diagnosis of pre-eclampsia and confers an increased risk to the mother and baby, but the absolute levels should not be used for clinical decision-making.

Urea and creatinine

Renal function is generally maintained in pre-eclampsia until the late stage. If urea or creatinine is elevated early in the disease process, underlying renal disease should be suspected. There tends to be a rise post-partum, which is of little significance as renal failure is uncommon in pre-eclampsia in the absence of haemorrhage, HELLP syndrome or sepsis.

Platelets

A falling platelet count is associated with worsening disease and is in itself a risk to the mother. However, it is not until the count is less than $100 \times 10^6/l$ that there may be an associated coagulation abnormality. A count of less than 100 should be a consideration for delivery, as this will tend to fall further.

Liver function tests

An AST level of above 75 iu/l is seen as significant and a level above 150 iu/l is associated with increased morbidity to the mother. A diagnosis of HELLP syndrome needs confirmation of haemolysis, either by LDH levels or by blood film. These tests are not generally done in the UK, and the diagnosis of HELLP is usually based on platelets and liver function tests (LFTs) alone (ELLP).

Fluid management

If delivery is planned, close fluid balance with charting of input and output is essential. A catheter with a urometer is helpful during delivery and in the immediate postpartum period. The use of continuous oxygen saturation monitoring with a pulse oximeter can demonstrate early signs of pulmonary oedema [15].

How should the fetus be assessed?

After an initial clinical assessment, a cardiotocograph should be carried out. This gives immediate information about fetal well-being and a reactive reassuring tracing suggests that the fetus is not in any immediate danger. Women in labour with severe pre-eclampsia should have continuous electronic fetal monitoring.

The main pathology affecting the fetus is placental insufficiency leading to intrauterine growth restriction (IUGR) in around 30% of pre-eclamptic pregnancies. If conservative management is planned, then further assessment of the fetus using ultrasound should be carried out. Ultrasound assessment of fetal size at presentation is a valuable one-off measurement to assess fetal growth, and can be informative for the decision to deliver, assessment of survival chance, and to inform the neonatal unit. Liquor volume should be assessed at the same time along with umbilical artery

Doppler waveform, using absent or reversed-end diastolic flow as a diagnostic criteria [19]. In the presence of normal liquor volume and umbilical Doppler waveforms, continuation of the pregnancy for an average of 15 days is possible if the mother is stable. If abnormalities of fetal assessment are found, prolongation for more than a few days is unlikely, although a course of antenatal steroids should still be attempted if required. Repeat assessment of liquor volume and umbilical artery Doppler waveform can be used along with cardiotocography to assess fetal well-being and optimize delivery.

Predelivery care
General measures

Initially, the woman should be managed in a high-dependency area, ideally with one-to-one midwifery care. After initial assessment, a decision has to be made about continued management, particularly the need for antihypertensive therapy, magnesium sulphate and antenatal steroids. If delivery is planned, the need for transfer because of fetal and/or maternal care should be considered. This management should be led by the most senior obstetrician present and the consultant should be called to attend. Close liaison with neonatal and anaesthetic colleagues is necessary, again at senior level.

An intravenous cannula should always be inserted, but fluid given with care. A urinary catheter is not always necessary, but may be helpful to monitor urine output over delivery and postpartum.

Antihypertensive therapy

A blood pressure greater than 160/110 mmHg requires treatment in the maternal interest and many authorities, including the author, recommend that a threshold diastolic blood pressure of over 100 mmHg should be used. Similarly, if the blood pressure is below 160/100 mmHg, there is no immediate need for antihypertensive therapy unless it is associated with other markers of severe disease, such as heavy proteinuria or disordered liver or haematological test results. In these situations, antihypertensive treatment is used to prevent a hypertensive crisis. Most women can be managed with oral therapy alone [15], with the preferred therapeutic agents being labetalol, nifedipine, hydralazine or Methyldopa (Table 24.3) [2].

Table 24.3 Antihypertensive therapy.

Labetalol

Oral dose of 200 mg repeated hourly as required

Daily dose range from 200 mg BD to a maximum of 400 mg qid

IV bolus dose 50 mg (=10 ml of labetalol 5 mg/ml) given over at least 1 min. Can be repeated every 10 min if required to a maximum dose of 200 mg.

The pulse rate should be monitored and remain over 60 beats per minute

IV infusion of neat labetalol at a rate of 4 ml/h via a syringe pump. The infusion rate should be doubled every half-hour to a maximum of 32 ml (160 mg)/h until the blood pressure has reduced and stabilized at an acceptable level.

Nifedipine

Oral dose of 10 mg repeated 6 hourly

After delivery initially this may be changed to the slow-release preparation given 12 hourly

Hydralazine

IV bolus dose of 5 mg with repeating 5–10 mg IV every 30 min until control is achieved to a maximum of 20 mg.

IV infusion of 0.5–10 mg/h IV to a maximum of 20 mg.

IM dose – intermittent doses of 5–10 mg up to a maximum of 30 mg

Methyldopa

Oral dose of 250 mg orally usually given three times a day. This can be increased to a 500 mg dose up to four times a day with a maximum daily dose of 2 g.

Labetalol

Labetalol has the advantage that it can be given initially by mouth and then, if needed, intravenously by bolus or infusion. Most women will respond to an initial 200 mg oral dose, which should lead to a reduction in blood pressure in about half an hour. A second oral dose can be given if needed an hour later. Regular daily medication can then be commenced. If there is no response to oral therapy, or if it cannot be tolerated, control should be by repeated IV bolus of labetalol followed by a labetalol infusion if required (Table 24.3). Labetalol should be avoided, if possible, in women with known asthma.

Nifedipine

If labetalol is contra-indicated or fails to control the blood pressure, then Nifedipine is an alternative or additive agent. This should be given as a 10 mg oral tablet. If it controls blood pressure it should be repeated 6 hourly initially, although it may be changed after delivery to a slow-release preparation which lasts 12 h. Blood pressure should be measured every 10 min in the first half hour after treatment, as often there can be a very marked drop in pressure. The previous voiced concern over interaction between magnesium sulphate and Nifedipine does not appear to be a clinical problem.

Hydralazine

Hydralazine has traditionally been the drug of choice in the acute situation, but a review has suggested that hydralazine may be less preferable compared with labetalol [9]. Although the evidence is not strong enough to preclude its use, it has largely been superseded by labetalol, which has the advantages of the oral as well as intravenous route. When using hydralazine there is an increased risk of hypotension, so the starting dose should be 5 mg IV and repeated as required. An infusion can also be used, as can the intramuscular route (Table 24.3).

Methyldopa

Methyldopa is still commonly used in the UK and throughout the world, and has been proven safe in long-term follow-up of the delivered babies. However, studies have suggested superior benefits of labetalol [6]. It is less effective in the acute situation, but may be the only drug available if others are contra-indicated or fail. If used, the starting dose is 250 mg orally, usually given three times a day. This can be increased to a 500 mg dose up to four times a day, with a maximum daily dose of 2 g.

Hospitals should have a guideline available outlining their drug of choice. It is important that attendant staff know how to give the drug and what effect to expect. Too often, too little drug is given with the resulting lack of benefit.

If the mother is easily stabilized and the fetus appears well, a prolongation of pregnancy of an average of 15 days is possible, as long as there is no other reason to deliver. In most cases a delay of 48 h is possible to allow the use of antenatal steroids in pregnancies under 34 weeks' gestation.

Table 24.4 Magnesium sulphate intravenous protocol.

Magnesium sulphate is given as a loading dose followed by a continuous infusion for 24 h or until 24 h after delivery, whichever is the later.

Loading dose

25 ml magnesium sulphate 20% IV over 25 min via a syringe pump at an infusion rate of 60 ml/h.

Maintenance dose

50 ml magnesium sulphate 20% IV via a syringe pump at an infusion rate of 5 ml/h. Each syringe should last 10 h.

There is no need to measure magnesium levels with the above protocol

Important observations

The following observations should be performed:
 (i) continuous pulse oximetry,
 (ii) hourly urine output (> than 100 ml in 4 h),
 (iii) hourly respiratory rate (should be >12/min),
 (iv) deep tendon reflexes.

The antidote is 10 ml 10% calcium gluconate given slowly intravenously over 10 min

Management of seizures (Table 24.4)

Usually, women will present after the convulsion has occurred, and sometimes it is diagnosed by history alone. However, if present during the convulsion, this is a medical emergency and its management should be subject to regular multidisciplinary training drills. The woman should be protected from injury during the convulsion and not left alone. Help should be summoned, including the anaesthetist and senior obstetrician. The usual assessment of airway, breathing and circulation is the primary approach, with the woman in the left lateral position and oxygen administered by face mask. The respiratory rate, pulse and blood pressure should be checked.

Magnesium sulphate is the therapy of choice, even in the acute situation, and diazepam and phenytoin should not be first-line drugs. This should be given by standard regime (Table 24.4). Since 97% of magnesium is excreted in the urine, the presence of oliguria can lead to toxic levels. If oliguria is present, further magnesium sulphate infusion should be withheld. Since magnesium is not being excreted, no other anticonvulsant is needed. Magnesium can then be re-introduced if urine output improves.

Recurrent seizures can be treated with either a further bolus of 2 g magnesium sulphate or an increase

Table 24.5 Causes of death in women in the MAGPIE study.

	Magnesium group	Placebo	Total
Cardiorespiratory failure	5	7	12
Stroke	3	2	5
Other	3	3	6
Renal failure	0	3	3
PE	0	3	3
Infection	0	2	2
Total	11	20	31

in the infusion rate to 1.5 or 2.0 g/h. If seizures persist, then alternative agents such as diazepam or thiopentone can be used, but prolonged use of diazepam is associated with an increase in maternal death and neonatal respiratory depression. If all therapy fails and convulsions persist, intubation and transfer to intensive care facilities for intermittent positive pressure ventilation may be needed.

The main side effects of magnesium are motor paralysis, absent tendon reflexes, respiratory depression and cardiac arrhythmia, but these are unusual with the 1 g/h dosage. If there is any concern, the antidote calcium gluconate should be given (Table 24.4).

Once stabilized, delivery should be planned, but a delay of several hours is allowable to allow full preparation, assuming that there is no acute fetal concern, such as a fetal bradycardia.

How should seizures be prevented?

Although it is clear that, in the presence of convulsions, magnesium sulphate is the drug of choice, its role in prevention of convulsions in severe pre-eclampsia is less clear. The MAGPIE trial has demonstrated that administration of magnesium sulphate to women with pre-eclampsia reduces the risk of an eclamptic seizure by 58% compared to placebo. Although the relative risk reduction was similar regardless of the severity of pre-eclampsia, the number needed to treat depended on the absolute risk. Therefore, its benefit is less clear in low-risk and premature presentations. In the trial, there was also a reduction in the rate of complications independent of the convulsions. The cases of death were similar in both groups except for the more unusual causes, for the developed world, of thrombosis and sepsis (Table 24.5).

It would seem that its benefit to women in the developed world is less definite. In the last 12 years, there has been a rise in the number of women dying of pre-eclampsia/eclampsia in the UK despite the use of magnesium. These have been mostly due to cerebral vascular accident. Therefore, in the UK, where the incidence of eclampsia is low, lowering blood pressure in severe pre-eclampsia should be the first-line therapy, not magnesium sulphate, as this is the main risk of death. Magnesium sulphate should be limited to those women who are being delivered and the blood pressure is poorly controlled or there are other concerning signs, particularly persistent headache. If used, the infusion should be continued for 24 h following delivery or 24 h after the last seizure, whichever is the later, unless there is a clinical reason to continue.

How should fluid balance be managed?

Pulmonary oedema is the second most common cause of maternal death (Table 24.2), often being associated with inappropriate fluid management. Since the main risk of pulmonary oedema is in the first 48 h postpartum, fluid replacement should be managed carefully throughout the intrapartum/postnatal period. Fluid expansion should not be used [8], and fluid restriction is associated with a good maternal outcome. Total fluids should be limited to 80 ml/h or 1 ml/kg/h. Urine output should be measured as part of the input/output assessment, but there is no need to maintain a particular output volume to prevent renal failure, as oliguria occurs in around 30% of women with severe pre-eclampsia and renal failure is rare. Fluid restriction should be maintained until there is a postpartum diuresis. If there is associated maternal haemorrhage, fluid restriction is inappropriate, but replacement should be given using some form of invasive monitoring. This is usually by central venous pressure monitoring, which needs to be used with care, as pulmonary oedema can occur even in the presence of a 'normal' CVP.

Thromboprophylaxis

Women with severe pre-eclampsia are at risk of venous thrombosis. Antenatally, in labour and postnatally, all patients should have thromboprophylaxis in the form of antiembolic stockings and/or heparin until they are mobile. Heparin administration is not a contra-indication to the insertion of an epidural catheter. However, low molecular weight heparin should not be given until 2 h after spinal anaesthesia and an epidural catheter should not be removed until 10 h after the last dose, because of the risk of an epidural haematoma.

Delivery guidelines

The decision to deliver is the most important factor in the care of a pre-eclamptic woman. Delivery should be 'on the best day in the best way'. Delay in delivery can help with stabilizing the mother, transferring the woman to another unit, use of steroids or even prolongation of the pregnancy for a period of time. However, delaying delivery could also increase the risk to the mother and her baby.

Gestation before 34 weeks

The timing, place and mode of delivery is the most important part of the care of the pre-eclamptic woman. If the gestation is less than 34 weeks and delivery can be deferred, corticosteroids should be given, although this decision needs to be constantly reassessed for any change in maternal or fetal condition. However, even 24 h of steroid therapy helps to reduce fetal respiratory morbidity and mortality. Conservative management at very early gestations may improve the perinatal outcome, but must be carefully balanced with maternal well-being. If the delivery decision involves transfer to another unit, it is important that the woman is stable prior to transfer (Table 24.6) and, if she is not, it is better to deliver in the base unit and transfer the baby postnatally, if required.

Gestation after 34 weeks

If the gestation is greater than 34 weeks, delivery after stabilization is recommended, as no benefit for mother or baby will be gained from delay except for transfer to a more appropriate unit.

The delivery

The timing, place and mode of delivery need to be carefully planned, involving all appropriate professionals. The aim should be to deliver, particularly premature infants, during normal working hours. The mode of delivery should be influenced by the presentation of the fetus, the fetal condition, and the likelihood of success of induction of labour after

Table 24.6 Preparation for transfer.

Prior to transfer the condition must be stabilized. The following is required.

1. Transfer should be discussed with appropriate consultant medical staff and all the relevant people at the receiving unit, e.g. the neonatal unit and neonatal medical staff, the resident obstetrician, the midwife in charge of the delivery suite, intensive care and the intensive care anaesthetist (where appropriate).
2. All basic investigations should have been performed and the results clearly recorded in the accompanying notes or telephoned through as soon as available.
3. Blood pressure should be stabilized at an acceptable level.
4. If the woman is ventilated, it is important to ensure ventilatory requirements are stable and oxygen saturations are being maintained.
5. Fetal well-being has been assessed to be certain that transfer is in the fetal interest before delivery. Steroids should be given if the woman is preterm.
6. Appropriate personnel are available to transfer the woman. This will normally mean at least a senior midwife, but may require an obstetrician or anaesthetist.

assessment of the cervix. Although a vaginal delivery is generally preferable, below 32 weeks' gestation caesarean section is preferable, as the success of induction is reduced. After 34 weeks with a cephalic presentation, vaginal delivery should be considered with the likelihood of a successful vaginal delivery being increased by the use of vaginal prostaglandins.

Antihypertensive treatment should be continued throughout, preferably orally and intravenous infusion used only if oral therapy fails. Epidural anaesthesia should be used for obstetric need and not as a method of controlling blood pressure. The third stage should be managed with 5 units Syntocinon given intramuscularly or slowly intravenously and not ergometrine or Syntometrine, as these can cause a sharp rise in blood pressure.

These women should receive high-dependency care and charts should be commenced to record all physiological monitoring and investigation results. To aid monitoring, an indwelling urinary catheter should be inserted and oxygen saturation should be measured by pulse oximeter and, if a CVP line is present, this should be measured continuously. All results should be charted as outlined.

Units should be moving to using Modified Early Warning Scores (MOEW) and these can be used in conjunction with these charts.

Anaesthesia and fluids

Generally, women with pre-eclampsia tend to maintain their blood pressure during regional blockade, and routine fluid loading is unnecessary and may add to fluid overload. If hypotension occurs, small doses of a vasoconstrictor can be used. Even at caesarean section, fluid replacement of greater than 500 ml of fluid, unless matched against blood loss, is not usually necessary. General anaesthesia should be avoided if possible, as intubation and extubation can lead to increases in systolic and diastolic blood pressure, as well as heart rate, bringing increased risk to the mother.

How should the woman be managed following delivery?

Most women that die do so after delivery. Therefore, although delivery is the start of the reversal process, the first 24–48 h are critical in the care management. Around 60% of women worsen within 24 h and the improvement in the maternal condition may not be seen until 48 h after delivery. Therefore, continued vigilance is required. Also both eclampsia and severe pre-eclampsia can present for the first time postnatally, so women with signs or symptoms compatible with pre-eclampsia should be carefully assessed and managed accordingly.

Woman should continue high-dependency care, and all results charted. Again, there should be some form of MOEWs scoring in place. Blood pressure and pulse should be measured regularly until stable, and then with lengthening intervals depending on the clinical condition. Although, initially, blood pressure may fall postpartum, it often rises again at around 24 h. Therefore, a reduction in antihypertensive therapy should be made in a stepwise fashion and titrated against measurements. Temperature should be measured four-hourly or whenever the patient complains of feeling hot. The respiratory rate should be measured hourly, especially if the women is on magnesium sulphate.

Postpartum fluid management

Pulmonary oedema is mostly a postpartum risk. Therefore, fluid restriction should continue until the natural diuresis occurs, which is sometime between 24 and 48 h postdelivery. If the woman is well enough to tolerate more than 80 ml/h oral fluids, IV fluids can be stopped and the restriction lifted.

If oxygen saturation falls below 95%, then medical review is essential. If the fluid balance is in positive excess for more than 750 ml since delivery, then 20 mg of IV furosemide should be given. If the positive fluid balance is less than this, then an infusion of 250 ml of 'Gelofusine' or similar can be given over 20 min, but if the urine output remains low over the following 4 h then 20 mg of IV furosemide should be given. If there is no diuresis and the oxygen saturation does not rise, then renal referral should be considered.

Cases requiring large volumes of replacement fluid such as fresh frozen plasma, blood or platelets can be problematical and need management by those experienced in these cases. It is never difficult putting more fluid in, but getting it out can be a real problem.

HELLP syndrome

HELLP syndrome may occur for the first time postpartum and is a reflection of the severity of the underlying disease. It requires no particular treatment apart from the normal supportive measures. Corticosteroids have been used in HELLP syndrome, but although they lead to a more rapid resolution of the biochemical and haematological abnormalities, there is no evidence that they reduce morbidity [13].

Ongoing care and discharge

Although late eclampsia has been reported up to 4 weeks postnatally, the incidence of eclampsia and severe pre-eclampsia falls after the fourth postpartum day. Therefore, most women will need inpatient care for at least 4 days following delivery. Careful review to ensure improving clinical signs is needed before discharge by a senior doctor. However, if all else is well, there is no reason why the woman cannot go home on antihypertensive treatment and be weaned off therapy as an outpatient. Sometimes, blood pressure can take up to 3 months to return to normal. However, evidence suggests that up to 13% of women with pre-eclampsia will have underlying renal problems or essential hypertension that was not suspected antenatally. Women with persisting hypertension and proteinuria at 6 weeks should be considered for further investigation.

References

1. Walker J J. Pre-eclampsia. *Lancet* 2000; **356**: 1260–5.

2. *Why Mothers Die 2000–2002. Report on Confidential Inquiries into Maternal Deaths in the United Kingdom.* London: RCOG Press, 2004.

3. Tuffnell D J, Shennan A H, Waugh J J S, Walker J J. *The Management of Severe Pre-eclampsia/Eclampsia.* London: RCOG, 2006.

4. Which anticonvulsant for women with eclampsia? Evidence from the Collaborative Eclampsia Trial. *Lancet* 1995; **345**: 1455–63.

5. The Magpie Trial Collaboration Group. Do women with pre-eclampsia, and their babies, benefit from magnesium sulphate? The Magpie Trial: a randomised placebo-controlled trial. *Lancet* 2002; **359**: 1877–90.

6. Magee L A, Ornstein M P, von Dadelszen P. Fortnightly review: management of hypertension in pregnancy. *Br Med J* 1999; **318**: 1332–6.

7. Brown M A, Buddle M L, Farrell T, Davis G K. Efficacy and safety of nifedipine tablets for the acute treatment of severe hypertension in pregnancy. *Am J Obstet Gynecol* 2002; **187**: 1046–50.

8. Duley L, Williams J, Henderson-Smart D J. Plasma volume expansion for treatment of women with pre-eclampsia. *Cochrane Database Syst Rev* 2000; **2**: CD001805.

9. Magee L A, Cham C, Waterman E J, Ohlsson A, von Dadelszen P. Hydralazine for treatment of severe hypertension in pregnancy: meta-analysis. *Br Med J* 2003; **327**: 955–60.

10. Magee L A, Elran E, Bull S B, Logan A, Koren G. Risks and benefits of beta-receptor blockers for pregnancy hypertension: overview of the randomized trials. *Eur J Obstet Gynecol Reprod Biol* 2000; **88**: 15–26.

11. Douglas K A, Redman C W. Eclampsia in the United Kingdom. *Br Med J* 1994; **309**: 1395–400.

12. Ferrazzani S, Caruso A, De Carolis S, Martino I V, Mancuso S. Proteinuria and outcome of 444 pregnancies complicated by hypertension. *Am J Obstet Gynecol* 1990; **162**: 366–71.

13. Martin J N, Jr, Rinehart B K, May W L, Magann E F, Terrone D A, Blake P G. The spectrum of severe preeclampsia: comparative analysis by HELLP (hemolysis, elevated liver enzyme levels, and low platelet count) syndrome classification. *Am J Obstet Gynecol* 1999; **180**: 1373–84.

14. Martin J N J, Thigpen B D, Moore R C, Rose, C H, Cushman J, May W. Stroke and severe preeclampsia and eclampsia: a paradigm shift focusing on systolic blood pressure. *Obstet Gynecol* 2005; **105**: 246–54.

15. Tuffnell D J, Jankowicz D, Lindow S W, *et al.* Outcomes of severe pre-eclampsia/eclampsia in Yorkshire 1999/2003. *Br J Obstet Gynaecol* 2005; **112**: 875–80.

16. Lewis G. (Ed). *The Confidential Enquiry into Maternal and Child Health (CEMACH). Saving Mothers' Lives: Reviewing Maternal Deaths to Make Motherhood Safer – 2003–2005. The Seventh Report on Confidential Enquiries into Maternal Deaths in the United Kingdom.* London: CEMACH, 2007.

17. Brown M A, Buddle M L, Farrell T, Davis G, Jones M. Randomised trial of management of hypertensive pregnancies by Korotkoff phase IV or phase V. *Lancet* 1998; **352**: 777–81.

18. Brown M A, Buddle M L. Inadequacy of dipstick proteinuria in hypertensive pregnancy. *Aust NZ J Obstet Gynaecol* 1995; **35**: 366–39.

19. Neilson J P, Alfirevic Z. Doppler ultrasound for fetal assessment in high risk pregnancies. *Cochrane Database Syst Rev* 2000: CD000073.

Chapter 25

Neonatal resuscitation and the management of immediate neonatal problems

Paul Mannix

The vast majority of newborn babies require no help in adaptation to their new extrauterine life. They rapidly clear lung fluid, create a functional residual capacity and breathe on their own within seconds of their birth. However, it is very difficult to predict the baby who will need resuscitation, and so I start this chapter with the comment that any person involved in the delivery of care to the pregnant woman should have an understanding of the principles of newborn resuscitation. This includes medical students on their obstetric attachment, student midwives in training, midwives, obstetricians and obstetric anaesthetists, as well as neonatologists and paediatricians.

De Lee stated in 1897 that 'there are three grand principles governing the treatment of asphyxia neonatorum: first, maintain the body heat; second, free the air passages from obstructions; third, stimulate respiration, or supply air to the lungs for oxygenation of the blood' [1]. Over 100 years later, these principles remain largely unchanged.

In this chapter, the principles and physiology of neonatal resuscitation are discussed using the animal models of Dawes and Cross from the 1960s and 1970s. The UK Resuscitation Council uses this physiology for the basis of its teaching for newborn life support. It uses a step-by-step approach to the assessment and onward management of the baby who has not achieved normal breathing in the moments immediately after birth. Special cases in which resuscitation is required, such as preterm babies, babies born in the presence of meconium-stained liquor, babies born at home and babies with congenital anomalies, and the management of some of the more difficult neonatal issues, such as persistent pulmonary hypertension of the newborn and the baby born with shock, are also described.

Prior to the 1950s, numerous techniques for the resuscitation of the newborn were advocated and employed, all with some degree of apparent success. These included insufflation of the stomach with oxygen [2], hyperbaric oxygen [3], rapid hypothermia [4], and the use of respiratory stimulants on the tongue [5,6].

In the 1960s and 1970s, physiologists such as Kenneth Cross in London, Geoffrey Dawes in Oxford and other neonatal physiologists undertook major studies to assess the effect of a hypoxic insult on the fetus [7–9]. Their seminal work allows a great understanding of what is happening in utero to a baby, and helps to guide our actions in the process of resuscitation.

They used pregnant animals and externalized the fetus. After they had inserted arterial and venous lines for monitoring the physiological parameters, they placed a saline-filled bag over the head of the fetus. They then rendered the fetus hypoxic by occluding the umbilical cord and made recordings until the fetus died or it had responded to resuscitation. Their findings were extrapolated to the human fetus and are represented on the figures used below to explain their findings.

Consider the graph in Figure 25.1.

If a fetus is rendered hypoxic (time 0 on Figure 25.1), it responds by increasing the rate and depth of its breathing pattern, as shown in the lines at the top of the graph – each vertical line representing a breath. After a period of time, the fetus loses consciousness owing to hypoxia of the cerebral tissues, and this results in a loss of control from higher breathing centres. The period of apnoea which follows is termed 'primary apnoea'. After a period of time, the spinal reflex centres come into play, because they are no longer being

---

Best Practice in Labour and Delivery, ed. R. Warren and S. Arulkumaran. Published by Cambridge University Press.
© Cambridge University Press 2009.

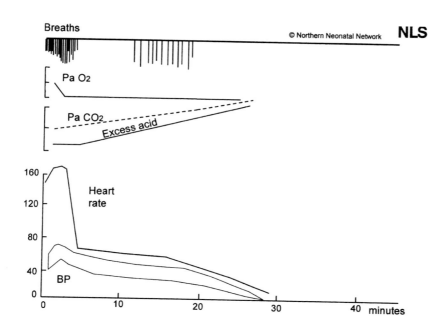

Figure 25.1 Diagrammatic representation of primary and terminal apnoea following the onset of acute total asphyxia at time 0

inhibited by the higher cerebral centres. This results in intermittent deep gasping respirations – each gasp occurring about every 6–10 s [8]. In the presence of continued hypoxia, this gasping will finally stop, and the fetus enters the phase of 'terminal apnoea'. Some like to call this phase 'secondary apnoea', but it deflects from the reality of the situation. This fetus *will* die unless someone in attendance at this delivery inflates the chest. As such, the more descriptive term 'terminal apnoea' should be used.

The next section in the graph relates to the oxygen, carbon dioxide and pH of the fetus. Clearly in this model, the animal has been rendered hypoxic. As such, the oxygen levels fall to a minimum and fail to respond to the rapid and increasing respiratory rate and fail to respond to the gasping. In the same way, the carbon dioxide levels begin to rise as the fetus is unable to dispose of the carbon dioxide produced. This carbon dioxide is converted to carbonic acid, which along with the increasing lactic acidosis from the hypoxia results in an excess of acid and a fall in the fetal pH. This fact is well known to those practising on a labour ward, and is the physiological basis behind the use of fetal scalp pH assessment to monitor fetal well-being during labour.

Turning to the cardiovascular responses in the hypoxic fetus, we see one of the ways in which the fetus differs from the adult. An adult rendered hypoxic for short periods would quickly develop cardiac

failure and suffer a cardiac arrest. The fetus, on the other hand, is designed to cope with the hypoxia associated with birth. Each time the uterus contracts, the flow of oxygenated blood from placenta to fetus is interrupted with the well-recognized consequence of a fetal bradycardia on the CTG. The same is seen in our animal model. The initial response to the hypoxia is an increase in the heart rate, but this is followed by a fall in the heart rate, not to zero as in the adult but to a rate of around 80 beats per minute (bpm). The heart relies on its stores of glycogen for an energy source during the hypoxic episodes, and only after a prolonged period of asphyxia does the fetal heart rate drop to very low levels and finally stop altogether.

By using other cardiovascular responses, the asphyxiated fetus aims to maintain its blood pressure. It diverts (redistributes) its blood flow away from non-essential organs (skin and splanchnic circulation) and sends it to vital organs (brain, heart, kidneys). As such, the baby who has experienced the longest period of intrauterine asphyxia will appear white and pale owing to this redistribution, the baby having vasoconstricted its peripheral circulation.

Finally, the heart can no longer continue without oxygen, and as the heart fails the blood pressure drops and the fetal heart stops.

That explains the background physiology to intrapartum asphyxia. The difficulty facing the person needing to resuscitate the baby is that they have no

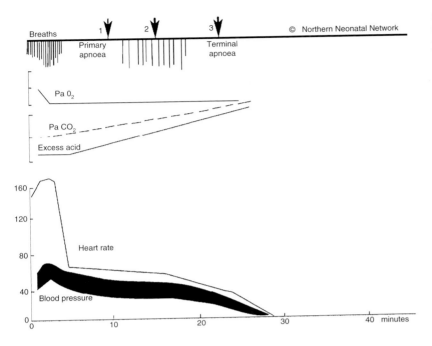

Figure 25.2 Diagramatic representation of primary and terminal apnoea following the onset of acute total asphyxia at time 0 with three time points marked

idea how far along this asphyxial timescale the baby has travelled. The baby born at each of the three arrows marked in Figure 25.2 present the same clinical findings – apnoeic, bradycardic and probably pale. The basis for the resuscitation of these babies is to start by performing the actions needed to resuscitate the baby at point 1 and if there is no response, move on to those actions needed for the baby at point 2, and so on in a stepwise manner, always assessing any change in colour, tone, respiratory effort and heart rate to the particular manoeuvre that was tried.

The first action in any resuscitation in the newborn, no matter how unwell the baby appears, is to get the baby wiped and dried and wrapped in warmed towels. It is far more difficult to resuscitate a cold, wet baby than it is to resuscitate a warm, dry baby.

Let us consider these babies born at different points along this asphyxial pathway and what they will need for resuscitation.

Let us consider the baby born in the primary apnoeic phase of asphyxia (Figure 25.3 – arrow 1 on Figure 25.2).

We know from the physiology we have just looked at that primary apnoea is always followed by gasping respiration. Therefore we know that this baby will gasp. If, at the point of gasping, this baby has a patent airway, it will be successful in getting oxygen into its lungs. This will quickly pass into the bloodstream and

as soon as it passes into the coronary arteries, the heart will respond with an increase in rate and the baby will turn pink. To all intents and purposes, the baby has resuscitated itself. We will have dried and wrapped the baby. We might have needed to open or clear the airway, but the rest was down to the baby.

Secondly, let us consider a baby who has been hypoxic for a little longer than the first baby who has now reached the gasping phase (Figure 25.4 – arrow 2 in Figure 25.2).

As with the previous baby, so long as the baby continues to take gasps and has an open and patent airway, it will resuscitate itself. The gasping will draw air into the lungs which, once absorbed into the bloodstream, will pass to the coronary arteries, resulting in an increase in the heart rate and the baby turning pink. Again, we will have dried and wrapped the baby before anything else, but this baby may take a little while to re-establish a normal respiratory pattern and may need some supportive ventilation breaths but, as with the previous baby, it has to all intents and purposes resuscitated itself.

Let us thirdly consider the baby who has taken its last gasp in utero and has been delivered in the terminal apnoeic phase (Figure 25.5 – arrow 3 in Figure 25.2).

This baby has now taken its last breath. If no action is taken, this baby *will* die. Owing to the fact

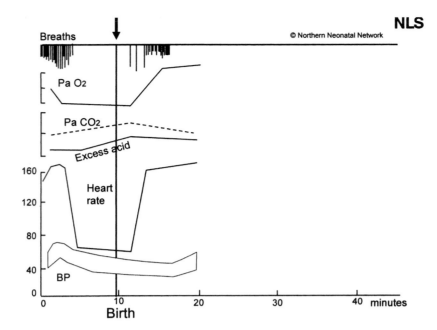

Figure 25.3 Diagrammatic representation of response to birth in primary apnoea

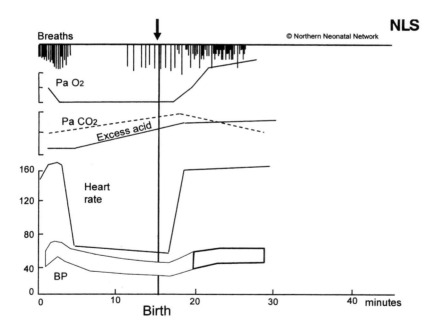

Figure 25.4 Diagrammatic representation of response to birth in gasping phase of intrapartum asphyxia

that the baby has never made an extrauterine breath, its lungs will still be full of fluid. When we start to resuscitate the baby we need to remember this. Having dried and wrapped the baby, the breaths we give need to be long and sustained in order to empty the alveoli of all of the lung fluid and allow the formation of a functional residual capacity.

The initial breaths are called inflation breaths and are normally given at 30 cm of water each for 2–3 s duration. We give five such breaths and are watching to assess if we achieve chest wall movement. It is not uncommon that adequate chest wall movement is only seen on the fourth and fifth breaths, as the first three breaths simply have been effective in pushing

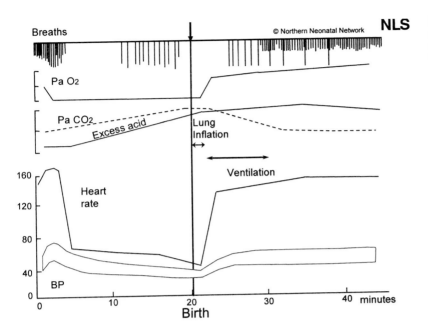

Breaths

© Northern Neonatal Network **NLS**

Pa O₂

Pa CO₂

Excess acid

Lung Inflation

Ventilation

160

120

80

40

0

Heart rate

BP

0   10   20   30   40   minutes

Birth

Figure 25.5 Diagrammatic representation of the physiological effect of lung inflation in a baby born in early terminal apnoea

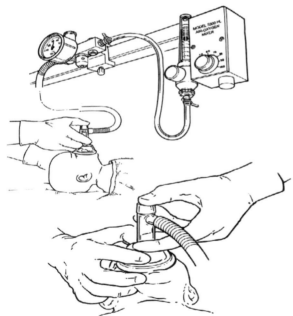

Figure 25.6 Head neutral position and correct hand position for use of T-piece and mask

that lung fluid out of the alveoli into the interstitial tissues and pulmonary lymphatics for drainage.

Inflating the chest using a bag and mask or a T-piece and mask is a skill which requires some learning, and it would be useful to practice this in your own delivery unit. We recommend the use of the soft-edged laerdal masks. The mask chosen needs to be the correct size – fitting over the nose and mouth but not extending below the chin or onto the orbits. The mask needs to be held in place by a downward pressure on the stem usually by holding the stem between the thumb and the forefinger. The middle finger can sit on the chin to allow support and to hold the head in a neutral position. The fourth and fifth fingers should rest on the jaw, making sure they are in contact with bone and not with the submandibular soft tissues. Pressure in the latter area will simply push the tongue up into the airway and make effective chest wall inflation more difficult by occluding the airway. If using a T-piece the correct hand position is shown in Figure 25.6.

If still unable to get the chest wall to move, ensure you are not overextending the neck. Once certain you are in the neutral position (Figures 25.6, 25.7 and 25.10), it may be appropriate to inspect the oropharynx by direct vision using a laryngoscope. When doing this one should be prepared to suction out any particulate material which may be occluding the airway (e.g. vernix, blood, meconium). It might also be useful at this point to insert an oropharyngeal (Guedel) airway, remembering that in the baby these are inserted in the same alignment as it will sit, unlike in the adult in which it is inserted and then rotated.

If you are still unable to effect chest wall movements, you will need to enlist the help of another.

277

In such circumstances, you can use two hands to achieve adequate airway control and hold the mask whilst your colleague provides the inflation in the bag or T-piece. With two people, it allows you to provide a forward movement of the jaw, pushing the angle of the jaw anteriorly to increase the pharyngeal space by moving the tongue forward, which is known as a jaw thrust. This is shown in Figure 25.7.

How do we know if the baby has responded to our inflation breaths? Well, consider the baby who gasped

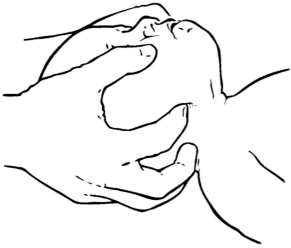

Figure 25.7 Double-handed jaw thrust with head in the neutral position

in the first two scenarios. If you remember, the measure of the baby responding was by finding an increase in the heart rate. There is no difference in this baby. Yes, it is further along the asphyxial pathway of our animal model, but adequate inflation breaths should result in an increase in the heart rate, as that air gets oxygen into the bloodstream and into the coronary arteries. You will see from Figure 25.5 that the lung inflation results in an increase in the heart rate although the baby has not yet established its own respiratory pattern. We need to provide shorter ventilation breaths for a short period of time after which we will see the baby begin to gasp. This gasping will then be interspersed with normal respiratory effort just like we had seen in the two previous scenarios.

Finally, let us consider another baby who has also reached the terminal apnoeic phase (Figure 25.8 – arrow 3 in Figure 25.2). This baby will not breathe for itself, and requires us to give five inflation breaths in order to oxygenate it and then allow an improvement in the heart rate. Let us consider that we have given the baby five inflation breaths and we are certain that we have seen good chest wall movement. Our assessment of effectiveness of the resuscitation thus far is to assess the heart rate, but in this case, there has been no increase. The heart rate is still at 40 bpm, for example. Why is this, and what do we need to do?

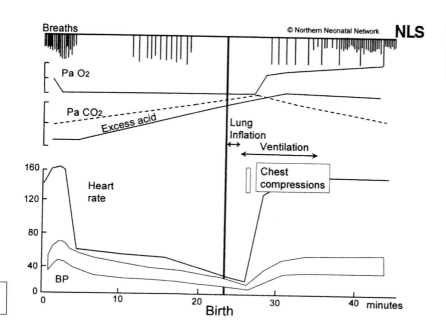

Figure 25.8 Diagrammatic representation of the physiological response to cardiac compressions in a baby born in early terminal apnoea who has not responded to lung inflation

the xiphisternum on a point one finger's breadth below an imaginary line drawn between the baby's nipples. The compressions should be about one-third of the depth of the chest to the baby's spine (Figure 25.9).

The compressions should be given in a ratio of 3:1 with short ventilation breaths. A total of 120 events in a minute should be the aim – but the quality of the compression and ventilation is probably more important than the quantity [10]. They should be continued for 30 s and then the baby reassessed. Hopefully, there will have been an increase in the heart rate and the baby will be becoming pink and active. If not, and one is happy that chest wall movement is effective and compressions are adequate, one should consider the use of drugs after gaining venous access via the insertion of an umbilical venous catheter (UVC). Such action would almost certainly be the domain of the neonatal team, but with more trainees spending some time in neonatal training posts or attending Newborn Life Support courses, it would not be inappropriate for an obstetrician, midwife or anaesthetist with some UVC experience to insert the line. One would consider using sodium bicarbonate, adrenaline and dextrose as part of the resuscitation. In babies remaining pale and bradycardic, one should always consider blood loss and in such cases, volume (O negative blood) can be life-saving.

All this can be summarized in the algorithm shown in Figure 25.11. This is the 2008 UK Resuscitation Council newborn life support algorithm for the resuscitation of the newborn baby.

Opening the airway

The neonate has a relatively large occiput and if the infant is floppy, this often results in the neck flexing the chin onto the chest wall, leading to obstruction of the airway. In such cases, one needs to be able to open the airway using simple manoeuvres. The simplest manoeuvre is the 'chin lift', which simply puts the newborn baby's head into a neutral position, opening the airway and allowing the baby to take in air if it is making any sort of respiratory effort (Figure 25.10). Note that in opening the airway, the baby's face should be parallel to the surface on which it is being resuscitated, with the eyes looking straight upwards. This is different from the adult position, where the neck is extended with the patient "sniffing the morning air". Figure 25.10 illustrates the correct position of the newborn baby's head to achieve the neutral position.

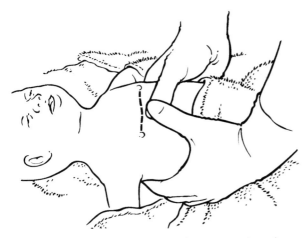

Figure 25.9 Position for two-handed chest compressions when standing at the side or foot of the baby

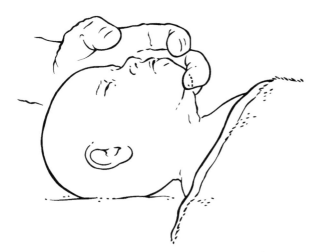

Figure 25.10 Placing of head in the neutral position using a chin lift

Well, what we can assume is that this heart has been too compromised by the episode of intrapartum asphyxia. It has failed to respond to the effective inflation breaths. This tells us that this baby requires a short (30 s) period of cardiac compressions in order to try and move blood from the pulmonary vasculature into the coronaries so that the oxygen given with successful inflation breaths can get into the coronaries and give the heart the bump-start it needs.

Chest compressions are best given with two hands encircling the chest wall. Fingers at the back, thumbs at the front. The thumbs should be on the lower third of

Newborn Life Support

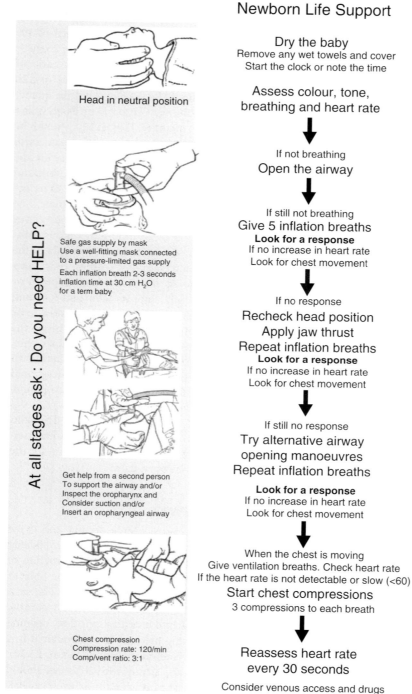

Head in neutral position

Safe gas supply by mask
Use a well-fitting mask connected
to a pressure-limited gas supply

Each inflation breath 2-3 seconds
inflation time at 30 cm H₂O
for a term baby

Get help from a second person
To support the airway and/or
Inspect the oropharynx and
Consider suction and/or
Insert an oropharyngeal airway

Chest compression
Compression rate: 120/min
Comp/vent ratio: 3:1

At all stages ask : Do you need HELP?

Dry the baby
Remove any wet towels and cover
Start the clock or note the time

**Assess colour, tone,
breathing and heart rate**

If not breathing
Open the airway

If still not breathing
Give 5 inflation breaths
Look for a response
If no increase in heart rate
Look for chest movement

If no response
**Recheck head position
Apply jaw thrust
Repeat inflation breaths**
Look for a response
If no increase in heart rate
Look for chest movement

If still no response
**Try alternative airway
opening manoeuvres
Repeat inflation breaths**

Look for a response
If no increase in heart rate
Look for chest movement

When the chest is moving
Give ventilation breaths. Check heart rate
If the heart rate is not detectable or slow (<60)
Start chest compressions
3 compressions to each breath

**Reassess heart rate
every 30 seconds**

Consider venous access and drugs

**If meconium present and
baby breathing well:**
Do not suction the airway
-baby floppy and not breathing well:
Consider inspection and suction
before inflation breaths

If breathing:
Reassess heart rate and monitor baby

**If heart rate is satisfactory or
increasing:**
Continue ventilation breaths at
about 30/min until the baby
is breathing adequately

**If heart rate is satisfactory or
increasing:**
Continue ventilation breaths
at about 30/min until baby
is breathing adequately

If the chest is not moving:
Recheck head position and
Repeat inflation breaths
If competent, consider intubation

If the chest is still not moving:
The airway is the problem

If the heart rate is increasing:
Stop compressions
Continue ventilation breaths
at about 30/min
until the baby is breathing adequately

Figure 25.11 Newborn Life Support Algorithm 2008

If this fails to allow air entry, one can consider the jaw thrust manoeuvres described above.

Whatever the condition of the baby at birth, it is vital to remember that the baby will be wet and have a large surface area to body mass ratio. These two issues mean that the baby will lose heat very quickly. A cold, wet baby is much more difficult to resuscitate than a warm, dry baby.

For the newborn term baby, it is important that the baby is wiped and dried and wrapped in warm towels as quickly as possible after birth, particularly if it has not established a normal breathing pattern. Remember particularly to dry the head and, if need be, place a hat on the baby's head. Premature infants are now placed into warming bags undried, which has shown to be an effective method of conserving heat for the baby. The use of a warmer bag is only advocated if the baby will remain under an overhead radiant heater which would allow the child to maintain warmth. If a radiant heater is not available, then even the premature baby should be towelled dry and wrapped in warm, dry towels using a hat in the same way as the term baby.

Resuscitation of the premature baby

The resuscitation of the premature baby should be performed along exactly the same lines as that for the term baby. The differences are the two highlighted earlier. Firstly, the baby tends to be placed in a warming bag directly and left under a radiant heater for maximum temperature control; and secondly, the initial inflation breaths given may be at a lower pressure to effect the chest wall movements than in the term baby. Data from the EPICure study showed that temperature on admission to the neonatal unit was directly related to outcome and that too many babies born at less than 25 weeks completed gestation were too cold [11]. Following these results, much work was done trying to improve the temperature of these fragile babies, and the use of warmer bags and overhead radiant heaters is now commonplace and has been shown to be highly effective [12]. One needs to remember that the premature infant is more fragile than the term baby, is more prone to hypotension and hypoglycaemia than the term infant, and has far less energy stores for the resuscitation. As a consequence, it will get colder quicker, take longer to rewarm, and due to the probable lack of surfactant, have less-compliant lungs and need more help in establishing their respiration. Most of the premature babies who are being resuscitated are babies who require stabilization rather than resuscitation [13]. The preterm baby who has undergone the same asphyxial events as the term babies described earlier is not likely to survive, and most of the babies where the neonatal team are involved in the resuscitation are those preterm babies who are born and show signs not only of vitality but also of viability.

This whole question may be considered in other parts of this book, but the recent publication by the Nuffield Bioethics Council does give some sensible guidance on which babies should or should not be resuscitated [14].

Meconium-stained liquor

The newborn baby is born with its bowels containing meconium. This is a mixture of sloughed-off cells and bowel secretions formed over the time that the fetus has been developing in utero. Babies who are nearing term may, in the presence of an asphyxial insult, evacuate their bowels and hence the liquor will appear meconium-stained. From the earlier physiology which we have described (Figure 25.1), it will be understood that if the baby reaches the gasping phase of asphyxia and the liquor contains meconium, then that fetus is very likely to aspirate the meconium into their lungs. There is little that anyone can do about this meconium even at the time of the delivery, and the job of the resuscitator under such circumstances is to try and prevent any further aspiration of meconium which may be in the nose and the mouth of the newborn infant.

The guidance about what to do for a baby born with meconium-stained liquor has become simpler since the advent of the newborn life support algorithms (Figure 25.11). The baby born in the presence of meconium who is active, pink and crying should be wiped and wrapped in the same way as we have already described, and should be watched for any signs of respiratory distress owing to the meconium which may have been aspirated prior to the delivery. For the baby who is born floppy and not breathing, once the baby has been gently dried and covered with a warmed towel, direct inspection of the oropharynx would be advocated with the use of a laryngoscope and any particulate material present in the mouth should be aspirated using a Yankauer sucker. Once this has been done, the resuscitation can proceed in the ways already outlined, with manoeuvring of the airway to make it patent and, if necessary, giving the sustained inflation breaths in order to effect chest wall movement and allow oxygenation of the blood passing into the coronary arteries. The practice of suction of the nose and mouth with the child's head on the perineum, or of splinting the chest at birth are no longer advocated in the UK, nor is there any need to be suctioning from the nose and mouth thin meconium-stained liquor once the child has established its own respiratory effort, as these have been shown to provide no benefit [15].

Babies born outside hospital

Some women choose electively to give birth in the comfort of their own home. When such a decision has been made, a plan is put in place with the midwifery teams caring for that mother and her unborn child so that the child can be delivered safely in the home. Occasionally, some of these babies may not establish normal respiratory effort, or the child may be born without the midwife being present. Furthermore, some women may deliver outside of hospital unplanned, and therefore it is important that people working in the field of obstetrics, maternity and paediatrics as well as other highlighted specialities should understand the basic principles of the resuscitation. In a hospital setting nowadays, we have developed resuscitaires which carry all of the equipment necessary for us to perform an effective resuscitation of the newborn baby but, in essence, all that is really required is a flat surface, some warmed towels and some light. We must remember that the baby born out of hospital, particularly if unexpected, is more likely to get cold and therefore attention to drying the baby with something which is available and getting them wrapped and kept warm is of vital importance. The airway manoeuvres described can be done very simply and if the child does not establish their own respiration then mouth to nose-and-mouth resuscitation can be given by someone who is present at the time of the delivery. This may be life-saving. One needs to pay particular attention to temperature control. Cold rooms need warming and draughts from windows need to be minimized in order to allow the maximum warmth to the baby. Instruction can be reasonably easily given to any other helper as to how to perform cardiac massage if it were indicated, and if one is calling for an emergency ambulance one

ought to be clear that the ambulance is required for a newborn baby so that paramedics with the correct skills can be sent to assist whoever else is involved in the onward resuscitation. Remember to cover the head, that a baby can be placed in direct contact with the mother in order to maintain warmth and that hot water bottles can be useful, but should not be in direct contact with the child's skin and would be better wrapped in a towel. It is also helpful to look at your watch to have an accurate assessment of the time of the birth of the child and how long any attempts at resuscitation have been continuing.

Babies with congenital abnormalities

With the improvements in fetal medicine scanning, it is unusual now to be presented with a baby with a major unexpected congenital anomaly. Babies born with Pierre Robin sequence are a particular risk, owing to the small mouth due to their mandibular hypoplasia. The insertion of a nasopharyngeal or oropharyngeal airway in these cases can be of great benefit, as it allows better passage of air into the pharynx.

In babies known to have a diaphragmatic hernia, it is always preferable not to provide mask inflation of the lungs if it can be avoided. Inevitably some of that masked gas will pass into the intestines and can compromise the aeration of the lungs. It would always be preferable to intubate such a baby if it was showing signs of respiratory compromise, but one must do what they are capable of doing and in the absence of someone trained in neonatal intubation it would be entirely sensible to offer inflation breath and onward resuscitation in the same manner as outlined earlier in the chapter.

Persistent pulmonary hypertension of the newborn (PPHN)

At birth the baby needs to change the flows of blood through its circulation. The first breath leads to a massive fall in the pulmonary vascular resistance and that coupled with the clamping of the cord and the relative increase in the systemic vascular resistance are the major factors which cause the change from the fetal to the neonatal/adult circulation. Failure for this to occur results in an inappropriately high pulmonary vascular resistance, a reduction in effective pulmonary blood flow, shunting of blood from the right to the left side through both the *foramen ovale* and the *ductus arteriosus* and a baby who remains blue. There are many conditions which can result in PPHN, some of which can be anticipated from a knowledge of the pregnancy and the labour. Such causes would include perinatal asphyxia, meconium aspiration syndrome, congenital pneumonia, pulmonary hypoplasia secondary to oligohydramnios, and congenital lung abnormalities. The presence of such a shunt can often be easily demonstrated by assessing the saturations on the right hand (preductal) and either foot (postductal). A difference of more than 10% would be considered as significant [16]. Persistent pulmonary hypertension has a quoted incidence of about 1 to 5 per 1000 births [17].

The immediate management of the baby at birth is the same and is in line with what has been outlined in the earlier pages of this chapter: wipe and dry the baby to keep them warm, open the airway and assess the response. If there is no respiratory effort, then you need to give inflation breaths and follow the NLS algorithm appropriately. Unfortunately in some of these babies they need more intensive resuscitation and onward care. The mainstay of the management is to try to reduce the effective pulmonary vascular resistance or to increase the systemic vascular resistance by artificial means to allow a reversal of the right-to-left shunts. The manoeuvres needed include sedation and paralysis of the baby, ventilation with 100% oxygen (FiO_2 1.0), alkalinization of the pH either by hyperventilation to reduce the $PaCO_2$ or by the use of $NaHCO_3$ and the use of pulmonary vasodilator agents such as Prostacyclin or Tolazoline. More recently, inhaled nitric oxide has become more widely available, and is a very useful addition to the pharmacopeia for this difficult condition.

Shock

We have stated that the baby who has undergone a significant period of asphyxia will appear pale owing to the vasoconstriction of their peripheral circulation in order to maintain their blood pressure. It is also important to remember that the baby who has lost blood will also appear pale. A history of antepartum haemorrhage or the presence of a retroplacental clot can be the important clue to the failure of a baby to respond to a well-performed resuscitation. If the baby has (i) good chest wall movements with mask ventilation, (ii) is having adequate cardiac massage, and (iii) has failed to respond to drugs, it is important to consider a loss of circulating volume as a possible cause. The baby should be given 20 ml/kg of packed red blood cells as a bolus. This can have a dramatic effect by providing the red cells to deliver the oxygen to the coronaries, allowing the baby to respond to the resuscitation being carried out.

Summary

It is often difficult to predict which babies will require resuscitation at birth. As a consequence it is of great importance that all staff involved in the management of pregnant women should have the basic skills required for basic neonatal resuscitation. The pathway follows a logical system based on an understanding of the physiology of intrapartum asphyxia.

The baby needs to be wiped and dried and kept warm. The airway needs to be opened by placing the head in a neutral position, and if breathing is not established then resuscitation with inflation breaths needs to be given. The success of the inflation breaths is determined by the response in the heart rate. Cardiac compressions may be needed if the chest wall has inflated but the heart rate has not responded. Drugs may be needed if the heart rate does not respond. In a small number of cases, the baby will need blood because they are hypovolaemic following a fetal–maternal bleed, massive APH or a retroplacental clot.

The vast majority of babies born need no resuscitation and of those who do require help, about 95% will have responded with an increase in heart rate within 1–2 min of effective resuscitation.

References

1. De Lee J B. Asphyxia neonatorum: causation and treatment. *Medicine (Detroit)* 1897; **3**: 643–60.

2. Akerren Y, Furstenberg N. Gastrointestinal administration of oxygen in the treatment of asphyxia in the newborn. *J Obstet Gynaecol Br Emp* 1950; **57**: 705–13.

3. Hutchinson J, Kerr M, Williams K, Hopkinson W. Hyperbaric oxygen in the resuscitation of the newborn. *Lancet* 1963; **ii**: 1019–22.

4. Cordey R, Chiolero R, Miller J. Resuscitation of neonates by hypothermia: report of 20 cases with acid-base determination on 10 cases and long-term development of 33 cases. *Resuscitation* 1973; **2**: 169–87.

5. Daniel S S, Dawes G S, James L S, Ross B B. Analeptics and resuscitation of asphyxiated monkeys. *Br Med J* 1966; **ii**: 562–3.

6. Barrie H, Cottom D G, Wilson B D R. Respiratory stimulants in the newborn. *Lancet* 1962; **ii**: 742–6.

7. Cross K W. Resuscitation of the asphyxiated infant. *Br Med Bull* 1966; **22**: 73–8.

8. Dawes G. *Fetal and Neonatal Physiology*. Chicago: Year Book Publisher, 1968; Chapter 12: 141–9.

9. Godfrey S. Respiratory and cardiovascular changes during asphyxia and resuscitation of foetal newborn rabbits. *Quart J Exper Physiol* 1968; **53**: 97–118.

10. Whyte S D, Sinha A K, Wyllie J P. Neonatal resuscitation – a practical assessment. *Resuscitation* 1999; **40**: 21–5.

11. Costeloe K, Hennessy E, Gibson A T, Marlow N, Wilkinson A R. The EPICure study: outcomes to discharge from hospital for infants born at the threshold of viability. *Paediatrics* 2000; **106**(4): 659–71.

12. Vohra S, Frent G, Campbell V, Abbott M, Whyte R. Effect of polyethylene occlusive skin wrapping on heat loss in very low birthweight infants at delivery: a randomized trial. *J Pediatr* 1999; **134**(5): 547–51.

13. O'Donnell C, Davis P G, Morley C J. Resuscitation of premature infants: what are we doing wrong and can do better? *Biol Neonate* 2003; **84**: 76–82.

14. Nuffield Council on Bioethics. *Critical care decisions in fetal and neonatal medicine: ethical issues.* November 2006. Available at: www.nuffieldbioethics.org/go/ourwork/neonatal/introduction

15. Vain N E, Szyld E G, Prudent L M, Wiswell T E, Aguilar A M, Vivas N I. Oropharyngeal and nasopharyngeal suctioning of meconium-stained neonates before delivery of their shoulders: multicentre, randomised controlled trial. *Lancet* 2004; **364**: 597–602.

16. Pearlman S A, Maisels J. Preductal and postductal transcutaneous oxygen tension measurements in premature newborns with hyaline membrane disease. *Pediatrics* 1989; **83**: 98–100.

17. Weigel T J, Hageman J R. National survey of diagnosis and management of persistent pulmonary hypertension of the newborn. *J Perinatol* 1990; **10**: 369–75.

Chapter 26

The immediate puerperium

Mahishee Mehta and Leonie Penna

The delivery of the baby is a point in the labour when the parents relax and begin to celebrate, but for the health professional continued vigilance is necessary as a number of problems can occur in the puerperium. The definition of what constitutes the immediate puerperium is not fixed. The puerperium describes the time following childbirth during which a mother's anatomy and physiology return to the prepregnancy state. The time that this takes is likely to vary between individual women, but is generally considered to be complete by 6 weeks after birth. In certain legal situations, the puerperium is considered to last for a longer time, with 12 months being used as the upper limit for the definition of postpartum psychiatric illness and late maternal death.

The risk of most puerperal complications is greatest immediately after birth, with the incidence of most problems falling with the time elapsed since delivery. The type of delivery that a woman has will influence her risk of puerperal complications, as will the presence of certain antenatal risk factors.

Women now spend much less time in hospital than previously, even after relatively complex deliveries. Discharge home should only take place when the risk of serious 'immediate' complications has passed, with high-risk women remaining under observation for longer to detect complications early and to institute appropriate management to reduce morbidity and mortality. Women with significant risk factors will usually remain in hospital to be observed for a period of time after delivery, but for low-risk women they may deliver at home or be discharged home within a few hours of delivery. In the UK, a midwife offers women a visit daily at home for 10 days after giving birth.

The postnatal check [1]

The following should be observed and reviewed in all postpartum women for 7–10 days after delivery.

Maternal observations

Temperature, pulse and blood pressure should be measured daily in low-risk women. Women with risk factors for sepsis or hypertension require more frequent observation, and thus will usually stay in hospital for 24 h or more. A low-grade rise in temperature is often seen in the normal puerperium related to normal physiological processes.

Uterus

The uterus should involute steadily after delivery with the fundus no longer palpable abdominally in most women after day 10. Although a woman may describe 'after pains', the uterus should not be tender on palpation. A high fundus or uterine tenderness need further review.

Lochia

Bleeding will continue for a number of weeks (mean duration is 24 days), with 13% of normal women still bleeding at 8 weeks. However, the lochia should remain the same or reduce with each postnatal day. An increase in amount of lochia, the passage of clots or an offensive smell is abnormal and requires medical review.

Caesarean section scar

The dressing should be removed to inspect the wound on day 2. Inflammation, gaping or discharge are abnormal and require further management.

Best Practice in Labour and Delivery, ed. R. Warren and S. Arulkumaran. Published by Cambridge University Press.
© Cambridge University Press 2009.

Perineal wound

The wound should be clean and have no gaping or inflammation. Advice to maintain good hygiene should be repeated if necessary.

Bladder function

All women should be asked if they are experiencing any difficulty in voiding and any reported problems such as a feeling of incomplete emptying require further investigation. Postnatal pelvic floor exercise should be recommended to all women, and this can commence immediately even if delivery was by caesarean section.

Bowel function [2]

All women who have delivered vaginally and especially those who had an operative delivery should be asked about bowel function, as many women experience some bowel dysfunction but do not report their symptoms. In the first few days some incontinence of flatus or faeces appears to be a common experience. Reassurance that in the majority of women this symptom will resolve should be given, but it is important to follow-up the symptoms on subsequent days to ensure that this is indeed the case, with referral to a perineal clinic if symptoms persist.

Many women (20%) will have constipation and require dietary advice (including maintaining a good fluid intake) or the prescription of a bulking agent such as Fybogel, or a simple laxative such as Lactulose. Haemorrhoids that were present antenatally or developed for the first time in labour may be troublesome. They do not resolve immediately, and 10% of women will continue to have haemorrhoids in the future. Dietary advice, simple analgesia and topical creams should be offered, with surgical referral for women who have thrombosed piles.

Thrombosis risk

The risk of thrombosis should be considered for all women regardless of their mode of delivery [3], with appropriate thromboprophylaxis measures recommended where any risk is identified (thromboembolic deterrent stockings, encouraging mobilization, and low molecular weight heparin).

Infant feeding issues (and breast)

Breastfeeding should be encouraged unless specific contra-indications exist (such as maternal HIV and certain medications). Any problems with infant feeding should be discussed with referral to a breastfeeding specialist if advice is required.

Emotional/mental state

Any problems that occurred during labour should be discussed to reduce anxiety that may result from this. An assessment of emotional well-being is essential in all women, with appropriate reassurance offered for minor symptoms whilst ensuring the more serious symptoms are referred to a perinatal psychiatrist.

Social issues

Women with complex social problems (such as drug dependency, domestic violence or child protection issues) should be identified and may require a longer stay in hospital to ensure that the appropriate support networks have been alerted prior to discharge.

Other issues

All women should be offered contact details of providers of expert contraceptive advice and should be advised to access this as soon as possible (ideally within the first week). If a woman may have difficulty doing this, appropriate contraceptive advice and prescription should be given before discharge from the maternity unit.

An appropriate dose (based on the postdelivery maternal kleihauer) of anti-D immunoglobulin should be offered to all non-sensitized Rhesus-negative women within 72 h following the delivery of a Rhesus-positive baby.

Women who were found to be seronegative on antenatal screening for rubella should be offered vaccination with MMR (measles, mumps, rubella) vaccine following birth.

Puerperal complications
Secondary postpartum haemorrhage

A haemorrhage occurring 24 h or more after delivery is defined as a secondary postpartum haemorrhage (PPH). It is rare, complicating only about 1% of deliveries. The underlying pathology is almost always retained placental tissue and/or uterine infection. Other causes are very rare, but include coagulation disorders and cervical malignancy. Retained placenta is less common following delivery by caesarean section, but can still occur even when the notes document that the cavity was checked.

In either pathology, the uterus will be poorly contracted ('boggy') and high.

Important clinical features suggesting infection include uterine tenderness, tachycardia and pyrexia. The bleeding of secondary PPH is rarely massive and unrelenting, so maternal compromise is unusual; evidence of shock suggests severe sepsis requiring urgent intervention.

Swabs to exclude infection are essential in all women with increased lochia, and an ultrasound scan can assist in excluding retained products of conception. This should be performed by an experienced sonographer to try to reduce the false positive rate, as it is difficult to distinguish between blood clot and retained placental tissue in the postpartum uterine cavity.

In all cases of secondary PPH, infection should be assumed to be present even in the absence of clinical signs, and intravenous antibiotics (usually a cephalosporin and metronidazole) should be commenced. If there are clinical suspicions or ultrasound evidence of retained products then uterine curettage should be arranged after commencing antibiotics (to reduce the risk of generalized sepsis and uterine perforation). Postpartum curettage should be performed by an experienced surgeon, as there are significant risks of perforation and of future Asherman's syndrome, especially if there is uterine sepsis. Suction curettage is recommended, with the avoidance of sharp curettage if possible. Routine uterotonic drugs should be administered following the procedure.

Pelvic haematoma

Perineal trauma due to a difficult vaginal delivery or inadequate perineal suturing may result in the formation of a haematoma. This may be vulval, vaginal or subperitoneal. Broad-ligament haematomas can also form, usually following delivery by caesarean section, especially following failed instrumental delivery. This is an uncommon problem with an incidence quoted as 1 in 500–900 deliveries.

Clinical features

Primary pelvic haematomas are complications of delivery and present in the first 24 h after delivery.

Depending upon the site and extent of the haematoma, the presentation of symptoms can either be immediate or be delayed. Vulval and lower vaginal haematomas are usually obvious on perineal inspection and digital examination, with evidence of an exquisitely painful swelling on the vulva or in the wall of the vagina. Smaller haematomas may present as an area of discoloration (bruising). Haematomas may form higher in the pelvis arising as a result of high vaginal lacerations, cervical lacerations and tears of the broad-ligament vessels. These types of haematomas are often described as subperitoneal, but postnatal pelvic haematomas may also be retroperitoneal, usually secondary to bleeding as a complication of caesarean section. Subperitoneal haematomas are more difficult to diagnose than vulval and vaginal problems, presenting with more non-specific symptoms, although pain is invariably a feature. The uterine fundus may be deviated and as the potential spaces can hold large volumes of blood, the woman may develop signs and symptoms related to blood loss. These subperitoneal haematomas should be suspected in cases of haemodynamically unstable patients.

Smaller, self-limiting haematomas may not be diagnosed immediately and present in the early postnatal period with low-grade pyrexia or bladder and bowel dysfunction. In rare cases a haematoma can develop as a secondary problem due to infection or pressure necrosis in the paravaginal tissues; these cases present later in the puerperium.

Management

A small vulval haematoma (less than 5 cm and not increasing in size) can be treated conservatively with an ice pack and prophylactic broad-spectrum antibiotics (cephalosporin and metronidazole). Attempted evacuation of small haematomas is not indicated, as the blood is usually compartmentalized or has tracked into the tissues so that attempted evacuation is unrewarding and causes more tissue trauma. In larger haematomas (more than 5 cm in size), surgical evacuation should be considered. This is advisable if the haematoma is fluctuant, there is significant pain, or the haematoma is increasing in size. Evacuation will allow the securing of haemostasis and closure of dead space. The problems in suturing vaginal tissues following the evacuation of a haematoma should not be underestimated, as the tissue is very oedematous and friable. Suturing is required for haemostasis with large vessels, but vaginal packing with gauze can be used to obtain haemostasis in smaller, more diffuse vessels. The pack should be retained for 24 h (bladder catheterization and good analgesia are essential) prior to removal.

Selective angiography and embolization may be an option in retroperitoneal haematomas. However, exploratory laparotomy with ligation of vessels or hysterectomy may be required to manage cases with unremitting haemorrhage.

Puerperal sepsis and endometritis

A potentially life-threatening condition, puerperal sepsis is an infection during the postnatal period, which may occur following a vaginal or caesarean delivery. It is most likely to arise from infection of the genital tract, usually originating within the uterus as an endometritis, but other sources include surgical wound infections, breast infections, bowel pathology and urinary tract infections. Rare cases of overwhelming sepsis due to other septic foci, such as pneumonia, can occur in the puerperium, and the clinician should remain alert to the possibility in any woman presenting with non-specific symptoms. The most common causative organisms are *Streptococcus*, both group A and group B. Staphylococci, coliforms, anaerobes, mycoplasma and *Chlamydia* can all cause puerperal infection. In obstetrics, clostridium and methicillin-resistant staphylococcus A (MRSA) rarely cause problems.

The incidence of sepsis varies worldwide, with much higher rates of life-threatening severe sepsis seen in the developing world. The rates in industrialized countries are low, and therefore clinicians need to consider it a possible diagnosis in order to avoid delay in detection and management. Although the rates are low, it remains a significant cause of maternal death, and there has been no reduction in the number of women dying from infection in recent years. Sepsis can occur after any type of delivery, but multiple vaginal examinations and positive genital tract cultures for anaerobic Gram-negative bacilli are risk factors.

Clinical features

Endometritis presents with offensive lochia, which may also be heavy, as inflammation in the placental bed will increase bleeding. There may be uterine pain with an increase in 'after pains' and uterine tenderness on palpation. Low-grade pyrexia may be present. High-grade pyrexia, rigors, tachycardia or a woman who is systemically unwell is likely developing puerperal sepsis and requires urgent evaluation and treatment. Endometritis is not the only cause of puerperal sepsis, but is the most common. Other causes include urinary tract infection and chest infection (usually post-general anaesthetic or in women with respiratory disease, but primary pneumonia can occur).

Sepsis is defined as the systemic response to infection manifested by two or more of the following signs or symptoms:
- temperature $>38°C$;
- heart rate >100 beats/min;
- respiratory rate >20/min or $PaCO_2$ <32 mmHg;
- white cell count $>17 \times 10^9$/l or $<4 \times 10^9$/l or $>10\%$ immature forms;

AND one of the following:
- bacteraemia on blood cultures;
- positive swab (vaginal or wound);
- positive urine culture.

In keeping with this definition, UK guidelines on postnatal care [4] recommend that sepsis in the immediate puerperium should be suspected in the presence of two or more of these signs and symptoms:
- fever $>38.5°C$ on one occasion or $38°C$ on 2 occasions 4 h apart;
- shivering or rigors;
- abdominal tenderness with no other recognized source of infection;
- uterine subinvolution;
- offensive or heavy lochia;
- tachycardia.

Management

When genital tract sepsis is suspected, investigations should include blood cultures, wound and vaginal swabs. A urine culture should also be performed. Broad-spectrum antibiotics should be prescribed covering both aerobic and anaerobic organisms. In cases where endometritis is suspected, an ultrasound scan (preferably transvaginal) must be performed to exclude the possibility of retained products of conception (RPOC) even if the placenta was considered complete or delivery was by caesarean section. If RPOC are confirmed, then surgical uterine evacuation by suction curettage should be arranged after initial doses of intravenous antibiotics have been administered to reduce the risk of worsening bacteraemia. As there is a risk of uterine perforation and postpartum haemorrhage, uterine evacuation should be undertaken by an experienced surgeon and uterotonic drugs should be given routinely to all cases.

Ogilvie's syndrome

Ogilvie's syndrome describes an acute pseudo-obstruction of the large bowel that occurs following caesarean section or caesarean hysterectomy. It has more rarely been reported after instrumental delivery and spontaneous vaginal delivery. It is a rare complication, but often goes undiagnosed, and in the 2000–2003 Confidential Enquiry into Maternal and Child Health report there were four maternal deaths related to Ogilvie's syndrome [5].

The condition is caused by an autonomic imbalance resulting in decreased motility in the distal colon with resulting distention of the caecum. If undetected the caecum may rupture, causing peritonitis.

The symptoms begin 2–12 days after delivery by caesarean section. Eighty percent of cases will have crampy, non-localized abdominal pain. Bowel movements will usually be reduced, but in some cases flatus and faecal fluid will be passed. Bowel sounds are not necessarily helpful, as some women will have normal or even hyperactive bowel sounds and others can have sounds suggesting obstruction ('tinkling'), or absent bowel sounds. The temperature will be normal, but tachycardia and a raised white cell count may be seen. The most universal finding is progressive abdominal distention. The diagnosis can be made on a plain abdominal X-ray, which may show caecal dilatation, but an abdominal CT scan is now the investigation of choice, as this will distinguish Ogilvie's syndrome from mechanical obstruction or volvulus and also indicate an abdominal bleeding or peritonitis.

If the caecal dilatation is less than 10 cm the woman can be managed conservatively, keeping her nil-by-mouth and instituting a convention 'drip and suck' regimen with intravenous fluids and a nasogastric tube. Any medication that could reduce colonic motility such as opiates should be discontinued. Careful review is required and other management options should be continued if there is no improvement after 24–48 h.

If there is no improvement, a surgical opinion should be obtained. Intravenous Neostigmine can be considered if mechanical obstruction has been excluded. This treatment is associated with a rapid clinical response with a reduction in abdominal distention within 30 min of treatment. The other main treatment option is endoscopic decompression, but this is usually reserved for patients who do not respond to Neostigmine, and is associated with a significant risk of recurrence after the initial decompression. A laparotomy is mandatory if a perforation or bowel ischaemia is suspected, or if a mechanical obstruction cannot be excluded by imaging. Bowel resection may be necessary with a temporary stoma formation [6].

Thromboembolism

Venous thromboembolism (VTE) remains the most common direct cause of maternal death in the UK, with the puerperium representing the time of greatest risk. Sequential reports of Confidential Enquiries into Maternal and Child Health [5,7] have highlighted failures in obtaining objective diagnoses and employing adequate treatment. The subjective clinical assessment of deep venous thrombosis (DVT) and pulmonary thromboembolism (PTE) is particularly unreliable in the puerperium, and thus the threshold for performing further investigations should be lowered in postnatal women presenting with symptoms that could be due to thromboembolic disease.

The risk of VTE in pregnancy is 1–2/1000. The majority of cases occur in the puerperium with a fivefold increase in the risk in postnatal women compared to antenatal women. PE in particular is much more likely to occur postnatally.

The incidence of VTE in women having caesarean section has fallen in the UK due to the more universal use of thromboprophylactic measures. However, there has been no decrease in the incidence in women delivering vaginally, and it is important that a risk assessment for VTE is performed for all women and thromboprophylaxis recommended for high-risk women [3].

Risk factors

- Previous VTE.
- Thrombophilia (congenital and acquired):
  - Factor V Leiden,
  - protein C deficiency,
  - protein S deficiency,
  - antithrombin gene variant,
  - antiphospholipid syndrome.

- Increased maternal age >35 years.
- Increased parity >4.
- Operative delivery.
- Excessive blood loss.
- Infection.
- Pre-eclampsia.
- Immobilization >4 days (to include paraplegia).
- Obesity BMI >30 at booking.
- Medical disorders (nephritic syndrome, myeloproliferative conditions, sickle cell disease).

Clinical features

- Leg pain and swelling (usually unilateral).
- Lower abdominal pain.
- Low-grade pyrexia.
- Dyspnoea.
- Chest pain.
- Haemoptysis.
- Maternal collapse (massive PTE).

Any postnatal woman with signs and symptoms suggestive of VTE should commence treatment with low molecular weight heparin (LMWH) without delay until the diagnosis is excluded by objective testing [8]. The only exception to this would be if there was a reason why treatment is strongly contra-indicated, such as active bleeding or a high risk if further bleeding were to occur. In this situation, intravenous unfractionated heparin (this has a shorter half-life and can be reversed with protamine sulphate) should still be considered with the risks of treatment weighed against non-treatment. Before anticoagulant therapy is commenced, blood should be taken for a full blood count, coagulation screen, urea and electrolytes and liver function tests.

A thrombophilia screen is not routinely recommended, as the immediate management of acute VTE is not influenced by the results. As pregnancy can give false positive results, if undertaken thrombophilia screens should be interpreted by a haematologist. In long-term management a thrombophilia screen will be required, but this can be arranged after the acute event.

Investigations should be arranged with minimum delay and local protocols should reflect this and be followed. Multidisciplinary input from obstetricians, physicians, haematologists and radiologists is recommended to optimize the management of suspected and particularly confirmed thrombosis [9].

Investigations

Compression duplex ultrasound is the primary diagnostic test for DVT. If ultrasound is negative and there is a low level of clinical suspicion, anticoagulant treatment can be discontinued and no further investigation is required.

If ultrasound is negative but a high level of clinical suspicion exists, the woman should continue anticoagulation until the ultrasound is repeated in one week or an alternative diagnostic test employed. If the repeat testing is negative, then anticoagulant treatment can be discontinued.

If there is any suspicion of iliac vein thrombosis (suggested by symptoms of back pain and swelling of the entire limb), then contrast or magnetic resonance venography should be used to confirm the diagnosis.

A simple initial investigation in an ambulatory woman with suspected PTE is to perform oxygen saturation measurements by a pulse oximeter at rest and after exertion (such as walking up a flight of stairs). Resting hypoxia or a fall of more than 3% after exertion requires formal arterial blood gases.

D-dimers are of limited value in the puerperium as they may be elevated as part of a healthy pregnancy. They can be performed for their negative predictive value (94%), as in a woman with a normal result the risk that a thrombotic event has occurred is low, and further investigation may be avoided unless the clinical suspicion is extremely high [9].

Where there is clinical suspicion of acute PTE, a chest X-ray should be performed. Compression duplex Doppler should be performed if this is normal. If both tests are negative but there is persistent clinical suspicion of acute PTE, a ventilation–perfusion (V/Q) lung scan or a computed tomography pulmonary angiogram (CTPA) should be performed. Repeat testing should be carried out where V/Q scan or CTPA and duplex Doppler are normal but the clinical suspicion of PTE is high. Anticoagulant treatment should be continued until PTE is definitely excluded.

A chest X-ray can identify other pulmonary disease such as pneumonia, pneumothorax or lobar collapse. However, the chest X-ray is normal in over 50% of women with subsequently proven PTE. Abnormal features caused by PTE include atelectasis, pleural effusion, focal opacities, or pulmonary oedema.

The choice of technique for definitive diagnosis (V/Q scan or CTPA) will depend on local availability and should be only made after a discussion with the radiologist.

The British Thoracic Society [10] recommends CTPA as first-line investigation for non-massive PTE in non-pregnant women; despite the absence of firm evidence about the pregnant woman, these guidelines are generally followed in the pregnancy and the puerperium. CTPA has potential advantages over V/Q scanning, including greater sensitivity and specificity for most PTE (although it may not identify small peripheral thrombosis). It has the additional advantage of identifying other pathologies, such as aortic dissection. The main disadvantage of CTPA is the exposure of a high radiation dose to the maternal breasts, which may be associated with a subsequent increased lifetime risk of developing breast cancer.

V/Q scan has a high negative predictive value and is associated with a substantially lower radiation dose to breast tissue.

Management of confirmed VTE

In the puerperium, women can be offered a choice of LMWH or oral anticoagulation with warfarin. Neither heparin (unfractionated or LMWH) nor warfarin is contra-indicated in breastfeeding, and women can be reassured accordingly. Treatment should be continued for up to 6 months. It is essential that treatment is monitored and outpatient follow-up arrangement should be made. Although routine monitoring of peak anti-Xa activity for women on LMWH is not essential except in women at extremes of body weight (less than 50 kg and more than 89 kg), or with other complications increasing recurrence risk (such as renal impairment or recurrent VTE), many local protocols recommend this to ensure the appropriate minimum dose is administered. Women taking warfarin need regular monitoring of INR and dose adjustment as necessary. A platelet count should be checked after 7–10 days of treatment to exclude heparin-induced thrombocytopaenia.

Management of acute massive PTE should involve a multidisciplinary resuscitation team including a senior physician, obstetrician and radiologist. If massive PTE is confirmed, immediate thrombolysis should be considered. In extreme circumstances where the maternal condition is very unstable (confirmed or incipient cardiac arrest), this can also be administered prior to confirmation of the diagnosis. Intravenous unfractionated heparin remains the preferred treatment in massive PTE due to the extensive experience of its use and its rapid effect.

Women should be counselled regarding the need for prophylactic LMWH in the puerperium of any future pregnancy and the need for thrombophilia screening once the treatment is finished to decide if antenatal treatment should also be recommended.

Postpartum hypertension

For physiological reasons the blood pressure rises in the first 48 h postpartum. This worsens the hypertension seen in women who have been hypertensive in pregnancy and labour, and may result in a previously normotensive woman having hypertension.

This blood pressure will resolve spontaneously and it is important to try to get the right balance between overtreating by starting an antihypertensive too early and prolonging a woman's stay in hospital due to observation of mild hypertension.

When hypertension is diagnosed, the woman should be reviewed. Her history should be reviewed for evidence of essential hypertension (including a borderline elevated first trimester blood pressure recording) and for evidence of pregnancy-related hypertension (including transient hypertension in labour). Symptoms of headache and abdominal pain are extremely rare, but should be sought to exclude more serious pathology.

If a woman has a blood pressure that is persistently above 160/100 mmHg, an antihypertensive should be commenced [5]. Methyldopa should not be prescribed due to its mood depressant effects, with Labetalol or Nifedipine being first-line choices. These drugs have the advantage that they are effective rapidly, so that discharge from hospital will be possible as soon as an effective dose has been reached.

Women should be advised to attend their primary care physician for a blood pressure review at 2 weeks postnatal, as a significant number of women will be able to stop treatment.

Perineal breakdown

A sutured episiotomy or tear may break down in the early puerperium. Early breakdown (within 48 h) indicates poor suturing technique or the development of a haematoma, but with the progress of time since delivery the chances of an infective aetiology increases. There are no studies to indicate the best management of perineal breakdown, and so a commonsense approach is required.

Table 26.1 Causes of postnatal headache [11].

Cause	History
Migraine	Antenatal history. May appear like CVA or infective cause
Subarachnoid haemorrhage	Sudden onset severe headache, possible hypertension, altered consciousness, confusion or coma
Cerebral thrombosis or haemorrhage (CVA)	Convulsions, specific neurological deficit (motor, sensory), altered consciousness
Cerebral venous sinus thrombosis	Severe headache, confusion, altered consciousness, coma, neurological deficit
Meningitis and other infective causes	Posture-related headache, neck stiffness, vomiting, photophobia, confusion, altered consciousness, convulsions, raised temperature, history of travel to malarial area
Raised intracranial pressure	Headache. May be associated with early morning headache and vomiting if cerebral oedema. Altered conscious level if severe
Imminent eclampsia	Pre-eclampsia, hypertension, visual disturbance
Encephalopathy	Underlying severe disease (liver or renal failure) or other metabolic problem with severe metabolic acidosis
Diabetic hypoglycaemia	Diabetic on insulin, confusion, coma
Puerperal psychosis or hysterical conversion	Altered and often paranoid behaviour, risk factors for mental illness, changing or non-specific symptoms
Dural puncture headache	Severe, postural, gradual onset, history of regional spinal anaesthetic, occipital/frontal headache, neck stiffness

A swab should be taken from the wound even if there is no clinical suggestion of infection. A purulent or foul-smelling discharge, sloughing tissues or spreading erythema all suggest infection, and antibiotics (a cephalosporin and metronidazole) should be commenced. In the absence of clinical evidence of infection, it is reasonable to wait for the result of the swab or to start 'empirical' antibiotics if the breakdown occurs more than 48 h after the original suturing. Flucloxacillin may also be required if the swab results show *Staphylococcus*.

The decision to resuture should be taken by a senior obstetrician, as it is unlikely to be of benefit unless the wound is completely free from infection. Healing by secondary intention results in slower healing, but the long-term results are the same as healing by primary intention.

Dural puncture headache

Postnatal headache may occur due to several conditions and all should be considered as part of the differential diagnosis (see Table 26.1) to avoid missing the diagnosis of a life-threatening pathology [11].

However, postdural puncture headache is the commonest cause, with an incidence of 0.2–4% in women having epidural/spinals [12].

The headache develops after inadvertent dural puncture during epidural analgesia in 80% of cases. It may also occur after spinal anaesthesia, but the incidence is less than 1% due to the use of smaller-gauge needles. Although multifactorial, the headache is primarily due to a spinal fluid leak from the dural puncture causing a reduction in intracranial pressure. Most instances of dural puncture should be recognized at the time, and thus the possibility of a postnatal headache can be explained to the woman.

Clinical features

The headaches usually occur within 1–3 days of dural puncture and last for 1–2 weeks, but may extend to a longer period. The headache is usually frontal or occipital in distribution and is characterized by its postural nature. It is intermittent in onset, severe in intensity and exacerbated by sudden movements, including sitting up from supine position, coughing, and any straining. Occasionally it may be associated with photophobia, neck stiffness, nausea and diplopia.

In these women it is necessary to exclude other differential diagnosis including meningitis, encephalitis, subarachnoid haemorrhage and migraine. Any atypical headache requires review by a neurologist with a view to CT/MRI scanning and lumbar puncture.

Management

Postdural headache will resolve spontaneously without treatment within 2 weeks in 80% of cases. Conservative management can be considered, but the length of the recovery period means that specific treatments are required in most cases. A rare complication of conservative management is the development of a sagittal vein thrombosis or a caudal vein tear. Symptoms of blurred vision or tinnitus (cranial nerve palsy) require urgent anaesthetic and neurological review.

The woman should be well hydrated. Constipation can exacerbate the symptoms and should be avoided with stool softeners and laxatives prescribed empirically.

Regular analgesia should be offered and prescribed on a regular basis. Paracetamol 1 g 6-hourly may be sufficient, but Diclofenac can be added depending upon the severity.

Caffeine benzoate and Sumtriptan are no longer recommended, as they are associated with a high incidence of side effects and the evidence that they are beneficial is limited.

A blood patch where 20–25 ml of autologous blood is injected into the epidural spaces (usually being administered 24 h after the initial puncture and with 1–2 h lying flat after the procedure) will result in instantaneous resolution of symptoms in 80% of postdural puncture headaches. A second blood patch will be successful in 80% of the cases that failed the first time. Women with a persistent headache after two blood patches are unusual, and the aetiology of the headache should be reviewed with further investigation arranged if there are any atypical features.

Backache, symphysis pubis pain and neuropraxia

Minor complications are very common after regional block anesthesia, but they are also very common after delivery without epidural or spinal. One UK study that reviewed the incidence of backache found that this occurred in 32–37% of women without epidural and 22–45% with epidural analgesia [13]. Thus women complaining of backache can be reassured

that it is unlikely to be related to regional anaesthesia but more likely to be pregnancy-related.

The pain from symphysis pubis diastasis sometimes persists into the puerperium, but will eventually resolve (usually completely). Reassurance, simple analgesia and physiotherapy should be offered until the symptoms abate.

Nerve injury can occur following a complicated delivery or as a rare complication of regional anaesthesia. However, a significant number occur in apparently straightforward spontaneous deliveries, with an incidence of 1 in 2600 reported for traumatic nerve injury in women without regional anaesthesia.

An anaesthetist should review all women with symptoms suggestive of a neuropraxia if a regional block was used, and involvement of a neurologist at an early stage is advisable. Recovery can be expected in all cases, so initial treatment is supportive with reassurance, physiotherapy and analgesia if necessary.

Urinary tract infection

Urinary tract infection is defined as bacterial count of more than 10^5 on two successive 'clean catch' urine samples or a single catheter sample. Common causative organisms for postnatal urinary tract infections include *E.coli*, *Proteus* and *Klebsiella* species. The reported incidence is between 2 and 4%. A history of past urinary tract infection, renal tract abnormality and bladder catheterization during delivery are the main risk factors.

Symptoms include dysuria, supra-pubic and loin pain, increased frequency of micturition and pyrexia (high or low grade). Urinary tract infections are a cause of puerperal sepsis.

Management

A urine sample must be sent for microscopy and culture. An increased oral fluid intake should be encouraged and intravenous fluids given to women who have a high-grade pyrexia, or to women who have a poor oral fluid intake. Antibiotic therapy should be guided by the results of microbiological investigation, but therapy should be commenced if there is a high clinical suspicion before the results of cultures are available. In postnatal women, a cephalosporin will cover most of the common causes of infection. For a suspected or confirmed infection in a woman who is systemically well, oral antibiotics should be prescribed; however, if pyelonephritis is suspected or the woman is systemically unwell, intravenous anti-biotics and fluid therapy should be commenced. In women with a confirmed recurrent urinary infection in the absence of risk factors (usually catheterization), an interval renal ultrasound should be arranged to exclude any underlying pathology such as renal calculi.

Urinary retention

Untreated voiding disorders can lead to subsequent long-term impairment of detrusor function. Risk factors include perineal pain, impaired sensation of bladder distention following epidural, prolonged second stage and instrumental delivery. Typical symptoms include difficulty in voiding and a feeling of incomplete emptying of the bladder. If there is urinary retention, lower abdominal pain due to bladder distention may occur. Examination should be performed after the woman has attempted to void. A palpable bladder confirms the diagnosis, but smaller residual volumes will require ultrasound to diagnose. If in doubt a catheter can be passed to assess the residual volume.

Management

Symptomatic enquiry regarding bladder function should be made of all postnatal women and any symptoms require further review. Adequate analgesia should be prescribed for perineal trauma and symptoms of bladder dysfunction, and a gentle vaginal examination conducted to exclude a vaginal haematoma in those with significant vaginal pain.

If the woman is not voiding adequately within 12 h of delivery, a urinary catheter should be passed. If a residual volume of 100 ml or more is found, an indwelling catheter should be left in place for 24 h. A catheter sample should be sent for microscopy and culture to exclude a urinary tract infection as a precipitating cause. The catheter can be removed after 24 h and the residual volume checked by ultrasound after the woman has voided. A further residual of more than 100 ml requires recatheterization for a longer period of time prior to a further trial of catheter removal. In cases of persisting problem, the advice of a uro-gynaecologist should be obtained [14].

Urinary incontinence

Urinary incontinence in the immediate puerperium is uncommon, with most problems presenting as an inability to void. Most women will find an improvement in symptoms that may have occurred in the late third trimester. A woman who complains of incontinence in the first week after delivery should have a mid-stream urine analysis to exclude infection. If the symptoms are severe, the possibility of an early vesico-vaginal or ureteric-vaginal (post-caesarean section) fistula should be considered; however, these are extremely rare in obstetric practice in the developed world. All women should be instructed in pelvic floor exercises and advised to perform these regularly, as they are known to reduce the risk of long-term incontinence problems.

Caesarean section wound infection, dehiscence and breakdown

There is debate about the definition of a wound infection following caesarean section. A true definition would include inflammation or discharge of pus from a wound with a positive bacteriological culture; however, in practice many diagnoses are based on clinical features alone as the swab culture is negative (often because antibiotics are commenced or given prophylactically prior to swabs being taken).

Organisms commonly implicated in obstetric wound infections include *Staphylococcus epidermidis* and *S. aureus*, *Enterococcus faecalis*, *Escherichia coli* and *Proteus*. Although resistant organisms are less common in obstetric practice than in other clinical areas, the possibility of an organism such as MRSA must not be overlooked, and should be suspected in a woman who had a prolonged stay in hospital before or after delivery.

Wound infections occur in 5–15% of caesarean section incisions. Obstetricians may be surprised by this incidence, but most wound infections are treated in the community after discharge from hospital.

Wound infections are more common if a haematoma occurs (risk factors include pre-eclampsia with low platelets, abnormal coagulation at time of LSCS, or maternal obesity), or in caesarean section with a higher infection risk (risk factors include intrapartum caesarean, prolonged rupture of membranes, and multiple vaginal examination in labour).

Wound infection following caesarean section usually manifests within 2 weeks, most commonly presenting on day 4–5. Symptoms include pyrexia, localized pain, erythema, induration and discharge from the wound. A prior diagnosis of a wound haematoma may have been made.

Necrotizing fasciitis is rare. It is usually a poly-microbial infection that results in progressive destruction of superficial fascia and subcutaneous tissues. It is reported as a rare complication (1–2%) post-caesarean section (and even more rarely in episiotomy repair). Initial signs on inspection of the wound may not suggest anything other than a simple wound infection, but the diagnosis should be considered if the level of pain reported appears excessive or in a woman who is systemically unwell. Bullous skin lesions may be seen and tissue crepitus occurs in 50% of cases. If the diagnosis is suspected, imaging by CT or MRI can help confirm the diagnosis and delineate the extent of the fasciitis.

Management

If a wound infection is suspected, a wound swab should be taken and sent for microbiological investigation. Adequate analgesia should be prescribed (non-steroidal anti-inflammatory drugs such as voltarol if not contra-indicated) whilst providing appropriate wound care. Many hospitals now have a tissue viability team, and it is important to involve them at an early stage to obtain the most up-to-date advice regarding wound dressing. The possibility that the wound will break down should be anticipated. Appropriate counselling should be offered to the woman. Antibiotic therapy should be guided by the results of microbiological investigation, but prior to the results of these being available a regimen that includes cover for anaerobic pathogens should be commenced (usually a cephalosporin and metronidazole).

The signs of wound breakdown may vary from a superficial dehiscence to a burst abdomen. A burst abdomen requires urgent closure under general anaesthetic. A non-absorbable suture such as nylon or a slow-absorbable suture such as polydiaxanone (PDS) should be used to close the rectus sheath. For a burst midline incision, a mass closure technique should be used with deep retention sutures. Infection may be a causative factor, but this is less likely with dehiscence occurring on day 1–2 postoperative. The skin should be closed with loose interrupted sutures, and in the presence of gross wound sepsis it should be left open and packed.

For superficial wound breakdown, resuturing is not indicated due to the high likelihood of the presence of infection. The wound will require packing to allow effective healing by secondary intention.

If a diagnosis of necrotizing fasciitis is made, surgical debridement should be undertaken as soon as possible, with excision of all necrotic tissue. Careful attention to haemostasis is essential, and the wound should be left open following debridement. Broad-spectrum antibiotics are required with treatment effective for *Pseudomonas* or MRSA, such as impenem or vancomycin, respectively. Although mortality from necrotizing fasciitis in a general hospital population is high, prompt diagnosis and management in a postnatal woman appears to be associated with a better prognosis.

Breast problems

Breast problems are common and may contribute to the decision to discontinue breastfeeding. Nipple soreness, engorgement, mastitis and poor milk production can be prevented by demand breastfeeding with proper infant positioning from the first feed [2].

Women who bottle-feed may complain of breast pain, engorgement and leakage of milk. These symptoms are self-limiting and subside as prolactin levels fall. For most women reassurance is all that is required, but fluid restriction, breast binding or as a last resort medication such as Cabergoline can be considered.

Fatigue and anaemia

Tiredness is a very common complaint after delivery that may persist for long periods, with as many as 50% of women reporting still feeling tired at 1 year [2]. There is an association of tiredness with postpartum haemorrhage most likely due to anaemia. A policy of screening all women for anaemia 48 h after delivery or those at high risk is recommended. Oral iron should be commenced in women with haemoglobin below 10.5 g/dl and the reasons for compliance and avoidance of excessive tiredness should be explained. Tiredness is multifactorial, and factors such as the birth of twins, older maternal age, poor partner support and a poorly sleeping baby may increase the incidence of symptoms.

Psychiatric disorders

Having a baby is a significant risk to the mental health of all women [15]. Women with a past history of psychiatric conditions are at greatest risk. A 50% relapse rate is seen in subsequent pregnancies in women who developed an affective disorder in a previous pregnancy. The incidence of any clinical postnatal depression is reported as 15–20%, with 3–5% of women experiencing moderate to severe depression. In women who experience mental illness for the first time in the puerperium, the diagnosis is usually an affective disorder ranging in severity from mild depression to full puerperal psychosis. Fortunately treatments for postpartum affective disorders are very effective, so that if promptly diagnosed they are of short duration and have a good prognosis.

In the UK, a recent guideline is the basis for management of antenatal and postnatal mental health issues [16].

Non-serious emotional disturbance

The majority of women experience some alteration in their emotional state between the third and tenth day postpartum. These are known as postpartum blues, or baby blues. Observational studies have estimated the prevalence of postnatal blues to range from 15 to 85%. The condition is related to postpartum oestriol levels. Age, education and parity do not alter the incidence of postnatal blues, but poor social support, a history of depression, or stressful life events may aggravate the condition. Commonly reported symptoms include fatigue, tearfulness, anxiety, depression, confusion, headache, insomnia and irritability. Symptoms of postnatal blues usually peak around 3–5 days after childbirth. They usually last for 48 h, responding to reassurance and do not deteriorate over the following days, in contrast to postnatal depression. Due to the transient and self-limiting nature of symptoms, medical intervention is not indicated. All antenatal and newly delivered women should be warned to expect symptoms and reassured that they will resolve quickly without treatment. This is to reduce the anxiety for women and their families when symptoms occur.

Caution is required in the use of the term 'postnatal depression,' as it is frequently misused by women and carers and is associated with significant negative connotations. In particular, it is commonly used as a label for any mental illness occurring postnatally. It is important to recognize that some changes in mental state and function are a normal part of the postnatal experience; such features may include sleep disturbance, tiredness, loss of libido and anxious thoughts about the infant. However, mild depression in the

puerperium is common and often goes undiagnosed. It usually has an insidious onset and commonly presents between 3 months to 1 year after childbirth. Psychological treatments are very effective and medication should only be recommended as a second line of management where reassurance and counselling fail.

Serious mental disorders

The 1997–1999 Confidential Enquiry into Maternal Deaths in the UK [17] reported that psychiatric disorders is one of the leading cause of maternal death, with over half of these deaths being due to suicide. Similar findings have been documented in subsequent CEMACH reports [5,7]. The majority (about 60%) of suicides in pregnant and postnatal women occur in the 6 weeks before delivery and the 12 weeks after delivery.

In the postnatal period, women are vulnerable to the same range of mental disorders as other adults. However, the nature and treatment of mental disorders developing in relation to pregnancy differ in a number of important respects [16].

- Postnatal-onset psychotic disorders may have a rapid onset with more severe symptoms than psychoses occurring at other times, and require prompt diagnosis and treatment.
- The effects of disorders at this time have an impact not only on the woman but also on her newborn, existing children and other family members (especially her partner, who has a significant risk of depression themselves). All these individuals must be considered in management.
- The risk/benefit analysis regarding the use of psychotropic drugs in relation to breastfeeding must be considered generally with a higher threshold for pharmacological treatment and a greater use of psychosocial interventions.
- Postpartum affective disorders are particularly sensitive to treatment, having a shorter duration and better long-term prognosis.

General management of all psychiatric puerperal illness

Risk factors for puerperal psychiatric illness should be evaluated in all women in the antenatal period, and referral of women to the perinatal psychiatric

Table 26.2 Drugs used in for puerperal psychiatric disorders.

Drug (group)	Uses	Comments
Antipsychotics	Puerperal psychosis	Risk/benefit analysis in individual cases needed
	Bipolar disorder (manic phase)	Infants should be monitored for adverse effects, feeding patterns and growth and development
	Schizo-affective disorders	
Lithium	Recurrent depression	High levels in breast milk
	Mania and hypomania	Do not routinely prescribe in breastfeeding
	Bipolar affective disorder	
Antidepressants	New episode of mild depression with history of severe depression	Most tricyclic antidepressants have a higher fatal toxicity index than selective serotonin reuptake inhibitors (SSRIs)
	Moderate depressive episode and a history of depression	Fluoxetine is the SSRI with the lowest known risk Imipramine, Nortriptyline and Sertraline are present in breast milk at relatively low levels
	Severe depressive episode	Citalopram and Fluoxetine are present in breast milk at relatively high levels
Benzodiazepines	Anxiety disorder	Excreted in breast milk
	Sleep disorders	Diazepam infant serum levels vary from 0 to 14%
		Neonatal adverse effects vary from none to sedation, lethargy and weight loss
Carbamazepine	Prophylaxis in bipolar illness	Excreted in breast milk
	Acute mania	Infant serum levels range from 6 to 65% of maternal levels.

team should be made if significant risk factors are identified.

Once a possible disorder is diagnosed, appropriate assessments should be made with an urgent referral to a specialist in perinatal mental health. This should be discussed with the woman and her family.

Psychological treatments

These therapies are recommended as a first line where possible [18].

- Self-help strategies (guided self-help, computerized cognitive behavioural therapy, or exercise).
- Non-directive counselling delivered at home (listening visits).
- Cognitive behavioural therapy or interpersonal psychotherapy.

Pharmacological treatments (see Table 26.2)

Medication for certain conditions is unavoidable, but the prescribing clinician should always remember

that the mother should remain able to care for her infant, and if breastfeeding should be encouraged to continue [19].

- Drugs with lower risk profiles for the mother and infant should be preferred.
- The lowest effective dose should be commenced and slowly increased, to limit dose-related side effects.
- Monotherapy should be used in preference to combination treatment.
- Therapy should be discussed with a neonatologist if a woman is breastfeeding a preterm, low birth-weight or sick infant.

Puerperal psychosis

This is the most severe form of illness, up to one-third of these patients are manic, and two-thirds suffer from depressive psychosis.

The onset is abrupt but rarely before the third postpartum day, with most women presenting around day five. Initial symptoms include restlessness, agitation, perplexity, confusion, fear, suspicion, insomnia, not eating and drinking, delusions about themselves and their babies, and there may be rapid deterioration. After 3–5 days, the disease manifests more clearly as a manic or depressive psychosis.

Management

Urgent referral to a psychiatrist is required, and if possible admission to a psychiatric mother and baby unit. Initial sedation with a neuroleptic agent is usually advised (usually chlorpromazine 50 mg 3 times a day increasing to 150 mg chlorpromazine 3–4 times daily). Other drugs used are haloperidol 5 mg twice daily or trifluoperazine 5 mg twice daily. Side effects include extrapyramidal symptoms. Electroconvulsive therapy is the initial treatment of choice in severe depressive forms, followed by antidepressants. Puerperal psychosis usually responds very quickly to treatment, with recovery within 2 weeks for mania and 4–6 weeks for depressive illness.

Relapses are common following initial treatment, and hence medication should continue for 6 months following recovery. The risk of recurrence is up to 50% following any subsequent delivery, with the highest risk of recurrence if the next pregnancy is within 2 years. For this reason, women should be advised to delay the next pregnancy for 2 years.

Severe postnatal depression

Severe depression requiring medication occurs in 3–5% of pregnant women.

In contrast to puerperal psychosis, depression has a slower onset, with severe forms (accounting for one-third of cases) usually presenting in the first 3 weeks. The other two-thirds of cases present later, 10–12 weeks postnatally.

The risk factors are largely psychosocial, with poor social support, a lack of confiding relationships and recent adverse life events increasing the risk. Untreated postnatal depression has been implicated in disturbed bonding, with adverse effects on the cognitive and emotional development of the infant.

Presenting symptoms include early morning awakening, lack of concentration, impaired appetite, indecisiveness, loss of interest in life, and feelings of guilt and incompetence. Thoughts of self-harm are common and should always be asked about and followed-up to ascertain the strength of these feelings.

Infanticidal thoughts are rare, but women sometimes exhibit obsessional type of fears that they may cause harm to their babies.

Management

Extra support and non-directive counselling should be instituted via available support networks (in the UK, health visitors are trained to do this). If moderate/severe depression is diagnosed, formal cognitive behavioural therapy or psychotherapy should be recommended. Antidepressant medication may also be considered, with prescription usually by a primary care physician. About half of women require referral to psychiatric services, but inpatient care is needed in only a very small number of women (although the need for this should always be considered). There is no evidence that any form of hormonal supplement is beneficial for any puerperal psychiatric problem.

References

1. Fraser D, Cullen L. Postnatal management and breastfeeding. *Curr Obstet & Gynaecol* 2006; **16**(20): 65–71.

2. Glazener C, McArthur C. Postnatal morbidity. *Obstet Gynaecol* 2001; **3**(4): 179–83.

3. RCOG. *Thromboprophylaxis during Pregnancy, Labour and after Vaginal Delivery. Green-top Guideline No. 37.* London: Royal College of Obstetricians and Gynaecologists, 2004.

4. MCE. *Routine Postnatal Care of Women and their Babies.* NICE clinical guideline 37, September 2007. National Collaborating Centre for Women's and Children's Health. Available at: www.nice.org.uk

5. Confidential Enquiry into Maternal and Child Health. *Why Women Die 2000–2002.* London: RCOG, 2004.

6. Kakarla A, Posnett H, Jain A, George M, Ash A. Acute colonic pseudo-obstruction after caesarean section. *Obstet Gynaecolo* 2006; **8**(4): 207–12.

7. *Confidential Enquiry into Maternal and Child Health. Saving Mothers' Lives 2003–2005.* London: RCOG, 2007.

8. RCOG. *Thromboembolic Disease in Pregnancy and the Puerperium: Acute Management. Green-top Guideline No. 28.* London: Royal College of Obstetricians and Gynaecologists, 2007.

9. Ashgar F, Bowman P. A clinical approach to the management of venous thromboembolism in obstetrics. *Obstet Gynaecol* 2007; **9**(1): 3–8.

10. British Thoracic Society Standards of Care Committee Pulmonary Embolism Guideline Development Group. British Thoracic Society guidelines for the

management of suspected acute pulmonary embolism. *Thorax* 2003; **58**(6): 470–83.

11. Grady K, Howell C. *Managing Obstetric Emergencies and Trauma: The MOET Course Manual*, 2nd ed. London: RCOG Press, 2007.

12. Yentis S, May A, Malhotra S. *Analgesia, Anaesthesia and Pregnancy: A Practical Guide*, 2nd ed. Cambridge: Cambridge University Press, 2007.

13. Russell R, Groves P, Taub N, O'Dowd J, Reynolds F. Assessing long term backache after childbirth. *Br Med J* 1993; **306**(6888): 1299–303.

14. Kearney R, Cutner A. Postpartum voiding dysfunction. *Obstet Gynaecol* 2008; **10**(2): 71–4.

15. Cantwell R, Cox J. Psychiatric disorders in pregnancy and the puerperium. *Curr Obstet Gynaecol* 2006; **16**(1): 14–20.

16. NICE. *National Collaborating Centre for Mental Health. Antenatal and Postnatal Mental Health.* February 2007. National Institute for Health and Clinical Excellence. Available at: www.nice.org.uk

17. RCOG. *Confidential Enquiry into Maternal Deaths. Why Women Die 1997–1999.* London: RCOG, 2001.

18. National collaborating centre for mental health. Depression – depression management in primary and secondary care: National clinical practice guideline No. 23. 2006. British Psychological Society & Gaskell www.nice.org.uk

19. Taylor D, Paton C, Kerwin R. *The Maudsley Prescribing Guidelines*, 9th ed. London: Informa Healthcare, 2007.

Chapter 27

Triage and prioritization in a busy labour ward

Tracey Johnston and Nina Johns

Introduction and definition

The term 'triage' originates from the French language, meaning 'to sort' or 'sift'. Within medical practice, the term has come to describe a system used to rapidly assess the clinical needs of large numbers of casualties and assign management priorities. Although initially introduced within military settings to deal with huge casualties in wartime, triage has become a daily management tool in certain healthcare settings. It is a procedure for assessment, and planning and delivery of emergency care when workload exceeds capacity. It is particularly useful in areas of high-flow patient care with diverse clinical needs, such as Accident and Emergency and the labour ward.

The primary aim of triage is to deliver the appropriate care to each patient with the correct urgency required, in the right order, with the resources available at that time, in the most efficient way – 'do the most for the most, in the right order'. Four categories exist within the basic triage structure; these indicate the need for clinical intervention rather than the severity of injury, and are described in Table 27.1. Those requiring immediate intervention need further prioritization, using the well-recognized ABC systems assessment: Airway, Breathing, and Circulation [1].

The end point of triage is the allocation of a priority to each case and a mechanical resource to carry out care to each individual. The optimal care is received when the most appropriate priority is set and resources are used most efficiently. It is essential that all cases are assessed before treatment is carried out, as resources may be allocated to one when another still awaiting assessment is in greater need.

The principles of trauma triage

To enable a better understanding of triage in obstetric practice, it is worthwhile to introduce the concept using trauma, and reminding ourselves of the A B C D approach.

A = Airway	An airway problem will result in death if not dealt with rapidly
B = Breathing	If the airway is clear but there is a problem with breathing this must be addressed before
C = Circulation	This covers cardiac output, control of haemorrhage, and volume and red cell replacement
D = Disability	Depends on the type and extent of injuries as well as management

The key to successful triage is to be able to assess patients rapidly and accurately, and thus allocate them to intervention correctly. In the trauma situation, simple observation of mobility and conversing with the patient can tell you volumes. If someone is able to walk they must have a patent airway, be able to breathe and have enough of a circulation to keep them upright. If they are not walking but can talk coherently, again they have a patent airway and are able to breathe and have enough of a circulation to perfuse the brain. If they are confused, one has to consider whether this is secondary to a circulation problem causing cerebral hypoxia. If they are not walking or talking, are they breathing or not? If they

Best Practice in Labour and Delivery, ed. R. Warren and S. Arulkumaran. Published by Cambridge University Press.
© Cambridge University Press 2009.

Table 27.1 Trauma triage prioritization.

Priority	Category	
1	Immediate	Requires immediate resuscitation or emergency treatment or may die
2	Urgent	Treatment may be delayed for a few hours
3	Expectant	Can tolerate a significant delay
4	Dead	Condition so severe unlikely to survive

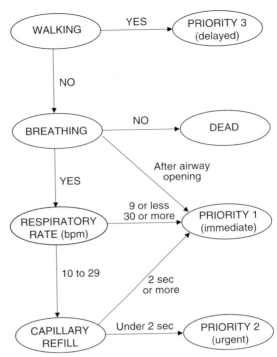

Figure 27.1 Algorithm for trauma triage [1] (reproduced with kind permission)

are breathing, their conscious level must be assessed. If they are unconscious, they have an unprotected airway which may rapidly progress to a priority 1 airway problem, and thus their airway must be secured quickly. If they are not breathing, the airway must be opened and, if breathing occurs, must be protected. If there is no breathing despite opening the airway, in the trauma situation they are probably dead. If this is your only patient, triage is not necessary because all resources can be directed to that patient. However, if there are numerous casualties and finite resources, it is difficult to justify using limited resources on someone who is very likely to die despite intervention and deprive someone else of treatment, who has a higher chance of survival. Figure 27.1 shows a useful algorithm for trauma triage [1].

Triage and prioritization in obstetrics

Whilst triage is an effective tool throughout medical practice, there are a number of specific difficulties within obstetrics that need to be considered. Prioritization on the labour ward must reflect constantly changing events. Not only do the numbers of patients within the department change, but also the clinical needs of those patients vary with time. Labour is a dynamic process which results in changes in both the maternal and fetal condition. As such, the urgency of treatment required will also change with time. Those with seemingly less urgent concerns will continue to labour and will need ongoing care. These individuals may then develop concerns requiring immediate priority over others, with unpredictable and unpreventable complications arising in normal labour. Regular reassessment of individual and departmental priorities is therefore essential.

The labour ward not only provides support for women in normal labour, it must be equipped to manage abnormal labour, life-threatening emergencies, severe maternal medical conditions, and acute surgical events. In addition to this, elective work on any labour ward, such as induction of labour and elective caesarean sections, also requires allocation of appropriate resources. The routine midwifery and obstetric care provided by the labour ward is coupled with high-dependency care, the management of surgical theatres, postoperative recovery, and assessment of unscheduled antenatal 'drop-ins' and admissions.

The majority of admissions to the labour ward are unplanned, with women attending from home, General Practice, hospital antenatal clinics, community midwifery clinics and other departments within the hospital. These admissions present with a spectrum of conditions, ranging from physiological labour to minor complaints unrelated to pregnancy, to acute emergencies. For those admissions that are planned, their progress of care will depend on the resources available and the emergency workload of the department. The workload on the labour ward is also linked to that of other departments, such as the neonatal

Table 27.2 Proposed obstetric staffing targets 2007–2010, reproduced with kind permission from Safer Childbirth [4], adapted from 'The Future Role of the Consultant' [14].

Category	Definition (births/year)	Consultant presence (year of adoption)				Specialist trainees (n)
		60-hour	98-hour		168-hour	
A	<2500	Units to continually review staffing to ensure adequate based on local needs				1
B	2500–4000	2009	–		–	2
C1	4000–5000	2008	2009		–	3
C2	5000–6000	Immediate	2008		2010	
C3	>6000	Immediate	Immediate if possible		2008	

intensive care unit and the postnatal wards. The inability of the neonatal unit to accept an admission of a preterm infant may necessitate an in-utero transfer out to another unit, taking time to organize and using valuable midwifery staff time to escort, while a lack of beds on the postnatal ward means that delivery rooms are blocked with postnatal women, and labour ward midwifery resources are used for their care.

Staffing

Co-ordination of these diverse clinical events requires appropriate numbers of medical and midwifery staff, with the relevant clinical skills and experience. There is clear evidence that one-to-one midwifery care in labour reduces intervention and improves women's satisfaction [2], but many units struggle to provide this. In the UK, almost three-quarters of Heads of Midwifery feel that their funded establishment is inadequate to cope with workload [3]. The number of midwives required to provide one-to-one care in labour depends on the case mix, with more midwives being required to provide care for women with complex pregnancies and those requiring emergency intervention. Appropriate midwifery staffing levels and the means to calculate the numbers required have been summarized recently in the joint document 'Safer Childbirth' [4]. One clear message is that women not in labour or requiring high-dependency care should not be seen or managed on the labour ward. For many units, however, to maximize the use of staff, particularly out of hours, this is exactly where they are seen. To improve use of labour ward resources, both in terms of staffing and physical space, these 'Category X' women should either be seen at home, or in a separately staffed area. This has led to

the development of maternity triage departments that see unplanned drop-ins or referrals.

As with midwifery staffing, the number of medical staff that should be allocated to the labour ward depends on the size of the unit and the complexity of the case mix. Again, Safer Childbirth [4] has addressed this in detail, looking at obstetric, anaesthetic and paediatric requirements with regard to UK practice. Table 27.2 summarizes the recommendations of this document with regard to obstetric staffing, but recognizes the financial implications of providing this.

Consultant input is essential for leadership, experience and teaching. Workload varies little over the 24 h period in the labour ward [5], and there is evidence that morbidity and mortality are increased overnight, when consultants are not routinely present [6,7]. Although it has always been presumed, evidence is emerging that demonstrates that consultant input reduces intervention [8] and improves outcomes [9]. Junior medical staff should be allocated to clinical tasks appropriate for their level of training, whilst learning new clinical and management skills with proper supervision. The move to competency-based training in the UK means that junior obstetric staff need to be directly supervised and observed when performing clinical interventions to allow assessment of their competencies, and this can only be carried out if the consultant is present at the time.

As most medical staff in the UK now work in a shift pattern on the labour ward, there is loss of continuity of care and an increased tendency to defer decision-making and intervention across shift boundaries. This increases the risk of a number of problems likely to occur at the same time, having to be dealt with by the on-coming shift who are unfamiliar with the patients. Changes in shift are ideally handled with effective handovers and regular ward rounds. In addition to medical staff, midwifery staff allocations should also be based on the midwives' experience and the woman's needs. During each shift a single senior midwife is needed to allocate midwifery staff appropriately, and to co-ordinate and supervise their practice. The 'shift leader' will provide all staff with a central and easily accessible person for advice and help, and is the essential point of contact and communication with medical staff. When workload demand exceeds the staff available, it is essential that this is identified early. Each unit should have an 'escalation policy' which can be implemented when demand exceeds resource, to allow mobilization of staff from other areas to manage the workload safely, and to allow redistribution of cases, such as cancelling elective work and discharging appropriate women home.

Space

Despite adequate staffing levels, physical resources such as delivery rooms, high-dependency beds and operating theatres are limited to a finite number. Once workload exceeds these resources, meticulous reassessment is required to organize which women can be transferred to antenatal or postnatal wards or discharged. Regular ward rounds by senior medical staff on both the antenatal and postnatal wards are also required to identify women and babies who can be discharged, allowing rapid transfer from the labour ward. It is essential to ensure that the service provided is safe, and the escalation policy should also address what happens when there are physically no beds in the department. Some units will choose to deliver appropriate women on the antenatal ward, whereas others will have arrangements with neighbouring units who will then take women for delivery when their own unit closes.

Surgical cases must be prioritized for the most efficient use of theatre time and personnel. Many units now perform elective operative obstetrics as a planned list with dedicated staff that are separate from those covering the labour ward, using a theatre that is not the emergency labour ward theatre. This clearly has cost implications, but has the huge benefit of ensuring that the management of obstetric emergencies is not being compromised by lack of staff or theatre space because of elective work. With regard to emergency work, simultaneous high-risk interventions should be avoided if possible. For example, a controlled amniotomy should not be carried out at the same time as fetal blood sampling on the department, as both may subsequently require immediate transfer to theatre for delivery by emergency caesarean section. Despite all this, there will be, on occasion, instances where emergency intervention is delayed because of theatre being blocked by another case, or staff not being immediately available. With meticulous planning and risk assessment to ensure that staffing and physical resources such as theatres are appropriate to the annual workload, and taking measures such as minimizing annual leave when high numbers of deliveries are predicted, or allocating extra staff to particularly high-risk elective cases, these incidences should be kept to a minimum, and we need to accept that very occasionally these things will happen. As part of serious untoward incident reporting, review of such cases should ensure that nothing different could have been done to avoid the event.

Workload

Obstetrics and midwifery is a speciality of peaks and troughs. All of us that work on the labour ward are aware of this, and resources must be in place to deal with these often unpredictable variations in workload. Staffing and space, and the role of an effective, accepted escalation policy have been discussed above. It is, however, essential to recognize that workload can be managed in the longer term. The number of deliveries expected in the future can be estimated by the number of women booked to deliver each month. Capacity can be calculated, and if the workload is predicted to exceed capacity, bookings can be capped. The effect of other influences should be assessed carefully, as one of the contributors to the problems experienced at Northwick Park, as described by the Healthcare Commission [10], was the impact of extra workload generated by the closure of a neighbouring unit.

Routine elective work on the labour ward, such as elective caesarean sections (in some units) and routine induction of labour, continues to occur in parallel with the unscheduled workload. However, for the labour ward to be managed effectively, the routine work must be limited, with finite numbers of cases each day. A central booking system or diary is essential to co-ordinate this. Ideally this should be held on the labour ward, but should co-ordinate with the antenatal wards and the central theatre office. This communication allows the wards and theatres to anticipate their workload and alter their staffing levels appropriately. Regular reports from the antenatal wards, with regard to the inductions in progress and potential transfers to the labour ward, also assist the shift leader to calculate changes in the workload on their department. This information can also be used to stagger clinical activities and interventions to avoid simultaneous problems occurring as a result – for example, delaying the commencement of an oxytocin infusion or administration of prostaglandins until another problem has been resolved. Furthermore, it must also be recognized that elective work can be postponed when there is excessive emergency work. Whilst it is disappointing for a woman to have her elective caesarean section postponed or her induction delayed, all women would want us to ensure safe conditions within the department.

General principles of triage and prioritization in obstetrics

As previously stated, the primary aim of triage is to deliver the appropriate care to each patient with the correct urgency required, with the resources available at that time, in the most efficient way and order. In pregnant women, assessment of the fetus immediately follows assessment of the mother. This may result in further conflicts in obstetric triage, as the fetal condition also needs to be considered. Whilst the fetus is best served by the resuscitation of its own mother, other mothers should take priority over unborn babies [11]. For example, assessment and resuscitation of an antenatal woman with an eclamptic seizure would take immediate priority over a fetal bradycardia in the same department. Difficulties on the labour ward, however, more commonly involve the management of multiple urgent problems rather than immediately life-threatening emergencies. The obstetric triage system therefore needs to provide a framework to prioritize several urgent problems, whilst maintaining the traditional structure for life-threatening emergencies. Sen and Paterson-Brown have outlined a comprehensive obstetric triage guide which provides such a framework [12] (Table 27.3). The categorization is slightly different in that there are five categories (see Table 27.3), and in the category 1 cases, instead of the

traditional A, B, C, D approach used for trauma, the D is replaced by F for fetal. In categories 2–5, they should be identified as a maternal problem (M) or a fetal problem (F), or both. By using this system, it becomes clear which problems need to be dealt with first, remembering that within the same category, a mother takes precedence over a fetus.

Additional to the skill of prioritization is the ability to allocate the most appropriately skilled member of staff to the individual patients. To achieve the most efficient use of the resources available, initial assessment of the labour ward requires detailed handover of the workload, together with knowledge of skills and experience of the staff on duty. Once the initial priorities have been defined and staff distributed appropriately, good communication, regular reviews and comprehensive ward rounds are needed to summarize and reassess the workload and changing priorities. Regular ward rounds also provide an opportunity to identify potential future problems and encourage positive decision-making, with clear plans outlined for each individual, including timing of examinations and stepwise decisions based on their findings, documented in the case notes. Problems tend to accumulate if decisions are deferred, resulting in simultaneous emergencies. Multidisciplinary ward rounds, including obstetric and anaesthetic medical staff and the midwifery shift leader, promote good communication between members of the team and enable planning of interventions which may require regional anaesthesia or analgesia, matched against the ongoing workload of the labour ward.

Within the systems of prioritization and triage in obstetrics there must always be the ability to deal with unexpected and unpredictable emergencies. Some obstetric emergencies can be anticipated, such as a large postpartum haemorrhage following a prolonged dysfunctional labour with oxytocin augmentation. If anticipated, these emergencies may be averted or, at least, planned for. For example, additional intravenous access prior to delivery and active management of the third stage with additional uterotonic agents can prevent or minimize postpartum haemorrhage. The outcome from other obstetric emergencies can be altered with swift identification of the problem and rapid intervention. For example, the use of continuous electronic fetal monitoring in women labouring after a previous caesarean section can identify scar complications early and allow rapid intervention and emergency delivery. For those rare obstetric

Table 27.3 Obstetric triage guide [12].

Category of obstetric priorities	Pathology	Examples
1. Immediately life-threatening	Airway obstruction (1A)	Laryngeal oedema (anaphylaxis/severe PET)
		Trauma
		Eclampsia (during/post fit)
	Breathing problem (1B)	Respiratory or cardiac arrest
		Pulmonary oedema (severe PET)
		Bronchospasm (asthma/anaphylaxis/AFE)
	Circulatory collapse (1C)	Massive haemorrhage (can be concealed)
		Uterine rupture
		Severe sepsis
	Fetal problems (1F)	Shoulder dystocia
		Terminal bradycardia (abruption/cord prolapse/uterine rupture)
2. Urgent (can deteriorate rapidly)	Maternal (2M)	Severe hypertension
		Unstable or ill diabetic
		Chest pain
	Fetal (2F)	Pathological CTG
		Chorioamnionitis
3. Semi-urgent attention needed (to prevent future disaster)	Maternal (3M)	Postpartum 'trickling'
	Fetal (3F)	Prolonged second stage of labour with a normal CTG
4. Can wait until other emergencies are under control	Maternal (4M)	Rupture of membranes with no contractions and normal CTG
	Fetal (4F)	Meconium staining of liquor in the presence of a normal CTG
5. Delay/postpone until things quieten down	Elective deliveries (5)	Elective CS/induction of labour with no maternal or fetal problem

emergencies which are often unpredictable, regular rehearsal drills and detailed departmental guidelines enable all staff to be familiar with the actions needed and their individual role.

Good communication on the labour ward is paramount, between patients, relatives and staff, and between members of staff. It is not possible to anticipate and recognize problems within individual delivery rooms without being fully aware of what is going on in that room. Ward rounds by the shift leader and medical staff should review each room occupied, although not all woman need to be reviewed personally unless clinically indicated. An update from the midwife looking after the woman is enough, as long as there is good ongoing communication with the shift leader. Following ward rounds, the labour ward board, detailing all the women on the department, should be revisited and the cases summarized. Potential problems should be communicated to the anaesthetic staff, theatre staff and the neonatal unit, as they also

Table 27.4 Clinical scenario A.

1	24 years, 28/40, Nulliparous chest pain and cough O$_2$ saturation 93% on air	7	32 years, G2P1 Previous stillbirth at 38/40 36/40, decreased fetal movements
2	28 years, 41/40, Nulliparous Cx 2 cm dilated at 02:30 Cx 3 cm dilated at 06:30, ARM	8	36 years, Nulliparous insulin-dependent diabetic Prostin induction at 38/40 Last BM 4.1, 90 min ago
3	18 years, 40/40, Nulliparous, transferred from birth centre, APH 150 ml	9	31 years, G3P2 Previous LSCS, followed by SVD Cx fully dilated at 06:30
4	27 years, para 1 SVD at 06:30 Awaiting suturing of second-degree tear	10	28 years, Nulliparous 31/40 dichorionic twins, IVF Painless PV bleeding
5		11	33 years, Nulliparous Cx 7cm dilated at 04:30 Cx 9 cm dilated at 07:30
6	22 years, G2P1 Cx 4 cm dilated at 05:30 Meconium-stained liquor Variable decelerations of FHR	12	34 years, G2P1 Maternal lupus BP 160/90, 1+ proteinuria Abdominal pain, no fetal movement
HDU1	37 years, Nulliparous 34/40 BP 175/112 3+ proteinuria, headache	HDU2	
Rec 1	33 years, para 1 Emergency LSCS at 9 cm dilated Vaginal bleeding, Estimated blood loss 1100 ml	Rec 2	35 years, para 3 Manual removal of placenta Oxytocin infusion, PR misoprostol Tachycardia HR 128 bpm

Notes: 08:30 Handover
2 elective LSCS – first case: maternal congenital heart disease, needs HDU
3 prostin inductions
Staff available:
2 ST1/2 (SHO)
8 Midwives – 3 senior who suture and cannulate
1 Shift leader midwife
1 Recovery nurse
1 ST 3–7 – obstetrics (registrar)
1 ST 3–7 – anaesthetics (registrar)
Anaesthetic and Obstetric Consultants available at 10am after Risk Management meeting.

form part of the team needed to co-ordinate safe practice. If this communication and teamwork is not well established it will lead to errors and conflicts between members of staff. For example, if the correct category of urgency for an emergency caesarean section is not communicated to the anaesthetist and theatre team, they may not attend quickly and delay the time to delivery. Both national and local enquiries looking at poor obstetric outcomes frequently highlight problems with communication being prominent in the series of events leading to the outcome. Multidisciplinary ward rounds, rehearsal drills and teaching sessions will help to improve teamwork and communication and should be encouraged. Clear lines of communication are required in emergencies, with calm and precise co-ordination from a single leading individual. These lines of communication can be established and practised during drills.

Clinical scenarios

The following clinical scenarios (Table 27.4 and Table 27.5) have been designed to represent the workload of a busy labour ward. Read through the tables as if you were receiving handover for your shift. Consider how you would prioritize the cases and how you would allocate the staff you have available, which are described at the bottom of the table. Initially the workload may seem impossible to manage, but use the obstetric triage system outlined in Table 27.3 then check your ideas with those suggested below.

Clinical scenario A

Having allocated a priority to all cases, staffing needs to be reviewed to allow staff allocation. The first priority when faced with a number of complex problems requiring intervention simultaneously is to ask

Table 27.5 Clinical scenario B.

1	22 years, Nulliparous transferred from birth centre Cx 9 cm dilated since 03:30	7	29 years, G2P1 Hepatitis B Cx 3 cm dilated at 06:30
2	38 years, Nulliparous undiagnosed breech Contracting 2:10 Cx 1 cm dilated 07:30	8	36 years, G10P8 Cx 6 cm dilated at 07:30 Thick meconium, fetal bradycardia of 90 bpm for 4 min
3	32 years, G3P2 Previous LSCS followed by SVD Cx 5 cm dilated at 06:30 Meconium-stained liquor	9	
4	31 years, Nulliparous prostin induction at 40+12/40 Cx 3 cm dilated at 04:00 Variable decelerations of FHR	10	24 years, Nulliparous 40+4/40 APH 200 ml
5	28 years, G4P2+1 33/40 Abdominal pain	11	33 years, G3P0+2 Previous stillbirth at 40/40 Prostin induction at 38/40 Awaiting ARM
6	34 years, Nulliparous 40/40, spontaneous labour Cx 4 cm dilated at 00:00 Cx 4 cm dilated at 04:00, ARM Cx 5 cm dilated at 08:00	12	41 years, G2P1 Dichorionic twins 34/40 Backache, small PV bleed
HDU1	35 years, para 1 Epileptic 2 seizures following spontaneous vaginal delivery	HDU2	
Rec 1	32 years, para 1 Forceps, third-degree tear PPH 1800 ml	Rec 2	29 years, para 2 Emergency LSCS for fetal tachycardia, prolonged SROM Pyrexial, HR 112, O$_2$ satn 93%

Notes: In theatre with LSCS + hysterectomy, massive PPH 3500 ml
08:30 Handover – 2 elective LSCS, 2 prostin inductions

Staff available:
2 ST 1/2 (SHO)
8 Midwives – 4 senior who suture and cannulate
1 Shift leader midwife
1 recovery nurse
1 ST 3–7 – obstetrics (registrar)
1 ST 3–7 – anaesthetics (registrar)
Anaesthetic and Obstetric Consultants available if requested.

available staff to attend. The consultant obstetrician and consultant anaesthetist should be contacted and asked to attend immediately (patient care has to take priority, so the meeting can continue without them, or be postponed).

1. The immediate priority is the woman in room 1 (priority 1B), who is hypoxic and needs full assessment and investigation for pulmonary embolus. She should be seen by the obstetric ST 1/2 as this is primarily a medical problem rather than an obstetric problem. She needs oxygen and anticoagulation with subcutaneous low molecular weight heparin, and investigations instituted to confirm the diagnosis. Midwife 1 should stay with her once medical staff have left.

2. The women in Recovery 1 and 2 are also an immediate priority (1C) as they may be haemodynamically unstable. The anaesthetic ST 3–7 should review the woman in Recovery 2 to try and determine the cause of the tachycardia, which is most likely to be hypovolaemia secondary to blood loss. He can institute initial resuscitation while Midwife 2 assesses the degree of blood loss and uterine tone, and sends off appropriate bloods. The obstetric consultant should see the woman in Recovery 1, who is being cared for by the recovery nurse, as she is still bleeding and may need to return to theatre for further examination, with or without a laparotomy.

3. The urgent maternal priority is in high-dependency bed 1 (priority 2M). The obstetric ST 3–7 can see her, assess the degree of severity of her pre-eclampsia and proceed to treatment of her hypertension. The anaesthetic consultant should

see this woman and institute invasive monitoring. Assessment of the fetal condition should follow stabilization of the mother, and initially this can be carried out by Midwife 3.

4. The urgent fetal priorities are in rooms 12 and 6 (priority 2F). The second obstetric ST 1/2 can review room 6, who is being cared for by Midwife 4, and assess the potential fetal distress and carry out a fetal blood sample. The concern in room 12 is both fetal and maternal. This woman is at high risk of a placental abruption and intrauterine fetal demise. Initially the shift leader can attend to auscultate the fetal heart. If it is present, the fetal priority changes, but the concern remains. She will need urgent obstetric review as soon as an obstetrician is free. If the women in recovery are stable and able to both be cared for by the recovery nurse, or returning to theatre, Midwife 2 can attend to this woman, otherwise Midwife 5 can attend.

5. The semi-urgent maternal priorities are in rooms 9, 10 and 3 (priority 3M). The woman in room 9 can be assessed by Midwife 6 initially, to confirm full dilation, review the continuous fetal heart rate monitoring and assess the progress in second stage. The midwife can then discuss her findings with the shift leader and obstetric registrar, to plan her further management. Review of the woman in room 3 can initially be carried out by Midwife 7. Assessment of blood loss, blood pressure, pulse and fetal condition can be established, as well as intravenous cannulation. One of the obstetricians can then subsequently examine the woman and diagnose the cause of antepartum haemorrhage when they are free. During this time, Midwife 8 can review the woman in room 10, assess the quantity of blood loss, the maternal and fetal conditions and establish intravenous access. If all is stable, the woman can then await review by obstetric staff once they are free, or be sent for a departmental ultrasound scan for placental localization.

6. The semi-urgent fetal priorities are in rooms 7 and 11 (priority 3F). The shift leader can see room 7, auscultate the fetal heart and commence electronic fetal monitoring. Once she has seen to room 10, Midwife 8 can assess the woman in room 11 in terms of uterine activity and assess the need for a further VE. If required, she can discuss

the need for augmentation of labour with the shift leader. In many units, augmentation with an oxytocin infusion in a nulliparous labourer can be started by the shift leader, without the immediate need for medical staff review. This can, however, be delayed if other women still need to be seen.

7. The other rooms, 2, 4 and 8, can now wait until the other emergencies are under control (priority 4M and 4F). The woman in room 8 can be reviewed by the shift leader, who can carry out BM monitoring and then ensure that the woman in room 2 is alright until a midwife is free to provide one-to-one care. The first available midwife or ST 1/2 can then suture the woman in room 4.

8. The elective work (priority 5) can be delayed until the labour ward is more composed.

It is clear from this that optimal care is not being delivered, as women in labour are not receiving one-to-one care, and resources are being utilized based on a priority of need. This principle is fundamental to triage. If staff are available elsewhere they should be asked to come and help out until the crisis is over (implement the escalation policy), and all elective work should be deferred until it is safe to continue.

Clinical scenario B

1. The immediate priorities are in theatre and recovery bed 2 (priority 1C). The case in theatre is already being managed by the night shift; however, they should be contacted to confirm that the situation is controlled and that any additional help is not required. If further help is needed, the consultant obstetrician and anaesthetist should be asked to attend. This patient will need a high-dependency bed once she is out of theatre. The woman in recovery bed 2, who is being cared for by the recovery nurse, appears to be septic; she should be assessed by the daytime anaesthetic ST 3–7 and transferred to a high-dependency bed for further treatment and invasive monitoring.

2. The immediate fetal priority is room 8 (priority 1F). The obstetric ST 3–7 should review this case. A fetal bradycardia in a multiparous patient in established labour may be due to rapid progress to full dilation. If this patient is in second stage she may need an instrumental delivery. Midwife 1 is

present to deliver if she progresses rapidly, or to assist the obstetrician if required.

3. The urgent maternal priorities are recovery bed 1 and room 10 (priority 2M). The obstetric ST 1/2 should assess the woman in recovery bed 1 with Midwife 2, as she has had a significant postpartum haemorrhage. Review of her blood pressure, pulse, repeat haemoglobin level and any ongoing blood loss will ascertain whether she is stable or requires further treatment. Midwife 3 should initially assess room 10. Assessment of blood loss, blood pressure, pulse and fetal condition can be established, as well as intravenous cannulation. The obstetric ST 1/2 can then subsequently examine the woman and diagnose the cause of antepartum haemorrhage.

4. The urgent fetal priority is in room 4 (priority 2F). The pattern of the electronic fetal heart rate monitoring needs to be identified and the woman needs to be examined to determine progress in labour. Midwife 4 should perform a VE to assess the stage of labour, and ask the obstetric ST 1/2 to review if there is suspected fetal compromise, with a view to fetal blood sampling.

5. It is difficult to prioritize the woman in room 5 based on the information available. The Shift Leader should quickly see this lady and prioritize her further after a rapid assessment. The abdominal pain may be something as simple as indigestion, in which case resources do not need to be allocated, or may be a massive abruption or preterm labour.

6. The semi-urgent maternal priorities are in HDU 1 and room 1 (priority 3M). The obstetric ST 3–7 should review the woman in high-dependency when he has finished in room 8. If this postnatal woman is stable with no further seizures, she can be transferred to the ward, as high-dependency will be needed by the case currently in theatre. Midwife 5 can assess the maternal and fetal condition in room 1. The obstetric ST 3–7 can then examine the woman when he has completed his assessment in HDU 1, and determine whether oxytocin or delivery is indicated.

7. The semi-urgent fetal priority is room 12 (3F). Midwife 6 needs to assess the maternal and fetal conditions and the degree of bleeding. If appropriate, she should gain IV access and send the appropriate bloods and commence fetal

monitoring. The obstetric ST 1/2 should then assess to determine the cause of the bleeding and rule out preterm labour when one is free.

8. Room 3 (priority 4F) and room 6 (priority 4 F/M) can now wait until the other emergencies are resolved. Midwife 7 can provide care and review the fetal condition in room 3. Midwife 8 can insert an intravenous cannula in room 6 and commence an oxytocin infusion after discussion with the shift leader, although this can be delayed until other priorities have been addressed.

9. Room 11 does not require care at the moment, and could be moved to the antenatal ward until the workload has settled. Similarly, room 2 does not require one-to-one care as she is not in established labour. Although she needs to be seen to discuss her options for delivery, this can be deferred and, again, she could be transferred to the antenatal ward in the meantime. Room 7 may need care. With the information available it is again difficult to allocate a priority as she may still be in the latent phase of labour, or may be contracting well and established. The Shift Leader should assess her further so she can be triaged properly.

As discussed above in relation to Clinical scenario A, the escalation policy should be implemented to draft staff in when appropriate. All elective work should be deferred until it is safe to proceed, and if possible moved out of the labour ward area. Even if consultant input is not immediately required, both the consultant obstetrician and the consultant anaesthetist can provide extra pairs of hands as well as support and guidance, and should be called to attend immediately. It is also clear that doing this as a paper exercise is somewhat artificial, as the labour ward is dynamic and the clinical situation changes all the time. What may be prioritized as requiring immediate intervention using up skilled staff can resolve quickly (e.g. the woman in room 8 delivers before the obstetric ST 3–7 attends), and cases which seem of a low priority may suddenly require immediate attention (e.g. the woman in room 3 ruptures her uterus with massive haemorrhage and a profound bradycardia).

In both the above scenarios there are a number of ways to prioritize the workload presented, and you may not agree with the suggestions given, but a systematic approach using a logical framework enables you to anticipate a likely series of events and allocate staff appropriately. Rapid and logical decision-making is a key skill in prioritization on a busy labour ward. As with most other skills in obstetrics, it can be taught, but there is also a degree of art and style which can only be improved by experience. We are all familiar with those we like to be on call with as things always seem calm and under control even when busy, and there are others who never seem to quite know what is going on even when relatively quiet. Triage is something we all practise every day on the labour ward, although this has rarely been taught formally. With the structures and approaches in this chapter, the art of triage can be formalized to a degree, with the aim of optimizing outcomes for both our patients – the mother and the baby.

References

1. Cox C, Grady K, Howell C. *Managing Obstetric Emergencies and Trauma. The MOET Course Manual*, 2nd edn. Oxford: RCOG Press, 2007.

2. Hodnett E D, Gates S, Hofmeyr G J, Sakala C. Continuous support for women during childbirth. *Cochrane Database of Syst Rev* 2007, **3**: CD003766. DOI: 10.1002/14651858. CD003766.pub2.

3. Royal College of Midwives. *RCM Annual Survey of Heads of Midwifery Service*. London: RCM, 2005.

4. RCOG. *Safer Childbirth: Minimum Standards for the Organisation and Delivery of Care in Labour*. London: RCOG Press, 2007.

5. *NHS Modernisation Agency. Findings and Recommendations from the Hospital at Night Project*. London: NMSHA, 2005.

6. National Patient Safety Agency, 2006.

7. Luo Z C, Karlberg J. Timing of birth and infant and early neonatal mortality in Sweden 1973–95: longitudinal birth register study. *Br Med J* 2001; **323**: 1327–34.

8. Olah K S. Reversal of the decision for caesarean section second in the vaginal stage of labour on the basis of a consultant assessment. *J Obstet Gynaecol* 2005; **25**: 115–16.

9. Murphy D J, Liebling R E, Patel R, Verity L, Swingler R. Cohort study of operative delivery in the second stage of labour and standard of obstetric care. *Br J Obstet Gynaecol* 2003; **110**: 610–5.

10. Healthcare Commision. *Investigation into 10 Maternal Deaths at, or Following Delivery at, Northwick Park Hospital, North West London Hospitals NHS Trust, Between April 2002 and April 2005*. London: Healthcare Commission, 2006.

11. Macdonald C, Redondo V, Baetz L, Boyle M. Obstetrical triage. *Canadian Nurse* 1993; **89**(7): 17–20.

12. Sen R, Paterson-Brown S. Prioritisation on the delivery suite. *Curr Obstet Gynaecol* 2005; **15**(4): 228–36.

13. Reid M. A formalized approach to obstetric–gynecologic triage. *J Emerg Nurs* 1993; **19**(1): 19–27.

14. Royal College of Obstetricians and Gynaecologists. *The Future Role of the Consultant: A Working Party Report*. London: RCOG, 2005.

Chapter 28

Risk management related to intrapartum care

Melissa K. Whitworth and Helen Scholefield

Introduction

Obstetrics, in particular intrapartum obstetrics, is very much a 'spectator' speciality. We perform a variety of procedures watched by the patient's birth partner and in no other area of medicine is clinician performance as open to the direct scrutiny of the patient's friends and family on a daily basis. Globally, pregnancy and childbirth are periods of high risk to maternal health. Annually, approximately eight million women suffer pregnancy-related complications and over half a million die. In developing countries, 1 woman in 16 may die of pregnancy-related complications compared to 1 in 2800 in developed countries. Tragically, most deaths are avoidable, the main causes are known, and more than 80% of maternal deaths could be prevented or avoided through actions that are proven to be effective and affordable, even in the poorer countries of the world. Key to reducing the risks associated with pregnancy and childbirth is the provision of high-quality care, and reduction of maternal mortality has been included in the Millennium Development Goals.

Alongside maternal mortality, the major fetal risk associated with the intrapartum period is stillbirth. Developed countries have an average intrapartum stillbirth rate of 0.6 per 1000 births. On the other hand, intrapartum deaths in developing regions are estimated at 9 out of every 1000 births.

Elimination or minimization of risk should be key to the practice of intrapartum obstetrics. The concept that when a mother comes into the healthcare environment she may suffer an adverse event which results in permanent injury or even death is not new. In the developed world, the extent of this problem and the underlying causes in terms of staff and healthcare provision failure are now attracting increasing

prominence. Medicine has always employed the central tenet 'first do no harm', and in many countries, a revolution in how to organize healthcare provision to minimize risks to patients is under way, driven by a desire to deliver the best possible clinical service.

Clinical governance is a framework through which organizations are accountable for continually improving quality of service and safeguarding high standards by creating an environment in which excellence in clinical care will flourish. It places an emphasis on local formulation of plans for delivery of care, taking into account available evidence with regards to best practice, and involving both staff and the patient groups who will benefit from improvements. Within clinical governance structures seven 'pillars' or key areas have been identified: patient and public involvement; audit; human resources; information and technology; research and effectiveness; education and training; and clinical risk management. It is clinical risk management relevant to the intrapartum period that this article will consider in more detail.

Putting it all in historical context

With publication of the Harvard Medical Practice study and the Institute of Medicine Report 'To Err is Human', patient safety and clinical risk management began in the last decade to formally enter mainstream obstetric and medical practice [1,2]. The former was an American retrospective review of 31,429 hospital records which attempted to identify and quantify adverse events caused by medical error. The obstetric cohort had a 1.5% adverse events rate and the rate of negligence was 38.3% [1]. A subsequent British study estimated the adverse event rate in obstetrics to be 4.0%, with 71% of events being preventable [3]. Whilst neither study provided data specific to the intrapartum period, the number of adverse events is clearly worrying. No such data are available for the developing world. A search of the medical literature (PubMed®) from 1997 to 2006 using the keywords of obstetrics and organizational culture; medical error; quality of health care; safety management or risk management reveals 4882 citations, almost twice the number published in the preceding decade. Whilst this gives an indication that patient safety and clinical risk policy have recently become more important within the practice of obstetrics, it gives no indication of the type and success of the developments occurring to promote that change.

It is acknowledged that many intrapartum adverse events recur. Examples of these are:

(1) misinterpretation of fetal heart rate monitoring with subsequent poor fetal outcome, such as fetal death or hypoxic ischaemic encephalopathy;
(2) third- or fourth-degree perineal trauma; and
(3) morbidity following shoulder dystocia.

The extension is that had lessons been learnt from the initial event, recurrences might or would have been avoidable. The processes of risk management have been introduced into healthcare in an attempt to address this dichotomy. In recent times, the term 'adverse event' has been replaced by 'clinical incident' in risk management parlance. Clinical risk management can be defined as organizational systems or processes that aim to improve quality of healthcare, and create and maintain safe systems of care whilst minimizing or moderating financial losses following an adverse outcome. Risk management addresses the various activities of an organization by identifying the risks that exist, assessing those risks for potential, frequency and severity, and eliminating those which can be eliminated. Given that many of the clinical incidents which occur in the intrapartum period are unpredictable and unavoidable, e.g. shoulder dystocia, one would perhaps consider them an irrelevance in risk management terms. However, clinical risk management is about far more than simply the prevention of clinical incidents. Reducing potential harm from clinical incidents by ensuring that management of unavoidable clinical incidents is optimum, through appropriate training and drills, is as important as event elimination.

What impacts do clinical incidents have?

The sequelae of clinical incidents may be physical, psychological or financial, and can affect patient, family and healthcare professionals. At their most devastating, intrapartum clinical incidents may result in maternal and/or fetal death and the psychological and social impacts are myriad. For example, there are many reports linking emergency caesarean section with postpartum symptoms of post-traumatic stress disorder. The physical consequences of intrapartum clinical incidents include dyspareunia, urinary and faecal incontinence, and loss of fertility.

Obstetrics is a 'risky' speciality. In the UK, more than half of the money paid out in clinical litigation settlements by the National Health Service (NHS) each year arises from obstetric problems which result in the birth of babies with significant brain damage. Although not always due to clinical error, a number of consistent factors contributing to these cases do involve negligence. The average sum awarded is around £1.5 million. The UK Government has targeted much of its healthcare legislation and policy development into improving patient safety [4].

In the United States between 1985 and 2005, specialist obstetric and gynaecological surgeons had the highest number of total closed claims and the third highest average expenses according to speciality. Over the period 2000–2002, obstetric and gynaecological surgeons saw their malpractice premiums increase by 22% as compared with an average rise of 15%. The American Medical Association has deemed that America is in the midst of a 'medical liability crisis', and there is a feeling amongst senior US obstetricians that this crisis threatens the speciality of obstetrics and gynaecology, with decreased interest amongst medical students and early retirement of established physicians.

The impact of clinical incidents on staff should not be overlooked. Thirty-eight percent of doctors who are sued suffer from clinical depression, and there is damage to morale and reputation. Staff can become so afraid of making another mistake they are unable to continue working in healthcare services, and move to other jobs where mistakes are unlikely to kill or harm someone.

Implementing clinical risk management relevant to the intrapartum period

A systematic approach to the implementation of clinical risk management in the intrapartum period can be divided into three distinct phases:

(1) risk identification,
(2) risk analysis, and
(3) risk control.

Each of these will be considered individually, but it must be remembered that risk management is a dynamic process and these will naturally overlap.

Risk identification

Possible approaches applicable to the intrapartum period include retrospective or prospective identification of clinical incidents or near misses; proactive identification of areas of service associated with risk; proactive identification of those patients at high risk; and formal risk assessment procedures.

Clinical incidents

Before we can learn from clinical incidents occurring in the intrapartum period, we need to develop systems whereby such incidents are reported prospectively. Whilst the initial studies looking at medical error/clinical incidents were retrospective in nature, retrospective identification of clinical incidents should not be used as the mainstay of risk management. It is a laborious, time-consuming task which should be kept for targeted projects, e.g. looking at areas in which under-reporting is suspected based on extrapolation from national statistics to a local level. Research shows that even when actual harm occurs, not all incidents are reported, and when no harm occurs, i.e. the incident is a close call or near miss, reporting rates are even lower. Whilst data specific to the intrapartum period are not available, a study looking at the maternity and baby notes of 500 deliveries in two UK obstetric units demonstrated that of 196 incidents, staff reported only 23%, with risk managers picking up a further 22%. The remaining 55% were only revealed as a result of the research. A questionnaire designed to explore reasons for low reporting rates identified that although most staff knew about the incident reporting system, almost 30% did not know where to find a list of reportable incidents. The main reasons for not reporting were high workload, fears that other staff members would be blamed, and a belief that the circumstances or outcome of a particular case did not warrant a report. An unwillingness to report patient safety incidents is obviously counterproductive to organizational learning, and highlights why a fair-blame culture must be developed. It is important that all staff are aware of how incident reporting takes place. Organizations must make it clear that the purpose of this is for the organization to learn from mistakes, and make changes that will reduce the risk of similar events occurring in the future, not for punishment of individuals. Failure to achieve this will seriously compromise the success of incident reporting.

Most incident reporting systems maintain two methods of documentation: a paper incident-report system coupled with a computerized database. Paper systems, whilst cheap to develop, have problems associated with them, including potential illegibility, confidentiality/security issues, loss of forms and slow processing. The benefits of a system in which incidents are reported via a networked, computerized form which feeds directly into a database have several advantages, including real-time data production, reduction in problems associated with confidentiality and security, and reduced workload for the risk management team. Whichever system is adopted, it must be audited on a regular basis to ensure that the required information is being captured.

Clinical incidents are usually reported using trigger lists. Suggested triggers for the intrapartum period are given in Table 28.1. It is essential that so-called near misses are included. These are events which could potentially lead to a serious adverse outcome, but for some reason did not. They provide an ideal learning opportunity, since as no one has been harmed they are less emotionally charged, and hence staff are less threatened by the investigation process. Identifying factors that combined to ensure that harm did not occur allows changes to be implemented that will reduce the chance of the near miss becoming an event in the future.

Risk assessment

Unlike clinical incident reporting, risk assessment aims to identify risks before incidents occur, and put into place procedures, barriers and other measures to reduce the risk. Intrapartum risk management cannot

Table 28.1 Trigger list of intrapartum clinical incidents.

Unexpected death	Maternal		Pulmonary oedema
	Intrapartum IUD		Shoulder dystocia
	Antenatal IUD >24 weeks' gestation		Cord pH at delivery of <7.00
Unexpected collapse	Maternal		Apgar <6 at 5 min
	Neonatal		Neonatal convulsions
Unexpected transfer to ITU/HDU	Maternal		Birth trauma major/minor
			Cord prolapse
	Neonatal		Antepartum/postpartum haemorrhage >1500 ml; and/or transfused
Missed diagnosis	Intrauterine growth restriction		Full dilatation caesarean section – no trial
	Fetal anomaly		Failed instrumental delivery/ manual rotation leading to caesarean section
	Breech		
	Misinterpretation of CTG		Failed instrumental delivery/ manual rotation second instrument successful
Medication errors – wrong	Drug	Infection	Wound
	Dose		Postpartum
	Patient		Septicaemia
	Time		Venepuncture site
	Route		UTI/chest infection >3 days after admission
	Not given		
Treatment/ procedure/clinical management	Cancellation/failure/delay (e.g. epidural/induction of labour/ caesarean section)	Communication problem	Within team
	>30 min from decision to delivery in caesarean section for fetal distress		Outside of immediate team
	Wrong/inappropriate treatment		With patient
	Guideline not followed/ available		Relative
			Consent
	Prolonged second stage		Patient records
	Eclampsia		ID problem
	Third- and fourth-degree tear		Admission/discharge
	Unplanned return to theatre	Staffing problems	Midwifery
	Ruptured uterus		Obstetric
	Hysterectomy		Other
	Caesarean section for second twin	Equipment problems	Failure
			Unavailable
		Other	

Practice tip 1 – Embedding clinical incident reporting into intrapartum care

- Achieve high reporting rates by having a quick to complete, easy to use trigger form.
- Incorporate incident severity grading and instructions on how to report into the trigger form.
- Make clinical incident reporting and analysis part of daily life on the delivery suite. In our unit, the delivery suite duty consultant facilitates a daily multidisciplinary educational review of any incidents that have occurred in the last 24–48 h. This is a visible way of demonstrating the importance we attach to learning from incidents, the systems approach to clinical risk assessment, and promotes a fair-blame culture.
- Encourage all staff to feel an integral part of the process by being involved in the grading and assessment of incidents occurring within the unit.
- Provide swift constructive feedback, both positive and negative, on clinical incidents in both group and individual settings, and where incidents require detailed follow-up endeavour to provide speedy individual copies of reports.
- Embedding reporting and assessment into the daily patchwork of work on delivery suite will enhance the profile of risk management and engage staff.

Practice tip 2 – Introducing risk assessment to a unit – workshop approach

- Using a series of workshops in which delivery suite personnel risk assess the delivery suite can introduce the concept of risk management to a unit and enthuse staff about the importance of risk management as a process.
- Participants are asked to identify before attending key risks they feel exist in (a) their area of work, (b) the delivery suite as a whole.
- Risks are recorded either using flip-chart/post-it notes, or for the more technologically advanced a PowerPoint™ slide.
- Things to consider include: personnel – staffing levels, skill mix, training; estates – environment; equipment – electronic fetal monitoring systems, infusion pumps, beds; practice – policies and procedures.
- Risks are then discussed by the group and the concept of risk rating introduced (see Table 28.2).
- Workshops can provide a wealth of information for risk management teams, as frontline staff offer a hands-on perspective to the risk assessment process.
- Staff can be asked to provide potential risk management solutions to the risks identified.

occur in isolation from maternal health in general. There are identifiable antenatal risk factors, e.g. obesity, which put women at higher risk of an adverse outcome during the intrapartum period. Proactive identification of these risks and appropriate antenatal management of them will reduce the likelihood of intrapartum problems. Risk assessment is a process which we informally perform during every clinical contact. It has its basis in the core elements of risk management. Wherever possible, risk assessments should be multidisciplinary. Possible methods of risk assessment are: workshops involving the multidisciplinary team; risk management team brainstorm; and lead clinician for delivery suite brainstorm.

Analysis of risk

There is little to be gained from collecting data on clinical incidents or performing risk assessment if the risks are not then collated and analysed. Key stages of risk analysis are (1) determining the consequences of the risk occurring, (2) determining the likelihood of the risk occurring, (3) ascribing a risk rating. A number of risk scoring systems are available, each with its proponents. Consistency of application is key. Reports should be considered as they are presented and trends identified.

Stage 1 – Determine the consequences of the risk occurring

For each hypothetical risk the consequences of it occurring must be determined, e.g. shoulder dystocia is a risk with potential consequences ranging from nothing to fetal death. Other examples of consequences might be injury/harm to patient, injury/harm to staff, damage to reputation or finances of hospital. The severity of each risk should be rated based on the consequences described and categorized as:

- insignificant,
- minor,
- moderate,
- major,
- catastrophic.

Table 28.2 How to determine a risk rating [16].

Likelihood	Consequences				
	Insignificant	*Minor*	*Moderate*	*Major*	*Catastrophic*
Almost certain	Significant	Significant	High	High	High
Likely	Moderate	Significant	Significant	High	High
Moderate	Low	Moderate	Significant	High	High
Unlikely	Low	Low	Moderate	Significant	High
Rare	Low	Low	Moderate	Significant	Significant

Stage 2 – Determine the likelihood of the risk occurring

To do this, standardized likelihood ratings should be used:

- almost certain,
- likely,
- moderate,
- unlikely,
- rare.

Stage 3 – Ascribe a risk rating

Based on consequence and likelihood ratings each risk should be ascribed a risk rating (Table 28.2). This will then allow prioritization of action planning to control the risks identified by the risk assessment. Risk control will be discussed in detail below.

The majority of clinical incidents will not require detailed analysis. For those that do, several methods have been established. The most frequently used systems are Root Cause Analysis (RCA), which has been adapted from processes used in high-risk industries, and Significant Event Audit, which was initially developed for general practice [5,6]. The most widely used RCA protocols recommend participation in the process of all staff involved in the incident. Attempts should be made to achieve this even if multiple Multi-professional review meetings are required. RCA is a technique for identifying the underlying organizational root cause(s) that can reasonably be identified, that management has control to fix, and when fixed will prevent (or significantly reduce the likelihood of) the problem's recurrence. In the UK, the National Patient Safety Agency (NPSA), established in 2001, aims to promote an open and fair culture across the NHS, encouraging all staff to report incidents and 'near misses', using an anonymized reporting system

to collect and analyse data. The NPSA has developed an online RCA toolkit which is free to access and which provides the user with guidance on how to perform RCA [7]. This is complemented by the Incident Decision Tree, which has been created to help NHS managers and senior clinicians decide whether they need to suspend (exclude) staff involved in a serious patient safety incident and to identify appropriate management action. The aim is to promote fair and consistent staff treatment within and between healthcare organizations.

Risk control

Whereas risk assessment is a process by which one can formally identify those risks which occur on the delivery suite and in the intrapartum period, risk control is the series of processes which aim to eliminate or minimize risk. Each risk will require a different set of control measures to address it. A worked example of intrapartum clinical risk management in practice is shown in Figure 28.1.

Processes involved in risk control include: induction, training, competence assessment, guidelines and protocols, communication and audit. Changes in delivery suite practice which have arisen as a result of clinical risk management are shown in Table 28.3.

Induction

All staff working in the complex and dynamic area of intrapartum care must be familiar with the procedures, policies and equipment used in the unit they are employed in, and have a good understanding of who to ask for assistance if they are unclear of their duties. Structured induction pathways should be employed to ensure that all staff, including temporary staff, are familiarized with the policies and guidelines used within the unit.

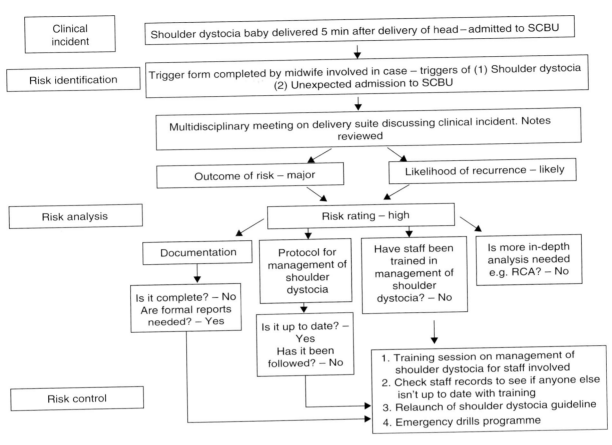

Figure 28.1 Intrapartum clinical risk management in practice- shoulder dystocia

Table 28.3 Examples of changes in delivery suite practice which have arisen as a result of clinical risk management.

Documentation aides	These facilitate the accurate recording of events whilst having the added advantage of improving the ease with which audit can be performed. Commonly used documentation aides include ones for the management of shoulder dystocia, obstetric haemorrhage and EFM.
'Specific event' box/bag	These are now commonplace on many delivery suites. Typical examples are ones for postpartum haemorrhage and eclampsia. Sophisticated boxes contain not only the drugs and clinical equipment needed to deal with the situation, but documentation aides to assist in accurate recording of the events.
PPH tray	Developed for the obstetric theatre environment, these contain a simple guide to insertion of a brace suture along with appropriate equipment.
Obstetric haemorrhage estimation charts	Developed and validated over the last two years, these vastly improve the accuracy of blood loss estimation, thereby reducing the risk of overtransfusion and transfusion-related complications [17].

Training and competence

Intrapartum healthcare is a risky business, but there was little appreciation of this during the formative years of most senior clinicians currently employed within obstetrics. The medical culture of 'see one, do one, teach one' does not fit comfortably with a patient safety agenda. Even within the present undergraduate and postgraduat curricula, scant attention appears to

Table 28.4 Training practices pertinent to intrapartum care.

Management of 1. Shoulder dystocia 2. Obstetric haemorrhage 3. Vaginal breech delivery 4. Cord prolapse 5. Eclampsia	These may be covered by in-house training or attendance on courses such as Advanced Life Support in Obstetrics or Managing Obstetric Emergencies and Trauma
EFM training	May be delivered in-house or using an accredited external training package
Obstetric emergency drills	These are covered in detail in Chapter 29

be paid to patient safety and risk management issues. We need to insist upon patient safety and risk management being a matter of good clinical practice at root, and reaffirm a commitment to these principles on a daily basis. Education of junior staff with regards to a no-blame culture, leadership, teamwork and good communication must be ongoing at all times.

Whilst training is not the same as competence, the two processes are closely interlinked. Each unit should have its own method of ensuring that clinical staff are competent to perform the tasks which their job plan assumes they are capable of. In particular, care must be taken with staff working in a unit for only a short period or those who are moving between different units during the course of their training. Training and its assessment differ between and within countries, but whichever system is used to assess competence it must be standardized to ensure fairness to staff, and fit for purpose in order to ensure patient safety. One can never remove all the risks associated with the delivery of a baby, whether this occurs as a result of a spontaneous vaginal delivery or an emergency caesarean section following an unsuccessful trial of instrumental delivery. However, there is good evidence that independent of the setting, practical, multiprofessional obstetric emergency training increases midwives' and doctors' knowledge of obstetric emergency management [8]. Examples of effective training practices are given in Table 28.4.

Guidelines

Throughout medicine, clinical guidelines are acknowledged as a key element in initiatives aimed at improving the quality and uniformity of clinical care. The number of guidelines developed and the rigour of the methods applied during development are hopefully continually improving. However, adherence to guidelines is poor in many disciplines, including obstetrics. In the UK in 2005, the healthcare commission was asked to review obstetric practices at Northwick Park Hospital because the number of maternal deaths in a three-year period was higher than expected [9]. Their review highlighted a number of areas where risk management practices were poor. In particular, many staff reported problems with the development, implementation and monitoring of guidelines, and they found evidence of staff using out-of-date guidelines. Guidelines must be simple to understand, up-to-date and easily accessible.

More recently, guidelines are being complemented by care bundles. A care bundle is a group of evidence-based interventions related to a disease or care process that, when executed together, result in better outcomes than when implemented individually. The selection of the evidence-based elements comprising the bundles should be based on sound science and local knowledge, and an agreement among clinicians that patients should receive all elements of care unless medically contra-indicated. Experience from the use of bundles in clinical areas, such as care of the ventilated patient, has shown that reliably applying these evidence-based interventions improves outcomes. With an aim to further improving intrapartum patient safety in the UK, the NPSA and the RCOG are developing care bundles for (1) management of placenta praevia following a previous caesarean section, and (2) electronic fetal monitoring (EFM). Careful evaluation of the implementation of such packages must occur.

Communication with the patient

In the intrapartum period the amount of time available to communicate with the patient can vary dramatically, but however long the consultation, effective communication is paramount. Communication skills which improve outcomes for patients include the following.

(1) Getting the full story from the patient's perspective – whilst obviously not applicable in the setting of an obstetric emergency, this is particularly important when reviewing previous deliveries, highlighting how good risk management in the antenatal period can impact on intrapartum care.

(2) Demonstrating 'acceptance' and empathy. These skills should be employed equally in the

emergency and routine setting and must become second nature to all clinicians. Even if a previous delivery was uncomplicated from an obstetric perspective, it may not have been from the patient's perspective.

(3) Being explicit about the structure of the interaction.

(4) Giving appropriate and timely explanations. Much of risk management pertains to effective communication.

(5) Involving the patient in explanation and planning.

(6) Making an agreed final plan with timescales and safety net.

The communication skills outlined above are based on a number of different models of consultation analysis. All require attention and should be developed from training onwards. Even in the setting of the obstetric emergency, it is still possible to communicate effectively with patients.

Communication between staff

This may occur verbally, through annotations in the patient record, by letter, or by electronic means. Whatever the method, patient confidentiality must be maintained. Different risks apply to different types of communication and record keeping. In the developed world the medical record is increasingly being transferred into electronic format. Good record keeping is an essential component of safe medical care, but there are risks associated with both written and electronic records. These risks can be reduced by using commonsense and vigilance. It is also useful to have knowledge of the legal requirements relevant to your department.

It is always interesting to review written medical notes, and good clinical risk management, in particular RCA, requires the regular assessment of events as recorded in the medical record. However, very few written medical notes stand up to detailed scrutiny. Problems commonly seen in handwritten records of the intrapartum period include:

- poor handwriting resulting in illegible entries;
- incomplete records as a result of using abbreviations/shorthand;
- lost or unavailable records;
- loss of records due to deterioration of print, e.g. problems with heat/light sensitive ink/paper used in some forms of EFM.

Some of these problems are equally applicable to electronic records, and the jury is still out as to which format has the advantage, although in the UK there is a large project underway to develop a single NHS electronic patient record system. Concern has been expressed that computerized records, particularly ones which employ a tick-box type format, do not give as high quality recording of consultations or events. However, electronic records should be easier to read, available when required, rapidly retrievable, and more easily analysed for audit, research and quality assurance.

Whilst it may be tempting to rush into electronic recording to enhance your ability to perform audit and quality assurance checks, care must be taken to ensure that the transition occurs as smoothly as possible. The period when dual records are being kept is the time of greatest risk, as information is often inadequately recorded in both electronic and written formats such that no comprehensive recording occurs. Time is a crucial commodity during many patient interactions, particularly in the high-pressure delivery suite environment, and where dual systems are being used another difficulty commonly encountered is that one group of clinicians uses the written record almost exclusively whilst others use only the electronic method. This leads to delays because two methods of recording need to be examined to obtain a complete picture of events. Many large obstetric units have now moved from hard copy EFM recording to electronic capture and storage. The well-documented problems with storage and longevity of paper EFM recordings have undoubtedly acted as an impetus in such a move, although little has been published about the success or otherwise of such transitions.

All clinical software programs should require the entry of a unique identifier along with an allocated individual password. Some systems currently in use are sophisticated enough to use fingerprint recognition techniques for authentication. Such safety mechanisms enable identification of individuals accessing and adding to the record. They do, however, represent a challenge in units in which there are a large number of temporary staff, e.g. locum doctors or midwives. These staff may find themselves unable to access key clinical data or perform basic clinical duties, such as prescribing/dispensing medication. Such problems must be addressed by induction procedures.

In the intrapartum period, particularly when dealing with an obstetric emergency, it is often impossible to record notes contemporaneously. Whichever format is used, staff must, however, ensure that they record in detail events they have been involved with, making clear the timescale of events and when the notes were written.

Audit

Medical audit has now become established as part of the regulatory and quality improvement systems in healthcare. Audit may take many forms, but at a local level audit is the means by which you can assess compliance with guidelines and protocols. The UKs Confidential Enquiry into Maternal Death (CEMD) is the longest-running example of national professional self-evaluation in the world, and is a clinical incident reporting system which has been used as a template worldwide. Since 1949, reports on maternal mortality in the UK have been published on a triannual basis [10,11]. Along similar lines, the Confidential Enquiry into Stillbirths and Deaths in Infancy (CESDI) was established in 1992 to improve understanding of how the risks of death in late fetal life and infancy might be reduced in the UK. In 2003, CEMD and CESDI merged to form the Confidential Enquiry into Maternal and Child Health (CEMACH). CEMACH undertakes detailed analysis of all reported cases to identify risks attributable to suboptimal clinical care. Recommendations for improving care are then made, an example of obstetric clinical risk management in practice. Over the first 50 years of the CEMD, substantial reductions were achieved in maternal deaths in the UK due to intrapartum complications such as haemorrhage [11]. Recent CESDI reports found suboptimal care in 75% of intrapartum-related fetal/neonatal deaths, and the most recent CEMD highlighted aspects of substandard care in 50% of women who died [11,12]. One of the main problems with this system of national recommendations is that mechanisms do not exist for ensuring recommendations are implemented. For example, the adoption of evidence-based guidelines for the management of women with severe pre-eclampsia was recommended in the 1997–1999 report, but a study in 2003 demonstrated that many units were continuing to use outdated protocols in this area [13,14]. However, at a local level, there are some examples in obstetrics of good risk management translating into better and safer care. The largest obstetric unit in the UK has seen an 11% decrease in number of clinical incidents in which the standard of care has been judged to have had room for improvement

since the introduction of a comprehensive risk management strategy [15].

The hierarchy of risk management

Many hospitals in the developed world have a clinical risk management team who enable the risk management policy of the hospital to move forward. In the UK, risk management specific to the intrapartum period would normally be the remit of a delivery suite or labour ward risk management review group, with the Chair of this group liaising with the hospital risk management team. This delivery suite risk management group should contain representation from senior and junior obstetricians, anaesthetists, midwifery staff and neonatologists. Other representation might include service users and community representation. The format of the risk management team meetings must be such as to encourage clinical incident reporting and the development of an open safety culture. Regular feedback from the clinical risk management team of both positive improvements and problem areas will undoubtedly help in this sphere.

Where do you go from here?

This will ultimately depend upon where 'here' is for your institution. Some units may have robust risk management procedures applicable to the intrapartum period, whilst others will undoubtedly have fledgling systems which require development over the next few years. Risk management in the intrapartum period requires the development of a blame-free culture within which mistakes, errors and near misses can be analysed objectively and preferably anonymously without staff worrying about adverse implications. It takes time to develop such a culture and a huge amount of effort is needed, particularly from senior staff, to ensure that all staff are empowered to participate in risk management processes. A risk management team must be developed, within which roles and remits are well defined. Staff within the team must be clear with regards to their responsibilities and familiar with all stages of the risk management process. Also essential to the risk management process are good links with and the involvement of service users. If data arising from them are properly collated and analysed, much can be learnt from complaints. The majority of labour wards/delivery suites will have a labour ward forum or a management committee responsible for managerial issues associated with intrapartum services. Such fora provide the ideal interface between the risk management team and the obstetric staff. Changes in practice arising from risk management assessments must be disseminated and examples of good practice highlighted.

Feedback to staff and keeping them engaged

If risk management is to be effective within a unit, all staff must be fully engaged in the process. In addition, it is essential that the intrapartum period, which undoubtedly is one of the riskiest times in pregnancy, is not looked at in isolation. Many intrapartum complications occur as a result of poor antenatal risk management. The ethos of effective clinical risk management should run through every aspect of care within the intrapartum period. Visible evidence of change in response to risk management recommendations is an important part of encouraging staff to participate. Staff can be encouraged to engage in the clinical risk management process by:

- inclusion of an outline of the risk management strategy in the induction process. This gives risk management an added degree of prominence and will encourage new staff to engage with the process;
- incentivizing staff to report clinical incidents by giving a prize to the top reporter of the month or year;
- giving formal positive feedback regarding clinical incidents which have been well managed. These can be put in staff portfolios and discussed at appraisal time;
- encouraging staff to openly discuss 'bad outcomes' and ways in which they feel things could have been managed differently; and
- encouraging the development of a no-blame culture.

Summary

Risk assessment is a tool that can be used prospectively and proactively to review risks. In many respects it is an early warning signal of where your main risks are, and helps prioritize those that need more immediate attention. Intrapartum risk management requires money and the development of a clinical risk

management team. Risk management needs to start at the very top of any organization and be embedded into every decision, clinical or non-clinical.

References

1. Brennan T A, Leape L L, Laird N M, et al. Incidence of adverse events and negligence in hospitalized patients. Results of the Harvard Medical Practice Study I. *N Engl J Med* 1991; **324**(6): 370–6.

2. Kohn L, Corrigan J, Donaldson M. *To Err is Human: Building a Safer Health System*. Washington, DC: Institute of Medicine, 1999.

3. Vincent C, Neale G, Woloshynowych M. Adverse events in British hospitals: preliminary retrospective record review. *Br Med J* 2001; **322**(7285): 517–9.

4. Ennis M, Vincent C A. Obstetric accidents: a review of 64 cases. *Br Med J* 1990; **300**(6736): 1365–7.

5. Pringle M, Bradley C P, Carmichael C M, Wallis H, Moore A. Significant event auditing. A study of the feasibility and potential of case-based auditing in primary medical care. Occasional Paper, *R Coll Gen Pract* 1995;70: **i-viii**: 1–71.

6. Clinical Risk Unit and ALARM. A Protocol for the Investigation and Analysis of Clinical Incidents. University College London, 1999.

7. Joint Commission on the Accreditation of Healthcare Organizations. Sentinel Event Root Cause Analysis tool Guide. Available at: www.npsa.org.uk (accessed 18 January 2008).

8. Crofts J F, Ellis D, Draycott T J, Winter C, Hunt L P, Akande V A. Change in knowledge of midwives and obstetricians following obstetric emergency training: a randomised controlled trial of local hospital, simulation centre and teamwork training. *Br J Obstet Gynaecol* 2007; **114**(12): 1534–41.

9. The Healthcare Commission. Investigation into 10 Maternal Deaths at, or Following Delivery at, Northwick Park Hospital, North West London Hospitals NHS Trust, Between April 2002 and April 2005. Available at: www.healthcarecommission.org.uk (accessed 30 January 2008).

10. Lewis G, ed. *Saving Mothers' Lives: Reviewing Maternal Deaths to Make Motherhood Safer – 2003–2005. The Seventh Report on Confidential Enquiries into Maternal Deaths in the United Kingdom*. London: The Confidential Enquiry into Maternal and Child Health (CEMACH), 2007.

11. Lewis G, ed. *Why Mothers Die 2000–2002: Sixth Report of the Confidential Enquiries into Maternal Deaths in the United Kingdom*. London: RCOG Press, 2004.

12. Confidential Enquiry into Stillbirths and Deaths in Infancy. *Project 27/28. An Enquiry into Quality of Care*

and its Effect on the Survival of Babies Born at 27–28 weeks. London: The Stationary Office, 2003.

13. Lewis G, ed. *Why Mothers Die 1997–1999: Fifth Report of the Confidential Enquiries into Maternal Deaths in the United Kingdom.* London: RCOG Press, 2001.

14. Whitworth M, Reid F, Arya R, Baker P, Myers J. Clinical guidelines in severe pre-eclampsia and eclampsia. *Clin Gov Int J* 2005; **10**(4): 291–9.

15. Scholefield H. Embedding quality improvement and patient safety at Liverpool Women's NHS Foundation Trust. *Best Pract Res Clin Obstet Gynaecol* 2007; **21**(4): 593–607.

16. MPS Risk Consulting. *The MPS Risk Consulting Approach to Clinical Risk Assessment.* Leeds: MPS Risk Consulting Ltd, 2006.

17. Bose P, Regan F, Paterson-Brown S. Improving the accuracy of estimated blood loss at obstetric haemorrhage using clinical reconstructions. *Br J Obstet Gynaecol* 2006; **113**(8): 919–24.

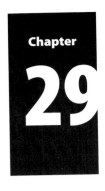

Chapter 29

Teamworking, skills and drills

Dimitrios M. Siassakos and Timothy J. Draycott

Background

Labour is usually normal, but a variety of emergencies can occur (Table 29.1). Many clinicians consider themselves trained to face such emergencies, when in reality they are not: in a recent study, 84% of trainees who had declared being confident of their competence in obstetric emergencies retracted their statements after simulation assessment [1]. Moreover, in a study of simulated shoulder dystocia, less than half the participants could complete delivery before training [2].

Some emergencies are common, but most much less so, and therefore it is difficult to learn by experience. The majority (64%) of trainees in a skills drills course had no experience of being in charge of real-life emergencies like shoulder dystocia, eclampsia or even PPH [1]. Pressures on the duration of training and the reduction in working hours as a result of the European Working Time Directive may result in clinicians of the future being even less confident in their practical skills, after even less time at the coalface.

Even when individual clinical experience is present, lack of communication and poor or non-existent teamwork have been identified as factors contributing to poor outcomes in national confidential enquiries [3] or litigation, where on average nine teamwork failures were identified per medico-legal case [4].

There has been a cultural shift away from striving for individual technical perfection to better team co-ordination and training, peer monitoring [4], and risk management. This has been reflected in the 'Safer Childbirth – Minimum Standards for the Organisation and Delivery of Care in Labour' paper, which recommends specific training in group dynamics for all those who are involved in the management of women in labour, or their babies [5].

The aviation industry has used Crew Resource Management (CRM) programmes to conduct such training and prevent teamwork failures. In accident and emergency departments, this has been successful in improving attitudes towards teamworking, improving team behaviours and reducing clinical error [6].

However, the same CRM methods ('MedTeams') have failed to achieve improvement in either real-life outcome or process measures when applied in labour ward settings [7]. Obstetric crises may be sufficiently different from other medical specialties or professions to require development of specific training and evaluation tools, rather than wholescale adoption of possibly inappropriate models from aviation or other medical contexts.

Moreover, it has been demonstrated that even in aviation (or other high-risk industries like nuclear power, offshore oil production or maritime), the only definite beneficial outcome from CRM training has been a positive reaction from trainees (Kirkpatrick level 1 [8]), with ambiguous results regarding higher levels (Kirkpatrick 2–4 [8]) of evaluation: knowledge, behaviour or outcome [9].

It seems that separate, non-context-specific teamwork training does not work, but integrated teamwork training does; 'full-mission' multiprofessional simulation per se appears to best suited to hone teamwork-related skills under conditions of ambiguity, time pressure, and stress, like obstetric crises [10]. A UK Department of Health-funded randomized controlled trial identified improvements in teamwork scores and markers of care after simulated eclampsia, even though additional teamwork training based on an aviation-derived CRM model once again conferred no additional benefit [11].

Using a modified version of Kirkpatrick's framework, we will summarize the existing evidence on

Best Practice in Labour and Delivery, ed. R. Warren and S. Arulkumaran. Published by Cambridge University Press.
© Cambridge University Press 2009.

Table 29.1 Obstetric emergencies suitable for rehearsals.

Emergency	UK incidence (approximate, per maternities)
Maternal collapse and perimortem caesarean section	0.03 per 1000
Seizures/eclampsia	0.5 per 1000
Cardiotocogram (CTG) interpretation	High rate of false-positives
Cord prolapse	1–6 per 1000
Breech delivery	30 per 1000
Shoulder dystocia	2–20 per 1000
Postpartum haemorrhage	Massive in 13 per 1000
Neonatal resuscitation	Common need

skills drills, across multiple levels of evaluation, and describe the active ingredients of effective teamwork training in obstetrics.

Evaluation of drills

Learning outcome

Satisfaction of learners

There is evidence that learners enjoy obstetric emergency training and feel more confident following it [12]. Multiprofessional teams taught using simulation are more likely to demonstrate sustained improvement in clinical management of the case, confidence, communication and transferable skills as well as knowledge of obstetric emergencies compared to teams taught with a lecture format [13].

Knowledge and skills

Healthcare professionals involved in obstetric care may be inclined to report high levels of competence in dealing with obstetric emergencies [14], but important knowledge gaps have been identified [Akande, pers. comm.; 15]. Obstetric emergency training may address such deficiencies; in the SaFE study, a definitive improvement in both knowledge and skills occurred after training [1], and was sustained for 6 and 12 months after training [16].

In another study, pretraining clinical performance was lower for drills requiring multiprofessional team effort (PPH, eclampsia) than for drills focusing on skills of the individual accoucheur (breech vaginal delivery, shoulder dystocia). Simulation performance increased by working in teams, even before training; the performance in either eclampsia or PPH was higher for the second pretraining drill than the first, regardless of whether the PPH station followed the eclampsia one or vice versa. Subsequent performance improved further with team-based simulation training, even though the scenarios were changed so as to avoid merely testing technical knowledge [1].

Attitudes

Behavioural changes are much more difficult to evaluate. Several tools and teamwork scales have been developed in the context of CRM or obstetric emergency training. Using such tools, simulation has been shown to improve learners' confidence and transferable communication skills [13]. However, most of the evaluation tools rely extensively on self-reporting, subjective assessments by observers, or both, with low correlation between the two methods [17].

Healthcare outcome: patient and organization

Obstetric emergency training can improve learners' satisfaction, knowledge, skills, and possibly team behaviour, but do these changes translate into better outcome for patients and healthcare organizations?

Patient outcome – safety

A retrospective observational study [18] has demonstrated improved perinatal outcomes in a large UK maternity unit after the introduction of 'in-house' obstetric emergency training: low Apgar scores (<7 at 5 min) and moderate, severe or total hypoxic–ischaemic encephalopathy (HIE) were all reduced by about 50%. There was also a 70% reduction of brachial plexus injuries and 30% decrease in litigation cases [19]. Similar results were noted in a large US unit, with a 16% drop in adverse outcomes and about a 50% reduction in total and high-severity claims [20], and in other Australian and UK units [15,21].

The common characteristics of these units, where improvement in outcome was demonstrated, were department-level incentives to train and 'in-house' training programmes with full penetration (100% of staff trained). These units also reported implementing several infrastructural changes that were suggested by their staff learners after participating in the training.

Cost-effectiveness

'In-house' simulation training is cost-effective [22]. It may also be less costly than attendance at external courses; in a UK unit, a recent calculation was £40,000 per annum for 'in-house' training versus £210,000 per annum for staff to attend external courses [19].

There is a potential for huge savings from litigation costs and insurance premiums by improving outcomes [20,23].

Patient satisfaction – humanity

Patient satisfaction is associated with efficient communication. It has been shown that a patient cared for by an obstetrician with a high number of previous lawsuits is more likely to report (s)he demonstrated deficient interpersonal skills. A study investigating claims in obstetrics and gynaecology reported that communication problems occurred in about one out of seven cases and adversely affected patients' and relatives' satisfaction and provoked concern for patient safety [24].

Training in obstetric emergencies can, per se, improve communication and subsequently patient satisfaction, and reduce litigation [19]. In the SaFE study there was a significant increase in every aspect of a patient-actress's perception of her care after training, whether she was cared for by a multiprofessional team or by an individual [25].

Safety and communication scores were significantly higher for teams trained 'in-house' with a patient-actress compared to teams trained at the simulation centre using a computerized patient mannequin. Other groups have also demonstrated that focusing on intrateam interactions and relying on simulation technology, whilst ignoring the patient perspective, may be detrimental to women's satisfaction. Designing obstetric training interventions to closely imitate the demands of real-life labour ward crises is more important for psychological fidelity than the technology of the equipment used [10].

Organizing drills

The UK NHS Litigation Authority mandate annual multidisciplinary skills drills through its Clinical Negligence Scheme for Trust (CNST) standards [23]. Similar recommendations are made by the Welsh Pool Risk, and in Scotland by CNORIS. Rehearsals allow new staff to familiarize themselves with their specific role in emergencies and permanent staff to maintain competence [5].

However, in 2003, only 51% of UK centres surveyed were conducting such rehearsals, and 14% were planning to develop them. Common causes for not undertaking skills drills were concerns about the impact on service provision and a perception of the training process as threatening or stressful [26]. We will discuss ways to alleviate such fears and maximize the benefit from drills.

Location of training

The emergency drills are best undertaken in a delivery room or another clinical area, as it provides the highest environmental fidelity. A suitable seminar room nearby should be used for lectures.

Delivery rooms may not always be available for use, but training in the true clinical environment enables local protocols and procedures to be tested and, if necessary, revised, thereby improving the system and creating a sense of general ownership.

The workload can be reduced in advance; for example, by limiting the number of elective caesarean sections. It may be best to leave the decision of which rooms will be used for each drill until the latest possible time, and remain flexible.

Course planning and administration

It is a good idea for the local training team to organize a planning meeting to allocate individual modules to specific trainers. The course programme can be finalized, equipment inventory discussed, and the trainers can practise the scenarios prior to running the courses so as to identify any problems.

In our unit, a practice development midwife administers the course. To ensure that staff are released to attend the training day, several dates may be arranged well in advance (ideally annually). All presentations, handouts and equipment may be stored centrally, and it is useful if trainers are familiar with each other's workstations and lectures, so that both trainers and workstations are interchangeable when necessary.

The programme should ideally change annually to maintain interest. Course manuals should be sent out to all participants prior to the course.

A database should be kept of all attendees for clinical negligence scheme assessments. Appraisals of consultants and trainee doctors and supervision schemes for midwives should identify non-attendees, and a mandatory session can be arranged at the end of the year. Certificates of attendance should be provided, and logbooks of training can be signed to increase motivation.

Access

Locally organized emergency training days should be available to both hospital and community staff. It is important to advertise and actively promote such days to the latter, particularly after recent trends to promote birth outside consultant-led units [27].

Scenarios

A drill briefing highlights actions the participants should undertake during the drills, e.g. obtaining and drawing up any appropriate drugs, and important safety information. This briefing should be read to the participants prior to the first drill and may be reinforced between drills, to avoid reinventing the wheel.

The scenarios should be simple and outline the immediate emergency action required. The participation in role play is a new experience for many healthcare professionals, and this is often the first obstacle to be encountered. Given time, participants overcome their initial embarrassment and appreciate the opportunity to actively take part in the scenario as part of 'the team'.

It works well to take one member of the team into the room first for a handover, whilst the rest of the team wait outside.

Facilitation

'In-house' trainers, 6–10 per day, should be enlisted. Adult learning is more sustainable when training has a clear focus on the process rather than the content of learning. Participants should feel welcome and relaxed and be encouraged to participate in the planning and evaluation of their learning. This is vital to the success of drills.

Objectives, feedback and assessment

Workshops should remain focused, and outcome-based training can achieve this. At the beginning of training sessions the learning objectives or the most common challenges should be identified. It may be useful to discuss difficulties and omissions identified from past learners, and aim to avoid the same mistakes.

Table 29.2 Pendleton's feedback rules.

Rule	
1	The team members say what they did well
2	The team members say what can be improved
3	The facilitator acknowledges what they did well
4	The facilitator states where they could improve

Specific checklists can help structure observation of clinical actions, and provide a useful starting point in the discussion and evaluation of management of the scenario [28].

Appropriate feedback to learners is as important as objectives. Learning is about having an experience, reviewing it, concluding and planning the future. Individuals with different learning styles may perform better in one or two stages of this circular process, but skills drills may help learners adopt a more balanced, mature style. For this to occur, there is a need for drills to incorporate both practical and reflective elements through constructive feedback that is directly linked to the outcome-based objectives. Pendleton's rules (Table 29.2) are useful, but several other feedback models exist.

So as to avoid intimidating authority gradients, a member of the group can provide feedback to the rest of the team, using the drill-specific checklist(s). Subsequently, group discussions with suggestions about what could be improved, altered or added can be facilitated by the drill leader together with the patient-actress.

Learners often perceive that they have performed very badly, so it is vital that positive actions are emphasized. We do not use formal assessment. It removes the threat of testing, may promote team ethos, and has led to both 100% staff participation and improved outcomes.

Evaluation sheets should be given to all participants, as their feedback can lead to both training and infrastructural improvements.

Patient-actresses

Drills tend to be more successful if the setting is as near to reality as possible [25]. Obstetric emergencies are unique in that there is significant audience participation; communication with women, their families and sometimes friends during acute management of the emergency is an essential skill.

Using a patient-actress, or integrating a patient-actress with a mannequin, is cheap, easy and effective

[28], and can increase the realism of the situation, enhance the communication between team members and women, and lead to improvement in communication scores as assessed by patient-actresses [25]. Therefore, it may be useful for the patient-actresses to give the team feedback after each drill.

A member of staff with experience of the emergencies portrayed can make an excellent patient. Alternatively, using a healthcare assistant as the patient-actor may be advantageous in giving them an insight into their role as part of the multiprofessional team when attending obstetric emergencies.

Equipment

The correct equipment must be available. If mannequins are used, a pregnant abdomen, bra and female wig add realism to the simulated scenario. In the PROMPT (practical obstetric multiprofessional training) course, props are used to increase the realism of the scenarios: blood-stained incontinence sheets, trousers that bleed, a pregnant uterus, life-size copy of O Rhesus negative blood bags stuck on to cardboard, a perineum with a prolapsed cord, etc. [28].

The level of fidelity of simulation is not as important as designing the drills to suit task demands in real life, and in many cases low-technology props may be as effective as more sophisticated equipment.

Pictorial guidelines can be used to facilitate visual estimation of blood loss [29], otherwise underestimation might occur in as many as 95% of obstetric haemorrhage cases [1].

Record keeping

A 'made-up' set of patient notes and partogram can be used at the handover in the delivery room, as an aide-memoir of the patient's history, and also to document the care given during the scenario.

Structured documentation proformas can be developed and used for both training and real-life emergencies. The team should allocate the role of scribe to one person during the drill. If necessary, this can be prompted by the trainer. Documentation, including the completion of clinical incident forms, should be discussed following the drill.

Teams and teamwork training

Teamwork is defined as the combined effective action of a group working towards a common goal. It requires individuals with different roles to communicate effectively and work together in a co-ordinated manner to achieve a successful outcome [28].

Theories of team effectiveness dictate that the outcome of teamworking is related to both the givens – task clarity and importance (clear, outcome-based objectives), group characteristics and size, organizational environment and culture – and the intervening factors of teams, like leadership, and communication. We will discuss these factors.

Team characteristics

A pragmatic size for a multiprofessional drill team is between four and six people, but there should be a compromise between the competing considerations of effective team size and volume of learners.

Participants should play their own role. Self-adhesive labels can be given to each team member so that it is easy to identify roles within each team. It is useful to run two stations for each scenario, so that one team participates in a drill prior to the lecture whilst the other team observes and then they swap for the drill after the lecture, alternating thereafter for different scenarios.

Friction between different health professions may prevent effective communication between health carers. Multiprofessional groups with doctors and midwives learning side-by-side may help prevent such friction. Skills drills are, by design, suitable for interprofessional learning, as the content is immediately relevant to both groups.

Interprofessional education does not necessarily mean professional socialization, though. Participants have reported higher rates of satisfaction in a two-day obstetric emergencies course compared to a one-day one [30]. Whether this was because the two-day course was less rushed, or whether the social activities planned for the evening after the first day improved interprofessional communication that reflected on satisfaction with training, was not established. A future trial may address this, by comparing performance after such courses, with or without social activities between study days.

Leadership

The benefits of skills drills may wane if training does not lead to the development of leadership skills [31]. Team leadership involves providing direction, structure and support for other team members. Leaders

Table 29.3 Measurement of team performance and communication skills in delivery room crisis simulation [32].

1	Clearly states situation (S)
2	Clearly states background (B)
3	Gives accurate assessment (A)
4	Requests recommended actions (R)
5	Repeats information back accurately
6	Calls for help appropriately
7	Clarity of requests
8	Requests directed to individuals
9	Double-checks data
10	Reports relevant information to team
11	Ensures team is in delivery room
12	Verifies team has correct information

vary in their level of expertise when involved in a particular emergency situation and in their readiness to lead. They may also vary in the profession; it is often the most senior obstetrician present, but may be the midwifery co-ordinator or anaesthetist. It is essential that the team leader is nominated and accepted by the rest of the team as early as possible, although the person leading may sometimes change during the drill.

Leadership is a complex skill. The team leader requires a certain amount of competence; however, it is unlikely that leaders possess all the abilities of every team member present (anaesthetic skills, for example). Leadership requires knowledge (provided with lectures and course material), but also communication and situational awareness.

Zabari *et al.* have developed a leadership and teamwork checklist that incorporates the SBAR (situation, background, assessment recommendation) communication tool, and can be used in delivery room crisis simulation to evaluate these skills [32] (Table 29.3). Alternatively, CRM training includes five statements to prevent disasters: (1) opening or attention getter, (2) state your concern clearly, (3) state the problem as you see it, (4) state a solution, and (5) obtain agreement [33].

Training in situational awareness using similar checklists, and also in voice projection and non-verbal communication, in addition to knowledge acquisition, may increase leadership quality and could be included in obstetric emergency courses. Learners

should be taught the philosophy of the 'non-participant' leader: try not to become engaged in practical tasks that can be undertaken by others. This allows the leader to take a step back and maintain a broader, 'helicopter' view of the unfolding crisis [28].

Communication among team members

Task clarification and leadership may not be adequate for team performance, if communication among the members of the team is ailing. Several obstacles to effective communication exist, particularly in settings involving different professions (midwives, doctors, nurses) and levels of seniority, as is the case in obstetric emergencies.

For effective communication, learners must be instructed that messages should be: (1) succinctly *formulated*, (2) *addressed* to specific individuals by eye or body contact or use of names, (3) clearly and concisely *delivered*, (4) *acknowledged*, and (5) *acted* upon. Checklists similar to the one developed by Zabari *et al.* can be used [32].

Communication training should include guidance on how to communicate problems to seniors. The 'two-challenge' rule by MedTeams, the recommendation to voice concerns and disagreements to seniors or leaders at least twice, is an example [33].

For each drill, team members should be assigned specific roles and responsibilities that are specified and clearly understood.

Safety culture

The knowledge, skills and attitudes that are essential for teamwork are critical for successful performance in 'high-reliability organizations' (HRO), settings that are hypercomplex, tightly coupled, hierarchical, time-compressed, and rely upon synchronized outcomes [34]. Maternity units uniquely demonstrate all of these characteristics: complex emergencies with frequently two patients to look after (mother and baby); tightly coupled events, when the decision–delivery interval of an emergency caesarean section depends on actions by every single member of the team; hierarchy within all involved professions; compressed decision-to-action intervals; and necessity for synchronized actions.

Organizations that provide maternity care could therefore function like HROs. Managers should support teamwork and enhance it through context-specific training. They should integrate emergency training into routine staff career development, appraisals, and certifications. Healthcare systems should recognize collective training as key to the development of the organization itself.

This culture appears not to be ubiquitous. In the SaFE study, questions regarding the perception of management's role in safety had the lowest scores across professional groups, reflecting a perception of negative attitude towards risk management. This attitude deteriorated after training in simulation centres, but not after local training (Akande, pers. comm.). This could reflect the fact that training in external courses can be perceived as paternalistic and driven by managerial targets rather than staff development needs, and cannot therefore create any sense of ownership.

On the other hand, there was an obvious positive impact of training, particularly if undertaken in the local setting, on job satisfaction and attitudes towards teamwork, and stress recognition. After 12 months, the improvement in attitudes towards teamwork was only sustained for healthcare professionals receiving training locally (Akande, pers. comm.).

This demonstrates how 'in-house' training of teams rather than individuals in managing obstetric emergencies is a major step towards a shared vision and a safety culture: blame the system, not the individual; safe solutions not fair blame; mixing and working together rather than placing individual performance under the microscope.

Integral versus additional teamwork training

A recent cluster randomized controlled trial [7] used a composite Adverse Outcome Index to study the impact of standardized CRM-based ('MedTeams') teamwork training, derived from aviation, on 11 measures of maternal and neonatal outcome in 7 US maternity units. Healthcare professionals (1307) were trained, but there was no difference before and after the intervention in any clinical outcome, or in 10 out of 11 process measures that were used to evaluate the quality of care.

In the UK, in the SaFE study there was no difference in clinical performance in drills, patient satisfaction, team knowledge, team behaviour, attitudes to stress recognition and safety climate, and between learners who had received additional teamwork training and those who were randomized to clinical training alone [11; Akande, pers. comm.]. There was also no difference in overall team performance, as measured by individual attitudes, global rating or content analysis, between the two groups; additional teamwork training failed to make a difference to either learning or clinical outcome, as measured by surrogate performance indicators.

It is possible that 'in-house' clinical training per se may improve teamwork, as members of the team bond and perform better, without the need for teamwork theories or non-context-specific team activities. Team formation can be described as occuring in four stages [35]: forming, storming, norming, and performing, but formation is rapid in obstetric emergencies. 'In-house' training may prepare 'shop-floor' teams for rapid transition to the performance stage once an emergency occurs: in an obstetric emergency course, teams performed significantly better on the second workstation than on the first, without any additional clinical or teamwork training in between [1].

Summary of lessons from experience

- Successful implementation of national guidelines requires safe local solutions.
- Ensure management supports changes and facilitates a sense of ownership by promoting local training.
- Reduce costs and ensure equal access by providing training 'in-house'. This develops a team of 'in-house experts', and ensures long-term sustainability.
- Encourage multiprofessional groups to participate in developing and running courses. This ensures that training is relevant to all staff, and becomes a true interprofessional learning experience.
- Mandate and confirm annual attendance of the course by all hospital and community, midwifery, obstetric and managerial staff.
- Use patient-actresses or integrated patient-actress–half-mannequin models, as they are cheap and provide high psychological fidelity.
- Teamwork training needs to be context-specific and integrated in the drills, rather than a separate activity.
- Using structured proformas is an effective way of reducing disparity in clinical interpretation and improving documentation.
- Make training fun. Consider a light-hearted quiz as an interlude during the day.

- Formal assessment is not necessary and may be detrimental to staff morale.
- Monitor clinical results. Feedback to staff. Improvement in outcomes is a great incentive to continue with training.

Conclusion – the future

Regular 'in-house' training, with or without high-fidelity mannequins or 'in-house' simulators, is probably the most effective method of training multiprofessional teams in acute settings like the labour ward. Local training appears to be more cost-effective. It can also consolidate behavioural changes, serve as a system for infrastructural changes, and lead to sustainable improvement in learning outcome and patient satisfaction. There is some evidence that it may also lead to improvement in neonatal and perhaps maternal outcome, as well as reduce litigation.

'In-house training' can provide quality: meet the development needs of staff, improve consumer outcome, and satisfy hospital management by reducing insurance and litigation costs.

The application of CRM methodology might improve the understanding of teamworking, but this has not been shown to translate into better obstetric outcome. Labour ward settings may be much more complex than cockpits in ways we do not, as yet, fully understand.

We may need to move beyond CRM and develop novel teamwork training methods, test them in simulation, compare them with real life, validate and refine them to ensure that they are applicable to labour wards and, why not, effectively generalizable to other healthcare teams.

Exciting developments keep emerging. The use of web-based or three-dimensional simulation and virtual or augmented reality programmes with haptic feedback are being developed for training in assisted delivery and obstetric emergencies [36].

Rigorous research is now urgently needed to validate both the available and the emerging training methods and their evaluation tools, and to confirm a sustainable difference in outcome.

References

1. Maslovitz S M D, Barkai G M D, Lessing J B M D, Ziv A M D, Many A M D. Recurrent obstetric management mistakes identified by simulation. *Obstet Gynecol* 2007; **109**(6): 1295–300.

2. Crofts J F, Ellis D, Draycott T J, Winter C, Hunt L P, Akande V A. Change in knowledge of midwives and obstetricians following obstetric emergency training: a randomised controlled trial of local hospital, simulation centre and teamwork training. *Br J Obstet Gynaecol* 2007; **114**(12): 1534–41.

3. Lewis G, ed. *The Confidential Enquiry into Maternal and Child Health (CEMACH). Saving Mothers' Lives: Reviewing Maternal Deaths to Make Motherhood Safer – 2003–2005. The Seventh Report of the Confidential Enquiries into Maternal Deaths in the United Kingdom.* London: CEMACH, 2007.

4. Risser D T, Rice M M, Salisbury M L, Simon R, Jay G D, Berns S D. The potential for improved teamwork to reduce medical errors in the emergency department. The MedTeams Research Consortium. *Ann Emerg Med* 1999; **34**(3): 373–83.

5. Royal College of Anaesthetists, Royal College of Midwives, Royal College of Obstetricians and Gynaecologists, Royal College of Paediatrics and Child Health. *Safer Childbirth: Minimum Standards for the Organisation and Delivery of Care in Labour.* London: RCOG Press, 2007.

6. Morey J C, Simon R, Jay G D, *et al.* Error reduction and performance improvement in the emergency department through formal teamwork training: evaluation results of the MedTeams project. *Health Serv Res* 2002; **37**(6): 1553–81.

7. Nielsen P E, Goldman M B, Mann S, *et al.* Effects of teamwork training on adverse outcomes and process of care in labor and delivery: a randomized controlled trial. *Obstet Gynecol* 2007; **109**(1): 48–55.

8. Freeth D, Hammick M, Koppel I, Reeves S, Barr H. Interprofessional Education Joint Evaluation Team. A Critical Review of Evaluations of Interprofessional Education: Commissioned by the Learning and Teaching Support Network Centre for Health Sciences and Practice; 2002.

9. Salas E, Wilson K A, Burke C S, Wightman D C. Does crew resource management training work? An update, an extension, and some critical needs. *Hum Factors* 2006; **48**(2): 392–412.

10. Beaubien J M, Baker D P. The use of simulation for training teamwork skills in health care: how low can you go? *Qual Safety Hlth Care* 2004; **13**: 151–16.

11. Ellis D, Crofts J F, Hunt L P, Read M, Fox R, James M. Hospital, simulation center, and teamwork training for eclampsia management: a randomized controlled trial. *Obstet Gynecol* 2008; **111**(3): 723–31.

12. Bower D J, Wolkomir M S, Schubot D B. The effects of the ALSO course as an educational intervention for residents. Advanced Life Support in Obstetrics. *Family Med* 1997; **29**(3): 187–93.

13. Birch L, Jones N, Doyle P M, *et al.* Obstetric skills drills: evaluation of teaching methods. *Nurse Educ Today* 2007 Mar 19.

14. Tucker J, Hundley V, Kiger A, *et al.* Sustainable maternity services in remote and rural Scotland? A qualitative survey of staff views on required skills, competencies and training. *Qual Safety Hlth Care* 2005; **14**(1): 34–40.

15. Thompson S, Neal S, Clark V. Clinical risk management in obstetrics: eclampsia drills. *Qual Safety Hlth Care* 2004; **13**(2): 127–9.

16. Crofts J F, Bartlett C, Ellis D, Hunt L P, Fox R, Draycott T J. Management of shoulder dystocia: skill retention 6 and 12 months after training. *Obstet Gynecol* 2007; **110**(5): 1069–74.

17. Morgan P J, Pittini R, Regehr G, Marrs C, Haley M F. Evaluating teamwork in a simulated obstetric environment. *Anesthesiology* 2007; **106**(5): 907–15.

18. Draycott T, Sibanda T, Owen L, *et al.* Does training in obstetric emergencies improve neonatal outcome? *Br J Obstet Gynaecol* 2006; **113**(2): 177–82.

19. Draycott T. Litigation, risk management and patient safety; a new approach to old problems. Forum on Maternity and the Newborn of the Royal Society of Medicine 2005; available at: www.rsm.ac.uk/academ/fmtm_n.php (accessed 12 December 2007).

20. Mann S, Marcus R, Sachs B P. Lessons from the cockpit: how team training can reduce errors on L&D. *Contemporary Ob/Gyn* 2006; 1–7.

21. Scholefield H. Embedding quality improvement and patient safety at Liverpool Women's NHS Foundation Trust. *Best Prac Res* 2007; **21**(4): 593–607.

22. Weinstock P H, Kappus L J, Kleinman M E, Grenier B, Hickey P, Burns J P. Toward a new paradigm in hospital-based pediatric education: the development of an onsite simulator program. *Pediatr Crit Care Med* 2005; **6**(6): 635–41.

23. NHS Litigation Authority. Clinical Negligence Scheme for Trusts: Maternity Standards. Criterion 4.1.1. 2006; available at: http://www.nhsla.com (accessed 29 May 2006).

24. White A A, Pichert J W, Bledsoe S H, Irwin C, Entman S S. Cause and effect analysis of closed claims in obstetrics and gynecology. *Obstet Gynecol* 2005; **105**(5): 1031–8.

25. Crofts J F, Bartlett C, Ellis D, *et al.* Patient-actor perception of care: a comparison of obstetric emergency training using manikins and patient-actors. *Qual Hlth Care* 2008; **17**(1): 20–4.

26. Anderson E R, Black R, Brocklehurst P. Acute obstetric emergency drill in England and Wales: a survey of practice. *Br J Obstet Gynaecol* 2005; **112**(3): 372–5.

27. National Collaborating Centre for Women's and Children's Health. *Intrapartum Care – Care of Healthy Women and their Babies during Childbirth.* Clinical Guideline. London: RCOG Press, 2007.

28. Draycott T, Winter C, Crofts J, Barnfield S. *PRactical Obstetric Multiprofessional Training (PROMPT) Trainer's Manual.* Bristol: PROMPT Foundation, 2008, in press.

29. Bose P, Regan F, Paterson-Brown S. Improving the accuracy of estimated blood loss at obstetric haemorrhage using clinical reconstructions. *Br J Obstet Gynaecol* 2006; **113**(8): 919–24.

30. Winter C, James M, Draycott T. *Developing a Training Package for Obstetric Emergencies.* Safer Healthcare; 2007.

31. Blakely T G. Implementing newborn mock codes. *Am J Maternal–Child Nurs* 2007; **32**(4): 230–5.

32. Zabari M, Suresh G, Tomlinson M, *et al.* Implementation and case-study results of potentially better practices for collaboration between obstetrics and neonatology to achieve improved perinatal outcomes. *Pediatrics* 2006; **118**: S153–S8.

33. US Army Research Laboratory. Emergency Team Coordination Course: Dynamics Research Corporation, 2004.

34. Baker D P, Day R, Salas E. Teamwork as an essential component of high-reliability organizations. *Hlth Serv Res* 2006; **41**(4 Pt 2): 1576–98.

35. Tuckman B. Developmental sequence in small groups. *Psychol Bull* 1965; **63**: 384–99.

36. Lapeer R. A mechanical contact model for the simulation of obstetric forceps delivery in a virtual/augmented environment. *Studies in Health Technology and Informatics: Medicine Meets Virtual Reality 13: The Magical Next Becomes the Medical Now* 2005 **111**: 284–9.

331

Cerebral palsy arising from events in labour

Julian Woolfson

The term 'cerebral palsy' represents a wide spectrum of neurological disability that includes brain damage or dysfunction as a result of genetic, biochemical, viral, and environmental causes. In addition, the fetus is uniquely susceptible to events in labour that cause it to become hypoxic or anoxic. These events include placental abruption, intermittently occluded or prolapsed umbilical cord, and uterine rupture. Most are unavoidable, but, rare as they may be, it is an essential part of obstetric care in labour to anticipate the unexpected and be prepared to deal with it.

However, there are other causes of intrapartum hypoxia, some of which are both avoidable and foreseeable. These include inappropriate obstetric or midwifery care; for example, uterine hyperstimulation as a result of injudicious use of oxytocin, or allowing the second stage of labour to go on for too long when the fetus is already showing signs of distress. Above all, at a time when intrapartum care is becoming increasingly complicated, with a decrease in the number of assisted vaginal deliveries as a result of deskilling and an increase in the number of women attempting a vaginal birth after a caesarean section (VBAC), the level of staffing – and the seniority of the personnel – in many hospitals is often inadequate for the 'new' obstetrics. Perhaps not surprisingly, this has resulted in a significant rise in the number of cases which end in litigation, whether the unfortunate outcome was avoidable or not.

The National Health Service (NHS) in the UK is vicariously liable for the actions of its medical, nursing, midwifery and ancillary staff and so all litigation in respect of negligence claims is technically against the NHS itself. This litigation is managed through the NHS Litigation Authority (NHSLA). According to data from the NHSLA, by 1995 there had been 12,000 medical negligence cases, with a net cost to the public of the UK of over £21 million. By 1998, only 3 years later, there had been over 16,000 claims against the NHS, of which almost 4000 were obstetric and gynaecologic cases. Cerebral palsy alone accounted for less than 10% of cases, but 38% of the total value; obstetrics and gynaecology in general accounted for 50% of the total value. By 2003, the annual NHS clinical negligence expenditure had risen from £1 million in 1974/75 (£6.3 million at 2002 prices) to £446 million in 2001/02.

Despite the creation within the NHSLA of the Central Negligence Scheme for Trusts (CNST), which sets and inspects risk management standards, the cost of litigation in all specialties rose significantly between 2004/5 (£502.9 million) and 2006/7(£600 million). Obstetrics alone accounted for around half of this.

The potential cost of open claims, that is to say claims which have not yet been resolved one way or another, are significantly higher. The value of open obstetric claims as at 31 March 2007 (£million) is shown in Table 30.1. The nature of these open obstetric claims against the NHS up to 31 March 2007 is shown in Table 30.2.

Many claims include allegations of negligence in respect of more than one of these categories. In all cases, however, the initial criterion for pursuing a claim is that the baby has developed cerebral palsy. Not all such cases will be related to the allegations made – the cerebral palsy may be due to other causes than mismanagement of the labour – but these are the starting points and, once started, the claims must be resolved by the Claimant (formerly known as the Plaintiff) withdrawing the claim, or the Defendant – the NHS, in most cases in the UK – making an admission of guilt, or resolving the case by negotiation (and the offer and acceptance of a reduced amount of

Best Practice in Labour and Delivery, ed. R. Warren and S. Arulkumaran. Published by Cambridge University Press.
© Cambridge University Press 2009.

Table 30.1 The potential value of open obstetric claims as at 31 March 2007 (£million).

Cerebral palsy	3296
Other brain damage	739
Erb's palsy	83
Developmental delay	77
Wrongful birth	33
Unnecessary pain	29
Others	23
Total	4280

Table 30.2 Open obstetric claims by cause as at 31 March 2007 (%).

Failure to respond to abnormal CTG	20.5
Failure to recognize complication	8.4
Failure to monitor, first stage of labour	8.0
Failure to monitor, second stage of labour	7.8
Failed or delayed diagnosis	7.7
Failed or delayed intervention	6.9
Application of excessive force	5.2
Other	35.5

money) without admitting liability or, in a very small number of cases, by going to court.

The legal process

For a claim to succeed, it is necessary for the Claimant to show two things. First, there must be a *breach of duty*, i.e. the care provided by the Defendant fell below a reasonable standard. Second, the Claimant must establish *causation*, i.e. it is necessary to show that the Claimant's damage was caused by that substandard care and that the damage would not have arisen but for the substandard care.

Establishing liability and causation rely on the evidence of experts in the appropriate fields. In a cerebral palsy claim there invariably will be an expert in obstetrics, an expert in midwifery (particularly in cases where the midwifery care is being criticized), an expert in neonatal care (to see whether any part of the damage may have been due to substandard resuscitation and/or neonatal care), a paediatric neurologist to establish the nature of the cerebral palsy and the

child's future needs, and a paediatric neuroradiologist to look at the CT and MRI imaging in order to determine the actual damage caused to the brain. Although both parties may occasionally agree to a single joint expert, particularly to consider causation, in the vast majority of cases there will be an obstetrician on each side.

The most important criteria for choosing an expert are first that (s)he must have been in active obstetric practice at the time of the child's birth and, second, that (s)he has no conflict of interest, that is to say they cannot have been involved in the clinical management and that they should not be related to or particularly close friends of the Defendant's doctors or midwives.

Types of cerebral palsy

Two principal types of cerebral palsy arise as a result of events in labour at term, although each case of cerebral palsy affects a child differently, and some have more than one form of cerebral palsy.

Spastic quadriplegic cerebral palsy is the commonest form of cerebral palsy and affects the body's ability to relax muscles, causing tightness and difficulties in movement. It is associated with parasagittal brain injury to the periventricular and subcortical white matter, which arises as a result of *prolonged partial hypoxia* during labour as a result of intermittent interruption to umbilical cord blood flow, maternal oxygenation or uterine blood flow for a period of at least an hour.

Dyskinetic or *athetoid* cerebral palsy affects the ability to control muscles, leading to involuntary and uncontrolled movements in the affected muscles. Children with this type of cerebral palsy have a disturbed sense of balance and depth perception, characterized by tremors or shaky movements. Dyskinetic cerebral palsy is associated with damage to the deep grey matter of the basal ganglia, and is usually the result of an acute-onset catastrophic reduction in fetoplacental perfusion and oxygenation when there is an umbilical cord prolapse or uterine rupture. It may also occur as a result of fetal acidaemia; for example, when the fetal anaerobic reserves have been exhausted. Sheep experiments and human observational data have shown that the fetus can withstand around 10–20 min of acute anoxia unscathed. If the asphyxia persists beyond 20 min, risk of fetal death increases, and beyond 30–35 min death is almost inevitable.

Unnecessary or inappropriate induction (e.g. for mildly raised blood pressure in a primigravida woman at term with a well-grown fetus) or augmentation of labour when the labour has progressed well until the second stage but then slows

↓

Prostaglandins and/or oxytocin used

↓

Induced or augmented labour is generally more painful than spontaneous labour

↓

Epidural more likely to be requested or offered

↓

CTG more likely to show fetal heart rate pattern abnormalities

↓

Shortage of midwives and/or unsupervised and inexperienced doctors physically present on the labour ward

↓

Failure to recognize when things are going wrong, either by 'standing back' and assessing the whole clinical situation or by recognizing that there is evidence of fetal or maternal distress

↓

Failure to act accordingly or in time

↓

Damaged mother/baby

Figure 30.1 The obstetric slippery slope

Cerebral palsy arising from events in labour

Inappropriate intervention in pregnancy and labour

There is no doubt that induction of labour has saved many lives, both maternal and fetal, and that augmentation of labour has significantly reduced the number of women that have been in labour for hours or days longer than they should have been. In this respect, the beneficial roles of drugs such as Syntocinon (oxytocin) and the various prostaglandins cannot be underestimated. However, they are powerful drugs and are capable of causing significant side effects when used inappropriately or incorrectly. These side effects include uterine hyperstimulation and, as a consequence of this, fetal hypoxia. It is – or should be – well known that oxytocic drugs such as Syntocinon must be used with particular caution when there is borderline cephalopelvic disproportion, secondary uterine inertia or pre-eclampsia. However, every year there are cases of fetal brain damage where the probable cause is inappropriate use of Syntocinon.

These generally come to light as part of the NHS complaints procedure or when the process of litigation is initiated. In some cases, the hyperstimulation and its effect on the fetal heart rate pattern have simply not been recognized or, worse, they have been recognized but ignored. In other cases, such is the enthusiasm for vaginal birth that caution has been over-ridden.

It is for all these reasons that induction and augmentation of labour should only be undertaken in appropriate circumstances, with the decisions being made by a doctor who is sufficiently experienced in obstetrics to understand the fundamental principles, risks and benefits of the intervention. All too often, however, the decision is not appropriately made and leads to the 'obstetric slippery slope' (Figure 30.1).

Failing to intervene in labour

(a) Failure to monitor the fetus appropriately

The fetal monitoring debate has run on for many years, as yet with no sign of universal agreement on whether and when to use a CTG rather than intermittent auscultation by means of Pinard stethoscope or

Table 30.3 Appropriate monitoring in an uncomplicated pregnancy [1].

For a woman who is healthy and has had an otherwise uncomplicated pregnancy, intermittent auscultation should be offered and recommended in labour to monitor fetal well-being.

[Recommendation grade A]

In the active stages of labour, intermittent auscultation should occur after a contraction, for a minimum of 60 s, and at least:
- every 15 min in the first stage
- every 5 min in the second stage.

[Recommendation grade B]

Continuous EFM should be offered and recommended in pregnancies previously monitored with intermittent auscultation:
- if there is evidence on auscultation of a baseline less than 110 bpm or greater than 160 bpm
- if there is evidence on auscultation of any decelerations
- if any intrapartum risk factors develop.

[Recommendation grade A]

Doppler-based technology. It is generally accepted that women with any of the traditional 'high-risk' indications should be monitored by means of continuous cardiotocography (CTG). These indications include induction or augmentation by means of oxytocin, a woman who has had a previous caesarean section and is now undergoing an attempt at vaginal birth (VBAC), twin pregnancies, women with preeclampsia or other medical problems, intrauterine growth restriction and, still in some units, breech presentation.

However, for those women classified as 'low risk', intermittent auscultation is considered to be sufficient. The recommendations set out in the Royal College of Obstetricians and Gynaecologists guideline 'The Use of Electronic Fetal Monitoring', published in 2001 and adopted by the UK National Institute for Clinical Excellence NICE) [1], are shown in Table 30.3. The Recommendation Grades are shown in Table 30.4.

All practising obstetricians and midwives know only too well that low-risk labours can and do become high risk, often quite quickly and without warning. In most cases, the change is recognized by an abnormal fetal heart rate pattern, detected by intermittent auscultation and managed appropriately, but in some cases it is not recognized until it is too late. This failure to recognize the change does not necessarily mean that the care was substandard, as there may be circumstances that are beyond control. These include the woman going to the toilet, rupturing her membranes spontaneously and the umbilical cord prolapsing, or when there is difficulty listening to the fetal

Table 30.4 Recommendation grades [1].

Grade	Requirements
A	Requires at least one randomized controlled trial as part of a body of literature of overall good quality and consistency addressing the specific recommendation
B	Requires the availability of well-conducted clinical studies but no randomized clinical trials on the topic of the recommendation
C	Requires evidence obtained from expert committee reports or opinions and/or clinical experience of respected authorities. Indicates an absence of directly applicable clinical studies of good quality

heart when the woman is distressed, moving about or on all-fours.

However, to these must be added those situations where there is inadequate staffing on the labour ward. As a result, a midwife may have to care for more than one woman at a time and, if there are emergencies requiring urgent intervention, there may not be sufficient numbers of adequately experienced medical staff. These situations, which are commoner than they should be, justifiably raise concerns about whether a CTG should be maintained in every labour, with a central monitoring station constantly manned by one or more experienced doctors or midwives.

The published guidelines are not always helpful. The perceived wisdom may be that intermittent auscultation is safe for low-risk women but, while the statistical analysis may indicate that it is safe, it does

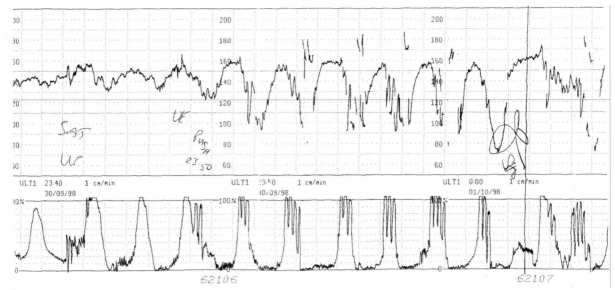

Figure 30.2 Second-stage CTG

not take into account the impact of the *consequences*, as opposed to the *probability*, of an adverse event occurring. For example, the risks of a spontaneous occult umbilical cord prolapse, or a small abruption, may be statistically low, but the consequences for the woman and her fetus may be grave if the event happens. In these situations, and usually with the advantage of hindsight, it is often asked why all labouring women are not monitored continuously by CTG, particularly when (again with hindsight) the problem would have been identified quickly.

This chapter is not the appropriate place to extend this debate, but one thing is certain: if a child who had been monitored during labour by means of intermittent auscultation is unexpectedly born asphyxiated and then goes on to develop cerebral palsy, which is confirmed to have arisen as a result of that asphyxia, it is more likely than not that litigation will follow. The allegations will include failure to carry out the intermittent auscultation properly (even if there is documentation in the records that intermittent auscultation was performed), failure to perform and maintain a CTG and, especially in today's world of rights, failure to give the woman the choice of whether to have continuous fetal monitoring from the outset. She would, of course, have to convince the court that she would have chosen to have continuous monitoring by CTG but, in resolving this, the court would have to consider her evidence against

that of the midwives or doctors with regard to what was said to whom, and when. Given that the woman is far more likely to remember what was said to her than the midwives or doctors, who care for many women, are likely to remember, it would not be surprising if a court found in her favour.

(b) Failure to respond to an abnormal CTG

Around 20% of all open obstetric claims (Table 30.2) concern failure to respond to an abnormal CTG. In theory, a failure such as this should never occur but, regrettably, it does. Sometimes the failure is that the response is delayed; in others, however, the failure arises because the doctor or midwife is too inexperienced to recognize that the fetal heart rate pattern is abnormal and that a response is needed.

One of the commonest such instances concerns the fetal heart rate pattern in the second stage of labour. Here, the fetal heart rate pattern can and frequently does show both early and late decelerations. An example is shown in Figure 30.2.

Providing that there is progress, with good descent of the fetal head to the point when it is easily visible, delivery can be anticipated quite quickly and so no intervention is required. In this particular case, however, which comes from the author's medico-legal files, the doctor, an SHO, wrote that the pattern 'was normal for the second stage of labour', when in fact what he should have said was that this sort of pattern

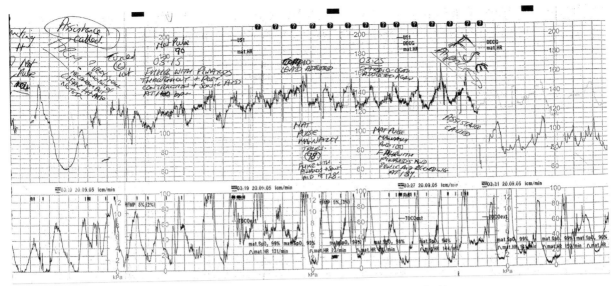

Figure 30.3 CTG recording the fetal heart rate, then the maternal heart rate, then back to the fetal heart rate

is *common* in the second stage of labour. The two are very different in terms of their role in interpreting the whole clinical picture but, having been told by the doctor that the pattern was 'normal', the midwife (who was also quite junior), the labouring woman and her partner were reassured and no action was taken. An episiotomy would have sufficed to achieve delivery sooner, but the labouring woman had expressed her strong desire not to have an episiotomy and so one was not performed. The baby eventually delivered normally, with a small vaginal tear, but he was in very poor condition, with Apgar scores of 0 and 1 at 1 and 5 min and cord pH of 6.9 (arterial) and 7.1 (venous). He required intensive resuscitation, including transfer to the Special Care Baby Unit, where he went on to develop signs of hypoxic–ischaemic encephalopathy (HIE).

He subsequently went on to develop athetoid cerebral palsy, which was confirmed on MRI to have been due to a circulatory collapse and profound cerebral hypoxia in the last few minutes before his birth. Litigation was commenced, but as the experts instructed by solicitors on both sides agreed that it was substandard care not to have at least performed an episiotomy or a simple lift-out forceps, and that delivery only 10 min earlier would have avoided his cerebral palsy, liability and causation were admitted and due compensation awarded.

A less common occurrence, frequently not recognized, is that the CTG reflects the labouring woman's

heart rate rather than that of the fetus. This only occurs when the fetal heart signal is being detected by an ultrasound transducer as opposed to a fetal scalp electrode and usually when the woman's position is changed. An example of this is shown in Figure 30.3.

Recognizing that the CTG is recording the maternal pulse relies on two things: first, the heart rate trace changes suddenly when the labouring woman is turned and, second, the maternal heart rate rises during a contraction whereas the fetal heart rate falls during the contraction (early deceleration) or after it (late deceleration). In the example shown in Figure 30.3, the change from fetal heart rate pattern to maternal heart rate occurs at around the time that the midwife calls for assistance and then changes the woman's position. It is clear from the annotations that the midwife suspected that the CTG might be recording the maternal heart rate and so she counted the maternal pulse, which she initially would have found reassuring.

However, after around 10 min more she appears to have recognized that what she believed was the fetal heart rate pattern (but was in fact the maternal heart rate) was showing what appeared to be late decelerations. At this point assistance was again requested and a fetal scalp electrode applied. The true fetal heart rate pattern, a bradycardia, was recognized and an emergency caesarean section performed. There was no undue delay, but by the time the baby was delivered there had been over 20 min of misleading information on the CTG, resulting in the true fetal heart rate pattern being obscured for long enough for the baby to become hypoxic and ultimately to go on to develop cerebral palsy. The issue in this case, should it come to litigation, would be whether there should have been a fetal scalp electrode earlier and failure of recognition of the maternal heart rate.

Failure to recognize complication

'Complication' in this context covers a wide range of possible events, including developing cephalopelvic disproportion, uterine hyperstimulation, uterine scar rupture in women undergoing VBAC, worsening pre-eclampsia, and delay in the first or second stage despite adequate uterine contractions. Properly managed, the chances of the fetus sustaining brain damage and subsequently developing cerebral palsy are small. However, when not properly managed the converse is true and, furthermore, if the child does develop cerebral palsy, then the injured child will probably have grounds for litigation.

Although they should have learned something about these potential complications, the combination of reduced exposure to acute obstetrics that has resulted from the reduction (particularly in UK medical schools) in the amount of time spent on the labour ward and the shortened hours now worked under the European Working Time Directive means that many junior doctors will be placed in positions of responsibility without sufficient understanding and experience to recognize complications. The abolition of the senior registrar grade in the 1990s removed at a stroke the senior labour ward cover, leaving a vacuum of senior, experienced presence on the labour wards which is only now beginning to be addressed by reconfiguration of services and increased consultant presence on the labour wards.

The pressure on the midwifery staff is correspondingly greater, particularly for those midwives in stand-alone midwifery units. Many of these units are geographically distant from tertiary (consultant) units and so there is an additional burden on the midwives, who must be able to not only recognize that the labour is becoming complicated, but must do so at a much earlier stage in order to allow sufficient time for the labouring woman to be transferred. In most cases they are successful, but when the complication arises too quickly, or is not recognized and the labouring

woman not transferred in time, an adverse outcome for the fetus will often result in litigation.

This will usually give rise to multiple issues, including informed consent about the risks of delivering in a maternity unit distant from medical assistance, the distance from the tertiary unit, the role of the ambulance services, and alleged delay in recognizing that a transfer might be necessary. There is also pressure on the tertiary centre, not least because if the fetus is stillborn or is born alive but goes on to develop cerebral palsy, the outcome is recorded against the place of delivery – in such cases the tertiary centre – rather than the place of delivery originally intended.

Application of excessive force

Every obstetrician, whether a trainee or a consultant, should be aware of the immortal words of Professor Sir Norman Jeffcoate, published in the *British Medical Journal* in 1953:

> It is in the case in which forceps have been applied, and in which unexpected difficulties are encountered, that tragedy may occur. Tragedy results from a train of human reactions, which have personal pride and prestige as their basis. We have all experienced them. The unexpected resistance to delivery is followed by a stronger pull and then removal of the blades to confirm the position of the foetal head. Further traction with little effect brings to mind the vision of a stillbirth. Now is the time to stop, but the patient and her relatives have been prepared for forceps delivery, not Caesarean section. Moreover, it requires much courage to admit to assistants, midwives and the onlookers that a mistake has been made and that vaginal delivery is not safe. The remote possibility of successful delivery spurs the obstetrician to renewed and more frantic efforts. Now he is seized with dread, casts caution to the wind, and ultimately he may or may not succeed in extracting a mangled foetus, the mother also being injured in one way or another.
>
> The situation is more dangerous if some progress is made than if the passage of the foetal head is completely obstructed. In the former case, the foetal head is crowded more and more into an ever decreasing pelvic diameter, with inevitable injury: in the latter it can come to no harm except from the pressure of the forceps themselves.
>
> One of the fears which drive the obstetrician to make frantic efforts is that the case may become one of 'failed forceps' – a label which, by tradition, involves everyone concerned with ignominy, and which itself can be responsible for bad obstetrics. How much better it would be if it were generally recognised that even the best exponents can make a mistake occasionally, and that failure to deliver with forceps is not so great a sin as a failure

to recognise defeat at an early stage. If the forceps are applied skilfully, no harm comes to the baby or to the mother, provided the attempts at extraction are discontinued immediately it becomes clear that there is greater difficulty than anticipated. All that is necessary is to have the courage to proceed to Caesarean section before the life of the foetus is jeopardised.

The same principles apply to the use of the ventouse, which in inexperienced hands (and particularly when used in the face of more disproportion than might have been recognized) may be just as dangerous.

Whichever instrument is chosen, if it is used inexpertly there can be extensive damage to the fetal head, resulting in intracerebral or intraventricular haemorrhage which, in turn, can cause cerebral palsy. It is therefore essential that trainee obstetricians are properly instructed in the use of forceps and the ventouse. They should also be supervised by a senior, more experienced obstetrician until he or she is satisfied that the trainee has sufficient dexterity and understanding of the fetal and maternal anatomy to be able to perform assisted vaginal deliveries unsupervised.

Failed or delayed diagnosis

It is commonly said – and probably true – that diagnoses are easiest made with hindsight. The reality, however, is that a diagnosis can and should be made in the majority of situations providing that the midwifery and medical staff are aware of what can go wrong, that they are suitably trained and that there are sufficient numbers of them available on the labour ward. The commonest 'failed' diagnoses are when a breech presentation is missed; when there is cephalo-pelvic disproportion present either as a result of a malposition or 'true' disproportion; when there is insufficient attention to the labouring woman's temperature, pulse and blood pressure; and, of course, when there are fetal heart rate changes that warrant further investigation or delivery.

The value of having senior, experienced midwives and obstetricians present on the labour ward cannot be overemphasized. Such presence will provide the less experienced staff with someone to whom they can quickly turn when they are uncertain of the clinical situation. However, there is an equally important role for the senior staff, namely being physically present and available for discussion, teaching, support and encouragement. Proper handover ward rounds for midwives and doctors *together* are an essential part of these processes, and are even more useful when they are led by senior midwives and obstetricians. Discussion of each woman's labour will include considering the potential pitfalls and problems, so that if/when a problem arises the less experienced staff will not only recognize it but will know what action to take.

Over the last few years it has become common practice in the UK to have regular 'drills' for situations such as shoulder dystocia, eclampsia, major haemorrhage and fetal distress. These drills have proven to be very useful and often life-saving. However, they are often held in isolation, away from the labour ward, when they would be best held on the labour ward and associated with teaching and retrospective case reviews. Again, the presence of senior midwives and obstetricians at these times is invaluable, not only because of their expertise, but because they set an important precedent: they are there, where they are needed. When there are medical students present, they should be part of the 'team' and should be encouraged to watch and assist in the management of labour.

Failed or delayed intervention

Here, the clinical situation has been recognized, but either no action is taken, or the action is taken but not soon enough. The commonest examples are delay in achieving delivery for fetal distress, whether by means of forceps or ventouse, or emergency caesarean section.

While it is a straightforward matter to record the time taken from decision to delivery, it is far more difficult to say whether the time taken was reasonable, mainly because there is no good 'yardstick' to set a standard. There have been many observational studies on decision–delivery times, not all of which agree with each other. Nevertheless, 30 min has been adopted as an audit standard, although the basis for arriving at this time is 'not clear, logical or evidence based' [2]. Nor is it achievable on a regular basis [3], or is there evidence that it makes a difference to the outcome other than that there is a non-significant trend to lower umbilical cord artery pH in babies delivered after 30 min by caesarean section [4]. However, the real difficulty in relying on a fixed time arises because there are two different types of fetal distress: *chronic* or *prolonged partial hypoxia* and *acute-onset hypoxia*. The urgency to deliver in the former is less than the latter.

The commonest causes of delay are transfer from the labour ward room to the operating theatre, the arrival of the anaesthetist and operating department assistant (ODA), and administering an appropriate anaesthetic. In most hospitals, these delays can be reduced to a degree, but there is little that can be done when, say, two emergency caesarean sections have to be done at around the same time.

Conclusions

It is impossible to underestimate the effects on a family of a child with cerebral palsy. Eventually, most families find their own ways of coping, particularly when the cerebral palsy was caused by something that was random, unpredictable and beyond anyone's control. But when the cerebral palsy arises as a result of events in labour, whether the labour is conducted at home, in a midwifery-led stand-alone unit, or a well-equipped consultant unit, there is an inevitable sense of grievance and anger that the staff in whom they trusted failed to avoid the damage to the baby. If the event was unpredictable, they will feel that the staff could and should have at least recognized what was happening and acted accordingly and in good time. However, if the event was predictable but unrecognized or, worse, actually caused by something that should (or should not) have been done, then their grievance and anger are far greater.

Understandably, the family will want to know in detail what happened, and why, and whether it was someone's fault and, if so, whose fault it was. In most cases, explanations are given and, where appropriate, apologies are offered; in the majority of these, such is the parents' distress and anger that there is disbelief and distrust. Attempted litigation will usually follow for a variety of reasons, including wanting to 'find out the truth', avoiding the same thing happening to someone else and, where necessary, to provide support for the disabled child.

The parents and family are not the only ones who suffer, although theirs is by far the greatest and most prolonged suffering. Although in the UK it is the NHS that pays, the doctors and midwives have to give evidence and face up to the possibility that they were responsible, singly or collectively, for what happened. Human nature being what it is, even if they are not guilty of negligence, many are so traumatized by the experience that they leave their professions, and often discourage others from joining those professions.

However, the most serious problem facing labour wards at the present is the lack of senior staff – medical and midwifery – present on the labour wards at all times. It is not sufficient for senior midwifery and medical staff to only 'be available' when rostered for labour ward duties: they should be physically present on the labour ward, taking teaching ward rounds and always supervising, training and teaching. This way, the more junior midwifery and medical staff can learn constantly.

Both the Royal College of Obstetricians and Gynaecologists (RCOG) and the CNST have published detailed guidelines and standards for staffing the labour ward. These could not be clearer: there should be consultant *presence* on the labour ward, not just cover. It is acknowledged that few maternity units can achieve this immediately, but a start should be made, initially by ensuring that when a consultant has a labour ward session it means that the consultant is on the labour ward, not in an office or generally around the hospital. The same must apply to senior midwives, who should also be present on the labour ward for their dedicated midwifery sessions, and not in an office or a meeting elsewhere.

Although implanting this policy will almost certainly reduce the number of inappropriate interventions, it will not prevent emergencies from occurring. But when they do arise, there will be experienced, senior staff available to deal with them. It would be naïve to say that there will never be any more cases of cerebral palsy as a result of events in labour, but the number will – and must – fall.

References

1. RCOG. Evidence-based Guideline Number 8, May 2001.
2. James J. Caesarean section for fetal distress. Editorial. *Br Med J* 2001; **322**: 1316–7.
3. Tuffnell D J, Wilkinson K, Berseford N. Interval between decision and delivery by caesarean section – are current standards achievable? *Br Med J* 2001; **322**: 1330–3.
4. Mackenzie I Z, Cooke I. Prospective 12 month study of 30 minutes decision to delivery intervals for emergency Caesarean section. *Br Med J* 2001; **322**: 1334–5.

Objective Structured Assessment of Technical Skills (OSATS) in obstetrics

S. M. Whitten and M. J. Blott

Background

The acquisition of technical competence in surgical procedures within obstetrics and gynaecology relied for many years upon the traditional model of 'see one, do one, teach one', with the trainee undertaking large numbers of procedures over a period of training which might extend for 7 years or more, working well in excess of 100 h a week. Trainees would often work for extended periods of time with a small number of trainers, thus allowing some degree of continuity to the process of assessment of practice. However, assessment of competence would be by means of unstructured observation by the trainer, in a subjective fashion, without a clear format and within an unspecified timeframe. Such methods of assessment are known to have poor test–retest and interobserver reliability [1]. Within the UK, the move towards reducing junior doctor working hours as part of the European Working Time Directive has seen a reduction in the total surgical training time from 30,000 to 6000 h [2], with a consequent reduction in the numbers of procedures actually undertaken as a junior doctor [3,4]. Further to this, the need to reduce working hours has seen the implementation of shift working patterns [5], with a consequent loss of the traditional firm structure and its ongoing high-intensity contact with individual trainers.

These changes in working patterns mean that for many trainees, sporadic contact with a large number of different trainers has become the norm. Assessment of competence in an individual procedure by an individual trainer might occur only occasionally within any given training post, depending on the working pattern and number of trainees and trainers within the training unit. The need for a valid formal assessment tool with good interobserver reliability was clearly needed if the challenges to achieving competency within this new training environment were to be overcome.

OSATS development within the Specialty Training Curriculum

Surgical training in the United States has involved a clinical skills laboratory assessment process for a number of years, albeit within a working environment which still involves a large number of training hours as a junior doctor. This objective structured method of assessment is used to assess a variety of specific surgical techniques including hysteroscopy, episiotomy repair, laparoscopic suturing and open bladder neck suspension [6–8]. Formalizing assessment in this way has been shown to have good construct validity and interrater reliability [6–10]. This method of assessment takes place in a 'dry' setting, away from the clinical environment, and thus does not allow for the inclusion of assessment of the overall clinical situation or decision-making skills that are important aspects within an individual's development of a competent practitioner. Furthermore, these methods require the presence of a dry laboratory setting with special equipment, and can be time-consuming and expensive. However, Winckel et al. have also demonstrated that a similar format of objective structured assessment could be developed for use in the operating theatre environment, with good construct validity and interrater reliability [11].

The development of the OSATS for use within obstetrics and gynaecology training has aimed to

---

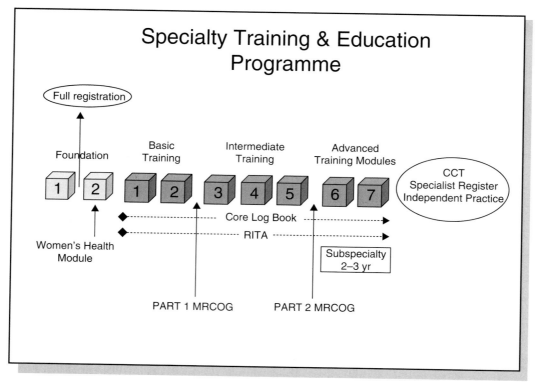

Figure 31.1 Specialty training in obstetrics and gynaecology

incorporate the structured format of technical skills assessment described above into the clinical environment, allowing this reliable method of assessment to be incorporated into a real-life setting, and to form part of the assessment process for determining competency of the trainee at all stages of training within the Specialty Training Curriculum.

The Royal College of Obstetricians and Gynaecologists implemented the current Specialty Training Curriculum in August 2007 as part of the implementation of the Modernising Medical Careers programme [12]. The curriculum is competency-based, with an anticipated training time of seven years to achieve competency as a fully independent practitioner. The curriculum is divided into three phases: basic, intermediate, and advanced training, with specific targets for each level framed in a modular programme of training (Figure 31.1). Basic training incorporates the first two years of specialty training, and requires the trainee to demonstrate, amongst other targets of training, technical competence in a number of surgical procedures, before being able to

progress to the next level of training [13]. Trainees will usually spend a year in each training unit within a defined region of training, and would be expected to demonstrate their continued competency for these key surgical procedures, alongside development of more complex technical and clinical skills as their training progresses.

OSATS format

The surgical procedures which are subject to assessment by OSATS as part of Basic Specialty Training are detailed below. Each is a commonly encountered and fundamental procedure within the clinical working environment of obstetrics and gynaecology within the UK. Trainees entering intermediate training would be expected to be competent in all listed procedures in order for them to work at a higher level of training, both in terms of further developing their own clinical competences and in time, in supervising their junior colleagues.

OSATS	(O = obstetrics; G = gynaecology)
• Fetal blood sampling	O
• Manual removal of the placenta	O
• Opening and closing the abdomen	O/G
• Operative vaginal delivery	O
• Caesarean section	O
• Perineal repair	O
• Diagnostic laparoscopy	G
• Diagnostic hysteroscopy	G
• Uterine evacuation	G

Each OSATS comprises two parts (See Figure 31.2).
1. a specific checklist of individual procedural steps,
2. an objective assessment of generic, transferable technical skills

The first part is judged by assessing each specific motor skill in combination with a cognitive function to produce a specific 'action'. Each action must be completed as part of the procedure. For each individual action, the trainee is judged to be either 'able to perform independently' or 'in need of help'.

The second part of the form requires the assessor to judge whether the trainee has demonstrated ability and competence at each of the seven generic domains common to all of the OSATS procedures, on a three-part structure – not able, some ability but needing development, and fully able.

Generic technical skills assessment domains

- Respect for tissue.
- Time, motion and flow of operation and forward planning.
- Knowledge and handling of instruments.
- Suturing and knotting skills as appropriate for the procedure.
- Technical use of assistants and relations with patient and the surgical team.
- Insight/attitude.
- Documentation of procedures.

The design of the OSATS form is spread over just two pages, incorporating space for the trainee to enter details of the level of complexity of each case, and for the assessor to enter feedback points for the further development of competence. The form is designed to allow the assessor to interpret the whole procedure as a series of specific domains, thus allowing the assessment to be objective and to enable specific areas for development to be pinpointed.

Trainees are advised to wait until they have undertaken each procedure a number of times before requesting a formal OSATS assessment. For an individual trainee, the portfolio of training documents progress through training, and this should incorporate evidence of progression at surgical skills as defined by the OSATS procedures. The trainee should be aware that, whilst full competence will be required to progress into intermediate training, demonstration of progression is inherent in the process of assessment of basic training, and it would be expected that each trainee will have undergone a number of OSATS assessments which are not fully 'signed off' before they are able to achieve full competency at each procedure. These should all be kept as part of the training portfolio. Educational supervisors will look for this evidence of progression as part of overall educational progress within the training programme.

Before undertaking an OSATS assessment, the trainee should feel able to perform the procedure competently under direct supervision and to have demonstrated this on several occasions before the first OSATS assessment. They should then request a formal assessment from a supervising clinical trainer. The trainee undertakes the procedure under direct observation and supervision by an assessor, who should complete the OSATS form with the trainee directly after completion of the procedure in order to provide an immediate source of feedback. Each area of the procedure should be assessed and documented as described above. The trainee and assessor then both sign and date the form once all the points have been discussed. A record of the date that each OSATS is signed off as completed in full should then be entered in the relevant section of the logbook module.

Trainees will proceed at different rates and the competency levels are the minimum that must be achieved prior to moving to the next stage of training. The OSATS form may be used to assess technical skills at differing levels of complexity; for example,

343

OPERATIVE VAGINAL DELIVERY

Trainee Name:		StR Year:		Date:	
Assessor Name:		Post:			
Clinical details of complexity/ difficulty of case **Instrument used:**					

	Performed independently	Needs help
	PLEASE TICK RELEVANT BOX	
Items under observation: opening		
Ensure patient and accompanying partner understand procedure		
Appropriate preoperative preparation: adequate analgesia, bladder empty		
Examination: engagement, position, station, caput, moulding, descent with contraction, pelvic size and shape		
Decision making: choice of instrument		
Correct assembly and checking of equipment		
Correct application of instrument		
Appropriate direction, force and timing of pull. Ensures head descends with traction		
Appropriate alteration of traction with delivery of head		
Protects perineum and assess need for episiotomy		
Checks for cord. Correct delivery of shoulders and body		
Delivery of placenta and membranes		
Checks for uterine laxity and vaginal trauma		
Estimated blood loss and manages blood loss		
Appropriate use of team		
Awareness of maternal and fetal well-being throughouts		
Comments:		

Examples of minimum levels of complexity for each stage of training

Basic Training — Uncomplicated. Non rotational
Intermediate Training — Rotational ventouse
Advanced — Rotational forceps/ventouse in theatre

Both sides of this form to be completed and signed

Figure 31.2 Example OSATS – operative vaginal delivery

GENERIC TECHNICAL SKILLS ASSESSMENT

Assessor, please ring the candidate's performance for each of the following factors:

Respect for tissue	Frequently used unnecessary force on tissue or caused damage by inappropriate use of instruments.	Careful handling of tissue but occasionally causes inadvertent damage.	Consistently handled tissues appropriately with minimal damage.
Time, motion and flow of operation and forward planning	Many unnecessary moves. Frequently stopped operating or needed to discuss next move.	Makes reasonable progress but some unnecessary moves. Sound knowledge of operation but slightly disjointed at times.	Economy of movement and maximum efficiency. Obviously planned course of operation with effortless flow from one move to the next.
Knowledge and handling of instruments	Lack of knowledge of instruments.	Competent use of instruments but occasionally awkward or tentative.	Obvious familiarity with instruments.
Suturing and knotting skills as appropriate for the procedure	Placed sutures inaccurately or tied knots insecurely and lacked attention to safety.	Knotting and suturing usually reliable but sometimes awkward.	Consistently placed sutures accurately with appropriate and secure knots and with proper attention to safety.
Technical use of assistants **Relations with patient and the surgical team**	Consistently placed assistants poorly or failed to use assistants. Communicated poorly or frequently showed lack of awareness of the needs of the patient and/or the professional team.	Appropriate use of assistant most of the time. Reasonable communication and awareness of the needs of the patient and/or of the professional team.	Strategically used assistants to the best advantage at all times. Consistently communicated and acted with awareness of the needs of the patient and/or of the professional team.
Insight/attitude	Poor understanding of areas of weakness.	Some understanding of areas of weakness.	Fully understands areas of weakness.
Documentation of procedures	Limited documentation, poorly written.	Adequate documentation but with some omissions or areas that need elaborating.	Comprehensive legible documentation, indicating findings, procedure and postoperative management.

Based on the checklist and the Generic Technical Skills Assessment, Dr .... has achieved/failed*
to achieve the OSAT competency

Needs further help with: * * *Date* *Signed (trainer)* *Signed (trainee)*	Competent to perform the entire procedure without the need for supervision Date Signed Signed

Delete where applicable, and date and sign the relevant box

Figure 31.2 (cont.)

the caesarean section OSATS may be used for assessing competency for a simple caesarean section or a complex caesarean section. The level of complexity should be indicated on the assessment form.

OSATS requirements

In order for the OSATS process to be formalized further within the curriculum, several key requirements have been determined by the Specialty Education and Assessment Committee of the RCOG to guide trainees undertaking specialty training, and their trainers.

- Two different assessors must be used for each type of OSATS procedure. The same assessor must not be used for all OSATS and a consultant must do at least one OSATS.
- The generic technical skills, not all of which will be relevant to every OSATS, will form an important part of the assessment process. It is anticipated that, to pass the OSATS, the majority of competences must be ringed in the middle or to the right of the generic skills assessment list. However, to be signed off for independent practice, the trainee must have the generic skill 'fully understands areas of weakness' within the generic skill of insight/attitude consistently ringed.
- Before the competences can be signed off in the logbook, each OSATS must have been successfully completed (i.e. every box ticked for independent practice) on at least **five** separate occasions.
- These numbers are indicative, such that where a trainer is satisfied that a trainee is competent, then it is entirely appropriate for them to sign off that competence recognizing that the number suggested in the curriculum is a guideline and benchmark for the majority.
- Trainees and trainers will need to provide evidence in support of competences signed off if the minimum number of OSATS has not been achieved.
- Once the trainee has been signed up for independent practice, it is recommended that, to demonstrate continued competency in an area, that the trainee undergoes an annual OSATS assessment.

OSATS in practice

Do OSATS work and are they practical in today's clinical environment? Both of these questions were

subject to intense scrutiny as part of the development of appropriate and fit-for-purpose assessment tools for the Specialty Training Curriculum. Trainees and trainers who were part of the consultation groups for development of the curriculum highlighted that any new assessment method would have to be fit for purpose and practicable in a busy working environment. Little research on OSATS in the clinical environment existed prior to their development for use within obstetrics and gynaecology; however, the evidence from 'dry' clinical skills laboratory settings as described earlier was encouraging, together with the feedback from development of OSATS-like assessments in the surgical operating environment by Winckel et al. [11]. With any new method of assessment, both applicability and familiarity with the process are likely to be important aspects to the overall success of the method in practical terms. In terms of user perception of usefulness, helpful data can be gained from assessment of the Objective Structured Assessment of Clinical Skills (OSCE) for medical students, now part of the assessment process in most medical schools in the UK. Zyromski et al. identified that 97% of students found the OSCE useful, and that students undergoing OSCE assessments were more likely to perceive the OSCEs' usefulness than those junior doctors who had not had direct experience of its application [14]. Pierre et al. found that 70% of students perceived the OSCE as a fair method of assessment [15].

Bodle et al. undertook a detailed investigation of trainee and trainer perceptions of the value and validity of OSATS for the assessment of surgical skills in the theatre environment as part of an RCOG-commissioned study during the development of the postgraduate training portfolio [16]. During a six-month period from October 2005 to March 2006 (during the development of plans for postgraduate training within the new curriculum), two deaneries piloted OSATS use for obstetrics and gynaecology (Yorkshire and Bristol). OSATS forms for two gynaecological procedures and four obstetric procedures, together with two feedback questionnaires – one for the assessee, one for the assessor – were distributed to all trainees and trainers. No additional training in the use of the OSATS forms was given. Feedback questionnaires using a five-point Likert scale asked participants to express agreement or disagreement with statements pertaining to OSATS in a number of domains.

Within this study, 38 trainees and 16 trainers provided feedback on the OSATS forms, completing 119 questionnaires in total. In terms of value of the OSATS as an assessment tool, 85% of trainee and 76% of trainer responses agreed or strongly agreed that OSATS would improve trainees' surgical skills. Stronger agreement was associated with the more junior grades, perhaps reflecting these trainees' familiarity with objective methods of assessment as part of current medical school assessment. Face validity was deemed to be good, with 80% of trainee and 76% of trainer responses agreeing or strongly agreeing with the ability of OSATS to assess surgical skills. Trainees differed from trainers in their perception of the practical application of OSATS, with 26% of trainee and 46% of trainer responses agreeing or strongly agreeing that it would be time-consuming and add to the burden of administrative work. However, in terms of the potential for OSATS to be applied as part of training on a formal basis, 76% of trainee and trainer responses agreed or strongly agreed that OSATS should become part of the annual assessment process for trainees.

The future

The use of OSATS as an assessment tool within obstetrics and gynaecology remains a developing area of work. At the time of writing, the new RCOG Specialty Training Curriculum has been in place for just over a year. Feedback from trainees and trainers is sought on a regular basis by means of direct enquiry at the time of Annual Assessment of Competency Progress, within trainee and trainer evaluation surveys, and through direct feedback and discussion within and between the Deanery Specialty Training Committees and the RCOG. Anecdotal experience within our own training unit suggests that effective completion of the OSATS form, carried out promptly at the end of an assessed procedure, should usually take no longer than 5–10 min. The structure of the forms to allow the same procedure to be assessed by multiple assessors should allow the trainee to acquire a developing portfolio of evidence as to their own progression of competency. In order for junior trainees to achieve this evidence, it is important that all those who are themselves competent practitioners for each skill (at both consultant and trainee level) commit to engagement with the process and support their trainees in the process of assessment and

feedback. As we move towards the conclusion of the reduction of junior doctors' hours programme within the European Working Time Directive, it will be important to continually assess the development of OSATS, alongside other forms of assessment, in determining how and when trainees progress through the training pathways on their way to achieving completion of training.

References

1. Reznick R K. Teaching and testing surgical skills. *Am J Surg* 1993; **165**: 358–61.

2. Chikwe J, de Souza A C, Pepper J R. No time to train surgeons. *Br Med J* 2004; **328**: 418–9.

3. Skidmore F D. Junior surgeons are becoming deskilled as a result of Calman proposals. *Br Med J* 1997; **314**: 1281.

4. Morris-Stiff G, Ball E, Torkington J, Foster M E, Lewis M H, Havard T J. Registrar operating experience over a 15-year period: more, less or more or less the same? *Surgeon J Roy Coll Surg Edinburgh & Ireland* 2004; **2**: 161–4.

5. Department of Health. *A Compendium of Solutions to Implementing the European Working Time Directive for Doctors in Training from August 2004.* London: HMSO, 2004.

6. Goff B A, Nielsen P E, Lentz G M, *et al.* Surgical skills assessment: a blinded examination of obstetrics and gynecology residents. *Am J Obstet Gynecol* 2002; **186**: 613–7.

7. Nielsen P E, Foglia L M, Mandel L S, Chow G E. Objective structured assessment of technical skills for episiotomy repair. *Am J Obstet Gynecol* 2003; **189**: 1257–60.

8. VanBloricom A L, Goff B A, Chinn M, Icasiano M M, Nielsen P, Mandel L. A new curriculum for hysteroscopy training as demonstrated by an objective structured assessment of technical skills (OSATS). *Am J Obstet Gynecol* 2005; **193**(5); 1856–65.

9. Swift S E, Carter J F. Institution and validation of an observed structured assessment of technical skills (OSATS) for obstetrics and gynaecology residents and faculty. *Am J Obstet Gynecol* 2006; **195**(2): 617–21.

10. Lentz G M, Mandel L S, Goff B A. A six-year study of surgical teaching and skills evaluation for obstetric/gynecologic residents in porcine and inanimate surgical models. *Am J Obstet Gynecol* 2005; **193**(6); 2056–61.

11. Winckel C P, Reznick R K, Cohen R, Taylor B. Reliability and construct validity of a structured technical skills assessment form. *Am J Surg* 1994; **167**: 423–7.

12. Department of Health. *Modernising Medical Careers. Operational Framework for Foundation Training.* London: HMSO, 2005.

13. RCOG (Royal College of Obstetrics & Gynaecology). *Report of the Basic Specialty Training Working Party in Obstetrics and Gynaecology.* London: RCOG Press, 2006.

14. Zyromski N J, Staren E D, Merrick H W. Surgery residents' perception of the Objective Structured Clinical Examination (OSCE). *Curr Surg* 2003; **60**: 533–7.

15. Pierre R B, Wierenga A, Barton M, Branday J M, Christie C D. Student evaluation of an OSCE in paediatrics at the University of the West Indies, Jamaica. *BMC Med Educ* 2004; **4**: 22.

16. Bodle J F, Kaufmann S J, Bisson D, Nathanson B, Binney D M. Value and face validity of objective structured assessment of technical skills (OSATS) for work based assessment of surgical skills in obstetrics and gynaecology. *Med Teach* 2008; **30**: 212–6.

Appendix

Maternity Dashboard : Clinical Performance and Governance Score Card

Ensure high quality safe care. Tool for Commissioners, Providers, Consumers and Regulators

This Appendix must be read in conjunction with Good Practice No. 7: *Maternity Dashboard: Clinical Performance and Governance Score Card*. It is an example card used by a London teaching hospital. (For best results, please print pages 7 and 8 on A3 paper as a double-page spread).

Category		Goal	Red Flag	Measure	Comment	Data Source	JAN	FEB	MAR	APR	MAY	JUNE	JULY	AUG	SEPT	OCT COMMENTS / ACTION THIS MONTH
Activity	**Organisation** Number ethnic group reps on Labour Ward Forum	4 reps	<2	Minutes	Aim for 4 but not guaranteed reps available – review 14ly	DATEX	2	2	2	2	2	2	2	2	1	
	Births Benchmarked to 5000 per annum	5000 (420)	>450	Births	If >900 over 2 month period, bookings to be capped	DATEX	379	363	426	431	451	418	426	427	420	Not all the booked patients are likely to deliver at SGH
	Scheduled Bookings Bookings (1st visit) Scheduled	5405 (450)	>500	Bookings (1st visit)	Tolerance 15%	DATEX	361	379	422	427	447	491	516	436	422	
	Instl Vag. Del. Ventouse & forceps	10–15%	<5% or >20%	Instl. Vag D'Birth	Tolerance 15%	DATEX	11.8	7.6	10.8	10.2	11.2	11.2	12.8	12.7	14.5	
	C-Section Total rate (planned & unscheduled)	<23%	>25%	C-section/Birth	If >30% then cap & refer to other provider	DATEX	25.5	23.2	23.4	22.5	23.5	19.3	21.7	25.14	23.6	Resident consultant cover was increased to 60 hours per week
Workforce	**Staffing levels** Weekly hours of consultant cover on labour ward	>60 hours	<44 hours	Hours	Per week	Labour Suite off-duty				43		43	56	46	54	
	Midwife/birth ratio	1:30	>1:40	W'TE/births		HCM	1:33	1:35	1:3	1:54	1:36	1:35	1:3	1:3		Under review
	Supervisor to midwife ratio	<1:15	>1:20			HCM	1:17	1:19	1:18	1:18	1:16	1:16	1:10	1:17		Under review
	Ed & training Prog : attendance	>90%	<90%		Review 6 monthly		90%								100%	100% New staff attended Skills & Drills/CTG/STAN Training on induction
Clinical Indicators	**Maternal Morbidity** Eclampsia	◆	◆	No. of patients		DATEX	0	0	0	0	0	0	0	0	0	
	ICU admissions in obstetrics			No. of patients		DATEX	0	0	1	0	0	0	1	0	0	
	Blood transfusions (4 units of blood)			No. of patients		DATEX	0	0	1	1	0	1	0	1	0	Uterine artery embolisation in April
	Postpartum hysterectomies			No. of patients		DATEX	0	0	0	0	0	0	0	0	0	
	Neonatal morbidity Number of cases of meconium aspiration			No. of patients		DATEX	0	0	1	0	0	1	1	1	0	
	Number of cases of hypoxic encephalopathy (Grades 2 & 3)			No. of patients		DATEX	0	0	0	0	0	0	0	0	0	
	Risk Management Number of SUIs	<1%	>3%	Ins Del/Birth	Investigations undertaken	Risk Dep	0.8	0.6	0.7	0.8	0.7	0.5	0.4	0.2	0.3	
	Failed instrumental delivery	<10 / month	>15 / month			Risk Dep	6	6	6	3	3	4	4	3	3	Possible Overdiagnosis/Mandatory training & Skills and Drills of Shoulder Dystocia
	Massive PPH >7l	<6 / month	>10 / month		0.5–1.5% of Deliveries	Risk Dep	6	6	6	6	6	6	5	6	6	
	Shoulder dystocia	<6 / month	>10 / month			Risk Dep										Individual training issues identified. Audit on 3rd-degree tear initiated.
	3rd-degree tear	<6 / month	>10 / month		<5% of Deliveries (RCOG)	Risk Dep	14	6	6	6	6	10	5	6	6	Ventouse hands-on one to one training for SpRs carried out.
	Complaints Number of complaints	<5 / month	>8 / month													
	Number of times unit closed for admissions in each month	<1 per month	>3 times per month													

Index

abdominal examination 7–8, 17

abdominal sepsis 176

abruption 70

acidaemia 45–6

acidosis 45

activated factor VII 169

acupuncture 26–7

acute chest syndrome (ACS) 234

acute illness, postpartum period
 171, 181
  adverse drug reactions 179
   anaphylactic/anaphylactoid
    reactions 179
   drug withdrawal 179
   toxicity/side effects 179
  air embolus 180
  amniotic fluid embolus 176
  cardiac disease 178
   aortic dissection 178
   arrhythmias 178
   myocardial infarction (MI) 178
  causes 171, 172
  epilepsy 180
  general anaesthesia 177
   aspiration pneumonitis 177
   atelectasis 177
   respiratory depression 177
  hypertensive disorders 175
  incidence 171
  management 172–5
   assessment 173–5
   resuscitation 173
  metabolic conditions 179–80
  peripartum cardiomyopathy
   (PPCM) 176
  postpartum haemorrhage 175
  presentation 171–2
  regional anaesthesia 177–8
  respiratory disease 178–9
   asthma 178
   pneumonia 179
  stroke/cerebrovascular accident
   (CVA) 180
  thromboembolic disease 176–7
   cerebral vein thrombosis 177

   pulmonary embolism 176–7
   vasovagal syncope 180–1

Addison's disease 236

adhesions, caesarean section and 114

admission cardiotocograph (CTG) 39

adrenal insufficiency 236–7

adverse drug reactions 179
  anaphylactic/anaphylactoid
   reactions 179
  drug withdrawal 179
  toxicity/side effects 179

adverse events *see* clinical incidents

air embolus 180

all-fours manoeuvre 137

amniocentesis, preterm prelabour
 rupture of membranes and
 212–13

amnioinfusion, intravenous
 resuscitation 71

amniotic fluid embolus 176

amniotomy 196

ampicillin, preterm prelabour rupture
 of membranes and 209–11,
 212–13

anaemia 295

anaesthesia 18, 31–7, 105
  asthma and 237
  changes in practice 77–8
  complications 112
  fetal reserve and 68
  general anaesthesia 35–7
   diminishing rates of 77–8
   failed intubation 35–7
   indications for 77
   myasthenia gravis and 238
   postpartum collapse 177
   preoxygenation 35
   pulmonary aspiration risk
    76–7, 177
   rapid sequence induction 35
  maternal position 33
  pre-eclampsia and 270

premedication 32–3
regional anaesthesia 33–5
  combined spinal epidural
   anaesthesia 35
  epidural anaesthesia 34–5
  increasing rates of 78
  postpartum collapse 177–8
  spinal anaesthesia 34
  vaginal birth after caesarean 246
 risk 31, 76–7
 selection of anaesthetic technique
  31–2

anal canal 183–4

anal sphincters 184
 injury 99, 182
  diagnosis 186–7
  follow-up 191
  postoperative care 190–1
  repair 188–90
  subsequent pregnancy
   management 191–3

anal triangle 183–4

analgesia 18, 26–31
 acupuncture 26–7
 asthma and 237
 hydrotherapy 26
 induction of labour and 202, 204
  with intrauterine death 205–6
 inhalational analgesia 27
  nitrous oxide 27
 regional analgesia 28–31
  complications and side effects
   29–30
  contra-indications for 28
  effects on labour 30–1
  establishment of 29
  heart disease and 228
  indications for 28
  low molecular weight heparin
   and 230
  maintenance of 29
  myasthenia gravis and 238
  patient-controlled 29
 support during labour 26
 systemic opioid analgesia 27–8, 78
  pethidine 27–8
  remifentanil 28

350

transcutaneous electrical nerve stimulation (TENS) 27
twin birth 126
anaphylactic/anaphylactoid reactions 179
antepartum haemorrhage (APH) 141–50
  aetiology 141
  causes of 142
  history 141
  management 141–2
  physical examination 141
  placenta percreta/accreta 146
  placenta praevia 142–6
  placental abruption 146–50
  vasa praevia 146
anti-shock garment 168
antibiotic therapy
  group B streptococcus eradication 212
  infective endocarditis prophylaxis 229
  preterm labour management 221–2
  preterm prelabour rupture of membranes 209–11, 212–13
  puerperal sepsis 288
  urinary tract infection 293–4
anticoagulation management 230–2
  metal heart valves and 231–2
  recurrent miscarriage and 230–1
  urgent delivery and 232
  venous thromboembolism prophylaxis 231
antihypertensive therapy 266–7
  hydralazine 267
  labetalol 267
  methyldopa 267
  nifedipine 267
antiretroviral treatment 239
aortic dissection 178
Apgar score, prolonged second stage of labour and 85
apnoea 273–4
  see also hypoxia
arrhythmias 178
arteriovenous malformations (AVM), cerebral 238–9
artificial rupture of membranes (ARM) 23, 196
asphyxia 66, 274–5
  see also hypoxia; resuscitation
aspiration of gastric contents 32–3, 76
  aspiration pneumonitis 177

practical obstetric considerations 76–7
asthma 178, 237
asynclitism 7
atelectasis 177
atonia 160, 162
atosiban 70, 220
attitude 7
augmentation see management
autocaval compression 68–9
backache 293
backache, regional analgesia and 30
Berry aneurysms 239
birth canal 1–3
Bishop score 9, 197, 198
bladder
  dysfunction, regional analgesia and 30
  injury 112, 249–50
  postnatal check 286
blood pressure measurement 264–5
blood sampling 162
  see also fetal scalp blood sampling (FBS)
blood transfusion 163–4
bowel
  injury 112, 249–50
  Ogilvie's syndrome 113, 289
  postnatal check 286
brachial plexus injury 100
  classification 139
    Erb's palsy 139
    Klumpke's palsy 139
    total brachial plexus injury 139
  shoulder dystocia and 138–9
  risk of 139
Bracht technique 120, 122
breast problems 295
breastfeeding 286
breech presentation 6, 116
  breech birth at term 116
  twin birth 127
    preterm breech 127–9
  vaginal breech birth 118–24
    assisted breech delivery 120–1
    Bracht technique 122
    conduct of breech birth 120
    conduct of labour 119–20
    contra-indications 119
    head entrapment 124

manoeuvres for delay in delivery of the arms 122–4
selection for 118–19
see also external cephalic version (ECV)
bupivacaine 29
caesarean section (CS) 104, 114–15, 241
  adjuncts to 112
  anaesthesia for see anaesthesia
  classification 104, 105
  complications 108, 112–14
    adhesions 114
    anaesthetic 112
    endometriosis 114
    fetal complications 112
    fistula formation 114
    future fertility 113–14
    haemorrhage , 112–13
    hernia formation 114
    infection 113
    keloid scarring 114
    paralytic ileus 113
    pelvic organ damage 112
    placenta praevia 114
    puerperal problems 294–5
    scar rupture 114
    thromboembolic disease 113
    wound 113, 294–5
  cord prolapse and 133
  fetal distress and 72
  heart disease and 228
  indications 104, 106–7
  intraoperative procedures 105–11
    delivering the baby 109–10
    delivering the placenta 110
    drains and closure 111
    patient preparation 105
    skin incision and peritoneal cavity access 108
    surgical principles 105
    uterine closure 110–11
    uterus exposure and entry 108–9, 110
  multiple birth 124–5, 127
    preterm breech 127–9
  postnatal check 285
  preoperative procedures 104–5
    blood tests/products 105
    consent 104–5
  rate 14
  scar dehiscence 59
  subsequent pregnancy management 241
    augmentation 246–7, 248
    data limitations 241
    delivery setting 246
    epidural anaesthesia 246

caesarean section (CS) (cont.)
    induction of labour 201–2, 246–7,
        247–8
    mode of delivery 241–6, 249
    monitoring in labour 246–7
    outcome of future pregnancies
        249
    uterine contractions 59
    see also elective repeat caesarean
        section (ERCS); vaginal birth
        after caesarean (VBAC)
    timing of 105
    versus operative vaginal delivery
        90–1
caput succedaneum 4
carbetocin 155, 164
carbohydrate solutions 79–80
carboprost 155, 229
cardiotocograph (CTG) 39–41, 43–4
    acting on a suspicious CTG 44
    failure to monitor appropriately
        334–6
    failure to respond to abnormal CTG
        336–8
    incorporating the clinical picture 45
    interpretation 44
    on admission 39
    see also electronic fetal monitoring
        (EFM); fetal heart rate (FHR)
        monitoring
cardiovascular disease see heart
        disease; thromboembolic
        disease
cell salvaging 169
cephalhaematoma 99
cerebral arteriovenous malformations
        (AVM) 239
cerebral palsy 332, 340
    arising from events in labour
        334–40
    application of excessive force
        338–9
    failed or delayed diagnosis 339
    failed or delayed intervention
        339–40
    failure to monitor fetus
        appropriately 334–6
    failure to recognize complication
        338
    failure to respond to abnormal
        cardiotocograph 336–8
    inappropriate intervention 334
    see also risk management
    causes 332
    negligence claims 332–3

types of 333
    dyskinetic or athetoid 333
    spastic quadriplegic 333
cerebral vein thrombosis 177
cerebrovascular accident (CVA) 180
cervical cerclage 222–3
cervical consistency 9
cervical dilatation
    labour progress 14
    nomogram/partogram 14–15, 19
        action line 15, 21–3
        alert line 15
    secondary arrest of (SACD) 19–20
cervical dilators 195–6
cervical effacement 9–10
cervical length measurement 198–9
    preterm labour prediction 219
cervical position 9
chest compressions 279
chest infection 113
chorioamnionitis 208
classical arm development 123
clinical governance 311
clinical incidents 311–12
    impacts of 312
    reporting 313–15
    triggers 314
    see also cerebral palsy; risk
        management
co-amoxiclav 221–2
coagulation failure 160
    see also inherited coagulation
        deficiencies
combined spinal epidural anaesthesia
        (CSE) 35
    sequential block 35
communication 305–6, 318–20
    among team members 328
    between staff 319
        feedback 321
    with patient 318–19
complication 338
    failure to recognize 338
    see also caesarean section (CS);
        puerperium; uterine rupture;
        wound complications
compression duplex ultrasound 290
compression sutures 165–6
computed tomography pulmonary
        angiogram (CTPA) 290–1

computerized records 319–20
congenital abnormalities 282
connective tissue disorders, uterine
        rupture and 254–5
consent, caesarean section 104–5
continuous positive airway pressure
        (CPAP) 234
contraction-associated proteins
        (CAPS) 6
contractions 6, 54–62
    abnormal patterns 60
    efficiency of 21
    electric and physical basis of 54
    fetal distress and 68
        intrauterine resuscitation 70
    induced labour and 59–60
    maternal characteristics and 59
    measurement of 24, 54–7
        external tocography 55
        internal tocography 55–6
        manual palpation 55
        maternal perception 54–5
        need for 54
        quantification 56–7
        uterine electromyography
            (EMG) 56
    normal labour 58
    parameters 55
    parity and 58
    previous caesarean section and 59
    see also labour; uterine activity
controlled cord traction (CCT) 154
convulsions see seizures
cord compression 68
    induction of labour and 203
    reducing 132–3
        bladder filling 133
        digital elevation 132
        maternal positioning 133
cord prolapse 69, 131–4
    definition 131
    documentation 134
    incidence 131
    management 132–4
        call for help 132
        delivery 133
        preparation for immediate
            delivery 132, 133
        recognition of prolapse 132
        reducing compression 132–3
    morbidity and mortality 134
    pathophysiology 131
    prediction 131
    prevention 131–2
    risk factors 131, 132

corticosteroid therapy
  preterm labour management
    221, 222
  preterm prelabour rupture of
    membranes 211

corticotrophin-releasing hormone
  (CRH) 5

cortisol 5

creatinine monitoring 265–6

Crew Resource Management (CRM)
  323, 330

cystic fibrosis 237

cytokines, preterm labour and 217

decelerations see fetal heart rate (FHR)

decision-making
  fetal distress 67, 73–4
  information filtering 74
  nature of in emergency situations 73

deep vein thrombosis see venous
  thromboembolism (VTE)

dehydroepiandrosterone sulphate
  (DHEAS) 5

depression, postnatal 296, 298
  management 298

diabetes 179–80, 234–6
  delivery and 234–5, 235–6
  gestational diabetes 236
  labour and 235–6
    induction of labour 201
  neonate management 236
  postpartum diabetic control 236
  pre-existing diabetes 234
  shoulder dystocia risk and 134

diaphragmatic hernia 282

dinoprostone 197
  administration 203

disseminated intravascular
  coagulation (DIC) 150
  stages of 150
  treatment 150

documentation
  cord prolapse 134
  shoulder dystocia 138

drills
  evaluation 324–5
    cost-effectiveness 325
    healthcare outcome 324–5
    learning outcome 324
    obstetric emergencies suitable
      for 324
  organization 325–7
    access 326

course planning and
  administration 325–6
  equipment 327
  facilitation 326
  location of training 325
  objectives, feedback and
    assessment 326
  patient-actresses 326–7
  record keeping 327
  scenarios 326

drug reactions see adverse drug
  reactions

dural puncture
  epidural analgesia and 30
  postdural puncture headache 30,
    292–3
    clinical features 292–3
    management 293

dystocia 19
  vaginal birth after caesarean 248
  see also shoulder dystocia

eclampsia 175, 262, 264
  definitions 262
  see also pre-eclampsia

elective repeat caesarean section (ERCS)
  comparative risks and benefits
    243, 244, 250
  data limitations 241
  determining the mode of delivery
    241–3
  timing of 249
  see also caesarean section (CS)

electrocardiogram see fetal
  electrocardiogram (ECG)

electromyography (EMG), uterine 56

electronic fetal monitoring (EFM) 38
  continuous 39–43
  failure to monitor appropriately
    334–6
  failure to respond to abnormal
    cardiotocograph 336–8
  indications for 40
  intermittent 39
  see also fetal heart rate (FHR)
    monitoring

electronic records 319–20

emergencies 323, 324
  training see drills

endometriosis, caesarean section
  and 114

endometritis 288–9
  caesarean section and 113
  clinical features 288
  management 288–9

engagement 10

epidural anaesthesia 34–5
  combined spinal epidural
    anaesthesia (CSE) 35
    sequential block 35
  dosing 34–5
  increasing rates of 78
  prolonged second stage of labour
    and 86–7
  side effects 86–7
  vaginal birth after caesarean 246

epidural analgesia 28
  accidental dural puncture 30
  backache and 30
  effects on labour 30–1
  patient-controlled (PCEA) 29
  see also analgesia

epidural haemorrhage 100

epilepsy 180, 237–8

episiotomy 185–6, 187–8
  in prolonged second stage
    of labour 88
  indications 185–6
  shoulder dystocia and 136
  see also perineum

Erb's palsy 139

ergot alkaloids 154, 164
  heart disease and 228, 229

error 311–12
  see also clinical incidents

erythromycin
  preterm labour management 221–2
  preterm prelabour rupture of
    membranes and 209–11, 212–13

examination 15–17
  abdominal 7–8, 17
  antepartum haemorrhage and 141
  pelvic 8–9
  pre-eclampsia 264
  vaginal 9, 17

excessive force 338–9

external cephalic version (ECV)
  116–18
  conduct of 117–18
  efficacy 116–17
  safety 117
  techniques to improve success 117
  twin birth 127
  uptake 117

facial nerve palsy 100

false labour 17

fatigue 295

feedback

feedback (cont.)
  from drills 326
  risk management 321
fentanyl 29, 78
fertility, caesarean section and 113–14
fetal distress 66
  causes 67–70
    abruption 70
    contractions 68
    cord compression 68
    cord prolapse 69
    failure to progress 68
    maternal positioning 68–9
    uterine rupture 70
    vasa praevia 69
  consequences of intervention 66–7
  decision-making 67, 73–4
  delivery 71–2
    caesarean section 72
    forceps or vacuum delivery 72
  fetal reserve 67
    assessment 67
  management 67–74
    non-technical skills 72–4
  see also intrauterine resuscitation
fetal electrocardiogram (ECG) 47–8
  ST segment analysis 47
    pathophysiological changes 47–8
fetal fibronectin see fibronectin, fetal
fetal growth restriction see intrauterine
  growth restriction (IUGR)
fetal heart rate (FHR)
  cord prolapse and 133
  hypoxia responses 274
  uterine rupture and 256
fetal heart rate (FHR) monitoring
  accelerations 41–2
  baseline heart rate 41
  baseline variability (BLV) 41
  categorization of FHR features 43–4
  continuous electronic fetal
    monitoring (EFN) 39–43
  cycling 42
  decelerations 42–3
    complicated variable
      decelerations 42
    early decelerations 42
    interpretation of 42–3
    late decelerations 42
    prolonged decelerations 42
    uncomplicated variable
      decelerations 42
  failure to monitor appropriately
    334–6
  failure to respond to abnormal
    cardiotocograph 336–8

intermittent auscultation (IA) 38–9
intermittent electronic fetal
  monitoring (EFM) 39
  Recommendation Grades 335
  sinusoidal trace 43–4
  twin birth 125–6
  see also cardiotocograph (CTG);
    intrapartum fetal surveillance
fetal pulse-oxymetry (FPO) 48–9
fetal reserve 67
  anaesthesia and 68
  antenatal factors 67
  assessment 67
fetal scalp blood sampling (FBS) 45–7
  interpretation of results 45
  lactate measurements 46–7
  problems with 46
fetal scalp stimulation tests 45
feto-maternal haemorrhage 147
fetus
  assessment in pre-eclampsia 266
  asynclitism 7
  attitude 7
  blood sampling see fetal scalp blood
    sampling (FBS)
  caesarean section complications 112
  injuries during operative vaginal
    delivery 99–100, 100–1
    cephalhaematoma 99
    intracranial trauma 100
    nerve injury 100–1
    scalp trauma 99
    skull fractures 100
    subgaleal haemorrhage 99–100
  intrauterine fetal demise (IUD) 201
    induction of labour management
      205–6
  lie 6
  position 6–7
    delivery in malposition of the
      fetal head 98
    occipito-transverse (OT) position
      of the head 98
    persistent occipito-posterior
      position (POP) 86
  presentation 6, 86
  skull 3–4
    caput succedaneum 4
    fractures during operative vaginal
      delivery 100
    moulding 3, 21
  see also fetal distress; fetal heart rate
    (FHR); intrapartum fetal
    surveillance
fibronectin, fetal
  preterm labour prediction 219

suitability assessment for induction
  of labour 199
first stage of labour 15–18, 20–4
  abdominal examination 17
  analgesia and anaesthesia 18
  breech delivery 119–20
  general examination 15–17
  initial assessment 15
  investigations 17
  mobility and posture 18
  practical aspects 21–3
  twin birth 126
  vaginal examination 17
fistula formation, caesarean section
  and 114
fluid balance management 269, 270–1
fluid infusion 162
forceps delivery 97–8
  classical forceps 97
  excessive force 338–9
  fetal distress and 72
  forceps application 97
  in malposition of the fetal head 98
  special forceps 97
  traction 97–8
  versus vacuum delivery 89–90
  see also operative vaginal delivery
gastroesophageal reflux 77
gemeprost 204
general anaesthesia see anaesthesia
genital tract sepsis 176
gestational diabetes 236
  delivery 236
  diabetic control 236
Glasgow Coma Score 175
group B streptococcus (GBS), preterm
  prelabour rupture of
  membranes and 211–12
  eradication therapy 212
haematoma see cephalhaematoma;
  pelvic haematoma
haemophilia 233
  delivery 234
  postnatal management 234
  treatment 233
haemorrhage
  caesarean section complications
    112–13
  epidural 100
  feto-maternal 147
  retinal 101
  subdural 100
  subgaleal 99–100

uterine rupture and 257
see also antepartum haemorrhage (APH); postpartum haemorrhage

haemorrhagic shock 149–50
anti-shock garment 168
shock index (SI) 169
see also postpartum haemorrhage (PPH)

head entrapment 124

headache
postdural puncture headache 30, 292–3
postnatal, causes 292

heart disease 227–9
acute postpartum illness 178
infective endocarditis 229
mode of delivery 228
monitoring during labour 229
postpartum haemorrhage and 229
regional analgesia and 228
timing of delivery 228

HELLP syndrome 266, 271

heparin *see* low molecular weight heparin (LMWH)

hepatitis B 239

hepatitis C 240

hernia formation, caesarean section and 114

high blood pressure *see* hypertension; pre-eclampsia

HIV infection 239
antiretroviral treatment 239
mode of delivery 239

hydralazine 267

hydration in labour 76, 81–2
carbohydrate solutions 79–80
isotonic sport drinks 79
oral intake 78–9
patient choice 81
rehydration 17

hydrotherapy 26

hyperstimulation 202–3

hypertension 262
antihypertensive therapy 266–7
blood pressure measurement 264–5
induction of labour and 200
postpartum 291
see also pre-eclampsia

hyponatraemia 180

hypotension, regional analgesia and 29

hypotonia 160

hypoxia 40, 42–3, 45
causes 332
ECG changes 47–8
negligence claims 332–3
pathophysiology, animal studies 273–4
see also asphyxia; cerebral palsy; resuscitation

hypoxic ischaemic encephalopathy (HIE) 258

hysterectomy
postpartum haemorrhage and 167–8
previous caesarean section and 249–50
uterine rupture and 257–8

immediate puerperium 285
see also puerperium

incident reporting 313–15
see also clinical incidents

induction of labour 195
care during 203–4
failed induction 203
options 204
indications for 199–202
diabetes 201
fetal growth restriction 200
hypertension 200
intrauterine fetal demise (IUD) 201, 205–6
isolated oligohydramnios at term 200–1
macrosomia 201
maternal request 201
prelabour rupture of membranes (PROM) 199–200
previous caesarean section 201–2
prolonged pregnancy 199
twin pregnancy 201
methods 195–8
artificial rupture of membranes 196
dinoprostone 197
mechanical methods 195–6
membrane sweeping 195
misoprostol 197–8
oxytocin 196–7
risks of 202–3
fetal heart rate abnormalities 203
hyperstimulation 202–3
increased analgesia requirements 202
increased operative delivery 202
prostaglandin side effects 202
uterine rupture 203, 254
with previous caesarean section 246–7, 247–8

suitability assessment 198–9
Bishop score 197, 198
cervical length measurement by ultrasound 198–9
fetal fibronectin 199

infection
caesarean section complications 113
wound infection 294–5
group B streptococcus (GBS) 211–12
maternal infectious diseases 239–40
genital herpes 240
hepatitis B 239
hepatitis C 240
HIV 239
myasthenia gravis and 239
perineal breakdown 292
preterm labour risk and 218
puerperal sepsis 288–9
urinary tract 113, 293–4
see also antibiotic therapy

infective endocarditis 229
prophylaxis 229

inflation breaths 276

informed consent, caesarean section 104–5

inherited coagulation deficiencies 233–4
delivery 234
postnatal management 234
treatment 233

insulin, sliding scale of, 235–6

internal iliac artery ligation 166–7

internal podalic version (IPV) twin birth 127

interventional radiology, postpartum haemorrhage 167

intracranial trauma 100

intrapartum fetal surveillance 38, 49
continuous electronic fetal monitoring (EFM) 39–43
accelerations 41–2
baseline heart rate 41
baseline variability 41
cycling 42
decelerations 42–3
fetal electrocardiogram (ECG) 47–8
fetal pulse-oxymetry (FPO) 48–9
fetal scalp blood sampling (FBS) 45–7
fetal scalp stimulation tests 45
intermittent fetal monitoring 38–9
admission cardiotocograph (CTG) 39
intermittent auscultation (IA) 38–9

intrapartum fetal surveillance (cont.)
  intermittent electronic fetal
    monitoring (EFM) 39
  sinusoidal trace 43–4
  see also cardiotocograph (CTG);
    fetal heart rate (FHR)

intrauterine fetal demise (IUD) 201
  induction of labour management
    205–6
intrauterine growth restriction
    (IUGR) 200
  pre-eclampsia and 266

intrauterine resuscitation 70–1
  amnioinfusion 71
  intravenous fluids 70–1
  maternal positioning 70
  oxygen 71
  potential responses 70
  stopping the contractions 70
  tocolysis 70

intravenous fluids, intrauterine
    resuscitation 70–1

intubation difficulties 32
  failed intubation 35–7

investigations 17

isotonic sport drinks 79

keloid scarring 114

ketones 78–9

Kleihauer–Betke test 147

Klumpke's palsy 139

labetalol 267

labour 1, 6–7
  breech birth 119–20
  diagnosis of 15
  fetal presentation 6, 86
  induction of see induction of labour
  initiation of 5–6
  management of see management
  mechanism 10–11
    descent 10
    engagement 10
    expulsion 11
    extension 10
    external rotation 11
    flexion 10
    internal rotation 10
  normal 14–15
  progress of 14
    diagnosis of poor progress 19–20
    fetal distress and 68
  stages of 10
    see also first stage of labour;
      second stage of labour; third
      stage of labour

true versus false labour 17
  see also hydration in labour;
    nutrition in labour; preterm
    labour

labour ward
  clinical scenarios 306–10
  communication 305–6
  space 303
  staffing issues 302–3
  workload 303–4
  see also teamwork; triage

lactate measurements 46–7

laryngeal nerve injury 100

latent phase 19
  augmentation in 23

leadership 327–8

Leopold manoeuvres 7–8

levator ani 184–5

lidocaine 35

litigation 332–3
  legal process 333
  see also cerebral palsy

liver function tests 266

lochia 285

Lovset's manoeuvre 122

low molecular weight heparin
    (LMWH) 229–30, 230–2, 291
  metal heart valves and 231–2
  recurrent miscarriage and 230–1
  regional analgesia and 230
  therapeutic dose 230
  urgent delivery and 232
  venous thromboembolism
    prophylaxis 231

McRoberts' position 135–6

macrosomia 134
  induction of labour and 201
  vaginal birth after caesarean
    and 249–50

magnesium sulphate
  seizure management 268
  seizure prevention 268–9

management 14
  anticoagulation see anticoagulation
    management
  augmentation 20–4
    active phase of labour 23
    breech birth 119–20
    duration of 24
    following previous caesarean
      section 246–7, 248
    indications 20–1

latent phase of labour 23
  prolonged second stage of labour
    avoidance 88
  twin birth 126
  uterine contractions and 59–60
  uterine rupture and 254
  when to augment 21
  key components of 20
  optimal uterine activity
    achievement 24
  previous caesarean section and 241
    see also elective repeat caesarean
      section (ERCS); vaginal birth
      after caesarean (VBAC)
  see also first stage of labour; second
    stage of labour; specific
    conditions; third stage of labour

maternal medical disorders 227
  Addison's disease 236–7
  anticoagulation management
    230–2
  asthma 237
  Berry aneurysms 239
  cerebral arteriovenous
    malformations 239
  cystic fibrosis 237
  diabetes 234–6
  epilepsy 237–8
  heart disease 227–9
  infectious diseases 239–40
    genital herpes 240
    hepatitis B 239
    hepatitis C 240
    HIV 239
  inherited coagulation deficiencies
    233–4
  myasthenia gravis 238
  obstetric cholestasis (OC) 240
  renal disease 240
  sickle cell disease 234
  thrombocytopenia 232–3
  thrombosis 229–30
  see also specific conditions

maternal morbidity see morbidity

maternal position
  anaesthesia and 33
  fetal distress and 68–9
  intrauterine resuscitation 70
  prolonged second stage of labour
    and 87
  reducing cord compression 133

Mauriceau–Smellie–Viet technique
    120, 121

meconium 18–19
  aspiration 281–2

medical disorders see maternal
  medical disorders

medical error 311–12
    see also cerebral palsy; clinical incidents; negligence claims
membrane sweeping 195
Mendelson's syndrome *see* aspiration of gastric contents
mental disorders *see* psychiatric disorders
metabolic acidaemia 45–6
metal heart valves 231–2
methyldopa 267
metoclopramide 33
mifepristone 205
misoprostol 155, 164
    heart disease and 229
    induction in intrauterine death 205
    uterine rupture and 254
mobility in labour 18
monitoring 335
    failure to monitor appropriately 334–6
        Recommendation Grades 335
    labour following previous caesarean section 246–7
    pre-eclampsia 265–6
    see also fetal heart rate (FHR) monitoring
morbidity 14, 66
    breech birth at term 116
    cord prolapse and 134
    operative vaginal delivery
        fetal trauma 99–100
        maternal trauma 98–9
        vacuum versus forceps delivery 89–90, 98
        versus caesarean section 90–1
    placenta praevia 142–3
        fetal 143
        maternal 142–3
    placental abruption 147
        fetal 147
        maternal 147
    preterm birth and 216–17
    shoulder dystocia , 138–9
        maternal morbidity 138
        neonatal morbidity 138–9
    uterine rupture 258, 259
    vaginal birth after caesarean 243
mortality 14, 38, 66, 311
    anaesthetic related 31
    causes of maternal death 173, 268
    cord prolapse 134
    multiple birth 124–5
    placenta praevia 143

placental abruption 147
postpartum haemorrhage 160
pre-eclampsia/eclampsia 265
preterm birth and 216–17
uterine rupture 258–9
moulding 3, 21
multiple birth 116, 124–9
    at term 124–5
    caesarean section 124–5, 127
        preterm breech 127–9
    induction of labour 201
    preterm labour risk 218
    vaginal twin birth 125–9
        after previous caesarean section 249–50
        birth of non-vertex second twin 127
        conduct of birth 126–7
        conduct of labour 125–6
        inter twin delivery interval 126–7
        selection 125
myasthenia gravis (MG) 238–9
    drug use and drug interactions 238
    neonatal 238
myocardial infarction (MI) 178
myomectomy, uterine rupture and 254
myometrial activity *see* uterine activity
necrotizing fasciitis 295
negligence claims 332–3
    legal process 333
    see also cerebral palsy
neonate
    congenital abnormalities 282
    management with maternal diabetes 236
    neonatal myasthenia gravis 238
    persistent pulmonary hypertension of the newborn (PPHN) 282–3
    premature 223
    resuscitation 134, 273–9
        babies born outside hospital 282
        meconium-stained liquor and 281–2
        opening the airway 279–81
        premature baby 281
    shock 283
    shoulder dystocia 138–9
    see also morbidity; mortality
nerve injury during operative vaginal delivery 100–1
neuropraxia 293
nifedipine 220–1, 267
nitroglycerin 70

nitrous oxide 27
nuchal arms 123–4
nutrition in labour 76, 81–2
    carbohydrate solutions 79–80
    isotonic sport drinks 79
    light diet 79
    oral intake 78–9
    patient choice 81
    see also aspiration of gastric contents
obesity, shoulder dystocia risk and 134–5
objective structured assessment of technical skills (OSATS) 341
    development with specialty training 341–2
    format 342–3
    future developments 347
    generic technical skills assessment domain 343–6
    in practice 346–7
    requirements 346
obstetric anal sphincter injuries (OASIS) 99, 182
    diagnosis 186–7
    repair 188–90
        follow-up 191
        postoperative care 190–1
        subsequent pregnancy management 191–3
obstetric cholestasis (OC) 240
occipito-transverse (OT) position of the fetal head 98
Ogilvie's syndrome 113, 289
oligohydramnios 200–1
operative vaginal delivery 93
    choice of instrument 101
    classification 93
    contra-indications 94
    fetal injuries 99–100, 100–1
        cephalhaematoma 99
        intracranial trauma 100
        nerve injury 100–1
        scalp trauma 99
        skull factures 100
        subgaleal haemorrhage 99–100
    indications 93
    induction of labour and 202
    maternal injuries 98–9
    prior assessment 88–9, 94–5
    training 101
    vacuum versus forceps 89–90
    versus caesarean section 90–1
    see also forceps delivery; vacuum delivery
opioid analgesia 27–8, 78

oral intake 17, 78–9
  patient choice 81
  see also hydration in labour;
    nutrition in labour

ovarian artery ligation 166

oxygen, intrauterine resuscitation 71

oxytocin 154, 196–7
  administration 204
  dosage 23–4
  intraumbilical 155
  postpartum haemorrhage 164
  prelabour rupture of membranes
    and 200
  prolonged second stage of labour
    avoidance 88
  twin birth 126
  uterine contractions and 59–60

pain relief 26
  asthma and 237
  induction of labour and 204
    with intrauterine death 205–6
  women's views of 26
  see also analgesia

paralytic ileus 113

partogram 14–15, 19
  action line 15, 21–3
  alert line 15

patient-controlled epidural analgesia
  (PCEA) 29

Pawlik's manoeuvre 8

pelvic devascularization 166–7

pelvic floor morbidity 99

pelvic haematoma 287–8
  clinical features 287
  management 287–8

pelvis 1–3
  examination 8–9
  inlet 1
  outlet 1–3
  shapes 1
  tilt 1

perineal repair see perineal trauma

perineal trauma 98–9, 182
  classification 185
  diagnosis 186–7
  management 182, 187–93
    first-degree tears 187
    follow-up 191
    postoperative care 190–1
    second-degree tears 187–8
    subsequent pregnancy 191–3
    third- and fourth-degree tears
      188–90

medico-legal considerations 193
postnatal check 286
prevention 193
tears 98–9
training 193
see also episiotomy

perineum
  anatomy 182
    anal triangle 183–4
    levator ani 184–5
    perineal body 184
    urogenital triangle 182–3
  assessment after birth 154
  postpartum breakdown 291–2
  see also perineal trauma

peripartum cardiomyopathy (PPCM)
  176

persistent occipito-posterior position
  (POP) 86

persistent pulmonary hypertension of
  the newborn (PPHN) 282–3

pethidine 27–8

Pierre Robin sequence 282

placenta
  delivery in caesarean section 110
  separation 153
    signs of 153–4
  see also retained placenta

placenta accreta/increta/percreta
  146, 158–9
  previous caesarean section and
    249–50
    pre-operative investigations 249
  see also retained placenta

placenta praevia 114, 142–6
  definition 142
  diagnosis 143–4
  fetal risks 143
  grading of 142
  management 144–6
    expectant management 144–5
    immediate delivery 144
    mode of delivery 145–6
  maternal risks 142–3
  prevalence 142
  previous caesarean section and 249
    pre-operative investigations 249
  screening 144

placental abruption 146–50
  clinical implication 147
    fetal risks 147
    maternal risks 147
  diagnosis 147–8
    ultrasonography 148
  grading of 146

management 148–50
  disseminated intravascular
    coagulation 150
  expectant management 148–9
  haemorrhagic shock 149–50
  immediate delivery 149
  postpartum haemorrhage 150
  renal failure 150
  subsequent pregnancy 150
  previous caesarean section
    and 249–50
  risk factors 146–7

platelet monitoring 266

postdural puncture headache
  30, 292–3
  clinical features 292–3
  management 293

postnatal check 285–6
  bladder function 286
  bowel function 286
  caesarean section scar 285
  emotional/mental state 286
  infant feeding issues 286
  lochia 285
  maternal observations 285
  perineal wound 286
  social issues 286
  thrombosis risk 286
  uterus 285

postnatal depression 296, 298
  management 298

postpartum collapse see acute illness,
  postpartum period

postpartum haemorrhage (PPH) 150,
  156, 160, 169, 175
  causes of 160
  haemodynamic changes 161
  heart disease and 229
  management 161–2
    activated factor VII 169
    anti-shock garment 168
    cell salvaging 169
    compression sutures 165–6
    direct uterine massage 165
    hysterectomy 167–8
    interventional radiology 167
    pharmacological treatment 164
    surgical management 164
    systematic pelvic
      devascularization 166–7
    tamponade or uterine packing
      164–5
  mortality 160
  prevention 158
  primary PPH 161
  resuscitation 162–4
  risk factors 157–8, 161

rule of 161
secondary PPH 161, 286–7
sepsis 176
shock index (SI) 169
tamponade test 168

posture in labour 18

pre-eclampsia 175, 262
  assessment 264
    blood pressure measurement
      264–5
    fetal assessment 266
    proteinuria measurement 265
  classification 264
  definitions 262
  diagnosis 262, 264
  management 266–9, 269–70
    antihypertensive therapy 266–7
    delivery 269–70
    discharge 271
    fluid balance 269, 270–1
    postdelivery care 270–1
    predelivery care 266–9
    problems 263–4
    seizures 268–9
    thromboprophylaxis 269
  monitoring 265–6
    fluid management 266
    liver function tests 266
    platelets 266
    urea and creatinine 265–6
    uric acid 265

prelabour rupture of membranes
    (PROM) 199–200
  see also preterm prelabour rupture
    of membranes (pPROM)

premature labour see preterm labour

premedication 32–3

presentation 6
  breech presentation 6
  prolonged second stage of labour
    and 86

preterm birth 216
  causes 217
  epidemiology 216, 217
  resuscitation of the premature
    baby 281
  sequelae 216–17
  vaginal birth after caesarean 249–50

preterm labour 216
  care of premature neonate 223
  long-term prediction of 219–20
    cervical length 219
    fetal fibronectins 219
    inflammatory markers 219–20
    risk scoring systems 220
  management 220–2

antibiotics 221–2
  cervical cerclage 222–3
  corticosteroids 221, 222
  tocolysis 220–1
mode of delivery 223
pathophysiology 217–18
prevention 222–3
  progesterone 222
risk factors 218–19
  demographics 218
  infection 218
  obstetric history 218
  psychosocial factors 218–19
see also preterm birth

preterm prelabour rupture of
    membranes (pPROM) 207–13
  amniocentesis role 212–13
  diagnosis 208
  group B streptococcal colonization
    and 211–12
    eradication therapy 212
  management 208–11
    antibiotic therapy 209–11
    appropriate setting for 208–9
    corticosteroid therapy 211
    timing of delivery 209
    tocolysis 211
  pathophysiology 207

primary dysfunctional labour
    (PDL) 19

prioritization see triage

progesterone 5
  preterm labour and 217
    prevention 222

progress of labour 14
  augmentation see management
  diagnosis of poor progress 19–20
  fetal distress and 68

prolonged pregnancy 199

prolonged second stage of labour
    see second stage of labour

prostaglandins 5–6, 164, 198, 200
  asthma and 237
  care during administration
    203–4
  options on failed induction 204
  previous caesarean section
    and 247
  side effects 202
    hyperstimulation 202–3

proteinuria measurement 265

psychiatric disorders 295–6, 296–7
  management 296–7
    pharmacological treatments 297
    psychological treatments 297

non-serious emotional disturbance
    296
postnatal depression 298
puerperal psychosis 297–8
serious disorders 296

puerperal psychosis 297–8
  management 298

puerperium 285
  complications 286–98
    anaemia 295
    backache 293
    breast problems 295
    caesarean section wound
      problems 294–5
    fatigue 295
    neuropraxia 293
    Ogilvie's syndrome 289
    pelvic haematoma 287–8
    perineal breakdown 291–2
    postdural puncture headache
      292–3
    postpartum hypertension 291
    psychiatric disorders 295–8
    secondary postpartum
      haemorrhage 286–7
    sepsis and endometritis 288–9
    symphysis pubis pain 293
    thromboembolism 289–91
    urinary incontinence 294
    urinary retention 294
    urinary tract infection 293–4
  postnatal check 285–6

pulmonary aspiration see aspiration
    of gastric contents

pulmonary embolism (PE) 176–7

pulmonary oedema 269, 270–1

pushing in labour 87–8

ranitidine 33

regional anaesthesia see anaesthesia

regional analgesia see analgesia

rehydration 17
  fluid infusion 162

remifentanil 28

renal disease 239–40

renal failure 150

respiratory depression 177

resuscitation
  neonate 134, 273–9
    babies born outside hospital 282
    meconium-stained liquor and
      281–2
    opening the airway 279–81
    premature baby 281

resuscitation (cont.)
  postpartum collapse 173, 174
  postpartum haemorrhage 162–4
  see also intrauterine resuscitation

retained placenta 156–9
  causes of 156
  management 156
    manual removal technique 156–7
    postpartum care 157
    postpartum haemorrhage
      prevention 158
    risk factors 156
      for postpartum haemorrhage
        157–8
    special circumstances 158–9

retinal haemorrhage 101

risk management 311, 313–20, 321
  context 311–12
  developments 320–1
  feedback 321
  hierarchy of 320
  resulting changes in practice 317
  risk analysis 315–16
  risk control 316–20
    audit 320
    communication 318–20
    guidelines 318
    induction 316
    training 317–18
  risk identification 313–15
    clinical incidents 313–15
    risk assessment 313–15, 316

ritodrine 220, 221

Root Cause Analysis (RCA) 316

Rubin I manoeuvre 136

Rubin II manoeuvre 136–7

rupture of membranes see artificial
    rupture of membranes (ARM);
    prelabour rupture of
    membranes (PROM)

safety culture 328–9

scalp stimulation tests 45

scalp trauma during operative vaginal
    delivery 99–100

scar dehiscence 59

screening, placenta praevia 144

second stage of labour 84
  duration 84–5
  prolonged 84–5, 91
    assessment prior to operative
      delivery 88–9
    avoidance 87–8
    causes of 86

epidural anaesthesia and 86–7
episiotomy and 88
operative vaginal delivery versus
    caesarean section 90–1
outcomes 85
vacuum versus forceps delivery
    89–90

secondary arrest of cervical dilatation
    (SACD) 19–20

seizures
  eclamptic 268–9
    management 268
    prevention 268–9
  epileptic 237–8

sepsis 176, 288
  puerperal 288–9
    clinical features 288
    management 288–9

shock, neonatal 283
  see also haemorrhagic shock

shock index (SI) 169

shoulder dystocia 134–40
  definition 134
  documentation 138
  incidence 134
  management 135–8
    after the birth 138
    all-fours manoeuvre 137
    call for help 135
    delivery of the posterior arm 137
    episiotomy and 136
    internal rotational manoeuvres
      136–7
    McRoberts' position 135–6
    recognition of shoulder dystocia 135
    Rubin II manoeuvre 136–7
    stating the problem 135
    suprapubic pressure 136
    symphysiotomy 137–8
    things not to do 138
    Woods' screw 136
    Zavenelli manoeuvre 137
  maternal morbidity 138
  neonatal morbidity and mortality
    138–9
    brachial plexus injury 138–9
  pathophysiology 134
  prediction 135
  prevention 135
  risk factors 134–5
    gestational age 135
    instrumental delivery 134
    intrapartum risks 135
    macrosomia 134
    maternal diabetes mellitus 134
    maternal obesity 134–5
    parity 135

previous shoulder dystocia 134
training recommendations 139–40

sickle cell disease 234

sinusoidal trace 43–4

skin incision 108

skull, fetal 3–4
  caput succedaneum 4
  fractures during operative vaginal
    delivery 100
  moulding 3, 21

sodium citrate 32–3

speculum examination 8–9

spinal anaesthesia 34
  combined spinal epidural
    anaesthesia (CSE) 35
  sequential block 35

spinal cord injury 101

staffing issues 302–3

starvation in labour see nutrition
    in labour

steroid therapy 237
  see also corticosteroid therapy

stroke 180

subaponeurotic haemorrhage 99–100

subarachnoid haemorrhage 100

subdural haemorrhage 100

subgaleal haemorrhage 99–100

support in labour 87

suprapubic pressure 136

symphyseal–fundal height (SFH) 7

symphysiotomy 137–8

symphysis pubis pain 293

synometrine 154–5, 164

syntocinon 164, 205
  heart disease and 228, 229
  regimens 198

systemic inflammatory response
    syndrome (SIRS) 176

tamponade, postpartum haemorrhage
    164–5

tamponade test 168

teamwork 323–4, 327–9
  communication among team
    members 328
  leadership 327–8
  lessons from experience 329–30
  safety culture 328–9
  team characteristics 327

team performance measurement
328
training 323–4, 330
integral versus additional training
329
lessons from experience 329–30
see also drills

technical skills *see* objective structured
assessment of technical skills
(OSATS); training

terbutaline 70

termination of pregnancy, uterine
rupture risk 254

third stage of labour 153
haemostasis 153
management 154–5
active management 154
caesarean section 154
errors 158
expectant management 154
uterotonic drugs 154–5
perineum assessment 154
placental separation 153
signs of 153–4
see also retained placenta
vaginal examination 154

thrombocytopenia 232–3

thromboembolic disease 176–7,
229–30
air embolus 180
amniotic fluid embolus 176
anticoagulation management
230–2
caesarean section complications 113
cerebral vein thrombosis 177
postnatal check 286
prophylaxis with pre-eclampsia 269
puerperal 289–91
clinical features 290
investigations 290–1
management 290, 291
risk factors 289–90
pulmonary embolism (PE) 176–7

thrombophilia screen 290

tocography
external 55
internal 55–6

tocolysis
external cephalic version and 117
intrauterine resuscitation 70
preterm labour management
220–1
preterm prelabour rupture of
membranes and 211
twin birth 126

training 341
emergency training *see* drills
operative vaginal delivery 101
perineal trauma 193
risk control 317–18
shoulder dystocia 139–40
teamwork 323–4, 330
integral versus additional training
329
lessons from experience 329–30
see also objective structured
assessment of technical skills
(OSATS)

transcutaneous electrical nerve
stimulation (TENS) 27

trauma
operative vaginal delivery 98–100
uterine rupture and 254
see also morbidity; perineal trauma

triage 300, 301
clinical scenarios 306–10
in obstetrics 301–2, 304–6
principles of 300–1

twin births *see* multiple birth

umbilical artery blood sampling 46

umbilical cord *see* cord compression;
cord prolapse

urea monitoring 265–6

ureteric injury 112, 249–50

uric acid monitoring 265

urinary incontinence 294

urinary retention 294
management 294

urinary tract infection
caesarean section complications 113
management 293–4
puerperal 293–4

urogenital triangle 182–3

uterine activity 4–5, 6
achievement of optimal activity 24
hyperstimulation 202–3
normal labour 58
quantification of 56–7
uterine activity units 57–8
see also contractions

uterine artery
catheterization 167
ligation 166

uterine electromyography (EMG) 56

uterine rupture 70, 252, 260
causes 253
classification 252–3

clinical features 255–6
antepartum rupture 255
intrapartum rupture 255–6
postpartum rupture 256
complications 258–9
maternal 258–9
perinatal 258
diagnosis 256–7
differential diagnosis 258
epidemiology 252
findings at time of laparotomy 256
management 257–8
mechanisms 255
risk factors 253–5
augmentation 254
congenital uterine malformation
254
connective tissue disorders 254–5
induction of labour 203, 254
obstructed labour 254
pregnancy termination 254
previous caesarean section 114,
246, 247, 253
previous uterine surgery 254
trauma 254
subsequent reproductive outcome
259–60

uterus
atonia 160, 162
closure 110–11
compression sutures 165–6
congenital malformation 254
exposure and entry 108–9
lower segment incision 109
midline and classical incisions 110
hyperstimulation 202–3
hypotonia 160
massage 165
packing, postpartum haemorrhage
164–5
postnatal check 285
see also uterine activity; uterine
rupture

vacuum delivery 95–7
fetal distress and 72
in malposition of the fetal head 98
traction 96–7
vacuum cup attachment 95–6
versus forceps delivery 89–90
see also operative vaginal delivery

vaginal birth after caesarean (VBAC)
augmentation 246–7, 248
comparative risks and benefits 243,
244, 250
contra-indications 243–5
obstetric complications 245
previous uterine incision 245
data limitations 241

vaginal birth after caesarean (VBAC)
(cont.)
definition of terms 242
delivery setting 246
determining the mode of delivery
241–3
epidural anaesthesia 246
fetal macrosomia and 249–50
induction of labour 201–2, 246–7,
247–8
intrapartum care 246
likelihood of success 245–6
monitoring in labour 246–7
preterm VBAC 249–50
short interdelivery period 249–50
twin gestation 249–50
see also caesarean section (CS)

vaginal examination 9, 17
after birth 154
vaginosis, preterm labour and
219–20
vasa praevia 69, 146
vasovagal syncope 180–1
venous thromboembolism (VTE)
113, 229–30
prophylaxis 231, 269
puerperal 289–91
clinical features 290
investigations 290–1
management 290, 291
risk factors 289–90

ventilation–perfusion (V/Q) lung scan
290–1
vesicouterine fistula 114
von Willebrand's disease (VWD) 233
delivery 234
postnatal management 234
treatment 233
warfarin 231, 232, 291
Woods' screw 136
workload 303–4
wound complications 113, 294–5
management 295
Zavenelli manoeuvre 137